NURSING SKILLS
and EVALUATION

NURSING SKILLS and EVALUATION

A Nursing Process Approach

SANDRA F. SMITH, RN, MS
DONNA DUELL, RN, MS

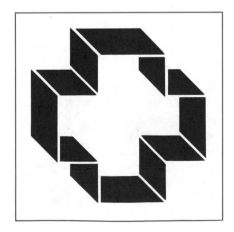

NATIONAL NURSING REVIEW
Los Altos, California

Project Director: Karen Hoxeng, RN
Cover Design: Russell Leong Design Group
Photography: Ronald W. May
Illustrations: Medical Graphics—Stephen M. Chapot, Lena Lyons
Dawn's Design
Composition: Hansen & Associates
Printing and Binding: Kingsport Press

Library of Congress Cataloging in Publication Data

Smith, Sandra Fucci.
  Nursing skills and evaluation.

  Bibliography: p.
  Includes index.
  1. Nursing. I. Duell, Donna J., 1938–
II. Title.
RT41.S583   610.73   81–22556
ISBN 0–917010–06–X   AACR2

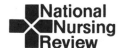
**National
Nursing
Review**

In the writing of this text, the authors and publisher have made every attempt to follow current nursing practice and to ensure that suggested diets, drug selection and dosages, and nursing procedures are up-to-date and conform with current recommendations and practices at time of publication. However, in view of new research conclusions, technological advancements, and government regulations, it is the responsibility of the nurse to be aware of any changes which may alter suggested drug and diet therapies or nursing protocols. The authors recommend that nurses and nursing students be aware of hospital and school policies regarding their role and responsibilities in performing nursing actions.

CONTRIBUTORS

Joan N. Althaus, RN, MSN, CCRN
Doctoral Candidate
University of San Francisco

Abby S. Bloch, MS, RD
Head Clinical Diet/Nutrition
  Specialist
Memorial Sloan Kettering Cancer
  Center

Barbara Devine Bode, RN, MN
Doctoral Program
University of Illinois

Christine Bolwell, RN, MSN, CCRN
Clinical Specialist
Sacramento, CA

Randy Caine, RN, MS
Assistant Professor
University of California,
  Los Angeles

Janet W. Cook, RN, MS
Assistant Professor
University of North Carolina

Lou Ann Emerson, RN, MSN
Assistant Professor
University of Cincinnati

Marsha Heims, RN, MS
Assistant Professor
Oregon Health Sciences University

Nancy Meyer Holloway, RN, MSN,
  CCRN, CEN
Clinical Specialist and Consultant
Orinda, CA

Jill D. Holmes, RN, MS
Clinical Specialist
Scripps Clinic and Research
  Foundation

Kathleen Kaplan, RN, MSN, CNM
Associate in Nursing
Columbia University

Sue Kelly, RN, MS
Supervising Public Health Nurse
County of Santa Clara

Patricia A. Kynes, RN, ET
Enterostomal Therapist
Mobile, AL

Terry W. Miller, RN, MS
Lecturer
San Jose State University

Susan D. North, RN, MS
Clinical Specialist
Johns Hopkins Medical Center

Sharon Dennis Raj, RN, MSN
Former Lecturer
San Jose State University

Judith A. Yanda, RN, MS
Clinical Specialist
Mission College

Mary G. Yarbrough, RN, MS
Assistant Administrator
O'Connor Hospital, San Jose

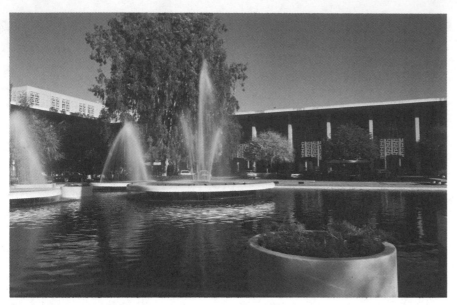

Stanford University Hospital

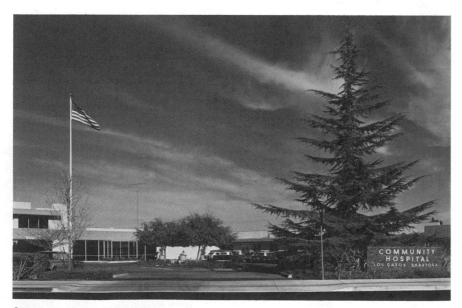

Community Hospital of Los Gatos

PREFACE

New techniques and technological advances continue to be developed and integrated into health care practice at a rapid rate. This trend is reflected in the expansion of the scope and character of nursing practice. Consequently, a wider range of nursing skills are required of the practitioner. These advancements, along with changes in the design and focus of nursing curricula, provide the rationale from which this book evolved. At a fundamentals level, this is a skills book; at a basic textbook level, it is a blend of theory and practice. Our goal has been to produce a book that is sufficiently comprehensive to be used by students for both initial learning and future reference.

Nursing Skills and Evaluation is designed for nursing students to assist them to master basic and advanced nursing procedures in the clinical areas. Basic concepts identified on Level I provide the foundation for the more advanced nursing skills described in the second, third and fourth levels.

The authors believe that an effective nursing skills book must be current, innovative, and relevant so that nursing students are able to master the many skills necessary for high quality nursing care. This book answers the need for a contemporary approach to teaching nursing skills and offers a conceptual framework for appropriate application to current nursing curricula. The challenge of presenting skills in both a conceptual and comprehensive format was formidable. We hope nursing students from all program levels will benefit from utilizing this text.

ACKNOWLEDGEMENTS

We would like to express our appreciation to all those who assisted us during the production of this book. Without them, the task of editing the manuscript and producing the illustrations would have been monumental.

Through the assistance and generosity of Stanford University Hospital and the Community Hospital of Los Gatos and Rehabilitation Center, Saratoga, we were able to conduct extensive photography in the appropriate clinical environment. We extend our thanks to Nancy Madsen, Joyce Miller, Jeanne deJoseph, Barbara Petree and June Olgilvie at Stanford University Hospital for their aid in coordinating our photography sessions. We acknowledge the efforts of Julian Ashton, and Sande Chapman, and Debbie Gaffri, also at Stanford. At the Community Hospital of Los Gatos, we thank Sally Talley, Fern Bolding, and Carol Thoryk for their help during the many hours we spent at their facility. We also thank El Camino Hospital where we obtained additional photographs.

We express our graditude to other individuals without whose assistance this book could not have been published: Lans Hayes of Mayfield Publishing Company for his initial encouragement and support; our friends and models, Ellen Troyer and Elizabeth Anderson; and our editors, Emily Henderson and Vi Sidre. Finally we wish to thank the many clients who consented to be photographed for the benefit of the students utilizing this text.

The never-ending task of proofreading was expertly handled by Pat Gundlock, Lois Dicus, and Laurie Lee all of whom are to be commended for their patience and fortitude in wading through mountains of pages. Our typists who graciously came to our rescue numerous times throughout the manuscript preparation were Suzanne Jansson, Robin Wiener, Tracy Duell, Jo Al Smith, and Jane Ericson.

We thank our special consultants who painstakingly read the manuscript and provided clinical expertise for the book: Joan Althaus, Elizabeth Anderson, Barbara Pratley, and Sally Talley.

Last, but by no means least, we would like to thank our families for putting up with "fast foods," endless hours and neglected household and interpersonal chores.

Sandra F. Smith, RN, MS
Donna J. Duell, RN, MS

INTRODUCTION

Nursing Skills and Evaluation presents a wide range of nursing skills in a conceptual framework. The components of the nursing process provide the format for the book. For the reader to utilize this book in the most effective way, it is important to understand how the authors organized the material and the format in which it is presented.

The conceptual aspect of this book is illustrated by the manner in which the content is structured: first by level, then by chapter, and finally by subject. The subjects are presented as actions, and the actions are discussed in terms of the Nursing Process. Level I, the most basic level of mastery for nursing students consists of four chapters. Each chapter includes learning objectives, an introduction, which provides the theoretical basis for skill performance, and guidelines for managing clients. The text defines basic concepts and then translates them into clinical reality. The clinical content consists of a series of nursing actions, and each action is presented in terms of the Nursing Process.

THE NURSING PROCESS

The Nursing Process is a term that describes the nursing activities necessary to successfully complete a nursing task. Similar to a problem-solving process, the key steps in the Nursing Process are assessment, planning, intervention and evaluation.

Assessment Assessment encompasses establishing a data base for a specific client. The nurse gathers information relevant to the client and then assigns meaning to this data. Assessment is a very critical phase, for all other steps in providing nursing care depend on the accuracy and reliability of the assessment process.

This book specifically defines the assessment component by describing the assessing activities that must be completed in order to effectively perform subsequent interventions. Each listed action is followed by a nursing assessment.

Planning The second step is planning. Other texts may include analysis as the second step but in *Nursing Skills and Evaluation*, the authors chose to combine analysis and planning. This step focuses on the goals which the student will identify for each action. These goals are based upon data interpretation and identification of client needs. Goal formulation is followed by the development of a plan of action for goal achievement. A very important step is the design of a strategy for goal completion. After strategy, another aspect of planning is selection of the materials or equipment necessary to complete the task and achieve the goal. Equipment is an essential consideration for skill performance; thus, it is an important aspect of planning in this book.

Intervention The third step in the nursing process framework is implementation or intervention. This step, labeled intervention in this text, explicitly describes the action component of performing a skill. Intervention involves initiating and completing those actions necessary to accomplish the identified goals. At this state, the text deviates from the traditional nursing process format and, maintaining the conceptual consistency, identifies all the interventions which may be appropriate for a given action. Thus, an action may include one, three or even five interventions.

Interventions are presented in a clear, concise step-by-step outline so that the student can understand specific actions in the order of their performance. This is important in order for the goal to be efficiently accomplished and the outcome of performance positive.

Evaluation The final phase of the Nursing Process is evaluation, determining the extent to which the identified goals were achieved. Evaluation is the examination of the outcome of the nursing interventions. This process is extremely important because, without this step, the nursing plan cannot be evaluated and adapted to the client's needs.

Because this final step of the Nursing Process is so critical to skill performance, the authors devised a specific approach to evaluation. This format will enable the student to evaluate the outcome and, concurrently, assess alternative actions that would result in positive outcomes or goal achievement. The text presents expected outcomes (evaluation of the identified goals) but additionally the reader is offered alternative clinical options to pursue if the goal is not achieved. These options are labeled Alternative Nursing Actions or simply ANA's.

A unique feature of this text is the identification of unexpected outcomes with alternative nursing actions. In any well-formulated plan, the strategies for goal achievement may go awry. If the unexpected occurs, alternative nursing actions are provided for the student to consider when reassessing the initial goals in relation to the outcome or when developing a new plan of action. This content, together with alternative nursing actions due to unexpected outcomes, will add a new dimension to students' learning and will make skill performance more than just a set of memorized, rote actions.

While the Nursing Process has provided the framework for this immense amount of nursing content, additional learning aids have been included: *rationale* for each skill performance to help the student immediately identify why the nurse would perform a certain skill; *clinical alerts* intended to call the student's attention to a critical situation or action; *nursing flags*, which are designed to emphasize specific aspects of client care; *nursing protocols* for appropriate situations which require that a specific protocol or sequence be followed in performance of a certain skill; *client teaching* when certain teaching principles are necessary for goal achievement; and, finally, *charting*, the completion of the evaluation process when the nurse records the client's responses to treatment or care.

The authors intend that nursing students will find this textbook relevant, useful, and adaptable to learning needs. Their intentions will be realized as nursing students find this book an effective learning aid and a valuable reference source.

ABOUT THE PUBLISHER

The publisher of this nursing skills textbook is National Nursing Review of Los Altos, California. Founded in 1976 by Sandra and Christopher Smith, NNR has earned a national reputation for assisting nursing students to prepare for the RN State Board Examinations. The company publishes nursing review textbooks and sponsors the *Sandra Smith Review*, a five-day, concentrated State Board preparation course offered twice per year in many cities throughout the United States.

If you would like to receive more information concerning review books, which can assist you throughout your nursing education, or review courses for RN State Board Examinations, please contact NNR at the address below.

National Nursing Review
342 State Street
Los Altos, California 94022

CONTENTS IN BRIEF

xiii

CONTENTS

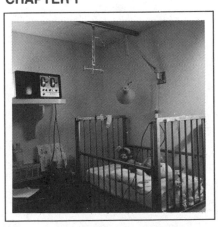

xvii

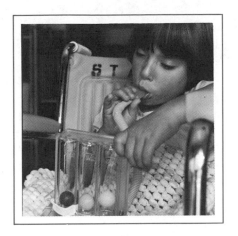

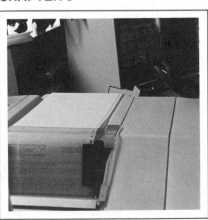

MAINTAINING INFECTION CONTROL: BARRIER NURSING   117   **CHAPTER 4**

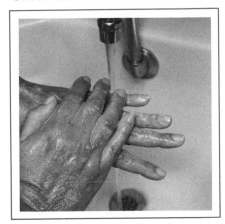

LEVEL II

MAINTENANCE OF HOMEOSTASIS

CHAPTER 5

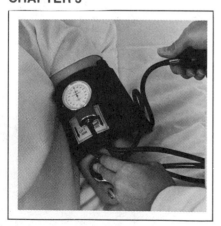

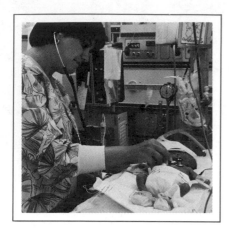

CHAPTER 7

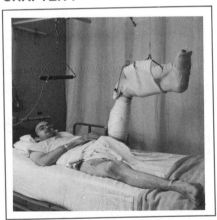

CHAPTER 8

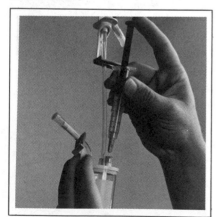

CHAPTER 9

ASSISTING WITH DIAGNOSTIC PROCEDURES   291

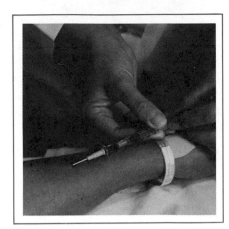

LEVEL III   **ALTERATIONS IN HOMEOSTASIS**

CHAPTER 10   **ALTERATIONS IN MOBILITY**   **317**

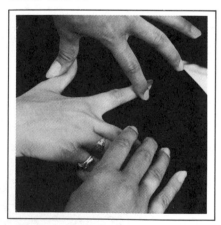

CHAPTER 11

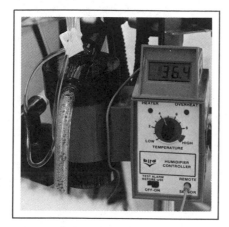

CHAPTER 12

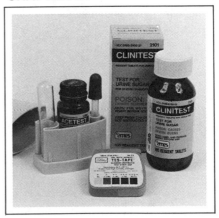

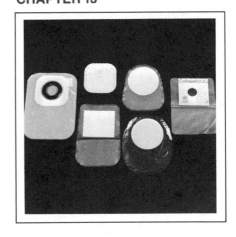

ALTERATIONS IN BOWEL ELIMINATION   427

CHAPTER 14

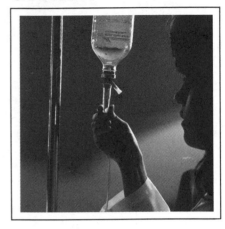

ALTERATIONS IN NUTRITIONAL STATUS   509

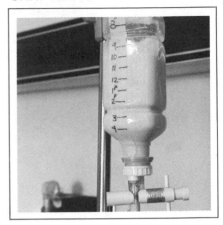

ALTERATIONS IN AERATION   545

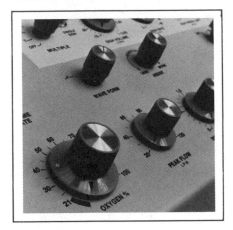

ALTERATIONS IN CIRCULATION   623

CHAPTER 17

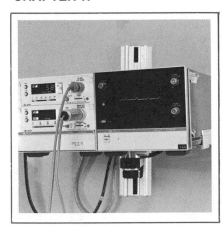

LEVEL IV	CRITICAL ALTERATIONS IN HOMEOSTASIS

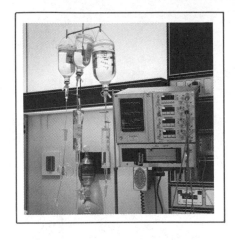

CHAPTER 19

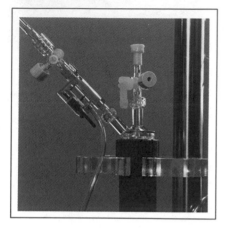

CHAPTER 20

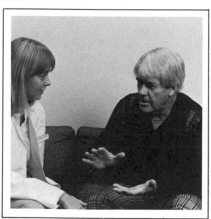

LEVEL I
Health Care Environment

CHAPTER 1
Adapting to the Hospital Environment

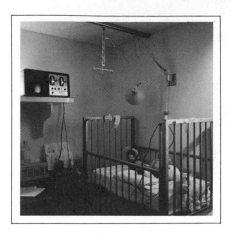

This chapter covers many of the elements essential to human adaptation to illness and wellness. It contains important characteristics that make up a healthful environment as well as a number of external conditions to which the client must adapt during illness.

HOLISTIC APPROACH TO MAINTAINING HOMEOSTASIS

As a nursing professional, one of your primary responsibilities is to make sure your clients have a safe and comfortable health care environment. It is your responsibility to help clients adapt to this environment in addition to health care in general.

From a holistic or total view, the term "environment" can generally be explained as the total of all the conditions and influences, both external and internal, that affect the life and development of an organism. As human beings we are constantly exposed to changing physical, biological, and social conditions. In order to survive, we continually assess our relationship to our changing surroundings. We also learn how to make adjustments that help us control and improve our environment. This complex process is called "adaptation."

Adaptation includes adjustments in all conscious and unconscious forms. People in most situations are able to control or adapt to their

LEARNING OBJECTIVES

Describe the characteristics that influence adaptation.
List the dimensions necessary for positive environmental adaptation.
Explain the sociocultural dimension of environmental adaptation.
Describe the admission and discharge procedures.
Identify guidelines for managing client care.
Outline the components of providing a safe environment.
Identify alternative nursing actions for expected outcomes.
Discuss the unexpected outcomes and the alternative nursing actions.

immediate surroundings. Usually the individual knows best how to adapt to the conditions that are specifically affecting him or her. Although no two people will respond to the environment in exactly the same way, common principles related to adaptation can be found in all human beings:

All adaptations are attempts to maintain optimum physical and chemical states, or homeostasis.

Individuals retain their own identity and uniqueness regardless of the degree of adaptation required.

Adaptation affects all aspects of human existence.

Human beings have limits in the process and degree of adaptation.

Adaptation is measured in relationship to time.

Adaptive responses to the environment may or may not be adequate or appropriate.

Adaptive attempts may be stressful.

The degree and process of adaptation varies from individual to individual.

Adaptation is an ongoing and continuous process about which the individual may be consciously or unconsciously aware.

Each of us adjusts to our immediate environment in a way that is unique to us. When this environment changes suddenly, for instance when we are hospitalized, we may not be able to adapt independently to our immediate surroundings safely and comfortably. It is at this point that assistance must be provided.

CHARACTERISTICS THAT INFLUENCE ADAPTATION

The characteristics that make all people unique also provide information about the process of adaptation to the environment. These factors must be considered when assessing clients' needs and ability to safely adjust to their immediate surroundings.

Age A client's age is a critical factor in the assessment process. Because terms such as "elderly" and "young" can be interpreted in many different ways, the health care provider may need to look at the client's developmental stage (physical and mental growth) rather than at the client's chronological age.

As people develop, sensory receptors help to process day-to-day events. Human beings learn how to protect themselves and how to adjust to changing needs through experiencing these events. During the learning process, young children may require entirely different precautions from teenagers. A thirty-year-old man who has learned through experience how to protect himself in a routine environment may not have adequate skills in an unfamiliar atmosphere.

The older adult often requires special assistance. Sensory impairments such as slowness of movement, poor vision or hearing, loss of balance, and even diminished acuity for taste and touch are not uncommon.

When impairments occur, interpretation of sensory messages is altered. This can result in a decreased ability to sense harmful environmental stimuli. The older person may not see or hear an approaching car, detect the taste of spoiling food, or move quickly enough to avoid falling.

Level of Consciousness The ability to perceive and react to environmental stimuli is closely related to level of consciousness. Adapting to a new or different environment requires learning through experience and possessing an awareness of the immediate surroundings. Making adjustments in the environment requires stimuli to travel over the sensory pathways of nerves to the central nervous system. In order to respond to stimuli, such as avoiding a burn from a hot object, motor neurons carry impulses to muscles to cause an involuntary reflex action, such as withdrawing the hand from hot water. Sensory impulses traveling to the cerebral cortex of the brain inform the person that this stimuli is potentially harmful. Voluntary movement then provides additional adaptation.

Consciousness is the state in which individuals are aware of themselves and their relationship to their surroundings. Unconsciousness indicates a lack of response or awareness of the environment. Levels of consciousness range from fully conscious to comatose. Difficulty in adapting to the immediate environment due to varying levels of consciousness can manifest itself in a variety of ways:

Distorted clients often view their environment in a fearful, distorted way. This can lead to extreme behavioral changes, self injury, or combativeness.

Neurologically injured clients may have decreased perceptions of stimuli, or none at all (such as heat, cold, pain, friction).

Partial or total paralysis inhibits movement and is accompanied by a loss of position sense (dangling limbs or poor body alignment).

Alterations in communication, sight, or hearing because of altered consciousness are barriers to sharing fears or concerns with others.

Fluctuating levels of consciousness create difficulty in promoting self-care and self-image because of an inability to follow directions.

Continuous assessment of changes in the client's level of consciousness is essential. Degree of awareness influences the type and amount of assistance the client will need while in less than familiar surroundings.

States of Illness Illness or injury causes a person to focus more intensely on him or herself. The very nature of disease or trauma requires the individual to use physical and mental energy to adapt to the situation and to become more egocentric. A client often cannot perform even the simplest daily activity. Fatigue or pain may render clients helpless. Assistance with activities such as bathing, eating, skin care, and elimination may be necessary.

When medications are used, side effects such as drowsiness prevent the individual from adequately assessing the environment. Perceptions may be distorted, and the client is more vulnerable to hazards.

Emotional stress and anxiety can occur in mild to acute degrees. While mild anxiety very often increases perceptual awareness, acute anxiety reduces perceptual awareness.

Because an individual is able to focus only on a specific amount of stimuli at one time, additional stimuli that may be equally important are not perceived. Potential environmental dangers are not processed. The client whose energy is focused on pain may not even hear instructions from the nurse. Depressed clients will also require assistance. Depression often results in slower than normal responses to stimuli. Alcohol, a central nervous system depressant, also causes dull, slow reactions to stimuli.

When pain, anxiety, illness, injury, weakness, medications, or even lack of sleep cause a decrease in sensory acuity, awareness of potential hazards is altered. The client may not be able to make the necessary biological, physical, or emotional adjustments to adapt to the immediate environment. Any of these conditions necessitates immediate assessment and action.

ECOSYSTEM DIMENSIONS OF ENVIRONMENTAL ADAPTATION

The conditions and influences that make up an environment can be divided into three basic categories: biological, physical, and socio-cultural. The biological dimensions of our environment include all living things, such as plants, animals, and micro-organisms. Water, oxygen, sunlight, organic compounds, and other components in which living things exist and develop make up the physical dimensions of an environment.

When we talk about the biological and physical dimensions together, we refer to both dimensions as an ecosystem, or the total of all living and nonliving things that are part of the chain of life.

As you become more aware of the factors that affect environmental adaptation, providing a safe and comfortable atmosphere for your clients becomes a greater challenge. As you assess your clients and help them adapt to the environment of a health care facility, you will want to consider the following essential elements: space, lighting, humidity, temperature, ventilation, sound levels, surfaces and equipment, a safe environment, food and water, waste disposal, time organization, privacy, individualized care, and information and teaching.

Adequate Space Everyone needs space in which to grow and develop. This space may consist of a room or an area as small as a shelf or corner. No matter what form space takes, individuals need to feel they have control over it – to be able to arrange it or decorate it to their liking.

Providing space for clients encourages stimulation and experimentation. Toddlers need the space of an area like a recreation room for discovery and motor skills, since playtime is their primary source of development. Adults often enjoy the social activities of a lounge, but

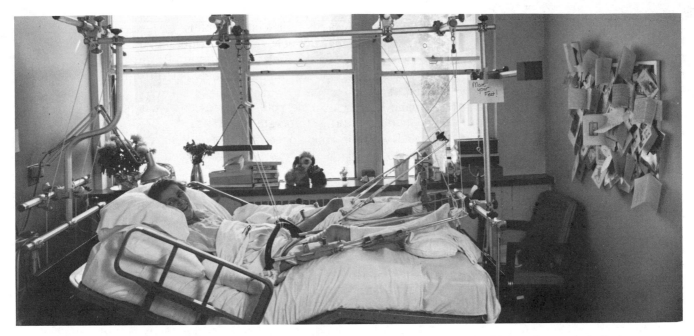

Provide area for personal effects.

may also require well-defined personal areas even if these areas are as simple as a bedside table or a bulletin board.

Natural and Artificial Light Light, like space, is necessary for growth and development. The production of vitamin D, a critical component of bone structure, occurs from ultraviolet radiation on the skin. Natural light also helps wounds heal. In a hospital setting, natural light can be used to decrease feelings of isolation and to encourage clients to continue their normal routine.

Whether natural or artificial, adequate light is essential for the preservation of sight, for safety, and for accurate assessments and nursing care. Because eye strain, as well as nervousness and fatigue can result from improper lighting, care should be taken to avoid glare, sharp contrast, and flickering lights.

Humidity and Temperature The ability to adapt to changes in humidity and/or temperature is directly related to comfort. Most people in this country are comfortable at a room temperature of 18.3° C to 25° C (65° F to 77° F) with the humidity at 30 to 60 percent. People in other cultures function equally well at lower or higher readings.

Conditions that may inhibit a person's ability to adjust to high temperatures include excessive physical work, dehydration, extremes in age (the very young and very old), decreased physical fitness, and inappropriate clothing. An individual who has difficulty adapting to high temperatures may experience a rapid rise in pulse rate, cramps, nausea, and vomiting. Severe inability to adapt to heat can result in heat stroke and death.

An individual who has difficulty adapting to lower temperatures may experience a change in behavior, depressed vital signs, and eventual unconsciousness. Hypothermia, an abnormally low body temperature, occurs when there is an imbalance between heat loss and heat production.

Extreme heat or extreme cold increases the incidence of infection and adds to discomfort. Temperatures in health care institutions can be regulated with air conditioners and dehumidifiers, although care should be taken to avoid drafts and excessive dryness.

Ventilation Particular attention should be given to assessing the movement of air within a client's immediate environment. An adequately ventilated room should contain a comfortable amount of moisture, be free of irritating pollutants, odors, or noxious fumes, and be at a tolerable temperature.

Adequate ventilation is especially important when more than one client is in a room. Other areas requiring optimum ventilation are operating rooms, delivery rooms, nurseries, isolation rooms, and sterile supply rooms.

A properly functioning ventilation system reduces airborne contaminants by regulating the amount of air movement within an enclosed area. When ventilation cannot be maintained by using doors and windows, mechanical devices such as fans or air conditioners may be used.

Comfortable Sound Levels Noise can be defined as any undesirable sound. The degree of noise that is comfortable is highly individual and related to past experiences. A businessman who lives on a busy street in a city may not adjust well to the absolute quiet he may experience at night in a hospital room. On the other hand, a farmer from a rural community may be disturbed by the slightest sound. Infants often sleep peacefully in an atmosphere of loud noise and confusion.

"Decibel" is the term used to describe the intensity of noise, or the measurement of the sensation produced by sound on the human ear. At close range, noise produced from heavy traffic, for example, has a decibel measure of 90, whereas a whisper at three feet has an intensity of 20 decibels.

At certain levels, noise is considered hazardous. Temporary or permanent hearing loss or damage can occur when noise is present for a prolonged time at intensities over 90 decibels. Other effects of sustained loud noise are muscle tension, increased blood pressure, blood vessel constriction, pallor, increased secretion of adrenal hormone, and nervous tension.

The pitch and quality of noise may also affect the client's environment. Unwanted sounds produced by sirens, traffic, and aircraft are often beyond the control of the health care provider. But noise within a hospital setting, especially loud talking, television, call systems, careless handling of dishes and other equipment, visitors, and excessive conversation at the nurses' station, can be controlled.

Nursing personnel should always be aware of the noise level and its effects on the client's well-being. Very ill individuals are often more sensitive to noise. Although too much noise can be a barrier to adapting to the immediate environment, absolute silence can be annoying and even frightening. Certain sounds can be reassuring because they represent activity or assistance to the client.

Clean Surfaces and Equipment   Today, most health care facilities are designed to be attractive, orderly, efficient, and clean. Since a person's outlook is strongly influenced by the surroundings, careful attention to appearance and cleanliness can assist with adjustment to the health care environment. Although it is essential to assess the routines and standards of cleanliness of each client, the health care provider may also have to teach the client how to organize and clean up. In some cases, instruction to the client may be critical to maintain or improve a health care condition.

The standards and routine cleaning procedures of the hospital are generally not a nursing function now because hospital housekeeping has become a specialized occupation requiring a background in microbiology, chemistry, epidemiology, and management. Maintaining an organized, clean environment, however, requires coordination by all health care providers.

Furnishings should be arranged to be physically comfortable, safe, and aesthetically appealing for the client. Adequate cleaning of the room should be done at a time of day which is coordinated with the client's needs so that the resulting sense of security adds to the client's ability to adapt adequately to the surrounding.

A Safe Environment   Providing a safe environment involves a number of people, including the client, visitors, and health care providers. Providing protection from hazardous situations and education about safety precautions is one of your most important responsibilities as a nurse.

Clients who are moved from their usual environment into one that is unfamiliar and often frightening may act in ways that are very different from their usual behavior. A threatening situation can interfere with the individual's adaptation to the immediate surroundings.

The design and decor of the client's room must satisfy two needs: client comfort and client safety. Tasteful, unobtrusive color helps to normalize the hospital room. Interesting color combinations and patterns generally appeal more to the senses than do the traditional white or green choices. Pictures, flowers, cards, colorful linens, and curtains can add variety and familiarity to a room.

Furniture should be comfortable, safe for the client, and convenient for the health care provider. All furniture and equipment should be movable. Beds are usually adjustable in height so that the client can get in and out of the bed safely. A step stool may be necessary for some people. For safety and a sense of security, adjustable side rails are essential on both sides of the bed. The head and foot of the bed may

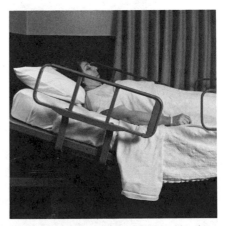

Side rails are placed in the UP position for all clients at night, and for clients at risk for falling during the day.

9

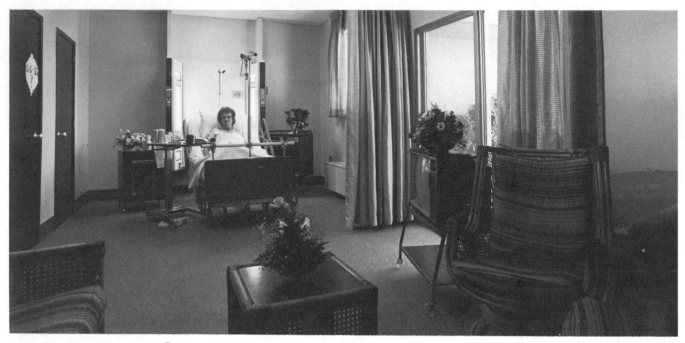

A comfortable environment.

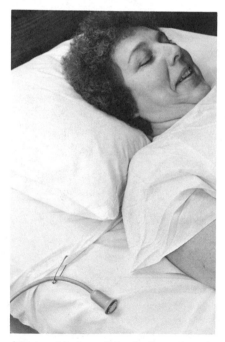

Attach call button within client's reach and instruct how to use if needed.

also be raised or lowered, depending on comfort or need. A mattress should be covered with a durable, waterproof casing. Some mattresses are made of specially designed foam rubber or filled with air or water depending on the physical need.

The overbed table is adjustable in height and slides over the bed to provide space for self-care activities or additional working surface for the nurse. The overbed table may also be used when the client sits in a chair. Small bed trays are sometimes convenient when the overbed table cannot be used. Bed trays are particularly useful for children in crib beds.

The bedside table, similar to a nightstand, holds the client's valuable or personal possessions in drawers. A cabinet section in the table can be used to store bathing or toiletry equipment, and the top provides space for the client's familiar items such as pictures or books.

A chair with firm back and arm supports should always be a part of the client's furnishing. Chairs should be made of durable, easily cleanable materials such as plastic or naugehyde. The client should be instructed to avoid contact between skin surfaces and the chair when sitting in a chair. A small towel or blanket can be placed under the client for this purpose.

A signaling system is also essential for the client to call for assistance. A signaling system may be an intercom, buzzer, electric light or hand-bell. Whatever device is available must be within a client's reach and ability to use.

The age of the client influences the specific safety precautions that need to be taken to provide a safe environment. For example, infants require constant supervision since they may attempt to put anything in their mouths or up their noses. The following sections discuss specific safety factors for different age groups.

Keep the following guidelines in mind when caring for infants:

Keep one hand on the infant when the infant is on an unprotected surface.

Never leave an infant unattended in a bath.

Keep crib rails up and crib mattress in a low position when infants are left alone.

Store objects that are small enough to put in the mouth, nose or ear in a safe place out of the infant's reach.

Inspect toys for buttons, staples, and sharp parts.

Secure cabinets and cupboards with childproof latches or locks.

Cover electrical outlets.

Block stairways with doors or gates.

Toddlers also require constant supervision and teaching. Safety precautions for toddlers include the following:

Secure all cabinets and closets.

Lock up dangerous solutions, medicines, alcoholic beverages, and caustic materials.

Put mechanical tools and electrical appliances out of reach.

Assess the child's room and toys for dangerous or harmful materials.

Pre-school age children can be taught more detailed aspects of safety. Fire precautions and guidelines for bathing should be stressed. Elementary school age children can usually protect themselves from hazards. They will require instruction on how to operate mechanical equipment, as well as information about fires and emergency exits.

Teenagers, adolescents, and adults should be given instruction about smoking, fire exits, and the use of special equipment. In addition,

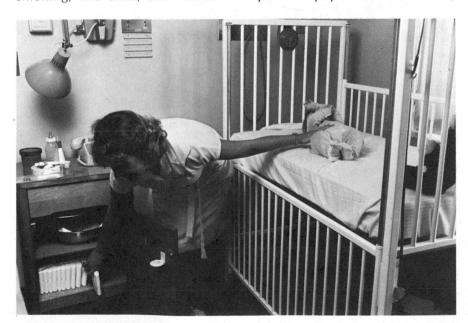

A safe environment.

11

general information regarding their safety during hospitalization should be explained.

Elderly adults are especially susceptible to injury from falls. Poor vision, decreased balance and stability, disorientation, or chronic physical problems such as arthritis contribute to the high incidence of falls among the elderly. Safety precautions for the elderly include the following:

Keep hallways clear of toys, scatter rugs, lamp cords, etc.

Provide adequate lighting.

Put necessary articles for personal hygiene and activities of daily living within easy reach.

Provide nonslip mats and handrails in bath tubs and showers.

Food and Water Fresh, healthful food and clean water, vital elements in an everyday routine, must be planned for and assured in appropriate amounts in health care facilities. While a client's well-being can be positively affected by the ingestion of the correct number of calories, fat, proteins, carbohydrates, minerals, vitamins, and water, it is well known that many people have nutritional habits that can negatively affect their well-being. A careful nutritional assessment is a critical step in helping the client adjust to the environment.

Safe Waste Disposal All waste products, whether contaminated equipment, human body wastes, garbage, soiled dressings, or refuse, must be disposed of in a way that prevents the spread of micro-organisms. Hospital wastes can be hazardous and highly infective. If wastes cannot be properly removed, the individual is at a risk and may not be able to adjust safely and comfortably to the surroundings.

Health care providers must be aware of the potential dangers to themselves as well as to their clients when disposing of waste materials. Most health care agencies have specific guidelines regarding the removal of various types of contaminated materials. Many of these guidelines have been established by experts (epidemiologists) knowledgeable in the detection and spread of diseases. The U.S. Public Health Service Center for Disease Control, the American Hospital Association, and State Departments of Health are some of the agencies that prepare guidelines for the disposal of dangerous products.

In some health care facilities, a position of Infection Control Nurse has been created to gather data on the type and frequency of various infections found in the hospital. Data about infections helps the Infection Control Nurse to locate the source of the problem, to predict its spread, and to identify the best method of prevention to decrease its recurrence. Many of the nosocomial, hospital-originated disease states, can be traced to inappropriate or careless disposal of wastes. Each health care provider plays a significant role in establishing a safe environment for the client by carrying out the recommended methods of waste disposal.

SOCIOCULTURAL DIMENSION OF ENVIRONMENTAL ADAPTATION

The first two dimensions of the environment, the biological and physical or ecosystem, refer to all living and non-living elements. The third dimension of an environment is sociocultural, which includes both past and present influences from the people and the culture surrounding the individual. Customs, religious and legal systems, and economic and political beliefs are all part of this environment. This dimension also involves responses and adjustments to the ideals, concepts, beliefs, activities, and pressure of various groups such as social clubs, peer groups, or colleagues.

Organization of Time How clients perceive and deal with time and the passing of time depend on their age, immediate situation, culture, and past experiences as well as their present physical and emotional condition. To a mother waiting for her child to return from surgery, hours seem like days. Small children generally do not have a well-developed sense of time. A three year old may act out feelings of abandonment when separated from a parent for just a few minutes. In an intensive care unit, time can be severely disrupted since health care activities continue around the clock. The ability to organize time is a critical element in adaptation. Helping clients assess and plan their time is one of the most important ways you can help them cope with their new surroundings.

Privacy Many people who enter a health care facility fear exposure and loss of identity. Providing privacy for a client is more than a luxury or a desirable condition. It is necessary and vitally important to the individual's attitude toward health care.

Clients should be given as much privacy as possible. Most individuals will give clues to the nurse about the degree of privacy that is comfortable. The client's culture, past experience, values, and age should all be considered when planning for privacy.

Hospital routines should be planned to promote privacy. If an embarrassing or upsetting situation occurs, the feelings of the client must be protected. People require time and space to think, organize, and reflect. Privacy is necessary for human development even at home. In the hospital, privacy is critical to the client's attitude and well-being.

Privacy can be promoted by drawing curtains or screens. Doors and window shades may also be used. Signs posted on room entrances give the client a sense of security from disturbances. This is especially important during physical exams, personal care, or emotional upset. Knocking or asking for permission to enter the client's room or area promotes mutual respect and enhances a sense of emotional space.

Privacy also extends beyond the physical need of the individual. Health status, conversation, and records are privileged information. A more trusting, therapeutic relationship will evolve if the client under-

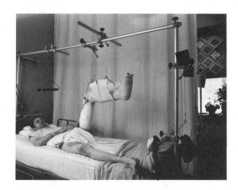

Draw curtain to ensure client privacy.

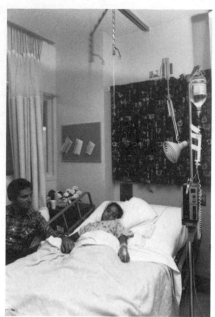

Individualized care.

stands that the confidences the client shares with health care providers will be used appropriately for his or her well-being.

Individualized Care   Providing an environment that is comfortable, safe, and individualized to meet the specific needs of a client is a challenging task. The client's adaptation to the immediate environment can either improve or interfere with the client's well-being. In order to assist the client in adjusting to the environment, a careful assessment of the situation should always include the person's usual routines, self-care abilities, cultural beliefs, and past experiences. To promote the best adaptation to a different environment, encourage as much independence as possible with each client. You may be required to use your resourcefulness, imagination, and ingenuity to assist the client through less than desirable periods. Open communication processes from client to staff are essential if positive adaptation is to occur.

Hospitalized clients also need emotional space. This form of space is that psychological area where the person can experience a sense of self. This is particularly difficult to achieve in a hospital setting when caretakers exercise control over many of the activities of daily living. It is important that the staff be aware of this element of space so that they can provide adequate privacy, quiet, and freedom of choice over all of the areas that the client can control. The staff must also be aware that the client never need relinquish total responsibility for his or her care.

Information and Teaching   The amount of information the client has about the environment and immediate situation directly affects the client's ability to safely and comfortably adjust. When the individual is given information and explanations about strange equipment, diagnostic procedures, or unfamiliar health care personnel, fears and feelings of helplessness can be reduced and a shared sense of responsibility enhanced. The client becomes more capable of asking questions and expressing concerns if prepared for unfamiliar occurrences.

Providing the client and the client's family, if appropriate, with information about the client's environment is the nurse's responsibility. As more people assume the role of consumers of health care, there is more demand for knowledge about aspects of health care. Including the client in planning and caring for him or herself promotes a sense of responsibility, independence and self-respect.

Teaching the client about various aspects of health care is one method of information-sharing. Over the years, the focus has changed from the professional staff doing everything for the client to helping the client be more independent. This change enables the client to adapt to the environment with guided assistance from health care providers. As the client learns about his or her own health care and becomes involved in meeting his or her particular needs, a sense of trust, responsibility and usefulness develops.

ADMISSION AND DISCHARGE FROM THE HEALTH CARE UNIT

The admission procedure for clients can be a negative experience if it is impersonal, mechanized, or impolite. It can be a positive step in health care if handled with attention and care. The impressions formed by the client during the admission process have a strong effect on his or her attitude toward the total care the client will receive. Because the admission procedure can be the initial introduction into the health care system, nurses should consider this process a key step in client care.

Adapting to the Role of Client All clients have needs that require discussion and planning as they take on the role of client in the health care setting. You must accept the client's perceptions of his or her new surroundings. Look for signs of anxiety that come from this encounter with a new environment. Be aware that anxiety is a natural reaction to an unfamiliar setting, to new procedures, and to new people. If, for example a client is extremely fatigued or overwhelmed by traveling and the admission procedure, you can help the client adapt to the surroundings, regain a sense of control and identity, and accept the changed circumstances.

Another way to assist the client to retain his or her identity and uniqueness is to communicate with the client as an individual. Ask questions and observe verbal responses as well as nonverbal cues. Provide ways to care for a client's personal possessions, clothing, and physical comfort so that the client adapts more easily to the change in environment and feels more secure and in control.

Be aware that the medical condition is only one part of the client's life and that the changes that have led up to admission affect other areas of the client's well-being. Clients may have concerns about new routines, financial matters, their families, or their future. By responding to a client's total needs at the time of admission, you can help the client establish a positive attitude toward the total care he or she will receive.

Acknowledge and accept any statements or behaviors the client uses to adapt to his or her new surroundings. Even though various cultures and groups differ in their responses to illness, and some responses may differ from your personal beliefs, acknowledge the client's individuality. Support the client's beliefs and behavior as long as they do not increase the risk of injury or illness. Be sensitive to any past health care experiences that may influence the client's feelings at the time of admission. A prior experience in a hospital may determine how a client responds to the current environment.

Admission to the Hospital The process of admitting a client to a health care facility will vary in institutions such as nursing homes, clinics, and hospitals. Regardless of the size or type of facility, the admission process is vitally important in order to provide safe, adequate care. Because the nurse-client relationship begins with admission, you should have a thorough understanding of the standard admission process.

If a client enters the hospital in an emergency situation, he or she may feel insecure or fearful because the client has had little time to make plans concerning family, travel, finances, or employment.

When the client arrives at the hospital, the first contact is usually with the admitting receptionist, who assigns a hospital number and interviews the client. If preadmission material was mailed to the client, it will be verified by the receptionist at this time; otherwise, the client must answer questions about age, address, financial or insurance status, next of kin, religion, employment, and consent for treatment. If the client cannot answer these questions due to age or condition, a relative usually gives the information. A parent or guardian must do this for a child.

During admission, clients may be requested to place valuables in the hospital safe or to send them home with their family. Clients also receive identification bracelets at this time.

Unless laboratory procedures are carried out in the client's room, the client will be directed or escorted to the hematology laboratory for baseline values on hemoglobin, hematocrit, complete blood count differential, and serological screening for syphilis. Depending on the policy of the facility, the client may then proceed to the electrocardiographic laboratory and to radiology to obtain a chest x-ray.

These procedures sometimes take several hours. Delays often result in physical and emotional strain for the client. When an alternative is offered, such as having laboratory procedures performed the day before admission, the client should be encouraged to use these options to decrease emotional and physical fatigue. More time can then be allowed on the actual admission day for adapting to the hospital environment.

Admission to the Nursing Unit When admission to the hospital is complete, the client is either directed to the nursing unit or escorted by a volunteer. The client may be met by a staff nurse assigned to admissions for that day or by the nurse who will be working with the client during the client's stay in the hospital. It is at this time that you must begin to assess your clients' needs and to plan for their care.

When you meet a client, introduce yourself and any other personnel who will provide care. Explain your role and functions to the client. Your initial contact will leave a lasting impression on the client, so try to present information in an uninterrupted, organized, and friendly manner. If there are other clients in the room, introduce them to the new client.

Tell the client about mealtimes, visiting hours, telephone use, requests for clergy, recreational and lounge use, physicians' visits, and other schedules. Some hospitals have printed booklets describing this information. The more information your client receives, the more control he or she has over the environment.

Help the client become familiar with his or her immediate physical space by showing the location and the operation of the intercom system,

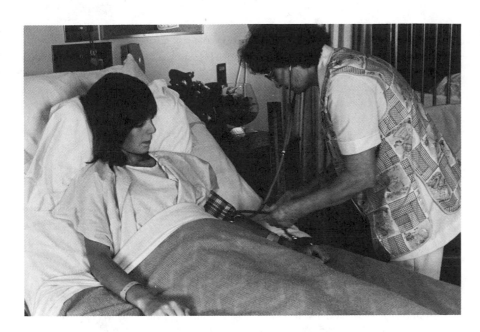

Admitting a client.

the location of the bathroom, and the operation of the call system inside the bathroom. If electric beds are used, show the client how to operate bed controls. You may also want to show the client how to operate the television and the radio.

Because clients may not be sure of their role while in the hospital, many hospitals have adopted versions of the American Hospital Association's *Patient's Bill of Rights*. This Bill includes the following rights: to obtain information about the client's illness or injury, to refuse medication or treatment, to participate in his or her own care, to know the rationale and/or risks of the treatment, and to receive courteous care. Make sure your clients understand their rights. Clear, uncomplicated explanations help them adapt to their new environment.

Once you have completed introductions and the environmental orientation, you may begin the nursing history and assessment to establish baseline data about the client's general condition. (See Chapter 6, Physical Assessment.) After completing the assessment, you may begin providing personal hygiene.

Discharge from the Health Care Unit When a client is discharged from a health care unit, preparations must be made to help the client transfer from a dependent role to a more independent role. Discharge from the hospital can be a welcome relief for the client, but it can also be a time of anxiety and fear. During this transition, the nursing staff can facilitate the process by being aware of individual client needs.

During the discharge process, you must take into consideration the physical, emotional, and psychosocial needs of the client and family. Your responsibilities for the discharge process will include assessing the

17

client's post-hospitalization needs and planning with the client and family to meet discharge needs. It is also important to communicate with appropriate health team members and community agencies. The final responsibilities of the discharge process will be terminating the nurse-client relationship, and evaluating the discharge process.

GUIDELINES FOR MANAGING CLIENTS

Assisting clients to adapt to the health care environment will decrease anxiety and enhance acceptance of health care.

- Assessment of the client's physical, emotional, and psychological needs provides data to help you anticipate any changes the client may experience in the new environment.
- Careful observation and assessment of the client's disabilities or limitations will help determine what changes the client may need to expect in this environment.
- Encouragement of both positive and negative emotions and feelings about the hospital environment will give you valuable information about the client's adjustment needs.

Adequate planning for discharge promotes a smooth transition for clients and families.

- Sufficient preparation time for the discharge process will increase your ability to communicate effectively with the client.
- Encouragement of the client's family or significant others in the discharge process will increase active involvement in meeting the client's needs after hospitalization.

ACTION: ADMITTING A CLIENT TO A HEALTH CARE UNIT

Rationale for Action
- To provide a comfortable and esthetically pleasing environment for the client
- To maintain asepsis by preventing the spread of microorganisms
- To provide the client with some control over the client's immediate environment

ASSESSMENT

1 Evaluate client's physical, emotional, and intellectual status.
2 Evaluate client's ability to adapt to the environment of a hospital unit. Observe for disabilities or limitations.
3 Assess client's condition and ability to orient to the nursing unit.
4 Assess the client's level of comfort or discomfort.
5 Determine client's understanding of his or her disease and the limitations disease imposes on client.
6 Complete the nursing history.
7 Conduct a total assessment, including height, weight, and vital signs.
8 Evaluate the results of lab values obtained on admission.

PLANNING

GOALS

- Client adapts to hospital environment with minimal distress.
- Client participates in his or her own plan of care.
- Client verbalizes his or her needs and feelings about hospitalization.

EQUIPMENT

- Admission kit for personal hygiene
- Thermometer
- Blood pressure cuff and stethoscope
- Urine container
- Rand or Kardex card and client care plan
- Client's chart

INTERVENTION: Admitting a Client to a Health Care Unit

1 Introduce yourself to the client and begin to establish a therapeutic nurse-client relationship.
2 Introduce the client to staff and to roommate, if present.
3 Explain equipment and hospital routines.
4 Obtain the client's health history.
5 Complete physical assessment of client.
6 Obtain the client's weight and height.
7 Obtain urine specimen.
8 Inform laboratory that client is available for chest x-ray and routine blood work if not obtained earlier.
9 Identify client's problem areas.
10 Begin client care plan.
11 Notify physician that the client has been admitted and obtain orders.
12 Reassess client's level of comfort and ability to adapt to hospitalization.
13 Complete client teaching for all unfamiliar procedures or interventions.
14 Fill out Rand or Kardex card and client's chart.

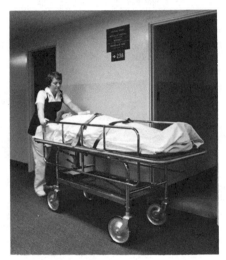

Seriously ill clients are admitted on guerneys.

EVALUATION

EXPECTED OUTCOMES

1 Client adapts to hospital environment. *If not*, follow these alternative nursing actions:
  ANA: Assess physiological and emotional basis for maladaption.
  ANA: Request consulting experts, i.e., client advocate, psychiatrist, social worker, etc.

19

Charting

- Admission procedures
- Adaptation to hospitalization
- Admission assessment data: height, weight, vital signs, physical assessment findings
- Nursing history
- Laboratory specimens
- X-rays

Rationale for Action

- To assist client to interpret environmental stimuli relevant to his or her safety
- To provide protection when states of illness decrease the individual's ability to receive and interpret environmental stimuli
- To promote levels of rest and comfort in a safe environment
- To enhance degrees of mobility in a safe environment

2 Client participates in his or her own plan of care. *If not,* follow these alternative nursing actions:

ANA: Elicit client's feelings (fears) concerning hospitalization.

ANA: Discuss with the client shared responsibility and the importance of participation in his or her care.

ANA: Keep the client informed even though he or she does not want to actively participate in the care plan.

ACTION: PROVIDING A SAFE ENVIRONMENT FOR CLIENTS

ASSESSMENT

1 Identify client's age, previous or chronic sensory impairments, previous level of mobility, ambulatory aids used, and general health history.
2 Assess client's present level of consciousness, orientation, mobility, and restrictions.
3 Review physician's plan of care.
4 Identify any impending loss of sensory or motor abilities due to illness or injury.
5 Assess preoperative and postoperative effect on client's physical, mental, and emotional states.
6 Assess the effect of sedation or anesthesia on client.
7 Evaluate client's ability to comprehend instruction about how to use potentially dangerous equipment.
8 Note medications previously and currently used as well as their desired effects.
9 Assess equipment to be used, noting additional safety precautions, e.g., heating pads, oxygen, etc.
10 Assess client's relationship with family or significant others.
11 Evaluate client's level of anxiety and ability to make judgments.
12 Assess client's reliability as an accurate health historian.
13 Observe client's verbal and nonverbal cues.

PLANNING

GOALS

- Client receives information regarding mechanical, chemical, and thermal safety precautions appropriate to his or her needs.
- Client's immediate environment is safe from potential mechanical, chemical, and thermal hazards.
- Client who smokes does so according to hospital policy.
- All electrical equipment is intact and operated safely.
- If oxygen is used, appropriate safety measures are in effect.
- Client is as comfortable as possible.
- All personal articles and call light are within easy reach of client.

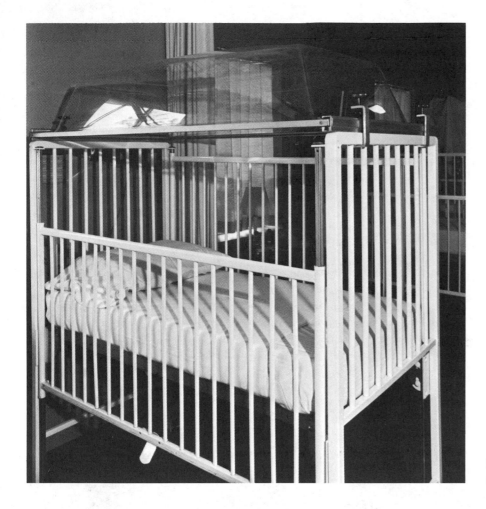

Hood prevents child from climbing out of bed.

EQUIPMENT

- Side rails
- Restraints
- Locks for movable equipment such as wheelchairs and guerneys
- Fire extinguishers
- Protective shields for x-ray
- Covers for heat and cold application devices
- Oxygen-In-Use signs

INTERVENTION: Preventing Mechanical Injuries

1 Put bed in low position when you are not in client's room.
2 Tell clients who are weak, in pain, or who have had surgery to ask for assistance before getting out of bed.
3 Make sure floors are free of debris that might cause clients to slip and fall. Spilled liquids should be wiped up immediately. Encourage housekeepers to use signs for slippery areas.

21

▶ Policies regarding the use of side rails vary from institution to institution. Side rails are most commonly used for individuals who are very young, very old, or unconscious, confused, or awakening from anesthesia or heavy sedation. In addition, blind clients, those with muscular or orthopedic disabilities, or on seizure precautions sometimes require side rails.

4 Check to see that client's unit and hallway are neat and free of hazardous equipment such as foot stools, electrical cords, shoes, etc.

5 Place articles such as call light, cups, etc., within client's reach.

6 Remind client and hospital personnel to lock wheelchairs and guerneys and to release the lock only after client is secure.

7 Keep side rails on cribs in the up position to protect clients. Keep side rails up for all confused, elderly, and surgical clients.

8 If restraints are necessary, follow these guidelines:

   a Use restraints for the client's protection, not for your convenience.

   b Review hospital policy or doctor's orders for the use of restraints.

   c Allow client as much freedom of movement as possible.

   d Always explain the purpose of the restraint to client or parent of a child.

   e Remember that restraints can cause increased anxiety and a feeling of decreasing self-image.

   f Remember that circulation and skin integrity can be affected by restraints. Frequently observe areas around the restraint for circulatory impairment or broken skin.

   g Pad bony prominences, i.e., wrists and ankles, beneath a restraint.

   h Attempt to make restraints as inconspicuous as possible for the client's sake as well as relatives and friends, who may be upset by seeing restraints.

Soft restraints prevent baby from interfering with therapeutic equipment.

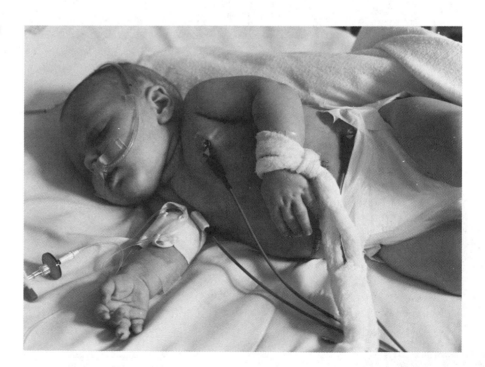

INTERVENTION: Preventing Drug Injuries

1 Keep all medicines in locked carts or cupboards.
2 Keep narcotics in double locked cabinets. Count all narcotics at the end of each shift.
3 Keep all poisonous solutions and materials in a secure area away from medicines.
4 Clearly label and separate topical medicines from parenteral or oral medicines.
5 Provide complete instructions to clients regarding medicines to be used at home. Make sure every physician involved with a client is aware of the medications the client is taking home.
6 Have another nurse check mathematical calculations for dosages of drugs such as heparin and insulin before administering them to clients.
7 Report any errors in the administration of medicines to the physician immediately. Complete a written report if required.

INTERVENTION: Preventing Thermal Injuries

1 Make sure that all electrical appliances are routinely checked and maintained.
2 Have all electrical appliances brought to the hospital by client (radios, electric razors, etc.) checked by the hospital maintenance staff.
3 When hot water bottles, heating pads, baths, hot compresses, and heat lamps are used, check the client frequently for burns.
4 When oxygen sources are used, post "No Smoking" signs and explain the combustible nature of oxygen to clients and families.
5 If smoking is allowed where oxygen is not in use, provide non-tip ashtrays. Inform clients and visitors about hospital's smoking regulations.
6 Store all combustible materials securely to prevent spontaneous combustion.
7 Make sure that all staff and employees participate in and understand fire prevention measures such as extinguishing fires and evacuating clients.

Clinical Alert
No client who is confused, under the influence of sedation, or incapacitated due to weakness or injury should be allowed to smoke without direct supervision.

INTERVENTION: Providing Safety for Clients During a Fire

1 Remove all clients from the immediate area to a safe place.
2 Follow institutional policy and procedure for type of fire prevention program and ringing the fire alarm to summon help.
3 Secure the burning area by closing all doors.
4 Shut off all possible oxygen sources and electrical appliances in the fire area.
5 If possible, employ the appropriate extinguishing method without endangering yourself.
6 Be familiar with the different types of fire extinguishers:

▶ To safely remove a client, make sure you know how to perform the following carries:
- Hip carry
- Pack strap carry
- Two-nurse seat carry
- Three-person carry
- Blanket pull carry

23

Class A

a Water type or soda-acid type

b Use on cloth, wood, paper, plastic, rubber, leather

c Never use on electrical fires due to danger of shock

Class B

a Foam, dry chemical, carbon dioxide

b Use on fires such as alcohol, acetone, oils, grease, paint thinner and remover

c Never use a class A extinguisher or water type on class B fires

Class C

a Dry chemical type, carbon dioxide type

b Use on electrical wiring, electrical equipment, or motors

c Never use a class A or class B extinguisher on a class C fire

7 Clear all fire exits.

INTERVENTION: Providing Safety for Clients Receiving Radioactive Materials

1 Review these guidelines:

a Increased time in the presence of a radioactive source increases exposure to radiation.

b Shields, such as lead walls or lead aprons, are used as a protective source.

c Exposure is greater the closer you are to the radioactive source.

d Radioactive material must be stored in lead-shielded containers when not in use.

2 If you or a family member are assisting with a radioactive procedure, put on a shield.

3 If a radioactive implant is used in a client, make sure all health care providers and visitors are protected with a shield. Limit their exposure to the client.

4 Keep track of how much time you spend in the presence of radioactive material.

5 Dispose of excreta carefully, according to hospital policy. Wear rubber gloves when performing this procedure.

6 Determine the type and amount of radiation used and its side effects and hazards.

7 Constantly assess and support clients who are undergoing radiation therapy. Bedrest, isolation, and unpleasant side effects are sometimes common.

EVALUATION

EXPECTED OUTCOMES

1 Client receives information regarding mechanical, chemical, and thermal safety precautions appropriate to his or her needs. *If not*, follow these alternative nursing actions:

ANA: Explain safety precautions to client and family.

ANA: Hold a conference with the individual responsible for disseminating safety information and elicit whether he or she is aware of the safety precautions. Ask why this information was not given to client.

ANA: Provide in-service program on safety precautions to staff members.

ANA: Work with other health care members to compile a pamphlet explaining safety precautions, which can be given to clients as needed.

2 Client's immediate environment is safe from potential mechanical, chemical, and thermal hazards. *If not*, follow these alternative nursing actions:

ANA: Notify appropriate hospital department, i.e., housekeeping, central supply, and ask them to rectify the situation.

ANA: Instruct nursing staff to check all potentially hazardous equipment carefully before using.

ANA: Report all malfunctioning equipment immediately to the proper department. Usually this is done through a written work order and a telephone call to the department.

ANA: Provide all staff members with the time to attend safety in-service seminars at least once a year.

3 Clients who smoke do so according to hospital policy. *If not*, follow these alternative nursing actions:

ANA: Explain to client why it is important to follow hospital routine for smoking.

ANA: Take smoking material away from client's bedside and place in nurses' station.

ANA: Set up smoking schedule with client when someone is available to stay with client. Explain schedule to client and leave schedule visible to client at bedside.

4 All electrical equipment is intact and operated safely. *If not*, follow these alternative nursing actions:

ANA: Report all frayed cords immediately and do not use equipment.

ANA: Check electrical equipment carefully before using with client.

ANA: Ensure that operating directions are clearly printed on or attached to the equipment.

ANA: If you are unfamiliar with the equipment's use, read operating directions, hospital procedure manual, or talk with central supply or maintainance personnel before using.

ANA: Do not use adaptor electrical plugs to plug in several electrical appliances. Instead, identify those devices which are essential and those which can be discontinued, i.e., television set, bedside lamp.

ANA: Make sure all electrical appliances are grounded properly before using.

5 If oxygen is used, appropriate safety measures are in effect, *If not*, follow these alternative nursing actions:

ANA: Ensure that Oxygen-In-Use signs are placed on door and on the wall over client's bed.

ANA: Instruct client and family on safety precautions.

ANA: Reinforce need for safety precautions with staff members.

6 Client is as comfortable as possible. *If not*, follow these alternative nursing actions:

ANA: Assess reason why client is uncomfortable.

ANA: Change position in bed.

ANA: Administer back care.

ANA: Take time to allow client to verbalize needs, and/or fears.

ANA: If above measures fail to make client comfortable, you may need to administer medication for pain or anxiety reduction.

7 Check to see that all personal articles and call light are within easy reach of client. *If not*, follow these alternative nursing actions:

ANA: Place all articles within easy access.

ANA: Instruct client not to reach for articles that are not easily accessible, but to call for the nurse.

ANA: Instruct client to always make sure he or she has the call light in reach before nursing personnel leave the room.

ANA: Frequently remind staff members to double check placement of equipment and call light before leaving client's room.

UNEXPECTED OUTCOME

The client, health care provider, or visitor experiences an accident or injury related to mechanical, chemical, or thermal trauma.

ANA: Provide immediate first aid or care.

ANA: Assess vital signs, and notify physician.

ANA: Report the incident according to institutional procedure. Incident reports are used to protect the injured individual as well as the health care providers and the hospital.

Charting
- Assessment notes
- Plans or needs about safety precautions
- Actual incidents involving mechanical, chemical, or thermal trauma
- Client education given

ACTION: DISCHARGING A CLIENT FROM A HEALTH CARE UNIT

Rationale for Action
- To prepare client for discharge
- To transfer client whose condition necessitates care at other facility
- To provide an environment, either home or another community agency or facility, that best meets the needs of the client

ASSESSMENT

1 Gather physical, emotional, and psychosocial information concerning client's discharge.
2 Evaluate disabilities and limitations that will extend after discharge.
3 Assess client's strengths.
4 Assess the degree of family involvement or activity in terms of client's present and future needs.
5 Determine the degree of involvement needed from community or support agencies.
6 Determine how much planning will be needed to facilitate discharge.
7 Determine areas where client teaching must be given.

PLANNING

GOALS

- Client verbalizes his or her feelings about discharge and identifies strengths and weaknesses.

- Client is aware of potential changes in environment and life style due to his or her disability or limitation.
- Client and family discuss how they can work together to help client maximize his or her potential.
- Client and family have information about community agencies and support systems which can assist them.
- Client knowledgeably discusses all points included in the nurse-client teaching including medications and self care.

EQUIPMENT

- Educational pamphlets
- Telephone numbers and information regarding clinic appointments or special groups such as stroke clubs
- Specific equipment needed upon discharge such as wheelchair or commode
- Medications
- Materials for dressing changes (if indicated) or antiembolic stockings

INTERVENTION: Planning for the Discharge

1 Verify discharge preparations or orders with physician.
2 Collaborate with appropriate health team members, i.e., dieticians, physical therapists, home health care team.
3 Order any equipment or supplies client will need to take home.
4 If necessary, initiate a referral to a community agency.
5 Coordinate time and day of discharge and mode of transportation with client and family or friend.
6 Identify the desired goals or outcomes for discharge planning.
7 Write discharge care plan for client's use.
8 Talk with client about the hospital stay and client's future expectations about health, health care, and needs.
9 Encourage client to verbalize fears and concerns.
10 Help client identify his or her strengths and weaknesses. Consider including adaptation to home environment if a disability will extend after discharge. Be alert for nonverbal clues.
11 Include family or significant others in discussions. Discuss how they can help the client to maximize his or her potential. Be alert for potential family crises brought on by client's discharge.
12 Discuss a planned involvement with a community agency, i.e., visiting nurse, with client and family when necessary.
13 Provide client teaching as needed. Supply written instructions, teaching aids, and supplies.
14 Provide family teaching as necessary.
15 Evaluate the client's and family's learning.
16 Provide time for physician-client communication concerning discharge.

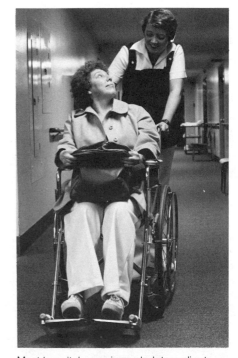

Most hospitals require ambulatory clients to be transported in a wheelchair to their mode of transportation at discharge.

INTERVENTION: Discharging a Client from a Health Care Unit

1 Make sure the physician's discharge orders have been written.
2 Review details of discharge with client. Give the client discharge care plan when appropriate.
3 Assist client with hygiene, dressing, packing, etc.
4 Review instructions and answer questions about medications, appointments, physical care, and supplies.
5 Terminate relationship with the client. Remember that each individual handles termination in his or her own way. Provide an opportunity for the client to express his or her feelings and impressions. Be alert for nonverbal expressions.
6 Follow your hospital's prescribed procedure for client discharge i.e., discharge time and method of leaving hospital unit.
7 If client is transferring to another health care facility, give client the discharge summary, interagency transfer data sheets, client care plan, discharge medications, and special equipment.
8 Document the client's discharge on the chart.

EVALUATION

EXPECTED OUTCOMES

1 Client verbalizes his or her feelings about being discharged and identifies strengths and weaknesses. *If not*, follow these alternative nursing actions:
ANA: Sit down with the client and listen to his or her verbalization about discharge. Allow enough time for termination.
ANA: Identify client's strengths and weaknesses as you perceive them in order to assist the client in his or her thinking about them.
2 Client is aware of potential changes in environment and life style due to his or her disability or limitations. *If not*, follow these alternative nursing actions:
ANA: Discuss possible changes in life style and environment with client and family.
ANA: Plan a home visit before discharge to determine alterations that might need to be done to accommodate client, i.e., doors widened, ramps built, and scatter rugs removed to allow wheelchair access.
ANA: Have the clergy, a social worker, or a member of the human support staff visit the client to help with his or her adjustment to an altered life style.
3 Client and family discuss how they can work together to help client maximize his or her potential. *If not*, follow these alternative nursing actions:
ANA: Discuss client's needs and future goals for health care individually with client and family to determine disparity in feelings and ability to handle the situation.

ANA: Obtain assistance from a psychologist, a social worker, or the clergy to help client and family work through the grief process and establish a therapeutic relationship.

4 Client and family have information about community agencies and support systems that can assist them. *If not*, follow these alternative nursing actions:

ANA: Identify which agencies would be most beneficial for client. Provide pamphlets about services, phone numbers, and persons to contact.

ANA: Have the discharge coordinator talk with client and family regarding appropriate agencies.

ANA: Refer client to a home health agency for assistance.

5 Client knowledgeably discusses all points included in the nurse-client teaching, including medication and self-care. *If not*, follow these alternative nursing actions:

ANA: Reinstruct client in areas of care that client does not fully understand.

ANA: Obtain printed information where possible as a means of providing information through another source.

ANA: Ask family to participate in teaching so they can reinforce information or carry out interventions as necessary.

ANA: Have client repeat information to you, to ensure accurate knowledge and understanding of information.

UNEXPECTED OUTCOMES

1 Client is discharged to an extended care facility (ECF).

ANA: Thoroughly explain why client needs to go to an ECF.

ANA: Provide time for client and family to deal with the loss of the client's independence and his or her previous role in the home setting.

ANA: Time permitting, arrange for the family to visit the ECF before final arrangements are made.

ANA: Ask a social worker to help you place client in an ECF.

ANA: Supply the ECF with appropriate documentation to ensure continuity of care.

2 Client doesn't understand the discharge process.

ANA: Repeat information as needed to help clarify unfamiliar terms or statements.

ANA: Directly involve the client's family as you teach the client about his or her required care.

ANA: Arrange for counseling or support groups to help family deal with anxiety and/or frustration.

3 Client wants to leave the hospital against medical advice (AMA).

ANA: Attempt to assess client's reasons for wanting to leave AMA.

ANA: Provide alternatives to leaving the hospital.

ANA: Do not force the adult client to remain in the hospital but do encourage discussion about the situation.

Charting

- Day-to-day preparatory activities such as teaching, return demonstrations, discussion with dietician, etc.
- Referrals to agencies, including dates, names, and specific contacts
- If specific discharge forms or client teaching sheets are used, record data using these forms
- Discharge data such as time, how discharged (ambulatory, wheelchair, ambulance, etc.), if accompanied by relative or nurse, and client's physical and psychosocial condition
- Discharge medications, special equipment, and materials taken home by client
- Client and family teaching completed
- Client's and family's comprehension of discharge and teaching

ANA: Notify the client advocate, a social worker, or the clergy to discuss situation with client.

ANA: If possible, consult your hospital's policies and procedures regarding leaving AMA before releasing client.

ANA: Have client sign AMA form, if possible.

ANA: If client will not sign AMA forms, call physician to obtain discharge orders.

CHAPTER 2
Adapting to Health Care

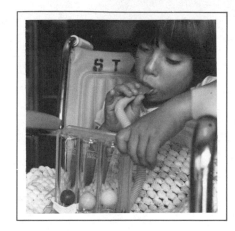

This chapter will present the skills associated with the physical aspects of daily care. In a conceptual format, these skills will encompass procedures important for assisting the client to adapt to health care in the hospital environment.

BASIC HEALTH CARE PROCEDURES

Clients enter the hospital environment because of an accident or acute illness requiring immediate care, or because the physician has recommended diagnostic procedures or surgery. The latter is commonly referred to as an "elective admission." Regardless of the reason, the client must rapidly alter everyday routines and activities of daily living. The client may be concerned about his or her health and well-being and may experience varying degrees of anxiety as a reaction to unfamiliar procedures, hospital personnel, and the hospital environment.

After the client has been admitted to the health care unit, many independent actions such as bathing, personal hygiene and general care may be curtailed by the nature of the illness and confinement. The client may require assistance with even the simplest of actions. Without therapeutic intervention, the total adaptation process may be put in jeopardy as additional physical problems occur.

LEARNING OBJECTIVES

Determine degree of personal hygiene assistance required by clients.
Identify guidelines for managing client care.
Describe methods of bedmaking which increase client comfort and prevent injury to nursing personnel.
Demonstrate safety awareness when caring for clients.
Identify appropriate comfort measures in assisting clients to regain health status.
Identify potential factors that contribute to the formation of decubitus ulcers.
Define components of individualized care that allow client to maintain self-image.
Describe nursing actions necessary to care for clients with prosthetic eye and contact lenses.
Identify alternative nursing actions for expected outcomes.
Discuss the unexpected outcomes and the alternative nursing actions.

Knowing when and how to intervene and performing skills such as bedmaking, bathing, personal hygiene, skin care and hair care will facilitate the process of adapting to the health care.

Bathing Bathing is accomplished in a variety of ways, according to the client's needs, condition, and personal habits. Bathing is necessary to cleanse the skin and to promote circulation. Baths may also be used as treatment to promote healing for a client with burns. Various types of bathing include:

Complete bed bath: The client is bathed entirely by the nurse due to physical and/or mental incapacity.

Partial bath: The client provides as much of his or her own bath care as possible, either in bed or at the sink. The nurse then assists by bathing any inaccessible areas.

Therapeutic bath: This bath is used as part of a treatment regime for specific conditions such as skin disorders, burns, high body temperature, and muscular injuries.

Oral Hygiene The condition of the oral cavity has a direct influence on an individual's overall state of health. Dental diseases require a "host" (the tooth and gum), an "agent" (plaque), and an "environment" (the presence of saliva and food, etc.). When plaque comes in contact with bacterial enzymes, carbohydrates, and acids, cavitation begins as the enamel of the tooth is decalcified. As food and plaque remain in the oral cavity, the possibility of dental decay increases. In the hospital the incidence of caries (cavities) can be decreased by use of a dentifrice containing fluoride, proper brushing and flossing and adequate nutrition.

Hair Care The appearance and condition of a client's hair can reflect his or her general physical and emotional health status, individuality and feelings of worth, and ability to care for him or herself. When complex medical care is required during illness or trauma, hair care is sometimes neglected.

Hair care is an important aspect of regular hygiene. To prevent damage to the hair, scalp, and surrounding skin, and to promote the client's sense of well-being, you should assess the condition of a client's hair. Following assessment provide basic hair and scalp care, shampooing, and shaving and deal with any special problems.

Foot Care The feet are especially susceptible to discomfort, trauma, and infection due to the amount of stress they must endure as well as to their distance from main blood supplies. Many problems can be avoided if proper foot care is taken. Some of the more common foot problems include:

Incurvated or ingrown toenails: The corners of the nail tend to press into skin, causing pain, ulceration, and infection.

Cracks and fissures between toes: This problem often occurs as a result of excessively dry skin.

Athlete's foot: Irritation characterized by itching, burning skin; caused by an easily transmitted fungus.

Corns: High calluses caused by pressure on toes, joints, or bony prominences.

Plantar warts: A virus manifested as a deep, often painful wart on the soles of the feet.

Calluses: Prominences that cause the epidermis to thicken over areas of pressure.

Decreased circulation to the feet: A problem which is often due to diabetes, vascular diseases, or to the constriction of major vessels to the lower extremities.

Infection due to poor nail care or cutting.

Excessive odor: A problem due to perspiration, the build-up of debris under nails and on skin, or poorly ventilated shoes.

Sports injuries/congenital deformities.

Perineal and Genital Care The perineum consists of the area between the thighs from the anterior pelvis to the anus. This area contains organs and structures related to sexual functioning, reproduction, and elimination.

Hygienic care involves cleaning the perineum and genitalia to prevent bacterial growth, which can rapidly increase in a warm, dark, moist environment. Perineal care is often provided as a routine part of bathing but may be required more frequently to prevent skin irritation, infection, discomfort, or odor.

All clients are susceptible to perineal irritation or infection. Those clients who are especially vulnerable are those who are immobilized, incontinent, debilitated, post-surgical, comatose, those who have metabolic and fluid balance disorders, or those who require systemic medications.

Skin Problems Skin types, colors, textures, and conditions are as different as each person's unique individuality. The condition of a client's skin will be determined by his health status, age, activity level, and environmental exposure.

The skin of an infant is often more sensitive and delicate than that of an adult because it has not been exposed to many of the elements of the environment. Most infants cannot tolerate strong soaps and lotions, and must be handled gently to avoid trauma. Another irritant to an infant's skin is urine. Young children will often have bruises, scrapes, and cuts on such vulnerable areas as the elbows, knees, hands, and chin.

Adolescents are affected by acne and have areas of increased oil secretion. Adults may have drier skin, especially as they age. Older adults cannot always tolerate harsh soaps because their skin is more delicate. They also require less frequent bathing and more lubrication with oil-rich creams and lotions.

Personal hygiene includes a variety of activities to promote cleanliness and to reduce irritation to the skin and mucous membranes. These activities generally consist of bathing, oral care, nail and hair care, perineal care, skin care, care of the feet, and care of the eyes, ears, and nose.

The need to provide personal hygiene will depend on each client's physical state and ability to care effectively for him or herself. Your first responsibility is to assess the client's level of ability. After gathering this data, you should assist the client as necessary, providing any teaching he or she may require.

GUIDELINES FOR MANAGING CLIENTS

A holistic approach on the part of the nurse is important to provide individualized care.
- Unfamiliar or life threatening hospital procedures can affect the client's adaptation to the health care system.
- Providing privacy when possible can protect the client from psychological distress associated with exposing his or her body to health care workers.
- Attention to the emotional-spiritual needs of the client is necessary to promote adaptation to the stressful hospital environment.

Daily care activities provide the nurse with an opportunity to do a total assessment and evaluation of the client as well as establish a working relationship.
- Careful and accurate assessment of client's skin and physical condition allows the nurse to plan individualized nursing care.
- Bathing and skin care promotes circulation, range of motion to immobilized joints, exercise to bedridden clients, and time to develop a relationship.
- Back care promotes comfort, relaxation, and a time for nurse-client interactions.
- Providing personal grooming increases the client's feelings of self-worth and self-esteem.

Rationale for Action
- To provide a clean comfortable sleeping and resting environment for the client
- To eliminate irritants to skin by providing wrinkle-free sheets and blankets
- To avoid client exertion by making bed while occupied
- To enhance client's self-image by providing a clean, neat and comfortable bed

ACTION: MAKING A BED

ASSESSMENT

1 Assess client's need to have linen changed.
2 Determine if client's present condition will permit a bed linen change.
3 Determine how many and what type of linens will be required.
4 Check client's unit for available linens.
5 Determine client's prescribed level of activity and any special precautions in movement.
6 Assess client's ability to get out of bed during linen change.

PLANNING

- Client is rested during and after bedmaking procedure.
- Client participates in the procedure, if able.
- Bed remains clean, dry, free of wrinkles or other skin irritants, and at a comfortable temperature.
- Skin remains free of irritation caused by contact with linens.
- Soiled linens are properly disposed of and do not promote cross contamination.
- Client is correctly aligned and feels physically and emotionally safe and comfortable.
- Nurse feels no stress to back or limbs during procedure.

EQUIPMENT

- Chair or table
- Linen hamper
- Linens (in order of use)
    bath blanket
    mattress pad
    bottom sheet
    rubber sheet or drawsheet, if needed
    incontinent pad, if needed
    top sheet
    blanket
    bedspread
    pillow case

PREPARING FOR BEDMAKING

1   Talk with client and explain how he or she can be involved in the procedure.
2   Explain the sequence for the procedure.
3   Arrange furniture and equipment, e.g., linen hamper.
4   Wipe chair or table before putting linen on it.
5   Wash your hands and collect linen.
6   Place linen on chair or table.
7   Remove call signal from linens.
8   Adjust the bed to a comfortable working height with side rails up. If client remains in bed, help him or her into a supine position.
9   Pull the curtain closed to provide privacy for client.

INTERVENTION: Making an Occupied Bed

1   Loosen top linens at the foot and on your side of the bed.
2   Lower side rail on your side of the bed. Keep side rail on opposite side in up position.
3   Remove spread and blanket. If they are to be reused, fold them and place on the chair.

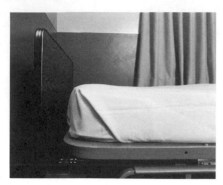

Mitered corners keep bed linens tight and wrinkle free.

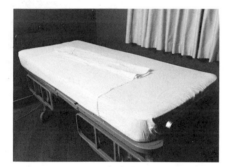

Tuck drawsheet in tightly. The drawsheet protects the bottom sheet. Absorbent pads may be placed under drawsheet.

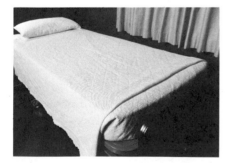

The top sheet and spread need to be pleated to allow room for client's feet.

4. Place bath blanket directly over client. Remove top sheet and place in linen bag.

5. Push mattress to head of bed. Center the mattress if necessary.

6. Help client move to the side of the bed, place in side lying position facing away from you.

7. Loosen bottom linens on your side of the bed.

8. Push dirty linen under, or as close as possible to client.

9. If mattress pad is not changed, smooth out wrinkles and recenter pad on the bed surface.

10. With client on the opposite side of the bed, place clean bottom sheet on mattress. Place the center fold of the sheet in the middle of the mattress with the end of the sheet even with the end of the mattress.

11. Unfold the bottom sheet and cover the mattress. Make sure the clean bottom sheet is underneath any used linen.

12. Tuck the top of the sheet under the head of the bed.

13. Miter the corner of the bottom sheet at the head of the bed.

14. Tuck the remaining side of the bottom sheet well under the mattress.

15. If client needs a drawsheet, center the drawsheet on the bed, fanfold half of the sheet under client. Tuck the sheet under the mattress. Smooth out wrinkles.

   a. If a pull sheet is needed, fold drawsheet in half or quarters. Position sheet in middle of bed. Fanfold half of the pull sheet under client.

   b. If incontinent pad is needed, fanfold pad and center it on bed under client's buttocks. Place the pad close to client for ease in pulling through to other side of bed.

16. Help client roll over to the other side of bed. Tell client why there is a hump of linen in the center of the bed. Make client comfortable.

17. Raise side rail.

18. Move linens to other side of bed within your reach.

19. Lower side rail and loosen bottom sheets.

Instruct client to roll over linen.

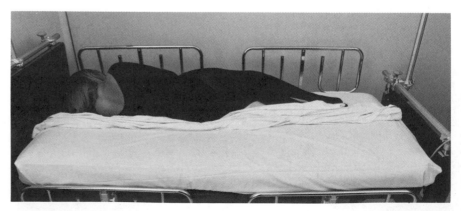

20 Pull dirty linen to side of bed and roll into a bundle at the foot of the bed or place linen in linen hamper. *Never* place dirty linen on the floor as cross-contamination occurs from this action.
21 Pull clean linen across mattress under client.
22 Miter the second top corner of the bottom sheet.
23 Tuck remaining bottom sheet well under the mattress. Gather sheet into your hand, lean away from the bed, and pull linens downward. Tuck sheet under mattress. If drawsheet is used, tighten and tuck it in the same way.
24 Help client into a supine position and adjust pillow.
25 Place top sheet, blanket, and spread over client. Leave a cuff of top sheet at the head of the bed.
26 Pull up all layers of linen at client's toes. Make a small pleat to allow room for client's feet.
27 Miter lower corners of bed.
28 Raise side rail.
29 Change pillow case.
30 Return bed to lowest position. Reattach call signal to linens. Position client for comfort.
31 Dispose of soiled laundry.
32 Wash your hands.

▶ If client is allowed out of bed, encourage him or her to ambulate or to perform personal hygiene activities while you are changing linens. If client must sit in a chair while the bed is changed, observe him or her carefully for fatigue or weakness. Do not leave client unattended if he or she is in a weakened state.

Clinical Alert

Clients who have spinal cord involvement, orthopedic injuries, burns, and other skin disorders or special tubes or drains may be required to move only in a specific manner. Check the Kardex for special instructions.

INTERVENTION: Making an Unoccupied Bed

1 Lower both side rails.
2 Loosen linen on all sides, including head and foot of bed.
3 Make up one side of the bed, then move to the other side of bed and make it. Follow appropriate steps for making an occupied bed.
4 Leave side rails down.
5 Leave bed open with linen fanfolded toward foot. If unit is vacant, leave top linen pulled up, covering bed.

INTERVENTION: Making a Surgical Bed

1 Wash your hands.
2 Bring linens to room.
3 Place the bottom sheet on the bed using the same method for making an unoccupied bed.
4 Place a drawsheet and absorbent pad on the bed.
5 Lay top sheet, blanket and bedspread over top of bed.
6 Fold up linen from foot, head and one side of the bed even with mattress.
7 Fold points from outside corners of bed on one side to meet at center of bed on opposite side.
8 Pick up center point of linen on side of bed next to you.
9 Fanfold linen to side of bed, to facilitate easy transfer of surgical clients.

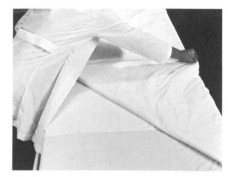

(a) Surgical bed: (Step 7).

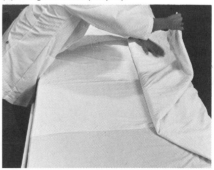

(b) Surgical bed: (Step 9).

EVALUATION

1 Client is rested during and after bedmaking procedure. *If not*, follow these alternative nursing actions:

ANA: Allow client to rest before any additional treatments are given.

ANA: Obtain assistance with bedmaking the next time.

ANA: Document the need for assistance with bedmaking for this client on his or her nursing care plan.

2 Client participates in the procedure. *If not*, follow these alternative nursing actions:

ANA: Ask another health care worker to assist you in making the bed.

ANA: If client will be out of bed for special treatment, procedure, or activity, wait until that time to make the bed.

3 Bed remains clean, dry, free of wrinkles or other skin irritants, and at a comfortable temperature. *If not*, follow these alternative nursing actions:

ANA: Check beds frequently when clients are known to be incontinent.

ANA: Place several incontinent pads under client to protect sheets from becoming soiled.

ANA: Following eating, ensure that bed is free of crumbs.

4 Skin remains free of irritation caused by contact with linens. *If not*, follow these alternative nursing actions:

ANA: Obtain hypoallergenic linen.

ANA: Place a sheepskin under client to prevent direct contact with sheets. Remember, however, that sheepskin can cause client to perspire, which could accentuate a skin problem.

5 Soiled linens are properly disposed of and do not promote cross contamination. *If not*, follow these alternative nursing actions:

ANA: Ensure that adequate linen hampers or bags are provided for the unit to prevent linen from being placed on the floor.

ANA: Remind health care workers to properly dispose of linens in hampers or bags and not on the floor.

ANA: Explain to ancillary employees how cross-contamination can occur when linen is not disposed of properly.

6 Client is correctly aligned and feels physically and emotionally safe and comfortable. *If not*, follow these alternative nursing actions:

ANA: Explain procedure thoroughly so client understands what is to be expected and is prepared for some discomfort caused by rolling over linen.

ANA: Assess client's position in bed before leaving the room.

ANA: Review activity level and any activities that could have the client out of bed during the day. Plan to make the bed when client is out of bed to reduce discomfort.

7 Nurse feels no stress to back or limbs during procedure. *If not*, follow these alternative nursing actions:

ANA: Make sure that bed is positioned for comfort of nurse while making bed.

ANA: Nurse has strain checked by physician and makes out incident report.

ANA: Nurse should attend safety inservice classes on preventing back strain for the future.

ANA: Remember, if client is heavy or difficult to move, obtain help with making the bed. Do not attempt to move the client by yourself.

UNEXPECTED OUTCOME

Client refuses to have bed made.

ANA: Assess reason for refusal. Client may be in pain or does not want to be disturbed.

ANA: Offer to make the bed at a later time.

ANA: Change only the pillow case and draw sheet, if client allows.

ANA: Beds do not need to be changed unless soiled or damp so allow client's independence if possible.

Charting

- Usually notation is made on Rand or Kardex
- Specific linens or equipment that cause discomfort for the client
- Special requirements for linens, e.g., certain detergents or elimination of starch
- Use of pull sheets, incontinent pads, or specified ways to keep bed dry

ACTION: BATHING THE CLIENT

ASSESSMENT

1 Assess client's need for bathing and other personal hygiene activities.
2 Check client's activity order. Note special precautions related to movement or exercise.
3 Assess client's ability to perform his own care. Determine how much assistance he or she will need.
4 Discuss client's preferences for the bathing procedure, bath and personal articles.
5 Check client's room for availability of bathing articles and linens.

PLANNING

GOALS

- Client's skin is free of excessive perspiration, debris, secretions and offensive body odors.
- Client's body positions have been changed and pressure points relieved.
- Client is more comfortable.
- Client has participated in bath procedure to best of his ability.
- During procedure nurse has had an opportunity to assess client's overall status, skin condition, level of mobility, comfort or pain.

EQUIPMENT

- Basin or sink with warm water (110° to 115° F or 43.3° to 46.1° C)
- Soap and soap dish

Rationale for Action

- To decrease the possibility of infection by removing excessive debris, secretions, and perspiration from the skin
- To promote circulation
- To maintain muscle tone through active or passive movement during bathing
- To prevent stasis of fluid in the lungs and to alternate points of pressure on the body by changing client's position during the bath
- To provide comfort for the client
- To improve the client's sense of self-worth

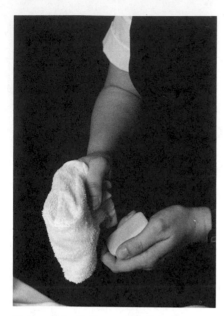

Make a mit with the washcloth before bathing client's face.

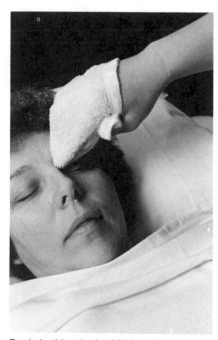

Begin bathing the bedridden client with the face. Use corner of washcloth to bathe eyes, washing from inner canthus outward and using a clean corner for the other eye.

- Personal articles, i.e., deodorant, powder, lotions
- Laundry bag
- Two to three towels
- Washcloth
- Bath blanket
- Clean pajamas or hospital gown
- Table for bathing equipment
- Shaving equipment for male clients

ADDITIONAL EQUIPMENT FOR INFANT'S OR CHILD'S BATH

- Tub or basin filled with warm water (100° F or 38° C)
- Two towels, one arranged like a diamond
- Washcloth
- Suction bulb
- Soap or cleaning agent
- Cotton balls
- Blanket
- Clean clothing

PREPARING FOR BATHING

1 Provide a comfortable room environment, i.e., comfortable temperature, lighting, etc.
2 Talk with client about plan for bathing to meet personal care needs.
3 Encourage client to bathe him or herself. This promotes exercise and a sense of self-worth.
4 Explain any unfamiliar methods or procedures regarding bathing.
5 Collect necessary equipment and place articles within reach.
6 Ask client if he or she needs to void or defecate before starting the bath.
7 Position the bed at a comfortable working height.
8 Assure privacy.

INTERVENTION: Bathing an Adult Client

1 Place bath blanket over client and over top linen. Loosen top linen at edges and foot of bed. Remove dirty top linen from under bath blanket, starting at client's shoulders and rolling linen down toward client's feet. Keep bath blanket in place over client. Place dirty linen in laundry bag.
2 Help client to the side of the bed closest to you. Keep the side rail on the far side of the bed in the "up" position.
3 Remove client's hospital gown. Keep client covered with bath blanket. Place gown in laundry bag.
4 Remove pillow if client will tolerate.
5 Place towel under head.
6 Make a mitt with a washcloth. Fold washcloth around your hand to prevent wet ends of cloth from annoying client.

7 Bathe client's face.

 a Wash around client's eyes, using clear water. With one edge of facecloth, wipe from the inner canthus toward the outer canthus. Using a different section of the washcloth, repeat procedure on other eye. Dry thoroughly.

 b Wash, rinse, and dry client's forehead, cheeks, nose, and area around lips. Use soap with client's permission.

 c Wash, rinse, and dry area behind and around client's ears.

 d Wash, rinse, and dry client's neck.

8 Remove towel from under client's head.

9 Bathe client's upper body and extremities. Place towel under area to be bathed.

 a Wash both arms by elevating client's arm and holding client's wrist. Use gentle strokes from the wrist toward the shoulder.

 b Wash, rinse, and dry client's axillae. Apply deodorant and/or powder if desired.

 c Wash client's hands by soaking them in the basin or with a washcloth. Nails can be cleaned now or after the bath.

 d Wash, rinse, and thoroughly dry client's chest, especially under breasts. Apply powder or cornstarch under breasts if desired.

10 Bathe client's abdomen. Using a towel over chest area and bath blanket, cover areas you are not bathing. Wash, rinse, and dry abdomen and umbilicus. Replace bath blanket over client's upper body and abdomen.

11 Bathe client's legs. Place towel under leg to be bathed. Drape other leg, hip, and genital area with bath blanket.

 a Carefully place bath basin on the towel near client's foot.

 b With one arm under the client's leg, grasp client's foot and bend knee. Place foot in basin of water.

 c Bathe client's leg, moving toward hip. Rinse and dry client's leg.

 d Wash client's foot with washcloth. Rinse and dry foot and area between toes thoroughly.

 e Carefully move basin to other side of bed and repeat procedure for client's other leg and foot.

12 Change bath water. Raise side rails when refilling basin. Check the water temperature before continuing with the bath.

13 During the bath, you should continuously assess each of the client's body systems. Careful attention should be paid to the verbal statements and nonverbal expressions.

14 Help client turn to a side-lying or prone position. Place towel under area to be bathed. Cover client with a bath blanket.

15 Wash, rinse, and dry client's back, moving from shoulders to buttocks.

16 Provide back massage now or after completion of bath.

17 Bathe client's genital area. Cover all body parts except area to be bathed. Place towel under client's hips.

 a For a female client: bathe from front to back. Use a different section of wash cloth for each stroke. Wash, rinse, and dry thoroughly between all skin folds.

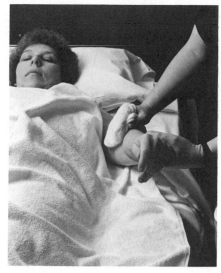

Place towel under the arm to keep bed linens dry when washing the upper extremities.

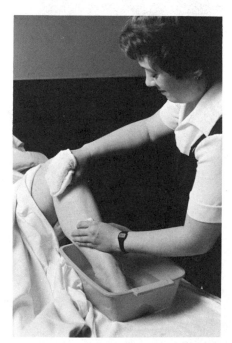

Place client's foot in basin, wash, then dry thoroughly before washing other foot.

b For a male client: carefully retract the foreskin on the uncircumcised penis. Wash, rinse, and dry gently and replace foreskin to its original position. Continue to wash, and dry penis, scrotum, and remaining skin folds.

18 Dress client in a clean hospital gown.
19 Clean and store bath equipment. Dispose of dirty linen.
20 Proceed with any other personal hygiene activities as needed.
21 Provide comfort and safety for client.
22 Wash your hands.

▶ Immerse an infant in a tub of water *only* after the umbilical cord stub has fallen off. Until it falls off, an infant should be sponge bathed.

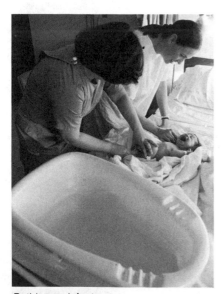

Bathing an infant.

INTERVENTION: Bathing an Infant or Child

1 Follow steps 1, 4, 5, and 7 in Preparing for Bathing (p. 40).
2 Wash your hands.
3 Test water temperature with your wrist or elbow.
4 Lift child onto table, using football hold.
5 Remove all clothing except shirt and diaper.
6 Cover child with towel or blanket. Keep your hand on the child at all times.
7 Clean child's eyes, using a cotton ball moistened with water. Wipe from inner to outer canthus.
8 Make a mitt with the washcloth.
9 Wash child's face with water.
10 Suction nose, if necessary, by compressing suction bulb *prior* to placing it in nostril. Release bulb *after* it is placed in nostril.
11 Wash child's ears and neck, paying attention to folds; dry all areas thoroughly.
12 Use a football hold when washing a child's head. Soap your own hands and wash child's hair and scalp, using a circular motion. Rinse child's hair and scalp thoroughly.
13 Place child on a towel with head facing the top corner.
14 Use the corner of the towel to dry the child's head with gentle, yet firm, circular movements.
15 Remove child's shirt or gown.
16 Remove and place closed safety pins in a safe area away from child. Remove diaper by picking up child's ankles in your hand. Wipe child's buttocks with diaper if necessary.
17 Pick up child and place feet first into basin or tub. Pick up infant by placing your hand and arm around infant, cradling the infant's head and neck in your elbow. Grasp the infant's thigh with your hand.
18 Wash and rinse the child's body, especially the skin folds.
19 Carefully remove the child from the water.
20 Dry child's body gently but thoroughly.
21 Wash child's genitalia.
   a For a female child: separate labia and with a cotton ball moistened with soap and water, cleanse downward once on each side. Use a fresh piece of cotton on each side.

b For an uncircumcised male child: do not force foreskin back. If it can be retracted, gently cleanse glans penis with a cotton ball moistened with soap and water.
   c For a circumcised male: gently cleanse with plain water.
22 Replace child's diaper and redress in new gown or shirt.
23 Provide comfort and safety by holding child for a period of time following bath procedure.
24 Wash your hands.

INTERVENTION: Bathing a Critically Ill Client

1 Follow steps in preparing for bathing.
2 Gather equipment: two bath blankets, Septi-soft soap, wash basin, washcloth, towel.
3 Place bath blanket in basin and soak bath blanket with very warm water.
4 Pour Septi-soft soap into bath blanket and work soap into bath blanket.
5 Wring out bath blanket.
6 Remove top covers from client and place wet bath blanket over client. Bath blanket extends from under client's chin down to feet.
7 Keep client covered with bath blanket while you rub anterior surfaces with your hands. Entire surfaces of legs and arms can be washed at this time.
8 After all body surfaces are washed, place dry bath blanket under client's chin. As you pull dry bath blanket down over client, remove wet blanket.
9 Dry client thoroughly.
10 Turn client on side.
11 Wash and dry back and buttocks with towel.
12 Give back rub.
13 Change bed linen.
14 Position for comfort.

EVALUATION

EXPECTED OUTCOMES

1 Client's skin is free of excessive perspiration, debris, secretions, and offensive odors. *If not*, follow these alternative nursing actions:
   ANA: Complete bed bath may need to be repeated more frequently to accomplish this goal.
   ANA: Reassess client's condition as necessary (for elevated temperature, presence of infection, etc.).
   ANA: Stronger deodorant soap may need to be used.
2 Body positions have been changed and muscles and joints have been exercised actively and/or passively during the bath. *If not*, follow these alternative nursing actions:

ANA: Check to see if pain medication is ordered and give prior to bath if exercise is painful.

ANA: Accomplish this objective later when client has had a chance to rest from the bath procedure.

ANA: Request assistance from a second staff member to avoid strain to client.

3   Client feels comfortable and does not complain of pain, fatigue, itching, or irritated or excessively dry skin. *If not*, follow these alternative nursing actions:

ANA: If bathing is exhausting client, do procedure on a shift when he or she will be able to rest more or do bath in segments.

ANA: Do not give complete bed bath if client is too tired or ill to tolerate. Bathing is rarely a case of life or death.

ANA: If client continues to complain of dry itchy skin, reassess for cause of complaint and/or request order for skin cream or alpha keri bath lotion.

ANA: If client has sensitivity to soap, use hypoallergenic soap or water for bath.

4   Client participates in bath procedure to the best of his or her ability. *If not*, follow these alternative nursing actions:

ANA: If client is unable to participate due to illness, do not request, force, or coerce. Client will only feel guilty taking your time.

ANA: If client is resistant to giving own bath, identify reasons for this behavior. Client may use this as a means of gaining attention from nursing staff. If so, plan to spend time with client after he or she completes the care.

ANA: If client is unwilling to participate, explain the positive benefits of exercise and movement.

ANA: If client is physically able but emotionally resistant, you may choose to allow this dependence to establish better rapport; however, foster independence by later encouraging client participation.

5   The nurse has assessed the integrity and condition of the client's skin and the level of mobility, comfort, or pain. *If not*, follow these alternative nursing actions:

ANA: If unable to complete overall assessment, return to client at a later time to do so.

ANA: Request client's cooperation by asking relevant questions to elicit necessary information.

UNEXPECTED OUTCOMES

1   Client is unwilling to accept complete bed bath.

ANA: Respect client's wishes and take other opportunities for assessment. Have client wash hands, face, and genitals. You should wash back and give back care.

ANA: Reexplain to client the purpose of a bath and request client participation.

Charting

- Client's overall ability to provide his or her own care
- Type of bath given, i.e., complete or partial and by whom, e.g., client, nurse, family member
- Condition of client's skin and any interventions provided for the skin, e.g., lotion, massage
- Client's concerns about bathing or self
- Documentation of client's educational needs; information shared with client or family members

2 Client is too shy to allow bath.

   ANA: Respect client's privacy and only wash areas client wishes you to do.

   ANA: Give assistance so client can do it by him or herself.

   ANA: Allow spouse or parents to give bath if this is more acceptable to client.

ACTION: ADMINISTERING EVENING CARE

ASSESSMENT

1 Review client's usual routines prior to sleep:

   a Usual time of sleep and length of sleeping period.

   b Personal hygiene routines.

   c Temperature of room and number of blankets, etc.

   d Anticipated elimination needs.

   e Religious or meditation needs.

2 Evaluate client's understanding and acceptance of safety precautions such as use of side rails.

3 Assess client's needs for comfort and security.

   a Dressings.

   b Medication.

   c Linen change or adjustment.

   d Positioning.

   e Television, radio, light.

   f Communication needs.

4 Assess physical and emotional status during evening care.

PLANNING

GOALS

- Client appears comfortable and ready for sleep in a safe, clean environment.
- Evening care has provided time for effective nurse-client communication and client has time to ask questions.
- Observations have been made regarding client's physical and emotional status and anticipated health care needs.

EQUIPMENT

- Towels, washcloth
- Clean linens if needed
- Basin of warm water, soap
- Dental items, i.e., toothbrush, dentifrice, denture cup
- Emesis basin, cup
- Fresh pitcher of water if allowed
- Skin care lotion and powder if desired

Rationale for Action

- To encourage a period of comfortable, uninterrupted rest
- To evaluate a client's present health status
- To provide time for client and nurse to review the previous day's events
- To provide time for client to communicate needs and questions regarding health care
- To provide the client with a clean, secure environment in which to sleep

- Personal care items, e.g., deodorant, moisturizers
- Bedpan, urinal, toilet paper
- Miscellaneous supplies as needed, e.g., dressings, special equipment

PREPARING FOR EVENING CARE

1 Explain the needs and benefits of evening care; discuss how the client can be involved.
2 Collect and arrange equipment.
3 Adjust the bed to a comfortable working height and assist the client into a comfortable position.
4 Assure privacy.

INTERVENTION: Providing Evening Care

1 Offer bedpan or urinal if client is unable to use bathroom. Assist with handwashing.
2 If client needs or requests a bath, provide assistance as needed.
3 Assist with mouth and dental care if necessary.
4 Remove equipment, extra linens, and pillows if possible. Remove stockings, ace wraps, binders, etc.
5 Change dressings. Perform any required procedural techniques.
6 Wash face, hands, and back. Provide back massage.
7 Assist with combing or brushing hair if desired.
8 Replace stockings, binders, etc.
9 Replace soiled linen, or straighten and tuck remaining linen. Fluff pillow.
10 Straighten top linens. Provide additional blankets if desired.
11 Remove any additional equipment. Place call signal and water (if allowed) within client's reach.
12 Administer medication if ordered.
13 Assist client into a comfortable position.
14 Make sure the client's environment is safe and comfortable.
15 Raise side rails, place bed in low position, and turn lighting to low.

INTERVENTION: Providing Back Care

1 Explain the purpose of a back rub, and ask client if he or she would like one.
2 Pull curtains or shut door to room to provide privacy.
3 Wash your hands with warm water.
4 Warm lotion by holding bottle under water.
5 Raise bed to comfortable height for you, and assist client into a comfortable prone or semi-prone position.

3 Client's skin shows no signs of dryness, flaking, itching, or burning. *If not*, follow these alternative nursing actions:

ANA: Obtain order for medication to prevent itching or burning.

ANA: If corn starch has been used, make sure it is completely removed before next application because it can cause skin break-down.

UNEXPECTED OUTCOMES

1 Skin breaks down and forms a decubitus ulcer.

ANA: Assess stage of ulcer.

ANA: Follow treatment for specific stage of ulcer. (See p. 134.)

ANA: Do not position on affected area.

2 Client cannot be positioned in a manner to avoid erythematous areas entirely.

ANA: Turn at least every hour.

ANA: Massage area very well with each change in position.

ANA: Use protocol for Stage I ulcer treatment on affected area.

ACTION: PROVIDING HAIR CARE

ASSESSMENT

1 Review general physical assessment findings.

2 Ask client if he or she has experienced loss of hair, tenderness of scalp, or itching.

3 Determine if client is able to perform own hair care. If unable, find out who usually assists client.

4 Observe client's hair and scalp, noting the following:

   a Texture.

   b Color.

   c Degree of thickness and hair distribution.

   d Degree of gloss or shine.

   e Dryness or oiliness.

   f Areas of irritation, rash, or scaliness on the scalp or surrounding skin.

   g Matting or snarls.

   h Pediculosis (lice).

5 Ask client about his or her usual hair care routines, products, and appliances.

6 Determine how and where hair care will be provided, i.e., in bed, on guerney, in wheelchair, etc.

7 Determine what instruction client needs about hair care.

PLANNING

GOALS

- Client's hair and scalp are clean with no subsequent irritation.
- Client is comfortable and not fatigued following procedure.
- Shaving is accomplished without cuts or discomfort.

Charting

- Client's skin condition: odor, temperature, turgor, sensation, cleanliness, integrity
- Client's mobility
- Turning frequency and client positioning
- Type of care given, e.g., massage, bathing
- Client's complaints about skin and/or decubitus ulcer
- Time and method used to obtain wound specimen

Rationale for Action

- To prevent irritation to the scalp and damage to the hair
- To help maintain client's existing condition of the hair and scalp
- To promote circulation to the hair follicle and growth of new hair
- To distribute oils along the hair shaft
- To promote self-esteem

EQUIPMENT

- Blunt end comb or pick
- Brush
- Towel
- Mirror
- Hair care products and/or ornaments

ADDITIONAL EQUIPMENT FOR SHAMPOOING

- Two bath towels
- Washcloth
- Shampoo
- Conditioner, if desired
- Hair dryer
- "Shampoo board" for clients confined to bed

ADDITIONAL EQUIPMENT FOR SHAVING

- Razor, specific to client's needs or wishes
- Shaving cream
- Aftershave lotion (optional)
- Two towels

▶ Shaving includes routine hair removal of any of the following areas:
- Removing unwanted facial hair
- Removing unwanted hair from the axillae and legs of women (depending on their cultural habits)
- Preparing skin for operations
- Removing hair from arms prior to the infusion of IV therapy to prevent discomfort from hair sticking to tape

PREPARING FOR HAIR CARE

1 Determine client's hair care needs.
2 Wash your hands.
3 Help client into a comfortable position to perform hair care.
4 Collect and assemble equipment.
5 Shampooing the hair can be accomplished in a variety of ways, depending on the client's usual routine and physical condition. In many institutions, a physician's order is necessary before shampooing a client's hair.
6 If possible, the easiest way to shampoo is to assist the client while he or she is in the shower. Caution should be taken to prevent the client from becoming overly tired or weak while in the shower.

INTERVENTION: Providing Routine Hair Care

1 Place all hair care items within reach.
2 Place towel over client's shoulders.
3 Brush or comb client's hair from scalp to hair ends using gentle, even strokes.
4 Style hair in a manner suitable to client.
5 Replace hair care items in appropriate place, and clean items as needed.
6 Wash your hands.

INTERVENTION: Providing Hair Care for Tangled Hair

1 Hold client's hair above the tangle to prevent discomfort.
2 Using a wide-toothed comb, gently comb tangle. Use short, gentle strokes.

3 You may also apply small amounts of vinegar or alcohol to client's hair to make combing the tangle easier.

4 Style client's hair in a manner that will prevent further tangling, e.g., a loose braid placed in an area that does not put pressure on the head is helpful.

INTERVENTION: Providing Hair Care for Coarse or Curly Hair

1 Comb hair in small sections to remove tangles.

2 Use a comb or pick to comb hair in small sections.

3 Apply a small amount of oil to dry or flaking areas of scalp.

4 Using a wide-toothed comb or pick, gently lift hair and smooth out evenly.

5 If braiding or cornrowing is desired, make small rows of braids close to the scalp in the client's choice of designs. (This type of braid is left in the hair for a longer period of time.)

INTERVENTION: Providing Hair Care for Beards and Moustaches

1 Ask client how he usually cares for his beard or moustache.

2 Observe client's skin underneath beard or moustache.

3 If necessary, comb or brush the beard or moustache.

4 With client's or family's direction, periodically trim client's moustache or beard with sharp scissors.

5 Shampoo beard or moustache as needed.

INTERVENTION: Shampooing Hair for Client in a Chair or Wheelchair

1 Have shampoo items readily available.

2 Drape one towel over client's shoulders and around neck. Place another towel within reach.

3 Pad the edge of the sink with a towel or bath blanket. Face client away from sink. Lock wheels of wheelchair.

4 Using washcloth to protect client's eyes, wet hair and gently make a lather with shampoo.

5 Rinse thoroughly and repeat if necessary.

6 Towel dry, add conditioner if desired, and rinse again.

7 Using a dry towel, pat hair dry and wrap turban style.

8 Use hair dryer if available.

9 Style as desired.

INTERVENTION: Shampooing Hair for Client on a Guerney

1 Position guerney with head end at sink.

2 Lock the brakes.

3 Put a pillow or rolled blanket under the client's shoulders to help elevate and extend the head.

4 Move client's head just beyond the edge of the stretcher to allow water to run off more easily.

5 Complete steps one through nine above.

INTERVENTION: Shampooing Hair for Client on Bedrest

1 If a shampoo board is available, place it under the client's head. This allows water and soap to run off into a basin at the side of the bed.
2 Complete step one through nine for shampooing a client confined to a chair.
3 If a shampoo board is not available, follow these guidelines:
   a Remove pillows so that client is flat on the bed.
   b Place a plastic sheet or plastic bed protector under client.
   c Roll a bath blanket or sheet and form a trough under client's head. Be sure to have trough directed over the edge of the bed.
   d Cover entire trough with a plastic sheet.
   e Adjust edge of trough to empty into a basin at the side of the bed.
   f Using pitchers of water, proceed with the routine shampooing procedure. Change bed linens and clothes immediately if they become wet.

INTERVENTION: Shaving a Client

▶ According to the hospital policy, be sure to have electric razor checked for safety aspects. Some hospitals do not allow clients to use their own electric razors.

1 Determine how the client usually shaves, i.e., use of blade or electric razor; use of special products.
2 Check to see if the client has excessive bleeding tendencies due to pathological conditions (hemophilia) or to the use of specific medications (anticoagulants or large doses of aspirin).
3 If not using an electric razor, complete these steps:
   a Apply a warm, moist towel to client's skin to soften hair.
   b Apply a thick layer of soap or shaving cream to shaving area.
   c Holding skin taut, use firm but small strokes in the direction opposite that of hair growth.
   d Gently remove soap or lather with a warm, damp towel. Inspect for areas you may have missed.

EVALUATION

EXPECTED OUTCOMES

1 Hair and scalp assessment are performed without complications. *If not*, follow these alternative nursing actions:
   ANA: Wait until client can tolerate assessment before completing procedure.
   ANA: Request family to assist if staff unable to assess condition of hair and scalp.
2 Client's hair and scalp are clean, comfortable, and styled according to client's preference. *If not*, follow these alternative nursing actions:
   ANA: If unable to complete procedure due to fatigue level, stop and allow client to rest and finish procedure.
   ANA: If scalp or hair is not clean, repeat procedure the next day.
3 After shampooing is completed, client is comfortable and rested. *If not*, follow these alternative nursing actions:

ANA: Allow for extended rest time without interruption until client is comfortable.

4 Shaving is accomplished without discomfort. *If not*, follow these alternative nursing actions:

ANA: Place warm towels on area to be shaved for fifteen minutes.

ANA: Apply more shaving cream.

ANA: Ensure that razor is sharp.

UNEXPECTED OUTCOMES

1 Extreme matting, snarling, blood, or nonremovable substances appear in client's hair.

ANA: Never cut a client's hair unless it is *absolutely* necessary. Check hospital policy regarding hair-cutting.

ANA: Secure family or physician permission.

2 Client is cut during shaving procedure.

ANA: Assess extent of cut and place clean towel on area with pressure to stop bleeding.

ANA: If cut appears to be more than a nick report to physician and fill out incident report.

Charting
- Documentation of hair care assessment and needs
- Shampooing method, outcomes, problems encountered
- Client's tolerance to hair care

ACTION: TREATING PEDICULOSIS

ASSESSMENT

1 Observe head (scalp), body (beard, eyebrows, arms, legs), and pubic areas for the following signs:
   a Small, hemorrhagic areas on the skin.
   b Scratches on the skin.
   c Habitual itching and scratching.
   d Insect-type bites or pustular eruptions behind ears or hairline.
   e Small, white dandruff-like particles.
2 Assess client's personal hygiene, living conditions, contact/exposure to others with lice, e.g., school age children, sexual partners, siblings.

Rationale for Action
- To remove lice from client's hair and prevent further skin problems such as impetigo or infection
- To remove cause of itching and intense need to scratch scalp
- To control spread to others

PLANNING

GOALS

- Lice are not present after treatment.
- Client understands the cause, treatment, and preventive measures regarding lice infestation.

EQUIPMENT

- Isolation bags
- Treatment solution as ordered, i.e., gamma benzene hexachloride (Kwell)
- Clean linen
- Fine-tooth comb
- Disinfectant for comb

INTERVENTION: Removing Lice

1 Remove and bag client's clothing and linens separately. Use isolation bags.
2 Notify physician and other health care providers.
3 Begin treatment as ordered by physician. Common treatment is gamma benzene hexachloride applied as a cream, lotion, or shampoo.
4 Apply solution and leave in place several minutes.
5 Rinse thoroughly.
6 Comb through hair with fine-tooth comb.
7 Repeat in 24 hours if necessary.
8 Disinfect comb and brushes with Kwell shampoo.
9 Sterilize equipment as prescribed.
10 Discuss the cause, treatment, and preventive measures regarding lice infestation with client and family.

EVALUATION

EXPECTED OUTCOMES

1 Lice are removed following treatment. *If not*, follow these alternative nursing actions:
  ANA: Repeat treatment in 24 hours.
  ANA: Recomb hair with fine-tooth comb to remove all nits.
  ANA: If axillary or pubic hair are infested, shaving should be done.
2 Client understands cause of problem and preventive measures. *If not*, follow these alternative nursing actions:
  ANA: Repeat information on level client can understand or ask family member to explain.

UNEXPECTED OUTCOMES

1 Kwell shampoo is left on too long a period of time.
  ANA: Observe for irritation or burning after rinsing out shampoo.
  ANA: If scalp is burned, notify physician for medication order.
  ANA: Do *not* repeat treatment until scalp is healed.
2 Other clients or staff become infested with lice.
  ANA: Isolate client's linen and personal hair grooming equipment to prevent spread of lice.
  ANA: Instruct client or staff on use of Kwell shampoo.

Charting
- Location of lice infestation
- Physician and health care providers notified
- Action taken and results
- Client teaching activities

ACTION: PROVIDING PERINEAL AND GENITAL CARE

ASSESSMENT

1 Review general assessment data about client.
2 Observe client for signs of perineal itching, burning on urination, or skin irritation. Ask client if he or she experiences any of these problems.

3 Assess client's ability to bathe him or herself and perform perineal care.

4 While providing privacy, assess the perineal/genital area for abnormal secretions, ulcerations, skin excoriations and sensitivity, drainage (amount, consistency, odor, color), swelling, enlarged lymph glands, catheter patency, and comfort.

5 Assess client's learning needs related to perineal and genital care.

PLANNING

GOALS

- Perineal care has been comfortably and effectively provided by either client or the nurse.
- Perineal area is clean, odor-free, and without irritation or excessive discharge.

EQUIPMENT

- Bath blanket or sheet
- Two bath towels
- Protective pad or plastic sheet
- Washcloth
- Three or more cotton balls (optional)
- Clean surgical gloves (optional)
- Bedpan (optional)
- Pitcher of warm water (optional)
- Antifungal/antibacterial solution (optional)

INTERVENTION: Providing Female Perineal and Genital Care

1 Check to see if specific physician orders are to be followed.
2 Talk with client about how she can perform care or assist with procedure.
3 Collect and arrange necessary equipment.
4 Provide privacy by closing door and pulling drapes.
5 Wash your hands.
6 Position client in a comfortable position. Perineal and genital care can be provided while client sits on a toilet or sitz bath, remains in bed in a supine position, or sits on a bedpan in a dorsal recumbent or semi-Fowler's position.
7 When care is given in bed, position client comfortably. Then wrap each of her legs with a bath blanket, folding the corners over the client's lower abdomen.
8 If possible, encourage client to bend her knees and separate her legs so that the perineal area can be cleansed.
9 Place a protective pad or towel and bedpan under client's hips.
10 The perineum is sometimes more comfortably and effectively cleansed by pouring warm water or a prescribed solution over the perineum while client is positioned on the bedpan.

Rationale for Action

- To decrease the growth of bacteria
- To remove excessive secretions
- To promote healing after surgery and vaginal deliveries
- To prevent the spread of micro-organisms for clients with indwelling catheters
- To increase comfort

11 Tell client what sensations she will feel as you perform the procedure.
12 Put on gloves if desired. Separate the labia with one hand to expose the urethral and vaginal openings. With your other hand, wipe from front to back in a downward motion, using warm water or soap and water and a washcloth or cotton balls. Be sure to use a different corner of the washcloth or a different cotton ball for each downward stroke.
13 Wash the external labia and anus.
14 Thoroughly pat dry with second towel.
15 Remove equipment and cover client.
16 Position client for comfort.
17 Wash your hands.

INTERVENTION: Providing Male Perineal and Genital Care

1 Check to see if specific physician orders are to be followed.
2 Talk with client about how he can perform care or assist with procedure.
3 Collect and arrange necessary equipment.
4 Provide privacy by closing door and pulling drapes.
5 Wash your hands and put on gloves if desired.
6 Cover client with bath blanket, exposing genital area as little as possible.
7 If the client has not been circumcised, retract his foreskin carefully to expose the glans penis.
8 Gently but securely hold the shaft of the penis in one hand.
9 Using a circular motion, start at the tip of the penis and wash downwards toward the shaft with soap and water. Do not repeat washing over an area without using a clean area of the washcloth.
10 Replace the foreskin over the glans penis.
11 Wash around the scrotum.
12 Wash the anus last.
13 Dry all areas thoroughly.
14 Remove articles and cover client.
15 Reposition client for comfort.
16 Wash your hands.

EVALUATION

EXPECTED OUTCOMES

1 Perineal care has been comfortably and effectively provided. *If not*, follow these alternative nursing actions:
    ANA: If client is uncomfortable with method, suggest sitz bath or bathtub if condition permits.
    ANA: If client is unable to assist with procedure or hold legs up, obtain help from other health care members.

2 Perineal area is clean, odor-free, and without irritation or discharge. *If not*, follow these alternative nursing actions:

ANA: Request order for medicated solution or powder to counteract irritation.

ANA: Request culture of discharge so appropriate treatment can be instituted.

UNEXPECTED OUTCOME

Client develops urinary tract infection.

ANA: Instruct client on proper technique for perineal care.

ANA: Instruct females to wash from anterior to posterior aspects of perineum, using different sections of cloth for each wipe.

ANA: Instruct male clients to wash from urethral opening down the shaft of penis.

Charting
- Assessment and care needs for perineal hygiene
- Client's level of understanding and teaching needs
- Perineal care provided and outcomes of care

ACTION: PROVIDING EYE CARE

ASSESSMENT

1 Ask client if he or she is using eyeglasses or contact lenses, has an artificial eye, or is experiencing any eye problems.
2 Observe client's eyes for symmetry and clarity.
3 Assess the skin surrounding client's eyes for excessive dryness, scaling, and irritation.
4 Observe eyelids for irritation, edema, crustation, sties, and lesions.
5 Observe client's tear ducts and sclera for inflammation and excessive tearing.
6 Assess client's pupils for response to light.
7 Observe client's eye movement or muscle action.

Rationale for Action
- To improve or maintain the client's vision
- To prevent irritation and infection
- To maintain or improve the client's appearance and self-esteem

PLANNING

GOALS

- The eyes and surrounding skin areas are clear, comfortable, and free of crustation.
- Client's vision is maintained or improved.
- Client's appearance reflects a positive self-image.

EQUIPMENT

- Water or normal saline
- Washcloth, cotton balls, tissues
- Sterile lubricant or eye preparations if ordered by physician
- Eye dropper or asepto bulb syringe if ordered by physician

PREPARING FOR EYE CARE

1 Determine client's eye care needs and obtain physician's order if needed.

63

2 Explain the necessity for and method of eye care to the client. Discuss how client can assist you.
3 Collect necessary equipment.
4 Wash your hands.

INTERVENTION: Providing Routine Eye Care

1 Use water or saline at room temperature.
2 Using the washcloth or cotton balls dampened in water or saline, gently wipe each eye from the inner to outer canthus. Use a separate cotton ball or corner of washcloth for each eye.
3 If crusting is present, gently place a warm, wet compress over the eye(s) until crusting is loosened.

INTERVENTION: Providing Eye Care for the Comatose Client

1 Cleanse the eyes using routine eye care method.
2 Use a dropper to instill a sterile ophthalmic solution (liquid tears, saline, methylcellulose) every three to four hours as ordered by a physician.
3 Keep client's eyes closed if blink reflex is absent. If eye pads or patches are used, explain their purpose to client's family. Do *not* tape eyes shut.

INTERVENTION: Providing Eye Care to a Client with Eye Glasses

1 Encourage client to wear eyeglasses as needed.
2 Clean glasses over a protected area, i.e., a towel. Holding glasses by the frame, gently wash the glass in tepid water. Use soap if necessary. Rinse thoroughly.
3 Dry and wipe lenses with a clean, soft cloth or lens paper.
4 Label eyeglasses with client's name.

INTERVENTION: Providing Eye Care to a Client with Artificial Eye

1 If possible, encourage client or family member to care for client's artificial eye.
2 If assisting with artificial eye care, utilize client's usual method for cleaning.
3 Gather equipment.
4 Wash your hands.
5 Remove eye prosthesis by depressing lower lid and sliding prosthesis out, or by using gentle suction with the rubber bulb of an eyedropper.
6 Flush empty socket with water or saline.
7 Clean prosthesis with soap and water. Rinse thoroughly.
8 Lift upper eyelid and slide prosthesis into place.
9 Wipe toward nose when prosthesis is in place.

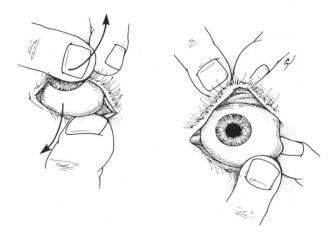

Removal of eye prosthesis.

INTERVENTION: Providing Eye Care to a Client with Contact Lenses

1 If possible, encourage client or family member to care for client's lenses.
2 If assisting with contact lens care, utilize client's usual method.
3 Wash your hands.
4 Place client in Fowler's position and place towel under client's chin.
5 Place the tip of your forefinger across the lower lid below its margin.
6 Place top of the forefinger of the other hand on the upper lid above its margin.
7 Assess for presence of lens.
8 Using a scissors motion, manipulate the two lids as the client closes, opens and rolls eyes.
9 Observe carefully when lens pops out to ensure you don't lose it.

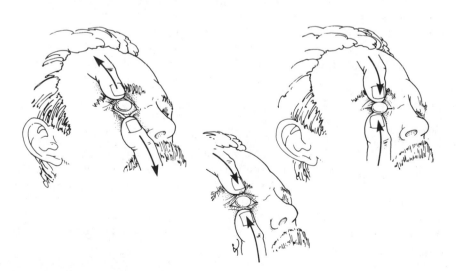

Removal of contact lens.

65

EVALUATION

EXPECTED OUTCOMES

1 Eyes and surrounding area are clear and free of crustation. *If not*, follow these alternative nursing actions:

ANA: Place warm, moist washcloth across eyes and leave in place for several minutes.

ANA: Moisten cotton applicator stick with sterile saline and gently twist the applicator stick over crusted surface to assist in removing crust.

2 Vision is maintained or improved. *If not*, follow these alternative nursing actions:

ANA: If eye problems exist, obtain ophthalmologist consult or eye clinic appointment.

Charting
- Documentation of eye assessment and eye care needs
- Method and outcome of eye care provided

ACTION: PROVIDING FOOT CARE

Rationale for Action
- To provide for specific foot care needs
- To encourage self-care and prevention of future problems
- To prevent infection, discomfort, deformities, circulatory problems and odor

ASSESSMENT

1 Review data from general physical assessment.
2 Observe the color of client's feet and lower extremities.
3 Assess temperature of each foot.
4 Note color, shape, condition, contour, and length of toenails.
5 Assess speed of color return when nailbed is depressed (capillary refill).
6 Inspect skin of entire foot (including corner of toes, between toes, and heels) for irritation, cracking, lesions, corns, calluses, deformities, and edema.
7 Assess mobility of ankle and toes. Footdrop or plantar flexion and rotation of feet can occur during prolonged bedrest.
8 Assess cleanliness of feet.
9 Inspect client's shoes for excessive wear, proper fit, etc.
10 During assessment, gather data from the client about level of comfort, pain, tenderness, etc.

PLANNING

GOALS

- Client's foot care needs have been satisfactorily met.
- Client's feet are clean, comfortable, warm, odor-free, adequately moisturized, and without cracks, lesions, or deformities due to prolonged immobility.
- Immobilized clients do not develop plantar flexion (foot drop).
- Client and family understand the importance of, and techniques for, proper foot care.

EQUIPMENT

- Basin of warm water
- Soap or emollient agent
- Washcloth
- Two towels
- Toenail clippers
- Nail file, emory board, pick, or orangewood stick
- Skin care lotion or lanolin

INTERVENTION: Providing Foot Care

1 Using assessment data, determine foot care needs based on client's condition.
2 Discuss procedure with client.
3 Collect necessary equipment.
4 Help client into a chair in a comfortable sitting position if possible.
5 Place towel or bath mat on floor in front of client. Place basin of warm water on towel.
6 Help client place feet in basin.
7 Add emollient agent to water, if desired.
8 Assist client with other personal hygiene activities while feet are soaking. Let feet soak for 10 minutes.
9 Using a washcloth, gently wash client's feet with soap and water.
10 Dry each foot thoroughly with a second towel. Dry between each toe.
11 Using nail clippers, cut straight across nails.
12 Clean underneath and on sides of nails using a file or orangewood stick.
13 If necessary, push back cuticles using an orangewood stick. Smooth rough edges with an emery board.
14 Apply lotion to entire foot focusing on callused or dry areas.
15 Assist client in putting on clean socks and shoes or slippers.

Place basin on the floor and allow client's feet to soak before completing foot care. Remember to dry thoroughly and powder unless otherwise instructed.

INTERVENTION: Using a Footboard

1 Assess client's ability to place feet in dorsal flexion. If unable to do so, or plantar flexion is continuous, provide a footboard.
2 Cover footboard with bath blanket to protect feet from rough surfaces.
3 Place footboard on the bed in a place where client's feet can firmly rest on it without sliding down in bed.
4 Observe legs to ensure that they are not in a flexed position when feet are against the board.
5 Tuck top linen under mattress at foot of bed, and bring linen up over the footboard to the top of the bed. Do not drape top linen over footboard as it can easily be pulled off the bed.

▶ Be sure to check the policy of your institution regarding the cutting of nails. Some health care facilities require that only a podiatrist (one who specializes in care of the feet) cut nails.

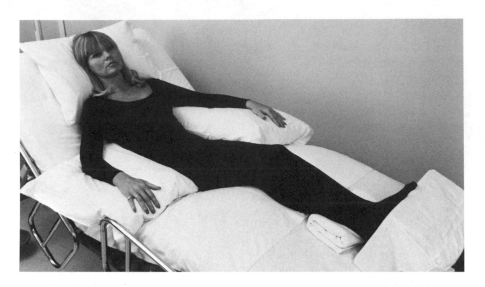

Footboard can be improvised if regular foot-board not available.

6 Put feet and ankles through range of motion exercises every four hours for clients on prolonged bed rest.

7 Observe heels and ankles frequently for signs of breakdown.

EVALUATION

EXPECTED OUTCOMES

1 Foot care has been given without complications. *If not*, follow these alternative nursing actions:

ANA: If client refuses foot care, provide equipment and instruction so he or she can complete it.

ANA: Suggest to physician that client requires care by podiatrist.

2 Client's feet are clean and appear free of complicating conditions such as excessive moisture, calluses, corns, blisters, abrasions, or infection. *If not*, follow these alternative nursing actions:

ANA: If excessive moisture is present, use moisture-absorbing powder.

ANA: Assess degree and type of condition and report to physician.

ANA: Instruct client in appropriate care of feet, especially if client is a diabetic.

3 Client and family understand the importance and techniques for proper foot care. *If not*, follow these alternative nursing actions:

ANA: Reinstruct client and family in foot care.

ANA: Have client or family member return a demonstration of foot care.

4 Footdrop (plantar flexion) is prevented. *If not*, follow these alternative nursing actions:

ANA: Help the client perform active and passive range of motion exercises at least twice every shift.

ANA: Apply splints or heel protectors when necessary.

ANA: Obtain order for physical therapy department to evaluate client.

UNEXPECTED OUTCOMES

1 Client has excessively dry, scaly skin, even after routine foot care.
   ANA: Alkali solutions such as Epsom salts or bicarbonate of soda may be helpful in softening skin and remaining scales. Repeated soaks are usually necessary.
2 Client has large calluses on feet.
   ANA: After soaking, rub a pumice stone or an abrasive material on the callused area. Calluses are *never* cut from the skin due to possible scarring to the epidermis.
   ANA: For diabetic clients, obtain services of a podiatrist.

Charting
- Initial assessment findings and overall status of client's feet
- Foot care needs and plans
- Care given and results of care
- Any abnormalities
- Involvement in client/family teaching

TERMINOLOGY

Bed-Making

Occupied bed: The client remains in the bed while it is being made.

Unoccupied bed: The client is out of the bed while it is being made.

Anesthesia (surgical, recovery) bed: A bed made in a specific manner for the client who is returning to the bed after having anesthesia or surgery.

Open bed: A bed being used by a client, the linens are folded down.

Closed bed: A bed not being used by a client, the linens are left to cover the bed.

Back-Care

Effleurage: Long stroking motions of the hands up and down the back. Hands do not leave skin surface. Pressure is light.

Tapotement: Alternate striking of fleshy part of hands on client's back as you move up and down back.

Petrissage: Pinching of skin, subcutaneous tissue, and muscle as you move up and down client's back.

Skin-Care

Acne: Skin condition due to irritation and infection of the sebaceous glands.

Bedsore: A synonym for decubitus ulcer or pressure sore. Area of cellular necrosis due to decreased circulation.

Blanching: A whitish hue to an area of skin.

Decubitus ulcer: A synonym for bedsore or pressure sore. Area of cellular necrosis due to decreased circulation.

Ecchymosis: Collection of blood underneath skin surface, bruise.

Emollient: Soothing, softening agent applied to body surfaces.

Epidermis: Superficial portion of skin.

Erythema: Redness of skin associated with rashes, infections and allergic responses.

Hyperemia: Influx of blood into an area causing redness to the skin.

Ischemia: Decreased, insufficient blood supply.

Lesion: An area of broken skin.

Necrosis: Cell death.

Pediculosis: Infestation of lice.

Pediculosis capitis: Head lice.

Pediculosis corporis: Body lice.

Pediculosis pubis: Crab lice.

Petechiae: Pinpoint reddish spots.

Purpura: Reddish-purple areas.

Shearing force: Layers of skin moving upon each other.

Turgor: The degree of elasticity of the skin.

Types of Beds When the client is confined to bed even for a short period of time, comfort is essential in order to promote rest and sleep. If the client is to remain in bed for an extended length of time all of his or her care and daily routines will be directed from bed. It will become the center of client's activity.

There are many different types of beds and related equipment available to meet the special health care needs of individual clients. The requirements of the basic hospital bed are discussed in ''Factors Affecting Environmental Adaptation-Secure Furnishings and Decor.'' Some of these special needs beds are described as follows:

Cribs and bassinets: Generally used for children and infants although larger crib-type beds are available for the adult client. Cribs are generally high from floor height to enable the nurse to work more easily with the client; therefore, side rails should *always* be up. Some institutions use a crib net or bubble top as an additional safety feature.

Stryker frame or foster frame: Generally used for individuals who are unable to move, such as with spinal cord injuries, and for clients who must be placed in the prone position, such as with decubitus ulcers. Canvas pieces are attached to a frame, which is placed over the client. It is then secured to the lower section of the frame so the client can be flipped over to the reverse position. The upper frame is then removed.

Circular frame: An electrically operated bed that is attached to a circular frame. The client can be placed in a variety of degrees with the support of an upper frame. The client can gradually be raised to a standing position or can be placed in the prone position. Circular beds can be operated by one person although it is strongly advised to use two people.

Recovery room bed: An adaptation of the basic hospital bed. This bed has the same features as the basic bed but is usually nonelectric. It is generally narrower and has side rails all the way around the bed instead of a head and footboard. It is easily movable and is occasionally used in intensive care units, labor rooms, and emergency rooms.

Water beds: Most commonly used for severe skin conditions such as decubitus ulcers or burns. Instead of the standard mattress, a specially designed heavy plastic casing is filled with water and serves as the mattress. It is used to create less pressure on weight bearing areas of the body.

Air beds: Instead of the standard mattress, a specially designed mattress automatically inflates and deflates to change areas of pressure on parts of the body.

Equipment Used with Beds   Aside from the standard types of equipment used on the basic hospital bed, specialized equipment can be added to meet the client's health care needs.

The footboard: Usually a solid support placed on the bed where the soles of the feet touch. It is secured to the mattress or bed frame. Footboards are used to prevent permanent plantar flexion (footdrop) and to exercise leg muscles. The footboard may also have side supports to help maintain proper alignment of feet.

The bed cradle: A device that is attached to the lower end of bed to prevent the bed linens from resting on the client's legs or feet. It is often used when a client has burns, ulcers, a wet cast, or specific circulatory diseases.

Balkan (overbed) frame: An overhead bed bar(s) that is used to support a trapeze, or a series of pulleys and weights used for traction equipment.

Hospital Bed Positions   Hospital beds are designed to adjust to a variety of positions according to the client's needs. Various positions are listed below:

Fowler's position: The head of the bed is at a 45-degree angle. Client's hips may or may not be flexed.

Semi-Fowler's position: The head of the bed is at a 30-degree angle; often used with cardiac and respiratory problems.

High-Fowler's position: The head of the bed is at a 90-degree angle; often used to achieve maximum chest expansion.

Trendelenburg's position: The mattress remains unbent, but the head of the bed is lowered and the foot is raised. "Shock blocks" may be used under the legs of the bed to achieve this position.

Reverse Trendelenburg's position: The mattress remains unbent, but the head of the bed is raised and the foot is lowered.

Contour position: The head of the bed and the foot of the bed are each raised slightly, causing a bend in the mattress.

Knee-gatch position: The lower section of bed under the knee area is raised slightly.

Sheets for Bed-Making

Full sheets: Regular full length flat sheets that can be used as the top and bottom sheet.

Contour sheets: Sheets that have elastic at each corner; fitted sheets.

Draw sheets: Sheets made of fabric, plastic, or rubber that are placed across the shoulder-to-knee area of the bed and tucked in on the sides.

Incontinent pads: Large, disposable pads that can be placed under the buttocks area, head, drains, or any place where excess moisture or fluid may collect on the bed.

Pull sheets: Sheets placed across the shoulder-to-knee area of the bed. The left side is untucked, wrinkle free, and folded under the client. Pull sheets are used to lift the client in the bed.

Levels of Personal Care

Complete care: The client requires total assistance from the nurse because the client is able to do little or nothing for him or herself. Complete bathing, skin care, oral care, nail and hair care, care of the feet, eyes, ears, and nose, and a total bed linen change are usually provided.

Partial care: The client performs as much of his or her own care as possible. The nurse completes the remaining care.

Early morning care: This type of care may or may not be a routine in some hospitals. If early morning care is provided, it is usually given by the night shift nurses. It may include bathing the hands and face, use of the bedpan or urinal, oral care, and other stimulating measures in preparation for breakfast.

P.M. care (H.S. care-hour of sleep care): P.M. care is usually provided to prepare the client for a relaxing, uninterrupted period of sleep. Activities include oral care, partial bathing, skin care and a soothing back massage, straightening or changing the bed linen, and offering the bedpan or urinal. The client should also be assessed for the need of food, drink, or medication before sleep.

O.R. care: Clients who will be undergoing surgery or diagnostic tests may be required to bathe the evening before. Partial bathing is sometimes allowed in the morning if time permits. If the client is not allowed to have anything by mouth, care must be taken *not* to allow swallowing of water or dentifrice while providing oral care. The client is usually given a clean gown. All dentures, hairpins, makeup, nail polish, contact lenses, and jewelry are removed and locked up. The client is encouraged to void before leaving for the operating room.

CHAPTER 3
Developing Therapeutic Communication Skills

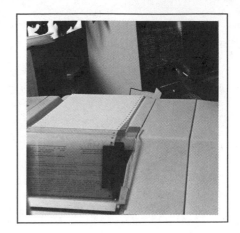

This chapter introduces the concept of communication in nursing practice. It is divided into three main sections, all of which deal with a different aspect of communication. The first section discusses therapeutic communication skills, verbal and non-verbal communication, anxiety and nurse-client relationship. The second section deals with client education. The third section — charting — comprises the written form of communication necessary for legal documentation and communication among health team members. It also includes a brief description of client care plans, incident reports and consent forms.

THERAPEUTIC COMMUNICATION

Communication Communication is the process of sending and receiving messages by means of symbols, words, signs, gestures, or other actions. It is a multilevel process consisting of the content or information part of the message and the part that defines the meaning of the message. Messages sent and received define the relationship between people. From the point of view of a learned skill, communication is intended to accomplish a defined goal. It is the transmission of facts, feelings, and meaning through the communication process.

The communication process forms one of the primary bases for administering all skills. Without clear communication the nurse cannot

LEARNING OBJECTIVES

Describe the components of a nurse-client relationship.
Define the communication process and list the factors that affect it.
List five examples of therapeutic communication or blocks to it.
List five examples of non-therapeutic communication.
Discuss what is meant by the interview-counseling process.
Identify and describe the five stages of anxiety.
Explain the main purposes of charting.
List the advantages and disadvantages of the three charting systems: source oriented, problem oriented, and computer assisted charting.
Discuss the purpose of completing an incident report.
List the goals of client education.
Identify at least three appropriate teaching strategies.

Phases in Nurse-Client Relationship Therapy

Initiation or orientation phase
- Establish boundaries of the relationship.
- Identify problems.
- Assess anxiety levels of self and client.
- Identify expectations.

Continuation or active working phase
- Promote attitude of acceptance of each other to decrease anxiety.
- Use specific therapeutic and problem-solving techniques to develop a working relationship.
- Continually assess and evaluate problems.
- Focus on increasing client's independence and decreasing client's reliance on the nurse.
- Maintain the goal of client's confronting and working through identified problems.

Termination phase
- Plan for the conclusion of therapy early in the development of the relationship.
- Maintain initially defined boundaries.
- Anticipate problems of termination:
    Client may become too dependent on the nurse. Encourage client to come independent.
    Termination may recall client's previous separation experiences, causing feelings of abandonment, rejection, and depression. Discuss client's previous experiences.
- Discuss client's feelings about termination.

assess, administer, or evaluate his or her actions in performing the skill. The principles of therapeutic communication form a basis for interviewing and counseling skills.

Nurse-Client Relationship Nurses are given the unique opportunity to share part of who they are with others who have asked directly or indirectly for assistance. It is within this interpersonal framework that the nurse-client relationship begins to develop and take on its individual characteristics.

Both individuals bring into the relationship their thoughts, feelings, sense of self or self-worth, behavior patterns, ability to adapt and cope, belief systems, and points-of-view about life and how they interact with it. Within all these complex variables, there is a commonly shared point at which the nurse-client relationship begins.

A nurse-client relationship may be defined as the interaction between the nurse and a client with shared therapeutic goals and objectives. Characteristics of the relationship include acceptance, honesty, understanding, and empathy of the nurse toward the client who is willingly or unwillingly seeking help. Generally, it is important for the nurse to view the client as a unique individual who is responsible for his or her own feelings, actions, and behaviors and who is an active participant in his or her health care program. The relationship will be more effective if the client shows a willingness to accept responsibility and actively participates in the therapeutic relationship. In psychiatry, however, this is not always possible, and the nurse must begin the relationship by accepting the level at which the client is able to participate. This, at times, is a difficult and frustrating process. The goal of relationship therapy is to assist the client to identify and meet his or her own needs. The nurse may assist the client in reaching his or her goal by demonstrating acceptance so that the client can experience the feeling of being accepted as an individual; by developing mutual trust through consistent, congruent nursing behaviors; by providing corrective emotional experiences to increase self-esteem; and finally by creating a safe, supportive environment. Some degree of emotional involvement and honest, open communication is essential throughout the relationship. The nurse must encourage the client to express within safe limits his or her feelings.

GUIDELINES FOR MANAGING CLIENTS

Basic propositions underlie the theory and components of the communication process.

- The foundation of the person's perception of him or herself and the world is the result of communicated messages received from significant others.
- Communication skills are learned as the individual grows and develops.
- Communication is a basic human need.
- A person cannot not communicate.

The communication process includes both verbal and nonverbal expressions and is affected by the following factors:

- The intrapersonal framework of the person
- The relationship between the participants
- The purpose of the sender
- The content
- The context
- The manner in which the message is sent
- The effect on the receiver

The nurse-client relationship is a therapeutic, professional relationship.

- The interaction occurs between two persons—a nurse, who possesses the skills, abilities, and resources to relieve another's discomfort, and a client, who is seeking assistance for alleviation of some existing problem.
- Basic acceptance of the value of the individual is a prerequisite for a nurse-client relationship.
- Awareness of the total client, including physical as well as emotional needs, is important.
- The nurse's understanding of his or herself, needs, and motives is important in the therapeutic process.
- Some degree of emotional involvement is required, but objectivity must be maintained.

Anxiety is a response to tensions and is experienced as a painful, vague uneasiness or diffuse apprehension.

- Anxiety is a form of energy whose presence is inferred from its effect on attention, behavior, learning, and perception.
- Anxiety is perceived subjectively by the conscious mind of the person experiencing it.
- Anxiety is a result of conflicts between the personality and the environment or between different forces within the personality.
- The causative conflicts and/or threats are undefined in the conscious mind of the person.

The amount or level of anxiety is related to both the degree of threat to the self and the degree to which behavior reduces the anxiety.

- Varying degrees of anxiety are common to all human beings at one time or another.
- Anxiety is always found in emotional disorders.
- Anxiety is easily transmitted from one individual to another.
- Constructive use of anxiety is healthy; it is often an incentive for growth.
- The greater the capacity to handle anxiety, the more control an individual has over his or her environment.

Rationale for Action

- To institute therapeutic rather than casual or non-goal oriented communication
- To transfer ideas from one person to another
- To create meaning through the process of communication
- To reduce uncertainty, and to strengthen the client's ego
- To affect or influence the client's physical, emotional and social environment
- To act effectively in relationships

ACTION: PROVIDING THERAPEUTIC COMMUNICATION

ASSESSMENT

1 Determine individual's ability to process information at the cognitive level.
2 Evaluate mental status data to establish baseline for intervention.
3 Evaluate ability of client to communicate on a verbal level.
4 Observe what is happening with the client here and now.
5 Identify developmental level of client so interaction expectations will be realistic.
6 Determine whether client exhibits primarily verbal or nonverbal behavior so you can relate to client on the appropriate level.
7 Assess anxiety level of client as anxiety will interfere with communication.

PLANNING

GOALS

- Therapeutic communication is initiated and maladaptive communication corrected.
- The client is assisted to meet own needs.
- The client experiences the feeling of being accepted.
- Mutual trust through consistent, congruent behavior is developed.
- Increased self-esteem of the client is promoted.
- A supportive environment for change is provided.

INTERVENTION: Utilizing Therapeutic Communication Techniques

1 Listen carefully, eagerly, actively, responsively, and seriously to what client says.
2 Acknowledge client without inserting your own values or judgments. Acknowledgment may be simple and with or without understanding. For example, in the response "I hear what you're saying," the person acknowledges a statement without agreeing with it. Acknowledgment may be verbal or nonverbal.
3 Use feedback to relay to client the effect of his or her words. This method helps keep client on course or alters course. It involves acknowledging, validating, clarifying, extending, and altering. Nurse to client: "You did that well."
4 Stay attuned to the harmony of verbal and nonverbal messages. This therapeutic process is known as mutual fit or congruence. For example, a client is crying, and the nurse says, "I want to help," and puts his or her hand on the client's shoulder.
5 Clarify client's message. Check out or make clear either the intent or hidden meaning of the message or determine if the message sent was the message received. Nurse: "You said it was hot in here. Would you like to open the window?"

6   Focus or refocus on client's statement. Pick up on central topics or "cues" given by client. Nurse: "You were telling me how hard it was to talk to your mother."

7   Validate accuracy of client's message. Nurse: "Yes, it is confusing with so many people around."

8   Identify and send back a message acknowledging the feeling expressed. This process, called reflection, conveys acceptance and great understanding. Nurse: "You distrust your doctor?"

9   Ask client open-ended questions. Asking questions that cannot be answered "Yes" or "No" or "Maybe" generally requires an answer of several words in order to broaden conversational opportunities and to help the client communicate. Nurse: "What kind of job would you like to do?"

10 Give client encouragement through use of nonverbal actions. Use body language to communicate interest, attention, understanding, support, caring, and/or listening in order to promote data gathering. Nurse: Nods appropriately as someone talks.

11 Restate the last few words the client says. Nurse: "You hear voices."

12 Paraphrase or reword what client has said. Nurse: "You mean you're unhappy."

13 Show interest and involvement without saying anything else. Nurse: "Yes . . ." "Uh hm . . ."

14 Use incomplete sentences to encourage client to continue. Nurse: "Then your life is . . ."

15 Keep your own verbalization minimal and let the client lead the conversation. Nurse: "You feel . . . ?"

16 Use broad opening statements to open communication. This process allows client freedom to talk and to focus on himself or herself. Nurse: "How have you been feeling?"

INTERVENTION: Preventing Blocks to Communication

1   Avoid internal validation (jumping to conclusions). Do not make an assumption about the meaning of someone else's behavior that is not validated by the other person. Example: The nurse finds the suicidal client smiling and joking and tells the staff, "Client is in a cheerful mood."

2   Do not give advice or tell client what to do. Giving your opinion or making decisions for client implies client cannot handle his or her own life decisions and that you are accepting responsibility. Nurse: "If I were you . . ."

3   Do not change the subject. Introducing new topics inappropriately is a pattern that may indicate anxiety. The client is crying and discussing his or her fear of surgery, when the nurse asks, "How many children do you have?"

4   Avoid responding in a way that focuses attention on the nurse instead of client. Nurse: "This sunshine is good for my roses. I have a beautiful rose garden."

5　Do not invalidate client's words by ignoring or denying client's presence, thoughts, or feelings. Client: "Hi, how are you?" Nurse: "I can't talk now. I'm on my way to lunch."

6　Avoid using cliches, pat answers, "cheery" words, advice, and "comforting" statements as an attempt to reassure the client. Most of what is called "reassurance" is really false reassurance. Nurse: "It's going to be all right."

7　Do not overload conversation by talking rapidly, changing subjects, and giving more information than can be absorbed at one time. Nurse: "What's your name? I see you're forty-eight years old and that you like sports. Where do you come from?"

8　Do not underload conversation by remaining silent and unresponsive, not picking up cues, or failing to give feedback. Client: "What's your name?" Nurse: Smiles and walks away.

9　Do not send verbal and nonverbal messages that contradict one another. Do not send two or more messages on different levels that seriously contradict one another. The contradiction may be between the content, verbal, nonverbal, and/or context (time, space). This contradiction is a double message. Client: "I like your dress." Nurse: Annoyed, frowns and looks disgusted.

10　Avoid value judgments. Do not give your opinion or moralize or imply your own values by using words such as "nice," "good," "bad," "right," "wrong," "should," and "ought." Nurse: "I think Dr. Steinberg is a very good doctor."

EVALUATION

EXPECTED OUTCOMES

1　Client develops the ability to assess and meet own needs. *If not*, follow these alternative nursing actions:
   ANA:　Reassess expectations of both client and nurse.
   ANA:　Redefine needs so both client and nurse are clear.
   ANA:　Increase emphasis on problem-solving ability of client.

2　Communication from client is improved so that it is clearer, more explicit, and centered on problem areas. *If not*, follow these alternative nursing actions:
   ANA:　Reassess client so that interactions are carried out on client's intellectual, emotional, and developmental level.
   ANA:　Redefine problem areas and maintain focus of communication on problems.

3　A supportive environment is created so that client can reduce anxiety level and experience change. *If not*, follow these alternative nursing actions:
   ANA:　Assist client to express feelings more effectively.
   ANA:　Assist client to develop more effective coping mechanisms by discussion of what behavior helps to reduce anxiety, role-playing, group therapy, etc.

UNEXPECTED OUTCOMES

1 Therapeutic communication is not achieved.

ANA: Eliminate blocks to communication from interaction style.

ANA: If a block does occur, recognize it.

ANA: Move to correct communication by utilizing therapeutic modes of communication.

ANA: Evaluate own process of communication during as well as after interaction.

2 Client's demanding behavior interferes with the therapeutic communication process.

ANA: Do not ignore demands; they will only increase in intensity.

ANA: Attempt to determine causal factors of behavior, e.g., high anxiety level.

ANA: Set limits to response patterns when client is demanding.

ANA: Control own feelings of anger and irritation.

ANA: Teach alternative means of getting needs met.

Charting
- Assessment data on client
- Identification of client needs
- Explicit goals of interaction
- Communication patterns of client
- Emotional state of client
- Expressed feelings and/or thoughts if relevant

ACTION: ESTABLISHING A NURSE-CLIENT RELATIONSHIP

ASSESSMENT

1 Determine the purpose of establishing a nurse-client relationship.

2 Consider the overall condition of client to determine if client will be able to benefit from a nurse-client relationship.

 a A specific relationship could feed into secondary gains of neurotic disorders.

 b An individual with chronic organic brain disorder would not benefit from a relationship per se.

3 Identify client expectations of a therapeutic relationship to determine if you will be able to meet these needs.

4 Examine your own feelings and expectations to evaluate potential ' impact on such a relationship.

5 Assess all components of communication, steps 1-7, in "Action: Providing Therapeutic Communication."

Rationale for Action
- To provide an environment where client can feel secure enough to alter behavior patterns
- To allow client to experience a positive, satisfying relationship
- To enable client to test out more adaptive ways to handle anxiety
- To provide a climate conducive to raising client's self-esteem

PLANNING

GOALS

- Therapeutic communication principles are utilized to provide a framework for change.
- Boundaries of professional relationship are maintained.
- Appropriate environment is established where therapeutic interaction can take place.
- Time is allocated to complete planned process of interaction.
- Termination of relationship is completed.

INTERVENTION: Developing a Nurse-Client Relationship

1 Assume the role of facilitator in the relationship.
2 Accept client as having value and worth as an individual.
3 Maintain relationship on a professional level.
4 Provide an environment conducive to client's experiencing corrective emotional experiences.
5 Keep interaction reality oriented, that is, in the here and now.
6 Listen actively.
7 Use nonverbal communication to support and encourage client.
   a Recognize meaning and purpose of nonverbal communication.
   b Keep verbal and nonverbal communication congruent.
8 Focus content and direction of conversation on client.
9 Interact on client's intellectual, developmental, and emotional level.
10 Focus on "how," "what," "when," "where," and "who," rather than on "why."
11 Teach client problem solving to correct maladaptive patterns.
12 Help client to identify, express, and cope with feelings.
13 Help client develop alternative coping mechanisms.
14 Recognize a high level of anxiety and assist client to deal with it.

EVALUATION

EXPECTED OUTCOMES

1 Principles of therapeutic communication are utilized. *If not*, follow these alternative nursing actions:
   ANA: Reevaluate own level of knowledge and understanding of communication principles and ask for consultation of a communication specialist (clinical specialist in psychiatric nursing).
   ANA: Practice removing blocks to communication by reviewing interaction, writing a process recording, or taping interaction with follow-up evaluation.
2 Boundaries of professional relationship are maintained. *If not*, follow these alternative nursing actions:
   ANA: Continue to set limits explicitly.
   ANA: Redefine limits and be consistent; if client cannot adhere to boundaries, reassessment is necessary.
3 The appropriate environment for interaction is established. *If not*, follow these alternative nursing actions:
   ANA: Change environment or time of interaction so milieu will be more conducive to the interaction.
   ANA   Continue with interaction, making explicit to client how difficult it is to communicate clearly in a confusing environment.
4 Termination of the relationship is completed successfully. *If not*, follow these alternative nursing actions:

ANA: Give client opportunity to fully discuss feelings of loss, rejection, etc.

ANA: Examine own feelings and attitudes so this will not recur.

ANA: Remember to allow adequate time for termination and begin the process early in the relationship.

UNEXPECTED OUTCOMES

1 Client refuses to participate in a nurse-client relationship.

ANA: Adhere to client's request and do not force or impose relationship therapy.

ANA: Continue to offer relationship therapy at intervals.

ANA: Suggest that another team member attempt to establish a relationship.

2 Nurse-client relationship degenerates into a social conversation.

ANA: Reevaluate the goals for the relationship and remind client of terms originally established.

ANA: Set firm limits and continually reexamine progress.

Charting

- Primary goals of nurse-client relationship and identified client needs
- On-going process of relationship therapy including client's expressed feelings, thoughts, etc.
- Client's behavior and changes in behavior, both positive and negative
- Cues to other team members on how best to relate to this particular client
- Data on how client is handling relationship as well as overall hospitalization

ACTION: COMPLETING THE INTERVIEW-COUNSELING PROCESS

ASSESSMENT

1 Determine purpose of the interview.
2 As the first step in therapeutic interviewing, assess client's total condition physical, emotional, spiritual, and social.
3 Observe accurately what is happening with the client here and now.
4 Be aware of your own feelings, reactions, and level of anxiety.
5 Assess client's communication patterns, behavior, and general demeanor.
6 Determine life situation of client.
7 Assess environmental conditions that may affect nurse-client interaction.

Rationale for Action

- To provide a framework for client to assess and change his or her behavior
- To determine life situation of client and establish goals for change in a positive direction
- To role model therapeutic communication and encourage client to communicate clearly
- To assist client to lower anxiety and substitute more effective coping mechanisms

PLANNING

GOALS

- The interview is goal-directed; that is, communication or transmission of facts, feelings, and meanings through words and gestures accomplish a defined goal.
- The environment is conducive to the interview process.
- Both nurse and client will agree implicitly or explicitly to conduct the interview.
- Purpose of interview is accomplished.
- There will be enough time to complete planned process or goals of interview.

INTERVENTION: Interviewing the Client

1 Provide a safe, private comfortable setting if possible.
2 Encourage client to describe perceptions and feelings.
   a Focus on communication but use indirect approach.
   b Use minimal verbal activity.
   c Encourage spontaneity.
3 Assist client to clarify feelings and events and place them in time sequence.
   a Focus on emotionally charged area.
   b Maintain accepting, nonjudgmental attitude.
4 Give broad, opening statements and ask open-ended questions to enable client to describe what is happening with him or her.
5 Use body language to convey empathy, interest, and encouragement to facilitate communication.
6 Use silence as a therapeutic tool; it enables client to pace and direct his or her own communications. Long periods of silence, however, may increase client's anxiety level.
7 Define the limits of the interview by determining the purpose for the interview and then structure the time and interaction patterns accordingly.
8 Never use interviewing techniques as stereotyped responses.
   a Use of such responses negates open and honest communication.
   b Use of structured responses is counterproductive, as it presents nurse as a dishonest communicator.
   c Interaction must be alive and responsive, not dependent on a technique for continuance.
   d Use "I" messages, not "you" messages. (For example, say, "I feel uncomfortable," not "you make me feel uncomfortable.")

Encourage client to describe perceptions and feelings.

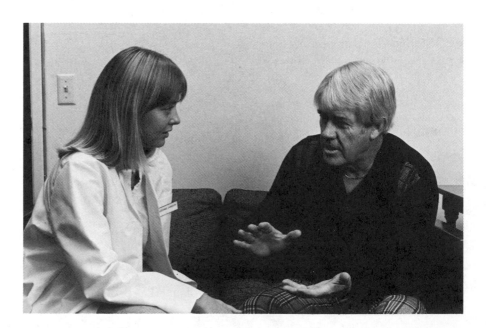

INTERVENTION: Guiding the Counseling Process

1 Be present and allow client to experience supportiveness.
2 Maintain consistency with flexibility to provide security.
3 Give information but not advice.
4 Assist client without persuading, admonishing, threatening, or compelling client to change attitudes, beliefs, or behaviors.
5 Use the interviewing process to facilitate accomplishment of a goal.
6 Use therapeutic communication skills such as active listening and empathic understanding.
7 Set limits and determine goals.
8 Enable client to make fullest use of potential within his or her current experience to develop new ways of coping with life situations.
9 Assist client to build more effective coping mechanisms:
  a Gather pertinent data.
  b Define the problem.
  c Mutually agree on working toward a solution.
  d Set goals.
  e Select alternatives.
  f Activate problem-solving behavior.
  g Evaluate and modify solution or goals throughout counseling process.

EVALUATION

EXPECTED OUTCOMES

1 The interview-counseling session remains goal-directed. *If not,* follow these alternative nursing actions:
ANA: Redefine specific established goals identified by nurse and client.
ANA: Continually examine the purpose of the interview-counseling session so you do not get sidetracked by unimportant issues.
ANA: Reevaluate the problem-solving process and modify as appropriate to client's problems and needs.
2 The environment is supportive and conducive to the communication process. *If not,* follow these alternative nursing actions:
ANA: Reassess needs and alter environment.
ANA: Change time of the interview-counseling session so environment is more appropriate.

UNEXPECTED OUTCOMES

1 Interview could not be completed because of client's behavior.
ANA: Acknowledge directly that client is unable to tolerate interaction at this time and open communication process to see if he or she can discuss problems.
ANA: After acknowledgement, set up new time for interview.
2 Client becomes verbally abusive during interview.
ANA: Do not respond in kind to abusive comments.
ANA: Try not to take abuse personally.

Charting

- Purpose of interview or counseling session
- Outcome of interview or counseling session
- Client behavior
- Client's expressed thoughts or feelings
- Future plans for repeat sessions
- Data that other team members will find useful in dealing with client

Rationale for Action

- To assist client to tolerate or manage anxiety more appropriately
- To assist client to develop more effective coping mechanisms
- To aid client in gaining a degree of insight into the source of anxiety
- To give client support in changing life-style patterns that cause anxiety
- To provide a nurse-client relationship as a means of assisting the client to handle anxiety

ANA: Interact with the client on a therapeutic basis.
  a Help the client examine his feelings.
  b Do not reject the client.
  c Give client feedback concerning your reactions to abusive comments.
  d Teach alternative ways to express his feelings.
ANA: Maintain a calm, accepting approach to client.

ACTION: MANAGING ANXIETY

ASSESSMENT

1 Assess client's degree of anxiety by determining client's ability to focus on what is happening to him or her in a situation.
  a Mild anxiety: client is able to focus realistically on most of what is happening within and to him or her.
  b Moderate anxiety: Client is able to partially focus on what is happening; focus is limited.
  c Severe anxiety: Client cannot focus on what is happening to him or her; focus is scattered.
2 Assess client's physiological reactions.
  a Increased heart rate
  b Increased or decreased appetite
  c Increased blood supply to skeletal muscles
  d Tendency to void and defecate
  e Dry mouth
  f Butterflies in stomach, nausea, vomiting, cramps, diarrhea
  g "Flight or fight" response
  h Tremors
  i Dyspnea
  j Palpitations
  k Tachycardia
  l Numbness of extremities
3 Evaluate client's psychological reactions.
  a Lack of concentration on work
  b Feelings of depression and guilt
  c Harbored fear of sudden death or insanity
  d Dread of being alone
  e Confusion
  f Tension
  g Agitation and restlessness
4 Determine which stage of anxiety client is experiencing.
  Ataraxia (absence of anxiety)
  a This state is uncommon.
  b It can be seen in persons who take drugs.
  c State indicates low motivation.

Mild

a Client's senses are alert.

b Attentiveness is increased.

c Motivation is increased.

Moderate

a Client's perception is narrowed and attention is selective.

b The degree of pathology depends on the individual.

c State may be detected in complaining, arguing, teasing behaviors.

d Anxiety may be converted to physical symptoms, such as headaches, low back pain, nausea, and diarrhea.

Severe

a All senses are gravely affected.

b Behavior becomes automatic.

c Energy is drained.

d Defense mechanisms are used to control anxiety.

e State cannot be used constructively by person.

f Psychologically, state is extremely painful.

g Nursing action is always indicated for this state.

Panic

a Individual is overwhelmed.

b Personality may disintegrate.

c The client may engage in wild, desperate, ineffective behavior.

d Client should be watched to prevent possible bodily harm to self and others.

e Client cannot tolerate panic state very long: client soon cannot control his or her behavior; client feels helpless; client is momentarily psychotic.

f Condition is pathological.

g Immediate intervention is needed: physical restraint, tranquilizers, nonstimulating environment, constant presence of nurse.

PLANNING

GOALS

- Behavior and/or symptoms related to anxiety are identified.
- Anxiety is decreased.
- Nurse intervenes when client is unable to cope through implementation of specific treatment plan, i.e., chemotherapy, 1:1, seclusion, restraints, and relaxation techniques, etc.
- Factors or persons who escalate client's anxiety are identified, and interventions are provided.
- Tolerance for anxiety is increased.
- More effective coping mechanisms for handling anxiety are developed.
- Client is assisted to channel anxiety-produced energy into constructive behavior.

INTERVENTION: Assisting the Client in Managing Anxiety

1 Identify anxious behavior and the level of anxiety that determines degree of intervention.
2 Remain with an anxious client.
3 Recognize anxiety in self.
4 Maintain appropriate attitudes toward client.
   a Acceptance
   b Matter-of-fact approach
   c Willingness to listen and help
   d Calmness and support
5 Recognize if additional help is required for intervention.
6 Provide activities that decrease anxiety and provide an outlet for energy.
7 Establish a person-to-person relationship.
   a Allow client to express feelings.
   b Proceed at client's pace.
   c Avoid forcing client.
   d Assist client in identifying anxiety.
   e Assist client in learning new ways of dealing with anxiety.
8 Provide appropriate physical environment.
   a Nonstimulating
   b Structured
   c Designed to prevent physical exhaustion or self-harm
9 Administer medication as directed and needed.

INTERVENTION: Managing the Aggressive or Combative Client

1 Observe client acutely for clues that the client is getting out of control.
   a Note rising anger — verbal and nonverbal behavior.
   b Note erratic or unpredictable response to staff or other clients.
2 Intervene immediately when loss of control is imminent.
3 Use a nonthreatening approach to the client.
4 Set firm limits on unacceptable behavior.
5 Maintain calm manner and do not show fear.
6 Avoid engaging in an argument or provoking the client.
7 Remove the client from the situation as soon as possible.
8 Attempt to calm the client so that he may regain control.
9 Be supportive and stay with the client.

EVALUATION

EXPECTED OUTCOMES

1 Interventions result in decrease of anxiety evidenced by client being more attentive and more alert and displaying more control of own behavior, i.e., client is able to sit with nurse rather than pace. Client is able to verbalize anxious thoughts. *If not*, follow these alternative nursing actions:

ANA: Assist client to use coping mechanisms by discussing with client the most effective methods he or she uses to lower anxiety. Institute role playing to highlight alternative actions and have client practice relaxation techniques.

ANA: Reevaluate medications client is taking and their effects on behavior.

2 Client is able to discuss anxious feelings. *If not*, follow these alternative nursing actions:

ANA: Assist client to identify feelings of anxiety.

ANA: Assist client to describe feelings of anxiety.

ANA: Encourage client to relate physiological symptoms of decreased anxiety.

3 Client is able to learn new ways of coping with anxiety. *If not*, follow these alternative nursing actions:

ANA: Assist client to raise tolerance level of anxiety by teaching intermediate measures of breathing techniques, relaxation methods, exercise programs, change in diet, etc.

4 Client is able to manage anxiety to the point where he does not become aggressive or combative. *If not*, follow these alternative nursing actions:

ANA: Summon assistance only when indicated; sudden involvement of many people will increase the client's agitation.

ANA: Use seclusion and/or restraints only if necessary.

ANA: Use problem-solving focus following outburst of aggressive or combative behavior to prevent recurrence:

a Encourage discussion of feelings surrounding incident.

b Attempt to look at causal factors of the behavior.

c Examine the client's response to stimulus and alternative responses.

d Point out consequences of aggressive behavior.

e Discuss the client's role of taking responsibility for his aggressive behavior.

UNEXPECTED OUTCOMES

1 Client becomes extremely defensive when nurse attempts to discuss coping mechanisms.

ANA: Avoid criticizing client's behavior and use of adjustment mechanisms.

ANA: Help client explore the underlying source of the anxiety rather than coping mechanisms.

ANA: Assist client at own pace in learning new or alternative adjustment patterns for healthier adaptation.

2 Client's anxiety level increases sharply during interaction with the nurse.

ANA: Use techniques to alleviate client's anxiety.

ANA: Use a firm supportive approach to explore any ineffective use of adjustment patterns.

Charting
- Level or degree of client's anxiety
- Behavior, thoughts or feelings that client expresses that indicate anxiety
- Degree of client's understanding, insight, etc., into source of anxiety
- Measures that nurse takes to assist client to lower anxiety
- Plans or goals that nurse and client establish to cope more effectively with anxiety

CLIENT EDUCATION

Client education as a legitimate process within the health care system had its "coming of age" during the 1970s. Factors contributing to this advancement of client education included a shift from the focus on treatment of acute, infectious, and curable diseases to the treatment of chronic, degenerative, noncurable diseases with multiple causes; increased involvement of consumers in their health care, including issues such as client's rights, informed consents, and client access to records; recognition of the cost benefits of client education; emergence of the self-care movement with its emphasis on the individual's responsibility for his or her state of health; and development of health education and client education theories through scientific research.

The goal of client education is to impact and influence behavioral changes by the individual that will promote the person's health status. The dynamics of human behavior and the forces that influence behavioral changes are highly complex, and there is simply no "one right way" to go about the process of educating clients in order to achieve this goal.

Learning Theories Since learning influences behavior, learning theories provide a framework for the education process. It is beyond the scope of this text to describe all learning theories, but two such theories provide a broad perspective. The cognitive theory emphasizes learning as an understanding of and insight into interrelationships involving perceptions, concepts, feelings, ideas; this type of learning also involves thinking and reasoning. Association theory, on the other hand, emphasizes learning by stimulus-response associations, and includes classical and operant conditioning, rote, and trial-and-error learning. While far apart in philosophy as to why and how learning occurs, proponents of both theories agree that behavior change is the outcome of learning and occurs as a result of practice. The nurse can choose to utilize those principles that are applicable to each teaching situation, whether it is use of behavior modification techniques (association theory) as part of a weight loss program or use of problem-solving games (cognitive theory) as part of group discussions for diabetics.

Goals of Learning The goals of learning can be classified as follows: cognitive (intellectual), affective (values, attitudes, feelings) and psychomotor (motor skills). These areas provide a framework for setting objectives and evaluating expected outcomes for specific teaching situations. They also assist in the decision making process for the use of different teaching strategies. (Refer to Table 1 for a summary of teaching strategies.) Of utmost importance is the recognition that the mere transmission of knowledge, such as a lecture, does not constitute learning. It is only one aspect. A change in the listener's attitude or value system must also occur before one's behavior changes, regardless of the knowledge one possesses.

The client teaching process is an important component of nursing care, although in actual practice many barriers to its realization exist. Some of these are created by nurses themselves. The description of the client education process as an action or skill within the nursing process provides a framework for the integration of both the nursing process and client-education within the practice of nursing.

ACTION: DEVELOPING TEACHING STRATEGIES

ASSESSMENT

1 Assess need for client teaching program.
2 Determine appropriate setting for individual client.
3 Identify client learning needs.
4 Assess knowledge and skill level of client.
5 Assess readiness and/or openness to learning.
6 Assess appropriate methodology for client teaching sessions.
7 Assess appropriate adjunctive materials, such as audiovisual aids, to enhance learning process.

PLANNING

GOALS

- Increased knowledge has positive effect on client's health status.
- The client's developmental stage, individual characteristics, prior knowledge, skills, and experiences support the learning situation.
- A more effective utilization by the client of the health care system results.
- Increased participation in the learning process enhances client self-esteem.

EQUIPMENT

- Room or suitable setting where teaching is to occur
- Teaching strategies
- Audiovisual equipment
- Charts and illustrations
- Written materials such as outlines or other handouts
- Equipment for demonstration and return demonstration
- Form such as a teaching Kardex or client chart to document when teaching is completed

INTERVENTION: Utilizing Methodology for Client Data Collection

1 Avoid judging client input to prevent client telling the nurse what client thinks the nurse wants to hear.
2 Utilize "how" questions to facilitate communication (more effective than "why" questions, which tend to set up a defensive reaction to the question).

Rationale for Action

- To acknowledge the impact of knowledge, values, and attitudes on health behaviors
- To acknowledge individual responsibility for health behaviors and health status
- To improve ability to make informed decisions affecting health status within health promotion and curative and maintenance activities
- To facilitate behavioral changes that are conducive to optimum health status

3 Utilize verbal and nonverbal behavior and congruence of both to provide important data.

4 Develop a questionnaire that can be completed by client or by nurse during the assessment interview.

5 Utilize observation skills.

6 Develop pretests and posttests to provide concrete evidence of change in client knowledge. (Example: "What would you do if . . . ?" questions provide good assessment of problem-solving abilities.)

7 Request demonstration of a skill previously learned or currently used to assess performance level.

INTERVENTION: Collecting Client Data

1 Identify personal characteristics.
   a Age/sex.
   b Educational level.
   c Marital status.
   d Family composition and living situation.
   e Ethnic group and cultural practices pertinent to learning.

2 Identify support systems available.

3 Identify values and attitudes toward self and others having his or her particular disease or condition.

4 Assess knowledge of anatomy and physiology (normal and disease-related) by specific questioning.

5 Evaluate capacity and ability to perform specific skills, including those previously learned.

6 Check knowledge of rationale behind specific skills.

7 Evaluate patterns of coping.
   a Past experiences of self and others in relation to the disease.
   b Perception by client of how ill he or she is at this time.
   c Reactions to stress and ways of managing anxiety.
   d Current level of self management:
   Where is client going?
   Is it working?
   If not, what is client willing to change or do differently?

INTERVENTION: Assessing Readiness to Learn

1 Determine client's physiological readiness.
   a Degree of physical comfort of client, such as lack of pain, level of alertness.
   b Acuteness of the illness and its influence on the client's ability to learn.
   c Environmental factors such as safety and supervision while practicing a new skill.

2 Assess client's psychological readiness.
   a Client's feeling state and its influence on receptivity to learning, i.e., an angry and hostile client is not going to hear much information until his or her anger is acknowledged or worked through.

    b Psychological barriers in the external environment and their impact.

    c Intellectual capacity and level of comprehension of client.

3 Evaluate client's motivational readiness.

    a Internal: self-directed, receives satisfaction from learning.

    b External: needs direction, guidance, and rewards from others.

    c Focus of control: belief about ability to control or influence one's environment.

INTERVENTION: Identifying Client Learning Needs

1 Utilize personal data and assessment to jointly determine learning needs of client.

2 Prioritize learning needs.

3 Review with client alternative resources available to meet learning needs.

4 Determine ability of facility or staff to meet learning needs.

5 Obtain verbal or written contract with client for educational program.

6 Refer client to other resources when appropriate.

INTERVENTION: Determining Appropriate Teaching Strategy

1 Consider the following factors when determining appropriate strategy:

    a Input from client about how he or she learns best.

    b Specific task or nature of the content to be transmitted and how it is best learned.

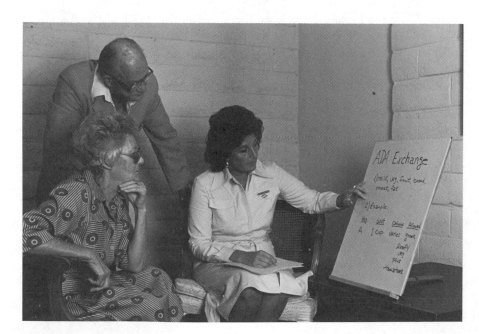

For client teaching to be effective, the nurse needs to provide a comfortable environment and identify client's level of understanding.

c Client attention span and retention ability.

d Teaching materials and resources available.

e Time, availability, skills, and abilities of staff; appropriate utilization of para-professional and professional staff.

f Participation by members of other health care disciplines as part of a team.

g Determination of most appropriate time for teaching.

2 Determine which type of teaching strategy will be effective in a given situation.

a Group process: use of principles from group dynamics, mental health, and other related fields to enhance learning/behavior changes in a small group setting.

b Lecture/discussion: presentation of content in a didactic fashion with opportunity for questions and interaction during or at the conclusion of the presentation.

c Demonstration/return demonstration: demonstration (videotape) by the instructor with practice by the learner and return demonstration of mastery of the skill.

d Role playing: assumption of roles by various participants/learners for the purpose of clarifying various aspects of a situation.

e Games: structured game situation with rules, etc., designed for the learner to accomplish specific educational objectives.

3 Select appropriate teaching adjuncts.

a Video-tape or video-cassette programs.

b Films.

c Slide and tape presentations.

d Programmed instruction materials.

e Books.

f Pamphlets and other written handouts.

g Diagrams, charts, and illustrations.

TABLE 1 USE OF TEACHING STRATEGIES ACCORDING TO TYPES OF LEARNING

TYPE OF LEARNING	TASK/CONTENT	TEACHING STRATEGIES
Cognitive	Facts	Lecture/Discussion
	Concepts	Audiovisual Aids
	Understanding	Written Materials
	Thinking	Problem-Solving Situations
Affective	Feelings	Group Process
	Attitudes	Role Playing
	Interests	Role Modeling
	Values	Games
	Appreciations	Active Participation in the
	Acceptance/Emotional	Learning Situation
	Adjustment	
Psychomotor	Motor Skills	Demonstration/Practice/
		Return Demonstration/
		Feedback
		Audiovisual Aids

INTERVENTION: Determining the Educational Setting

1 Choose an appropriate setting based on selected teaching strategy and available facility space.
2 Evaluate types of setting most appropriate to individual client and client's learning needs.
3 Consider an informal setting.
  a Spontaneous teaching interactions between nurse and client can occur at any time in any setting.
  b Usually no formal plan or evaluation tool is utilized.
4 Consider a formal setting.
  a Teaching is carried out in a specified area of the facility such as an in-service classroom.
  b Teaching can occur independently such as with audio-video programmed instruction modules or in a group setting.
  c Formal plan for the teaching program includes written goals, objectives, teaching strategies, content, and evaluation method.

INTERVENTION: Developing an Evaluation Tool

1 Utilize assessment of client educational level in developing type of tool to be utilized.
2 Evaluate types of tools for evaluation.
  a Pretest/posttest: measures changes in knowledge level, attitudes, values, etc.
  b Questionnaire: completed by client to report attitudes, certain behaviors, and, most frequently, level of satisfaction with the teaching program.
  c Physiological tracers: determined prior to teaching episode to be the criterion of measurement of success, i.e., changes in blood pressure values after teaching program for hypertensive clients.
  d Direct observation of behavior changes: report of level of performance during return demonstrations.
3 Choose an evaluative tool based on the goals and objectives of the teaching program.

INTERVENTION: Implementing the Teaching Strategy

1 Gather teaching materials appropriate for client's learning needs and teaching strategy.
2 Sit down with client in designated setting.
3 Specify behavioral objectives of the program.
4 Clarify or reclarify contract, agreements, or expected outcomes with the individual or group.
5 Assess teaching situation for any modifications needed and adjust plans accordingly.
6 Verbalize (teach) content to client(s).
7 Utilize appropriate communication skills.

8   Request feedback (evaluation interchange) during teaching process and utilize to make modifications as indicated or as appropriate.
9   Restate major principles or concepts in content.
10 Adhere to agreed-upon starting and ending times; negotiate any changes.
11 Provide closure to teaching situation by summarizing and reiterating agreements made, actions to be taken, or subsequent events to follow.
12 Provide positive reinforcement if not done previously.
13 Terminate teaching session by establishing time for next client contact.
14 Do postassessment of your own participation and plan for corrections and/or improvements in presentation.

EVALUATION

EXPECTED OUTCOMES

1   Client's knowledge regarding his or her health status has increased. *If not*, follow these alternative nursing actions:
    ANA: Reassess client for barriers to learning.
    ANA: Reevaluate testing tool and appropriateness for client.
    ANA: Problem-solve with the client as to next step to take.
2   Client's ability to make informed and effective health-related decisions, based on accurate information and awareness of self, has improved. *If not*, follow these alternative nursing actions:
    ANA: Assist client in realistically taking responsibility for ineffective decisions without guilt and shame attached.
    ANA: Assist client to identify those areas in which he or she is willing to make changes and support client's development of a plan of action.
    ANA: Refer to other resources such as mental health therapy as appropriate.
3   A more effective utilization of the health care delivery system has been promoted. *If not*, follow these alternative nursing actions:
    ANA: Assist the client to problem solve the issue.
    ANA: Identify possible barriers and ways in which to deal with them.
    ANA: Complete new interventions based on this assessment.

UNEXPECTED OUTCOMES

1   Client's health status has not improved as a result of teaching program.
    ANA: Immediately assess impact of teaching to determine if it or other factors are influencing health status.
    ANA: Determine what aspects of teaching program were not successful and complete a full evaluation.
    ANA: Revise parts of program and restructure for individual client needs.

Charting
- Topics or subjects covered as a part of client education process such as: medications, procedures, dietary plan, activity restrictions or follow-up care
- What information or tools were sent home with client
- Degree of client's participation in the teaching activity
- Progress in meeting the expected outcomes and/or course objectives
- Emotional response to the learning process

2 Client is hostile to teaching program.

    ANA: Assess basis for hostility and attempt to discuss with client.

    ANA: Suggest to client that another nurse begin teaching program.

CHARTING

Next to direct client care, charting is one of the nurses' most important functions. Charting, the process of recording vital information, serves many important purposes:

Charting communicates facts, figures, observations, etc., to other members of the client's health care team.

Charting assists supervisory personnel to evaluate the staff nurses' performance on a day-to-day basis for specific clients.

Charting provides a permanent record for future reference which may become a legal document in the event of litigation or prosecution.

Charting—A Method of Communication In communicating your observations and actions, charting helps to ensure both quality and continuity of health care for your clients. Information recorded by you becomes a valuable data base for nurses on subsequent shifts. Then, when you reassume responsibility for the client, you can determine what events occurred during prior time periods. In addition to the client's attending physician, other personnel interested in the chart may include the infection control nurse, discharge coordinator, utilization review personnel, or other hospital staff specialists who are checking on the client's progress or lack of positive reaction to treatment.

The client, as an individual, should receive individualized attention which focuses on his or her specific needs. As these needs are identified by each member of the health care team, they can be communicated to the others. Since nurses have the greatest amount of direct client contact, it is appropriate for the nurse to coordinate the important function of charting.

Charting provides one means for assessing the quality and effectiveness of nursing care. Head nurses, team leaders, and supervisors use nurses' notes as a basis for staff evaluations. Because charts are documented descriptions of nursing actions, the quality of nursing care may be evaluated on the basis of the quality of nurses' notes.

Complete and accurate charting is essential to protect both the client and the nurse. Since charting describes nursing interventions and their outcomes, other health care personnel can determine if subsequent treatment should be changed. Frequently, a client's reaction time is nearly as important as the reaction itself; therefore, accuracy of time observations becomes an integral part of the charting process.

A client's record includes all charting and becomes part of a legal document. Should a client's hospital record be introduced in court, the notes become a legal record of the care provided by each nurse. Legally, care that is not recorded is considered to be care that was not provided. It is necessary, therefore, to chart all care that you *do* provide, as well as any care that you *do not* provide.

The legal requirement for charting is found in state laws and/or professional requirements. For example, Title 22 of the California Administrative Code states, "Each inpatient medical record shall consist of at least the following items: nurses' notes which shall include but not be limited to the following: concise and accurate record of nursing care administered, record of pertinent observations including psychosocial and physical manifestations as well as incidents and unusual occurrences, and relevant nursing interpretation of such observations, name, dosage and time of administration of medications and treatment. Route of administration and site of injection shall be recorded if other than by oral administration. Record type of restraint and time of application and removal. The time of application and removal shall not be required for soft tie restraints used for support and protection of the patient."

The Manual of the Joint Commission for Accreditation of Hospitals states, "The plan of care must be documented and should reflect current standards of nursing practice . . . Documentation of nursing care shall be pertinent and concise, and shall reflect the patient's needs, problems, capabilities and limitations . . . Nursing interventions and patient response must be noted."

The Charting Process The format of the chart varies from hospital to hospital. Most important is the content of the notes. First, your notes should describe the assessment that you completed at the beginning of your shift. This information provides a baseline for changes that may occur later in the client's condition. If there are no such changes, this fact should be entered as the final note. Some hospitals require that all parts of the assessment be documented; others require that only abnormalities be documented.

As your shift progresses, you should always include certain items in your notes, including changes in the client's medical, mental, or emotional condition. Nurses are well attuned to medical changes, such as shock, hemorrhage, or a change in level of consciousness; however, the nurse may overlook subtle emotional changes. Anger, depression, or joy should also be documented, because these emotions often are indications of the client's response to his or her illness. Recording these changes is absolutely necessary if other nurses are to act appropriately during subsequent shifts. You should also chart if *no* changes occurred in the client's condition so that treatments can be modified as necessary. Normal aspects of the client's condition should be noted also.

Reactions to any unscheduled or p.r.n. medications must be recorded. Because each medication is given to meet a specified need, the client's response or lack of response must be recorded to document whether the need was met. To complete this part of the entry, note the time the medication was given, the problem for which the medication was designed, and the expected solution. For example: "7 pm. Client c/o abdominal incisional pain after ambulation. Medicated with Dem-

Time	Medications/Treatment	Observations	Signature
7 PM		CLIENT COMPLAINED OF	
		INCISIONAL PAIN FOLLOWING	
		AMBULATION.	
	DEMEROL 50MG. IM	GIVEN RUOQ	R. Janson RN
8 PM		CLIENT STATES PAIN IS	
		RELIEVED.	R. Janson RN

COMMUNITY HOSPITAL

NURSES' NOTES

Client Information

erol, 50 mg, IM." When the effects of the medication are known, write another note: "8 pm. Client states pain has been relieved."

Finally, it is important to record the client's response to teaching. These notes may describe return demonstrations, verbalization of learning, or resistance to instruction. Because most teaching takes place over a period of days, record both what you taught and how the client responded. Then, other nurses will know whether to repeat the previous instruction, reinforce it, or start a new topic.

Frequently, repetitive aspects of nursing care, such as vital signs and intake and output, are recorded on flow sheets. If flow sheets are used, you need not repeat the same information in your notes. An exception would be an abnormal measurement that is a part of a larger assessment. For example: "Client c/o sharp abdominal pain. BP-78/50. P-136. Skin cold and diaphoretic. Nasogastric tube draining bright red bloody fluid with small clots."

Charting and the Nursing Process The nursing process provides the framework for decision-making throughout all phases of nursing care. The components of the nursing process are assessment, planning, implementation (or intervention), and evaluation. This cycle is applied by the nurse both to routine situations and critical care emergencies.

It is important to relate the nursing process to charting because, for experienced nurses, the process may become only a mental exercise. The nurse "thinks through" the situation, makes decisions, takes action,

97

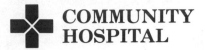

COMMUNITY HOSPITAL

CLINICAL RECORD

DATE																					
HOSP DAY/POSTOP DAY																					
TIME				0200	0600	1000	1400	1800	2200	0200	0600	1000	1400	1800	2200	0200	0600	1000	1400	1800	2200

KEY	PULSE	TEMP. C	TEMP. F
	140	40.6	105
	130	40.0	104
	120	39.4	103
	110	38.8	102
	100	38.3	101
	80	37.7	100
	80	37.2	99
	70	36.6	98
	60	36.1	97
	50	35.5	96

BLACK — PULSE & RESPIRATIONS
RED — TEMPERATURE

| RESPIRATIONS | | | | | | | | | | | | | | | | | | |
| BLOOD PRESSURE | | | | | | | | | | | | | | | | | | |

HEIGHT	WEIGHT			WEIGHT			WEIGHT		
	BREAKFAST	LUNCH	DINNER	BREAKFAST	LUNCH	DINNER	BREAKFAST	LUNCH	DINNER
DIET — TYPE									
% CONSUMED									

INTAKE & OUTPUT	0600-1400	1400-2200	2200-0600	0600-1400	1400-2200	2200-0600	0600-1400	1400-2200	2200-0600
INTAKE HOURS									
Oral									
IV									
Blood - Plasma									
Other									
8 Hr. Total									
Output									
Urine									
Emesis									
Stools									
GI Suction									
8 Hr. Total									
24 Hr. Intake									
24 Hr. Output									
SIGNATURE									

DATE:

CLINICAL RECORD

CLIENT CARE PLAN

Date	Client Problem	Deadline Date	Expected Outcome	Health Team Action
2/1/82	LGE. DRAINING ABD. WOUND	2/10/82	WOUND DRAINAGE DECREASED AND GRANULATION OBSERVED.	1. PLACE ON LT. SIDE c̄ CHUX UNDER HIPS AND ABD.
				2. IRRIGATE WOUND c̄ 50cc ½ NS AND ½ H₂ O₂. USE CATHETER TIPPED SYRINGE.
				3. PACK WOUND c̄ 60 cm IODOFORM GAUZE.

Client Care Plan

and then observes the results. Unless the entire process is recorded on the client care plan and documented in the chart, the next nurse who encounters a similar situation with the same client is deprived of important and potentially valuable background data. The second nurse, without knowing the full background, may repeat the entire process resulting in a loss of valuable time and an increase in client discomfort. When similar nursing interventions completed by different nurses have the same positive results, the client will experience a feeling of reassurance that may not be achieved if each nurse attempts a totally different set of interventions to reach the same objective.

The client, in a strange environment with unknown people doing unfamiliar and often uncomfortable things, often tries to find reassurance in any type of routine. The client soon expects a certain procedure to be done by the same person in the same way and at a predictable hour. Changes in the procedure are often upsetting to the client. It is imperative that the steps of any procedure, especially those that are complicated or personalized to the client, be documented in detail on the client care plan so that each nurse will do it the same way. However, the detailed description of how to perform a dressing change is written in the client's care plan, not in the nurses' notes. For example, the dressing change of a client with a large draining abdominal wound would have the following information documented on the client care plan:

Place client on L side with chux under hips and abdomen. This position is uncomfortable for client, so ease him into it; do not hurry.

Remove old dressing, noting location of drainage, quantity, color, and smell.

Irrigate wound with approximately 50 cc ½NS and ½ H_2O_2 using a catheter-tipped syringe. Catch solution in emesis basin.

Very gently (client is sensitive) pack deep area in distal wound with approximately 60 cm Iodoform gauze.

Cover entire wound with 10 cm × 10 cm pads (8–10) followed by ABDs (Surgipads) using double thickness at distal ⅓ of wound and single thickness on proximal ⅔.

Secure dressing with Mongomery straps, changing ties. When tying straps, client prefers them to the side.

The nurses' notes would describe the amount, color, consistency, and odor of the drainage. In addition, the amount and type of irrigating solution and type of abdominal dressing would be noted. It is important to add a statement as to the client's tolerance of the procedure.

Types of Charting   The three main charting systems are source oriented, problem oriented, and computer assisted charting. The most common system is the source-oriented chart, so named because the information is organized and presented according to its source. For example, there are separate sections for doctors' progress notes, nurses' notes, respiratory therapy notes, etc. To obtain a complete "picture" of the client, one must read through all sections and piece together the separate bits of data. This may be a time-consuming process and the result may not produce an accurate or complete assessment of the client.

A second system for chart organization is the problem-oriented medical record. In this system the chart is based on the problem list—all problems, present or not, identified with that client. Using the problems as reference points, each person giving care charts progress notes on the same sheets. In this way assessment of a specific incident by everyone concerned (MD, RN, dietician, enterostomal therapist, etc.) is in the same location and the client's overall picture can be easily seen.

The third and newest type of organizing data is computer-assisted charting. This type of charting constantly updates information from many sources. For example, physiological measurements are recorded and updated on the computer terminal at least hourly.

The information is easily retrievable by the nursing personnel as questions arise. Reference material for common nursing problems ensures quick reference and easily retrieved information in order to provide safe nursing care.

Source-Oriented Systems Charting   Systems charting is a common and efficient way of organizing client information in source-oriented nurses' notes. An outline of the systems to be reviewed, and sometimes specific subheadings for each, is established. Medical units may use one type of system for nurses' notes, while critical care may use another.

At the beginning of the shift the nurse performs a physical assessment on each client to determine the client's current status. This information becomes the initial systems charting. When changes occur, they are noted with the time under the appropriate system. If no changes occur during the shift, no other charting of this type may be necessary.

To record all pertinent client information, several flow sheets are used in conjunction with the systems form. One flow sheet is the vital signs sheet, which contains information such as temperature, pulse, blood pressure, respirations, urine output, hemodynamic monitoring values, infusion rates of vasoactive drugs, and daily weights. Other flow sheets may include a medication and an intake and output record. Special sheets such as neurological monitoring sheets and diabetic sheets are used as necessary.

Source-Oriented Narrative Charting Narrative charting is based upon chronology rather than systems. Information is charted in chronological order regardless of the subject of the note. For example, the nurses' notes for a client could appear as follows:

0735   Client c/o dull aching pain in RLQ incisional area.

0745   Medicated with Demerol 50 mg IM.

0820   Tolerated full liquid diet well. Ate all of meal.

0845   RLQ dressing changed. Incisional area clean, without edema or erythema. Scant serous drainage on dressing.

0930   Ambulated in hall without assistance.

Hospitals usually have maximum time requirements for this type of note, with common parameters being every two or three hours. While there may be a requirement for frequency of charting, there usually is not one for charting content. This leads to the primary deficiency of narrative charting; it is very easy to chart without specifying why the client is in the hospital or what is the client's overall condition. Note the example above. Why is the client in the hospital? What is the client's general condition? How is the client progressing?

When using narrative charting, an assessment should be performed at the beginning of the shift and as needed thereafter. When assessment is the initial entry in narrative charting, subsequent entries are more relevant and understandable. This combination of assessment and narrative charting is the best technique to ensure that adequate information about the client is recorded for all personnel who utilize nurses' notes.

Problem-Oriented Medical Records The second major type of charting is the problem-oriented medical records, or POMR. This system differs from source-oriented narrative charting not only in format but in philosophy. Problem-oriented medical records focus on the client's status rather than on the source of the information, i.e., department or member of the health care team who is originating the information. Narrative charting typically consists of doctors' progress notes, physical therapy progress notes, nurses' notes, respiratory therapy progress notes, etc.

Neurological Flow Sheet

COMMUNITY HOSPITAL

Client Information

PROGRESS NOTES

Date	Note progress of case, complications, change in diagnosis, condition on discharge
2/1/82	S UNABLE TO DETERMINE WHEN VOIDING. STATES "HAS NO FEELING" WHEN VOIDING.
	O VOIDS 30-50 CC q 1-1½ HRS.
	A URINARY FREQUENCY POSSIBLY RELATED TO CVA.
	P PLACE ON COMMODE EVERY HR. AND INCREASE TIME TO EVERY TWO HRS. CHECK WITH M.D. ABOUT ORDER FOR URINE CULTURE AND SENSITIVITY. L. Janson R.N

With POMR, only one set of progress notes is used, and all personnel caring for the client record their data on this set.

In its purest form, a POMR consists of five distinct parts: the data base (initial assessment), problem list, initial plan, progress notes, and discharge summary. The data base is made up of information from and about the client that is used to develop the problem list. Because the POMR system is systematic and well-defined, the data base consists of specific types of data, including the chief complaint (why client came to the hospital), personal and family medical history, allergies and reactions, medications taken at home, physical assessment, mental and emotional assessment, and lifestyle.

Development of a complete data base requires skill and practice. Basic features of client interviewing and physical assessment are covered in other sections of this text, but a few tips and reminders may help to sharpen your skills. First, select a time mutually acceptable to both you and the client. Know how much time you have for the interview and whether the client has scheduled appointments or tests. Be aware of the client's physical and emotional comfort, the physical environment of the interview location, and pending meal times. Second, consider how your questions might affect the client. Phrase questions that will cause the client to explain the answer — a "yes" or "no" is not sufficiently informative. Do not make the client defensive by being judgmental about his or her actions. Clients who believe you do not approve of their actions often will withhold potentially important information. Third, avoid leading statements. Many clients try to respond in an agreeable manner. For example, "Don't you . . .." statements may be answered by "No, of course not." Also, avoid using medical jargon unfamiliar to the client. Some words you use daily may be unknown to your client. The client will answer what he or she *thinks* you asked to

DATA BASE CARD

Name: _____
Age: _____ Sex: _____ Religion: _____
Admit Date: _____ Onset: _____
Notify: _____
Relationship: _____
Address: _____
_____
Telephone Number:
Home: _____
Work: _____
Allergies: _____
Med/Surg History: _____
_____
_____
_____
_____
_____
Social History: _____
_____

avoid showing his or her ignorance. This situation may result in an invalid data base because the data is incorrect.

After completing the data base, the nurse next defines the client problems for the problem list. A "problem" is any difficulty that the client cannot handle by him or herself — the client needs assistance from someone on the health care team. The difficulty may be a physical symptom, such as pain or infection; an emotional problem caused by fear of impending surgery or worry about a family member; or a social problem, such as loss of job and income or inability to live independently at home. Problems are usually defined as active (acute or chronic) or inactive (resolved). Active problems may also be potential — not yet present but likely to occur. Examine the following list of problems and see if you can determine how to categorize them.

Upper GI bleeding, 3 days' duration	Active
Children, 2 and 5 years old, at home with father	Active
Possible skin breakdown	Active-Potential
Appendectomy 1954	Resolved
Asthma since childhood	Active-Chronic

Medical diagnoses are included on the problem list if they are definite. If they are only tentative, the client's symptoms should be put on the list until the actual diagnosis is made. Of course, many of the symptoms may qualify as nursing diagnoses since they can be defined as interfering with the client's sense of well-being. For example, ascites or decreased ROM L knee would be nursing diagnoses.

The categories of the POMR closely approximate the steps in the nursing process. The data base and problem list equate to assessment; the initial plan to planning; the progress notes discuss intervention; and the discharge summary is an evaluation.

Nursing Problem List

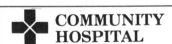

COMMUNITY HOSPITAL

NURSING PROBLEM LIST

Date Problem Began	Prob. #	Problem	Date Resolved	Date Recurred
2/1/82	1	URINARY INCONTINENCE		
2/1/82	2	LEFT SIDED WEAKNESS		
2/5/82	3	REFUSES TO EAT	2/9/82	
2/6/82	4	REDDENED COCCYX	2/12/82	

PATIENT CARE PLAN

DATE	PROBLEM	EXPECTED OUTCOME	DEADLINE	NURSING ACTION
6/20	Potential skin breakdown on coccyx and hips due to weakness and decreased mobility	Skin pink and intact	6/30	1 Turn from side to back to side q2h on even hours 2 Heat lamp to areas q4h for 15 min. 8-12-4-8-12-4 3 Clean sheepskin under client at all times 4 Put nothing between client and sheepskin 5 Massage bony areas for 3 min. each time client is turned 6 Encourage client to eat all of protein diet 7 Force fluids to 2500 cc q24h. Offer fluids q2h while awake and q4h at night

After you complete the data base and start the problem list, you then formulate your initial plan, called the patient care plan (PCP). For each major problem or group of problems, the PCP should include the following information: date, problem, expected outcome, deadline, and nursing actions.

Several basic ideas must be remembered when writing PCPs. First, always identify the cause of the problem because this will help determine the appropriate nursing actions. For example, the nursing actions for the problem "difficulty coughing and clearing airway due to pain after a thoracotomy" will be different from those for the problem "difficulty coughing and clearing airway due to myasthenia gravis."

Second, the expected outcome (EO) should be something that you can observe or the client can say or do. For example, you cannot be sure that the client understands the signs and symptoms of hyperglycemia; however, you can know for sure that the client can list six signs and symptoms of hyperglycemia. To know if an EO has been reached, it is necessary to write it so that anyone working with your client can readily identify the EO when it happens.

Third, the deadline indicates your estimate of when the problem should be solved using the indicated nursing actions; however, if you do not meet your deadlines, you should check them to see if they are realistic. Also, check your nursing actions and make certain they are complete and most appropriate for that specific problem.

Finally, nursing actions must be very specific so that their results can be determined and evaluated. Phrases such as "turn frequently" are too vague. Directions such as "q1' or q2' WA (while awake) and q4' at night" are not explicit enough to let the nurse know what alternative was preferred.

In the POMR system, one set of progress notes is used by everyone. This means that all members of the health care team write their observations on the same part of the chart. The entries on the problem list are always numbered, so when the nurse, physician, and the respiratory therapist all refer to problem 3 in their progress notes, everyone knows that they are referring to shortness of breath related to congestive heart failure.

Within the well-organized POMR system, progress notes have a specific format, usually called SOAP or SOAPIER. These acronyms translate as:

Subjective: client's symptoms and own description of problem
Objective: factual data, e.g., intake and output, vital signs, drainage, etc.
Assessment: your conclusions about the problem
Plan: what you decide to do about the problem
Implementation: your nursing interventions
Evaluation: how the implementation worked
Revision: how you plan to change the PCP if improvement is needed

When writing progress notes, remember that a separate SOAP note is needed for each problem. You should not combine problems. It is not always necessary to include the I, E, and R portions of the note; however, always include the S, O, A, and P parts, even if the client does not supply subjective statements. The I, E, and R can be included under the P section.

The discharge summary, the final step in the POMR system, includes both a summary of the client's hospitalization and documentation of client teaching. SOAPIER notes are again used as the charting format, and a summary should be written for each problem on the problem list. If the problem is fully resolved during hospitalization, that fact and the date it occurred (from the progress notes) is all that is necessary. The discharge summary is not a day-by-day account of the client's stay, but a short review. It is beneficial to include specific highlights such as the highest serum glucose level or the highest temperature, but all the values need not be included. Remember, a separate SOAPIER note should be written for each problem that is not fully resolved at the time of the discharge.

All invasive procedures, surgical interventions, and major diagnostic tests should be listed and the results outlined. Braces, equipment, and supplies (for dressing changes, catheterizations, etc.) should be included in the summary. If the equipment or braces are difficult to use or apply, it is helpful if pictures or diagrams are included. Client teaching completed, discharge medications, and specific teaching regarding the medications should also be documented.

Referrals to other health care services should be identified with the name of the agency and the contact person listed on the chart. If clients are being discharged to other health care facilities or to a visiting nurse, it is helpful if they receive not only a copy of the discharge summary, but a copy of the last client care plan. This provides for a smooth transition of care from one health care setting to another.

Because of the many changes necessary when implementing POMR, hospitals often use only part of it, or are changing to it in stages; therefore, it is common to find situations in which parts of several systems are in use. For example, SOAP nursing notes may be used while the remainder of the chart is source oriented, or doctors use the problem list and SOAP progress notes while nurses use systems charting for nurses' notes. Although progress is rather slow, it appears that many more hospitals will adopt the POMR system, not only for its format and ease of use, but also for its completeness in documenting client care.

Computer-Assisted Charting   Computers have become a valuable tool in documenting client care. One common system focuses on the client's physiological parameters. With input from various monitoring devices such as an arterial line and a Swan-Ganz catheter, the computer can automatically determine and frequently update many pieces of data, including hematology and chemistry tests, ABGs, cardiac output, and DE, VS, CVP, and PA pressures to name only a few. These results can be viewed on a VMT (video matrix terminal similar to a TV screen) or printed out on paper. The VS and hemodynamic data are continually updated, and many of the lab tests can be updated at least every hour.

Another type of computer system records, stores, and retrieves many pieces of data about the client that must be communicated throughout the hospital in order for the client to receive optimal care. For example, when a client is admitted and the physician enters orders into the computer, many things automatically happen. The dietary department is notified of the diet needs, pharmacy is notified of medications and IVs that were ordered, CSR is notified of special equipment needs, and the laboratory is notified of required tests. It is no longer necessary for the nurse to make out and deliver requests for all these departments, and then arrange for delivery or pick-up of the desired item. This has been a basic and broad overview of some of the functions of the Technicon Medical Information System (MIS), which is gaining popularity throughout the country.

At each nursing station in a hospital using this system, there are several computer terminals. These consist of VMT, a keyboard, and a light pen. The VMT shows a matrix-like TV picture, which the nurse can select using the light pen. These matrices are grouped together in a logical order so that general categories of information can be recorded. The nurse records the information by pointing the light pen at the proper word/phrase and pressing a button on the pen. With three quick taps on the button, the nurse can record "Client admitted ambulatory from the emergency room." If the client speaks only Spanish, she would tap "Client speaks" and then type in "Spanish" using the keyboard just below the VMT. All the pertinent information obtained while admitting the client and doing the initial physical assessment can easily and quickly be recorded using only the light pen and typing in data such as "How does the client feel about hospitalization." The admitting sheets the nurse takes to the bedside correlate to the information on the matrices, so that the data is easy to transfer and nothing is omitted.

Hospitals usually have programs that contain special matrices such as "The Nursing Master Guide." This is an example of a matrix that only lists other matrices that may be needed. Much of the routine care a

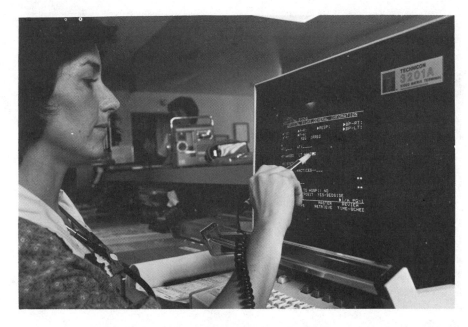

Light pen is used to record information into computer terminal.

nurse gives can be charted rapidly and completely in a matter of seconds using this and associated matrices.

When the nurse has completed charting, she taps "Review" and the VMT automatically displays all the data. At this time, the nurse can make corrections, additions, or deletions using only the light pen and the keyboard. If the data displayed is correct, the nurse taps "Enter," the data becomes a permanent part of the computer record for that client, and a hard copy is printed out to be put in the chart. In case you're worried about mistakes that are "entered," there are also ways of retrieving and changing them. It is easy to see the logical progression of the charting process. Also, the matrix titles act as gentle reminders of what needs to be charted.

When the client is to be discharged, the nursing discharge summary is completed. This shows not only the client's physical condition but also the status of client teaching and follow-up plans. Again, it is simply punched or tapped on the terminal and the data is displayed.

In addition to making the charting of client care and the communication between departments much simpler and less time consuming, the computer provides reference material for common nursing problems. For example, a matrix may show the signs and symptoms associated with diabetes mellitus. If the nurse is unsure of the signs and symptoms of the different forms of this disease, they can easily be found in the computer, and if needed, can be printed out and put in the chart. In this way, the nurse can quickly update him or herself about the client's condition and thereby provide optimal care.
optimal care.

As in many professions, use of the computer in nursing and medicine is becoming more common and its possible uses are rapidly expanding. If learning the skills of computer use is viewed as a challenge and the

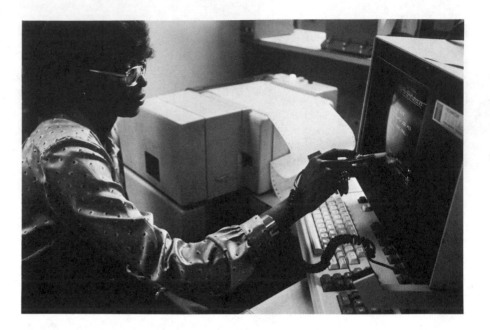

Printed hard copy of computer record is sent to unit to be placed in client's chart.

reward is more efficient nursing care and less time spent on paperwork, the learning time will have been well spent.

Client Care Plans Client care plans assist in communicating relevant information to all members of the health team and contribute to the goal of achieving continuity of care.

The Joint Commission states that a nursing care plan should be instituted within one hour after admission to the hospital.

An efficient way to start this process is for the unit manager/ward clerk to place a client care plan on each new client's Kardex card.

The two accepted types of client care plans are the individualized care plan and the standard care plan. Individualized care plans contain the mutually agreed upon goals set by the client, family, and health team members. Specific directions are written to define how these goals can best be achieved. The usual care plan format contains a problem list, a health team action section, and expected outcomes with deadline dates. Standard care plans are widely used to provide a guide for client care. The standard care plan identifies those problems relating to all clients having a specific medical condition. The health team actions include routine preventive nursing interventions. Because few clients can be classified as "standard," the standard care plans are usually accompanied by an individualized care plan.

For example, if a 22-year-old female client is admitted to the hospital for a total abdominal hysterectomy, she would not be classified as a "standard client." Most women who need a total abdominal hysterectomy are not 22 years old.

A typical standard care plan lists major potential problems and their assessment, treatment, and preventative nursing actions. For the 22-year-old female client described above, the standard care plan would look similar to the following example:

Date	Usual Problem	Expected Outcome	Deadline	Health Team Action
10-25-81	Potential urinary retention due to pain	Voiding qs s̄ residual urine	q. shift	Monitor I&O q 4hrs Force fluids to 2500 cc q/day Assist to commode or BR q4 hours

An individualized care plan would take into account that the client is of childbearing age. Following the initial physical and psychosocial assessment, information would normally be recorded on the care plan to assist the client in coping with this traumatic surgery. The client's ability to cope may relate to the reason for her surgery and whether she now has children or desires to bear children in the future.

The individualized care plan assists the staff to understand the client's feelings, requests for care, likes, and dislikes, and thereby to provide continuity of care, as shown by the following example:

Date	Usual Problem	Expected Outcome	Deadline	Health Team Action
10-25-81	Client depressed due to inability to have children	Client able to express feelings openly	q. shift	1 Allow ½ hour each shift for client to ventilate about inability to have children 2 Establish trust relationship by being non-judgmental and allowing client to express feelings and ask questions. Give client accurate information

Computer Matrix

```
MATRIX NO.3201      HOSP. NO.01    01/05/82    
DYNAMIC MATRIX

        GENERAL ADMIT NOTES                    01
                                               02
*CLIENT ADM:      /GUERNEY                      03
   AMB   /WC  /AMBULANCE   FROM EMERG RM         04
         FROM--                                 05
                                      **        06
(PRIMARY LANGUAGE OTHER THAN ENGLISH)           07
CLIENT SPEAKS--                       **        08
(CLIENT HAS:) (LOCATED AT:) (HOME) (HOSP)       09
   GLASSES                    **     **         10
   CONT LENSES                **     **         11
   HEARING AID                **     **         12
   CANE                       **     **         13
   CRUTCHES                   **     **         14
   WALKER                     **     **         15
   DENTURES                   **     **         16
   PROSTHESIS                 **     **         17
   --              (HOME) UPPER  U&L            18
   --              (HOSP) LOWER  PARTIAL        19
                   *ADMIT VITAL SIGNS           20
--------------------------------------------
```

```
MATRIX NO.1347      HOSP. NO.01    01/05/82    
DYNAMIC MATRIX

     NSG MASTER GUIDE - GENERAL                 01
RN/LVN-------------------------------           02
*VS-RESULTS,OBSV        *GEN REPORTING          03
*VS-OBSV ONLY           *GEN RPTG-SURG          04
*DIET,FLD BAL                                   05
*UNIT TESTS/EXAMS       *IMMED POST-OP:         06
*HYG,ACTIV,SAFETY       *ADMIT NOTES            07
*PROCEDURES                                     08
                        *MISC DATA              09
*BASIC CARE NEEDS                               10
*PHYSICAL ASSESS        *SPECIAL OBSV           11
*TEACH/DISCH PLANS                              12
                        *READY FOR THE OR       13
*UNSCHED,MISC MED       *TO THE OR              14
*MED FOLLOW-UP                                  15
                        *NSG DISCH SUMMARY      16
*IV,BLD BEGIN           *NSG TRANS SUMMARY      17
*IV,BLD END             *EXC CHARTING           18
*IV,BLD GEN OBSV                                19
*IV,NO.0---             *CHANGE SPECIALTY       20
--------------------------------------------
```

KARDEX/RAND CLIENT CARE PLAN

CLIENT EDUCATION PROGRAM			DISCHARGE CRITERIA	DISCHARGE PLAN	Addressograph
	DATE		PLAN:		
	Start	Finish	Stroke Rehab Eval _____	Discharge Coordinator	
Diabetic _____			Cardiac Rehab Eval _____	Date Involved _____	
Coronary _____			SOCIAL SERVICE	Home _____	
Other _____			Date Involved _____	ECF _____	
_____			Comment:	OTHER _____	

Date	Client Problem	Deadline Date	Expected Outcome	Health Team Action

Client Care Plan Data Base Information

A complete nursing care plan includes a section on client teaching. The plan should list specific items to be taught. When the teaching is completed, the nurse should update the plan with a summary of material covered. Health team members are then aware of the entire teaching program.

The term, "health team action," is used because all members of the health team are responsible for contributing to the care plan. For example, the dietician keeps other health team members aware of the client's special nutritional needs. The respiratory therapist identifies the most effective method of assisting the client to cough and deep breathe.

To be most useful, the information contained in the care plan must be specific. For example, the care plan for positioning a client most comfortably should document the exact procedure, step-by-step, instead of a vague reference "to position the client in a comfortable position." Care plans become a permanent part of the client's chart. For this reason they must be written in ink. Resolved problems should be crossed out using a colored felt tip pen. Care plans are updated on a routine basis (generally every 24 to 48 hours or as the client's condition changes). They document both current and resolved problems for which the health care team has planned and provided care.

Incident Reports (IR) Incident reports serve three main purposes: to help in documenting quality of care, to identify areas in which in-service education is needed, and to record the details of an incident for possible legal use.

With some staff nurses IRs have a poor reputation, and perhaps with some justification. When something goes wrong, and a nurse is told to "make out an IR," many nurses assume that IRs are a form of punishment for real or alleged misdeeds.

Although IRs should be completed regularly with any unusual occurrence, and may, on occasion, be used as a form of reprimand, they are no more or less than what their title suggests: a report of an incident.

As a tool for documenting quality of care, IRs inform the quality assurance coordinator and the head nurse of areas in which practice on

INCIDENT REPORT

COMPLETE IMMEDIATELY FOR EVERY
INCIDENT AND SEND TO ADMINISTRATOR

_____
HOSPITAL NAME

ADMINISTRATOR:
**Please forward to
Hospital Attorney**

_____
CITY

FOR ADDRESSOGRAPH PLATE
_____

CONFIDENTIAL REPORT OF INCIDENT (NOT A PART OF MEDICAL RECORD)

PATIENT_____ AGE_____ SEX_____ ROOM_____
(LAST NAME)   (FIRST NAME)   (M OR F)

ADMITTING DIAGNOSIS _____ DATE OF ADMISSION _____

ATTENDING PHYSICIAN _____ DATE OF INCIDENT _____ TIME_____ M

WERE BED RAILS UP? _____ WAS SAFETY BELT IN USE?_____

WAS PATIENT RATIONAL _____ HI LO BED POSITION_____

SEDATIVES _____ DOSE _____ TIME _____ ⎧ GIVEN WITHIN 12
                                                                                  ⎨ HOURS PREVIOUS
NARCOTICS _____ DOSE _____ TIME _____ ⎩ TO INCIDENT

TIME DOCTOR WAS CALLED _____A.M._____P.M.   TIME RESPONDED_____A.M._____P.M.
                                    (I.E., HOUSE PHYSICIAN-RESIDENT-INTERN-ETC.)

I NOTIFIED DR. _____TIME_____ M   BY_____

NURSE'S ACCOUNT OF THE INCIDENT (INCLUDE EXACT LOCATION)

_____
_____
_____
_____
_____

LIST PERSONS FAMILIAR WITH DETAILS OF INCIDENT - AND OTHER PATIENTS IN THE SAME ROOM

NAME _____ ADDRESS _____
NAME _____ ADDRESS _____
NAME _____ ADDRESS _____

HISTORY OF INCIDENT AS RELATED BY PATIENT _____

_____
_____
_____
_____

DATE OF REPORT _____   _____
                                                SIGNATURE OF NURSE OR SUPERVISOR REPORTING
_____

DOCTOR'S REPORT OF PATIENTS CONDITION (FROM PROGRESS REPORT) _____

_____
_____
_____
_____

ORIGINAL TO HOSPITAL ATTORNEY

Incident Report

the unit needs improvement. For example, there may be an increase in the number of clients who fell out of bed. Further research may show that because the census is up, the staff is very busy and is forgetting to reposition clients' overhead tables. In their attempt to get their water, kleenex, etc., more clients are falling out of bed. The problem solution may be to speak with the staff regarding the consequences of this action and, as a group, find a mutually acceptable way of preventing this type of incident from recurring.

IRs also suggest and document the need for in-service education. For example, when an unusual number of IRs are written regarding a new piece of equipment, the head nurse may conclude that the staff, especially those on evening and night shifts, needs instruction on operating this equipment properly and effectively. Another example would be an increase in IRs regarding IVs that are behind or ahead of schedule. This might indicate that the nurses do not know how to apply and regulate the IV pump correctly. Solution of this problem would be to conduct a series of classes for all shifts in which the operation of the IV pump is discussed and hands-on practice is given. Such classes could be given by someone in the hospital's in-service education department or by a representative of the manufacturer of the IV pumps.

Incident reports may also record the details of an occurrence for possible legal use. In some hospitals incident reports are called unusual occurrences and cover any situation that prevented the client from having a normal recovery. These incidents could include non-nursing actions such as returning to surgery for control of bleeding or having chest tubes inserted for a pneumothorax. In most situations, though, IRs pertain to nurse/client activities.

When completing an IR with possible legal implications, it is doubly important to record all details of the incident. It is not easy to recall details of the care you gave a client one or two months ago. Frequently, lawsuits are not filed for months or even years after an incident, so it is essential that you record important details promptly.

Information to record on the IR includes general details of the incident, the client's response, your action or reaction to the incident, and a list of other personnel who were aware of the details of the incident. Often there is space on the IR in which to record the physician's report of the client's condition following the incident. To fill in the section regarding the physician's report, the nurse later copies the doctor's progress notes from the chart onto the IR.

Upon completion, IRs are forwarded to the unit head nurse and then to nursing administration. Information from the report that is of interest to inservice education or quality assurance departments can be obtained at this time. Ultimately, the IR will be passed along to the hospital's legal department to be retained indefinitely in the event that legal action is later initiated on behalf of the client.

Consent Forms When an individual enters a hospital, some of the person's basic legal rights are affected. In order that these rights are not violated, the client must give permission (consent) for all treatment. If

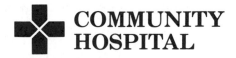 **COMMUNITY HOSPITAL**

AUTHORIZATION FOR AND CONSENT TO SURGERY, ADMINISTRATION OF ANESTHETICS, SPECIAL DIAGNOSTIC OR THERAPEUTIC PROCEDURES

Date _____ Time _____

Your admitting physician is _____, M. D.

Your surgeon is _____, M. D.

1. The hospital staff and facilities assist your physicians and surgeons in the performance of various surgical operations and other diagnostic and therapeutic procedures. These surgical operations and special diagnostic or therapeutic procedures all may involve calculated risks of complications, injury or even death, from both known and unknown causes and no warranty or guarantee has been made as to result or cure. Except in a case of emergency or exceptional circumstances, these operations and procedures are not performed upon clients unless and until the client has had an opportunity to discuss them with his/her physician. Each client has the right to consent to or refuse any proposed operation or special procedure (based upon the description or explanation received).

2. Your physicians and surgeons have determined that the operations or special procedures listed below may be beneficial in the diagnosis or treatment of your condition. Upon your authorization and consent, the operations or special procedures will be performed by your physicians and surgeons and their staff. The persons in attendance for the purpose of administering anesthesia or performing other specialized professional services, such as radiology, pathology and the like, are not the agents, servants or employees of the hospital or your physician or surgeon, but are independent contractors performing specialized services on your behalf and, as such, are your agents, servants, or employees. Any tissue or member severed in any operation will be disposed of in the discretion of the pathologist, except _____ and those body parts specified as donor organs.

3. Your signature opposite the operations or special procedures listed below constitutes your acknowledgement (a) that you have read and agreed to the foregoing, (b) that the operations or special procedures have been adequately explained to you by your attending physicians or surgeons and that you have all of the information that you desire, and (c) that you authorize and consent to the performance of the operations or special procedures.

Operation or Procedure

_____

_____

Signature _____   Signature _____
                         Client   Witness

(If client is a minor or unable to sign, complete the following): Client is a minor, is unable to sign because

_____

_____

                  Father   Guardian

_____

                  Mother   Other person and relationship

Surgical Consent Form

consent is not obtained, the hospital, doctor, and/or nurse may be charged with committing "battery" against the client. Battery, as defined by law, is an "offensive touching" of the client. This could include injection or any breaking of the skin's surface, x-rays, insertion of tubes, etc.

Before you panic and attempt to get a consent signed for the client's next blood pressure, you should know that routine nursing care is "consented to" when the client signs the "Conditions of Admissions." Also, certain procedures such as injections, intubations, dressings, etc., are treatments ordered by the physician and agreed to by the client. If the client has listened to the explanation of a specific procedure and agreed to allow the procedure to be carried out, he or she is giving implied consent; however, the client has the right to refuse any treatment. In that case the physician must be contacted regarding alternative actions.

When discussing the formal written or explicit consents, the two key activities are obtaining and witnessing consent. Obtaining consent is not a nursing function because it includes the explanation of what will be done, the risks of the procedure to that client, alternative procedures, and probable outcomes. This information should be given by the doctor.

The nurse's role is to witness the signing of the consent. When the consent form is presented to the client, it should be explained and the client should be encouraged to read it thoroughly before signing. Occasionally, a nurse is asked to explain or expand the physician's presentation. Acceptable practice is for the nurse to clarify, define a medical term, or add more details to physician's initial information. If the nurse feels that the client does not really understand what is going to occur, it is the nurse's responsibility to notify the doctor to give further explanation before the client signs the consent. An easy way to determine what the client understands is to ask the client to repeat back the physician's explanation. Under ordinary circumstances, only one witness to signing the consent is necessary. The witness does not have to be an RN, just someone over the age of eighteen.

There are many rules and regulations governing consents. If you have questions about them, consult the consent manual for your hospital, or a supervisory person. There are several important situations in which more information may be needed. One relates to the competency of the client. Generally, the client must sign personally, and spouses are no longer able to sign for the client. Permanent incompetence usually involves legal action to assign someone else as conservator. Temporary incompetence may be the result of hospital treatments such as drugs or anesthetics. When a narcotic or sedative has been given, at least four hours lapsed time is required before the client is considered competent to sign a consent. A second situation concerns the client who is a minor. The age of consent varies according to state and also according to specific situations such as emancipation (being away from the family and supporting self) and the type of medical problem (reportable diseases or pregnancy). An associated problem may arise when deciding who can legally sign for a minor. A third situation concerns emergency treatment: who can give consent if the client is unable, and what must be done if consent cannot be obtained when withholding treatment could result in grave danger to the client.

Proper use of consents can be a complicated process; however, if the nurse follows a few basic guidelines and, when appropriate, seeks assistance, consents will continue to be a source of protection for both the client and the nurse.

CHAPTER 4
Maintaining Infection Control: Barrier Nursing

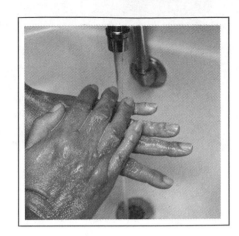

In this chapter, you will learn how to identify common hospital procedures that can precipitate nosocomial infections (infections acquired while in the hospital that were not present or incubating at the time of admission). You will also learn how to prevent and reduce these infections through planned nursing interventions that emphasize aseptic techniques. Ten percent of all clients enter the hospital with clinical infections. Another five percent acquire infections during their hospital stay. Barrier nursing is concerned with the prevention and reduction of infections.

ANATOMY AND PHYSIOLOGY OF THE BODY'S NATURAL DEFENSES

An individual's ability to resist infection is determined by the status of the body's defense mechanisms and by the person's general health. Factors that contribute to susceptibility to infection include altered nutritional status, stress, fatigue, disease, drugs, metabolic functions, and age. The body is protected against infection by immunities, by the inflammatory process, and by anatomical barriers that include the skin and mucous membranes.

BARRIERS TO INFECTION

When the integrity of the skin is broken, both resident and transient flora or bacteria have a direct route to the internal tissues of the body. To prevent the spread of infection, the body's internal defense mechanisms mobilize and begin clearing and repairing the damaged site. How quickly a wound heals depends on the degree of vascularization in the injured area, the location and cleanliness of the wound, and the degree of tissue damage.

The second way the body resists infections is through immunity. Natural immunity is inherited. Acquired immunity occurs after an individual has been exposed to a disease or infection.

The third way the body resists infection is through the inflammatory process. Inflammation involves utilization of metabolic energy, increased blood flow to the inflamed area, and, in many cases, drainage of inflammatory debris to the external environment.

When an area becomes inflamed, cells at the site activate the plasmin system, the clotting system, and the kinin system. The result of all of these systems is the release of histamine, which creates increased vascular permeability around the injured site, and the release of chemotaxic agents, which summon phagocytes into the vascular and tissue spaces. Phagocytes are connective tissue cells which combat and prevent infection by ingesting harmful microorganisms.

Alterations in the Body's Natural Defenses Any alteration in the body's natural defenses increases the probability that an infection will occur. Given the proper circumstances, almost any organism can be the cause of a significant hospital-related infection. Some of the variables that help determine which organism emerges as the pathogen are the virulence and number of organisms, the exposure and attachment of the organism to a susceptible site, and the duration of the client's exposure to the infectious challenge. The inherent health and immunologic status of the client are also major factors in determining whether an infection occurs.

Alterations in the skin barrier include any physiologic break in the integrity of the skin. Intentional breaks are caused by the use of percutaneous catheters and needles and by surgical procedures. Unintentional causes of skin breakdown include the development of decubitus ulcers and traumatic wounds.

CONDITIONS PREDISPOSING INFECTION

Certain conditions and invasive techniques predispose clients to infection because the integrity of the skin is broken or the illness itself establishes a climate favorable for the infectious process to occur. Among the most common are surgical wounds, changes in the antibacterial immune system, or alterations to the body.

Surgical Wounds From 40 to 65 percent of the clients who enter general hospitals are admitted as surgical clients. Approximately one half of these clients will have surgery, and out of this population, 8 percent will develop a postoperative wound infection. It has been documented that the longer a person is hospitalized prior to the surgical procedure the greater the risk of post-surgical infection. Other factors that influence infection rates are duration of time in the operating room, time surgery is done (between midnight and 8:00 a.m. is period of greatest risk) and whether the client has post-surgical drains in place. It would be well for the nurse to be aware of those conditions which increase the risk of post-surgical infection so that preventative steps (additional showering with antiseptic solution before surgery, prolonged scrubbing, clipping versus shaving hair at surgical site, etc.) can be taken.

Alterations in Antibacterial Immune Mechanisms   There are three categories of abnormalities in antibacterial immune mechanisms: those affecting inflammatory responses, those affecting phagocytic functions, and those affecting opsonins (humoral immunity).

Anything that interferes with the migration of phagocytic cells to the area of contamination or with the physical contact of phagocytes and bacteria will enhance the development of an infection. Examples of such interferences include deficient blood supplies, the presence of ischemic or dead tissue, sutured material, foreign bodies, and hematomas. Vasopressor agents, radiation injury, uremia, severe nutritional deficiencies, and steroid therapy inhibit the synthesis of antibodies and other essential proteins.

Clients with severe thermal injuries and severe nutritional deficiencies have abnormalities involving the number of neutrophils collected at the site of an inflammatory response and defects of bactericidal chemotaxic capacity. Clients with Hodgkin's disease have a specific defect in cell-mediated immunity.

Genetic inabilities to synthesize complement components or specific antibodies can cause abnormalities in opsonins. Burn clients may have complement inactivated by a circulating substance released by the damaged tissue. Without complement, lysis of cells and destruction of bacteria cannot take place.

Alterations in the Respiratory Tract   Common alterations in the respiratory tract that facilitate the development of an infection include endotracheal intubation, tracheostomy, and bronchotracheal suctioning.

The bronchi and trachea are so sensitive to foreign matter that they initiate the cough reflex whenever irritation occurs. Ciliated, mucus-coated epithelium lining the trachea and lungs aid in clearing the respiratory tract of bacteria and mucus by the beating motion of the cilia. Intubation by-passes the cough reflex and compromises the effectiveness of this action. Although the trachea is usually considered sterile, it does not remain sterile after 48 to 72 hours of intubation. Infections associated with endotracheal intubation include pneumonia, tracheitis, and purulent bronchitis.

Catheters placed directly into the trachea can force pathogenic microorganisms into the respiratory system. In addition, catheters can damage the mucous lining of the respiratory tract, further compromising the effectiveness of its clearing mechanisms.

Alterations in the Genitourinary Tract Instrumentation, including catheterization of the bladder, and complicated obstetric delivery after prolonged confinement in bed are two procedures that introduce potentially pathogenic bacteria into the genitourinary tract. Acute urinary tract infection and pyelonephritis often occur after the use of a catheter or cystoscope.

The most common alteration is the placement of an indwelling urinary catheter. Research has demonstrated that significant bacteriuria develop in only 2 percent of the clients who have a single "straight" catheterization (in and out) to empty a distended bladder. Although bacteriuria may be considered benign and will resolve after removal of the catheter (sometimes augmented with antibiotic therapy), bacteriuria following catheterization may result in symptomatic cystitis and, occasionally in acute pyelonephritis, chronic pyelonephritis and persistent asymptomatic bacteriuria.

Invasive Devices Predisposing to Infection Most nosocomial septicemias occur as a result of significant alterations in normal host defenses. These infections may be primary (caused by direct introduction of microorganisms into the bloodstream) or secondary (arising from an infection at another site, such as the urinary tract).

The use of IV therapy greatly increases the risk of introducing harmful microorganisms. Of the thirty-two million clients admitted to hospitals each year, almost eight million receive some form of IV therapy. The incidence of septicemia in clients receiving IV therapy varies from zero to 8 percent, with an even higher incidence when plastic catheters are used.

Septicemia may also be caused by the introduction of microorganisms from contaminated fluids, infected venesection sites, or foci of septic thrombophlebitis as a complication of using an indwelling IV catheter.

Infusion-related sepsis is also associated with contaminated infusion fluid, which may be contaminated either during manufacturing (intrinsic contamination) or during hospital use (extrinsic contamination).

Infusion phlebitis is a common sequela of IV therapy. Although phlebitis does not always represent systemic infection, its presence connotes an eighteen-fold increased risk of related sepsis as compared with no phlebitis. Approximately one half the clients who have catheter-related sepsis will develop phlebitis.

Infected Venipuncture Sites The wounds made by a percutaneous stick at the venipuncture site may become contaminated and infected, providing a reservoir of bacteria that move along the catheter into the bloodstream.

Organisms that travel down the catheter will ultimately reside in the thrombus, which is almost uniformly present on a catheter tip. Around the thrombus, bacteria are shielded from the immune response, and antibiotics, and grow undisturbed. When these microorganisms attain a critical level of colonization, they seed the bloodstream and cause bacteremia.

Total Parenteral Nutritional Therapy Total Parenteral Nutrition Therapy (TPN) is a means of achieving an anabolic state in clients who would otherwise be unable to maintain normal nitrogen balance. Problems with IV-related sepsis in TPN are the same as those seen in conventional IV therapy, only greatly magnified.

Because clients on TPN are critically ill and malnourished, catheters are left in place for long periods of time. The hypertonic solution used with these clients supports the growth of a wide variety of organisms, especially fungus, to a greater extent than conventional IV solutions.

Implanted Prosthetic Devices Commonly used implanted prosthetic devices include artificial cardiac valves, synthetic vascular grafts, orthopedic prosthetic joints, neurosurgical shunts, cerebrospinal fluid pressure monitoring devices, permanent artificial arteriovenous fistulas for hemodialysis, intraocular lenses, and breast and penal implants. Most infections associated with prosthetic devices do not respond well to antimicrobial therapy. These infections usually require removal and replacement of the prosthesis.

Infections that result from prosthetic devices are usually introduced during surgery, either as a contaminant on the prosthesis itself or during the surgical procedure. The implant may also be colonized from the bloodstream prior to endothelialization. Once the device has been covered with endothelium, it is relatively resistant to blood-born bacterial colonization.

GUIDELINES FOR MANAGING CLIENTS

The primary purpose for performing interventions associated with infection control is to establish and maintain asepsis so that infection can be prevented. As you perform interventions, refer to these guidelines.

- Clients with severe underlying diseases are most likely to develop nosocomial infections. It is essential to know the epidemiology of the disease to control its spread in the hospital.
- Invasive procedures that by-pass natural body defenses predispose the client to the development of infection.
- Barrier nursing should be practiced at all times to protect hospital personnel as well as clients. Barrier nursing is directed at isolating the infective agent, not the client.
- Clients become colonized by endogenous flora in the hospital after 72 hours. This type of flora tends to be highly resistant to antibiotics.

The mechanisms by which antimicrobial agents promote infection include:

- Increasing the susceptibility of clients to colonization with nosocomial microflora.
- Selecting and concentrating antibiotic resistant organisms on or in the host.

Admission histories are an important adjunct in identifying potentially contagious clients as they enter the hospital. Initiation of appropriate isolation techniques need to begin immediately.

- Sources of common contact between clients should be limited in the hospital environment, i.e., dressing carts, ice buckets, collection buckets for emptying urine.
- Hand washing before and after contact with each client is the single most important means of preventing the spread of infection. The major source of cross-contamination among clients is direct transmission of microbes by the staff's hands.
- When recommended procedures cannot be followed, all personnel must be aware of the increased risk to clients.

ACTION: USING ISOLATION EQUIPMENT

Rationale for Action
- To prevent spreading endogenous and exogenous flora
- To reduce the potential of transferring organisms from the hospital environment to the client
- To protect hospital personnel

ASSESSMENT

1 Identify appropriate times for handwashing.
2 Identify type of protective clothing required for barrier nursing.
3 Identify epidemiology of the disease to determine how to prevent infection from spreading.

PLANNING

GOALS

- Isolation environment remains free of contamination.
- Personnel working with isolation clients remain free of infection.
- Clients who are in a medically compromised state remain free of infection.

EQUIPMENT

- Soap and running water
- Antimicrobial cleaning agent
- Isolation cart containing mask, gown, gloves (sterile and/or clean), plastic bags, isolation tape
- Paper towels
- Sterile brush or sponge
- Sterile towel
- Cards indicating type of isolation to be followed

▶ When hands remain moist, they tend to gather and support more organisms from the environment. When hands are not dried thoroughly, they tend to become red and cracked and may eventually become infected.

INTERVENTION: Washing Your Hands

1 Wet your hands.
2 Place a small amount of soap on your hands. (Soap need not be antimicrobial.)
3 Rub your hands vigorously, keeping your fingers pointed down to facilitate mechanical removal of organisms.
4 Wash your hands for 30 seconds.
5 Clean under your fingernails with an orange-wood stick.

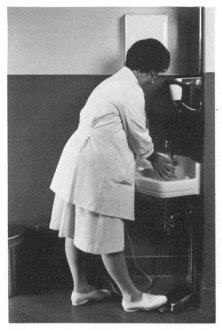
Wet hands thoroughly.

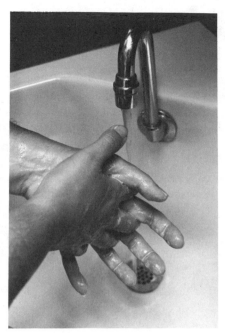
Keep fingers pointed down during hand-washing.

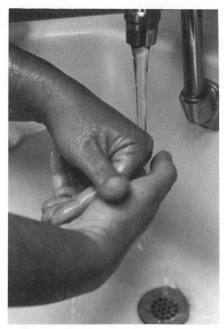
Wash for at least 30 seconds.

6 Rinse your hands under running water, keeping your fingers pointed downward.
7 Dry your hands with a paper towel.
8 Turn off water faucets, holding handles with paper towel.

INTERVENTION: Completing a Surgical Hand Scrub

1 Wet your hands.
2 With your arms held up in front of you, begin to scrub by cleaning your fingernails with a plastic or orange-wood stick.
3 Next, scrub your hands for four to five minutes with either an iodophor or a hexachlorophene or chlorhexidine antiseptic. (70 percent alcohol may be used also.)
4 Dry your hands with a sterile towel.

INTERVENTION: Using Clean Gloves

1 Wash and dry your hands.
2 Open glove wrapper.
3 Pick up glove, one at a time, by folded wrist edge.
4 Slip fingers in openings and pull glove up to wrist. Repeat step with second glove.
5 If you are wearing a gown, place gloves so that they cover gown wristlets. If you are not wearing a gown, place gloves so that they cover your wrists.

123

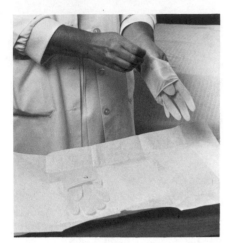

Lift glove up and away from sterile package to prevent contamination.

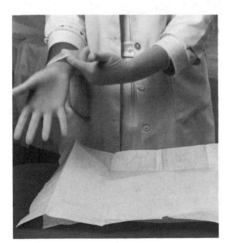

Maintain sterility while gloving, by allowing only sterile surfaces to touch.

6 Remove gloves by pulling them over your wrists and fingers until each glove is turned inside out.

INTERVENTION: Using Sterile Gloves

1 Wash and dry your hands.
2 Open glove wrapper, keeping both package and gloves sterile. Open wrapper from the middle of the package outward.
3 With your nondominant hand, remove the first glove by grasping the section that has a folded edge. Lift the glove up and away from the wrapper. Be careful not to touch the inside of the package or any part of the glove except the inner surface of the cuff.
4 Slip your dominant hand into the glove opening. Gently pull the glove into place with your nondominant hand, touching only the folded up cuff. Don't worry if you have difficulty easing your fingers all the way into the glove. After you have placed both gloves on your hands, you can move your fingers into place.
5 With your dominant, gloved hand, remove the other glove from the package, making sure you touch only the folded cuff. Lift this glove up and away from the wrapper.
6 Place your ungloved fingers into the new glove opening. Gently pull the glove over your hand as before.
7 Adjust both gloves, remembering to touch sterile surfaces with sterile surfaces.
8 Keep both sterile gloves in front of you above your waist level so that you can see them at all times and thus prevent potential contamination.

INTERVENTION: Putting on a Gown

1 Hold gown so that the opening will be in the back when you are wearing the gown.
2 Put the gown on by placing one arm at a time through the sleeves. Pull the gown up and over your shoulders.
3 Lap the gown around your back, tying the strings at your neck. (These ties are considered clean.)
4 Lap the gown around your waist, making sure your back is completely covered. Tie the strings around your waist. (These strings are considered dirty.)
5 To remove the gown, untie the waist strings first. (Remove gloves and mask, if applicable, now.)
6 Next untie the neck strings bringing them around your shoulders so that the gown is partially off your shoulders.
   Using your dominant hand, pull the sleeve wristlet over your nondominant hand. Repeat this procedure, using your nondominant hand to pull the sleeve wristlet over your dominant hand.
   Grasp the outside of the gown through the sleeves at the shoulders. Pull the gown down over your arms.

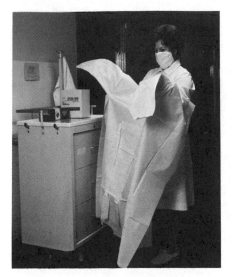

Put on isolation gown and mask before gloves when entering isolation room.

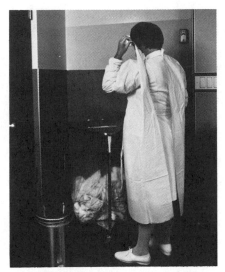

Untie neck string and pull gown over shoulder in preparation for leaving isolation room.

▶ Protocol for Protective Isolation Clothing
1 Gown
2 Cap
3 Mask
4 Gloves

9   Hold both gown shoulders in one hand. Carefully draw your other hand out of the gown, turning the arm of the gown inside out. Repeat this procedure with your other arm.

10 Hold the gown away from your body. Fold the gown up inside out.

11 Discard the gown if it is disposable. If the gown is reusable, place it in the appropriate container.

12 Wash your hands. Use a paper towel to turn off the water.

13 Put on new gown each time you enter an isolation room.

INTERVENTION: Using a Mask

1   Position mask to cover your *nose and mouth*.

2   Bend the nose bar so that it conforms over the bridge of your nose.

3   If you are using a mask with string ties, tie the top strings on top of your head to prevent slipping. If you are using a cone-shaped mask, tie the top strings over your ears.

4   Tie the bottom strings around your neck to secure the mask over your mouth. There should be no gaps between the mask and your face.

5   To remove the mask, untie the strings. Be sure to touch only the strings since they are considered clean.

6   Discard the mask in a trash container.

INTERVENTION: Removing Items from an Isolation Room

1   Close the contaminated bag inside the isolation room.

2   Set up a new bag for continued use.

▶ If you wear a mask outside a respiratory isolation room, discard the mask in a trash container immediately outside the isolation room. *DO NOT WEAR MASKS AROUND YOUR NECK.* Masks are contaminated with organisms from the air and from your breathing.

Clinical Alert
All items used for the care of a client in isolation are considered contaminated and should be double bagged and marked "Isolation" to protect the environment.

▶ Disposal Precautions

Secretion: Client should be instructed to expectorate into tissue held close to mouth. Suction catheters and gloves should be disposed of in impervious, sealed bags.

Excretion: Strict attention should be paid to careful handwashing; disease can be spread by oral-fecal route.

Blood: Needles and syringe should be disposable. Used needles should *not* be recapped. They should be placed in a puncture-resistant container that is prominently labeled "Isolation." Specimens should be labeled "Blood Precaution."

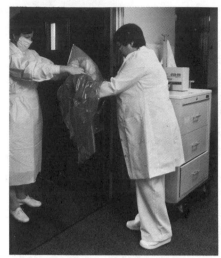

Prevent spread of microorganisms by double-bagging.

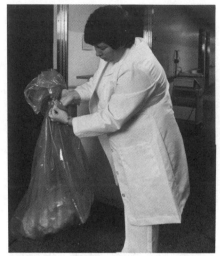

Close bag securely and clearly label as ISOLATION.

3 Have someone *outside* the room hold a clean bag with the top of the bag cuffed over his or her hands. If no one is available to help, assemble a clean bag in a hamper stand before you go into the isolation room.
4 Position the hamper stand outside the room for easy access.
5 Place the contaminated bag into the clean bag in the hamper outside the room. Be careful not to contaminate the outside of the clean bag.
6 Close the clean bag and mark it "Isolation." (Many hospitals use color coded bags to indicate isolation contents.)

INTERVENTION: Removing a Specimen from an Isolation Room

▶ Protocol for Leaving Isolation Room

1 Untie gown at waist.
2 Take off gloves.
3 Wash hands.
4 Take off cap.
5 Untie gown at neck.
6 Pull gown off and place in laundry hamper.
7 Take off mask.
8 Leave room and wash hands.

1 Before entering an isolation room mark a specimen container with the client's name, the type of specimen, and the word "Isolation."
2 Collect the specimen and place it in a plastic bag, using the same two-person approach as in double bagging contaminated items. Use clear bags so that laboratory personnel can see the specimen easily.
3 Label the clean bag with the word "Isolation," and then take the bag to the laboratory. (Affix a laboratory slip if appropriate.)

INTERVENTION: Transporting Client Outside Isolation Room

1 Explain procedure to client.
2 If client is being transported from a respiratory isolation room, tell him or her to wear a mask for the entire time the client is out of isolation. Clients being transported from a strict isolation room should wear a mask and a cap.

3 If client is being transported from a wound and skin, gastrointestinal, strict isolation, or protective isolation room, cover the transport vehicle, i.e., wheelchair, guerney, with a clean sheet *before* you enter the room.
4 Help the client into the transport vehicle. Cover the client, from shoulders down, with a sheet.
5 Tell the receiving department what type of isolation the client will need and what precautions hospital personnel should follow with the client.
6 When the client returns to the original isolation room, help him or her into bed. Cover the transportation vehicle with a sheet and remove it from the room.
7 Instruct all hospital personnel to wash their hands before they leave the area.

INTERVENTION: Removing Large Equipment Items from an Isolation Room

1 Wash equipment with an antimicrobial agent. (Washing is preferred to spraying.)
2 Cover equipment with a plastic bag.
3 Take bagged equipment to the decontamination area of central supply for further decontamination and processing.

TABLE 1 ISOLATION PROTOCOL

TYPE OF ISOLATION	PRIVATE ROOM	HANDS	GOWNS	MASKS	GLOVES	ARTICLES
Strict Isolation	Closed door	Wash when entering and leaving	All persons entering room	All persons entering room	All persons entering room	Double bag, discard or wrap before disinfection or sterilization
Enteric Isolation	Necessary for children only	Entering and exiting	For direct client contact	Not necessary	While in contact with articles contaminated with fecal material	Double bag, disinfect or discard if contaminated with urine or feces
Wound & Skin Isolation	Desirable but not essential	Wash when entering and leaving	For direct contact with infected wound	During dressing change only	While in direct contact with infected wound	Special precautions for instruments, dressings, linen
Respiratory Isolation	Closed door	Wash when entering and leaving	Not necessary	All persons entering room	Not necessary	Disinfect if contaminated with secretions
Protective Isolation	Closed door	Wash when entering and leaving	All persons entering room	All persons entering room	All persons having direct contact with client	No special precautions

EVALUATION

EXPECTED OUTCOMES

1 Isolation environment remains free of contamination. *If not*, follow these alternative nursing actions:

ANA: Assess whether the isolation technique is carried out appropriately.

ANA: Review the isolation technique with all members of nursing staff.

ANA: Identify if the proper isolation procedure was carried out for specific problem.

2 Personnel working with isolation clients remain free of infection. *If not*, follow these alternative nursing actions:

ANA: Examine barrier nursing techniques.

ANA: Report situation to employee health department for treatment.

ANA: Contact the infection control practitioner for consultation.

3 Clients who are in a medically compromised state remain free of pathogens. *If not*, follow these alternative nursing actions:

ANA: Advise physician of client's condition.

ANA: Contact the infection control practitioner to review clients in need of protective isolation procedures.

ANA: Identify alterations in protocol that promoted the infectious state.

ANA: Review isolation procedures with all nursing personnel.

UNEXPECTED OUTCOME

Outbreaks of disease occur in isolation environment.

ANA: Identify cause of outbreak and contact the infection control practitioner for consultation.

ANA: Examine handwashing and barrier nursing practices.

ANA: Present inservice education program on isolation technique to increase personnel's awareness of appropriate procedures.

Charting
- Type of barrier nursing being practiced
- Client's reactions to sensory deprivation
- Specimens sent to laboratory
- Breaks in technique written up on incident report

ACTION: CARING FOR WOUNDS

ASSESSMENT

1 Identify type of dressing needed, e.g., occlusive, nonocclusive, non-adhering, wet-dry, medicated.
2 Assess level of pain associated with wound and dressing change.
3 Determine if infection is present.
4 Assess need for culture and sensitivity of wound drainage.
5 Identify any isolation requirements.
6 Identify epidemiology of disease or wound source to prevent spreading of infection.

Rationale for Action
- To prevent infection and cross contamination
- To absorb fluid and provide a dry environment
- To immobilize and support a wound
- To assist in removal of necrotic tissue
- To apply medication
- To obtain a wound culture without contaminating the specimen
- To promote granulation wound healing

PLANNING

GOALS

- Wound granulates and healing process occurs.
- Wound is free of pathogenic microorganisms.
- Purulent drainage in wound decreases.
- Sterility is maintained during dressing change.
- A noncontaminated specimen is collected for culture.

EQUIPMENT

- Sterile pre-packaged dressing(s) as needed
- Tape, micropore, paper, or Montgomery tie tapes
- Disposable suture removal kit for disposable scissors and forceps
- Sterile gloves
- Clean gloves
- Cleansing solution as ordered, e.g., betadine, hydrogen peroxide
- Plastic bag
- Tray (if setting up sterile field)
- Sterile towels (at least four)

ADDITIONAL EQUIPMENT FOR IRRIGATING A WOUND

- Culture transport swab with transport media
- Anaerobic transport media with swab
- Sterile irrigation solution at 90° F to 95° F (32° C to 35° C)
- Sterile Robinson catheter
- Sterile asepto syringe
- Sterile graduate
- Sterile basin
- Chux
- Sterile gloves

ADDITIONAL EQUIPMENT FOR IRRIGATING AN OPEN WOUND

- Sterile forceps
- Bag
- Sterile gloves
- 3 percent hydrogen peroxide
- Sterile normal saline
- Fine-mesh gauze (plain or iodophor)
- Wide-mesh gauze (plain, petroleum, or antimicrobial)
- Sterile gauze pads
- Tape or Montgomery straps

ADDITIONAL EQUIPMENT FOR IRRIGATING A DRAINING WOUND

- Same items as above, except fine- and wide-mesh gauze
- Sterile cotton applicators
- Sterile safety pin
- ABD dressings

▶ Wound healing occurs in four phases.

Injury: At the time of injury, blood fills the wound and clots. Cellular debris from the epidermal and subdermal layers also fills the wound.

Inflammation Within a day, the wound edges become inflamed and swell. Phagocytes ingest cellular debris and bacteria, decreasing clot size. Epidermal cells and granular tissue begin to fill the space left by the clot.

Proliferation: About two days after the wound, epidermal cells cover the area. Fibroblasts begin reforming dermis.

Reformation: By the seventh day, epidermal integrity is restored. Fibroblasts proliferate, producing collagen. Blood vessels, lymphatics, and other connective tissue are being replaced. This process continues until healing is complete.

▶ Guidelines for Sterile Field

- Never turn your back on a sterile field.
- Avoid talking, coughing, sneezing, or reaching across a sterile field.
- Keep sterile objects above waist level.
- Do not spill solutions on the sterile field.
- Open all sterile packages away from the sterile field to prevent crossover and contamination.

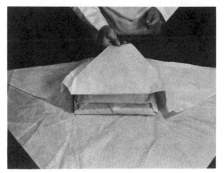

Do not cross over a sterile field when opening a sterile package.

INTERVENTION Preparing a Sterile Field

1 Gather equipment from supply area.
2 Clean off overbed table.
3 Place tray on overbed table or on another surface close to table.
4 Wash your hands, using aseptic techniques.
5 Place sterile towel packages on overbed table or on another surface close to the table. Place packages so that first wrapper edge can be opened away from the sterile area.
6 Using both hands, pick up the two side edges of the first wrapper and open them away from the middle of the sterile field.
7 Unfold the last edge toward you, without touching the wrapper.
8 Using pickup forceps or your hands, pick up one edge of the sterile towel and move away from the table. Gently shake the towel away from the sterile area.
9 When the towel is open, use your other hand to pick up the two edges that are away from you.
10 Lower the towel onto the tray or bedside stand so the towel is furthest away from you. Then lay the towel down on the tray by bringing it toward you, covering the entire tray. (Always work away from the sterile field to prevent crossing or bending over the sterile field.)
11 Repeat the same steps with a second sterile towel.
12 If solutions for cleansing the skin are required, place sterile medicine cups on the tray near one side.
13 Take the cap off the antiseptic bottle.
14 Pour a small amount of antiseptic solution into a medicine cup that is not on the tray to keep lip of the bottle free of contaminated particles.
15 Pour the antiseptic solution (with the label in uppermost position) from the side of the bottle directly into the medicine cup. If any solution drops onto the sterile field, you will need to set up a new sterile field since it will be considered contaminated.
16 If you have transfer forceps, use them to open sterile packages of dressing material. Place dressing material in the center of a sterile towel. (The outer 2.5 cm of the sterile towel's edge is considered contaminated, so do not allow dressing material to touch these edges.)
17 If you do not have transfer forceps, open sterile dressing packages with your hands, pulling back at the place indicated on the wrapper.
18 Hold onto the dressing with your thumb and forefinger at the folded edge of the wrapper. With your other hand, fold the top flap of the wrapper over your hand to expose the dressing.
19 Gently drop the dressing on the center of the sterile towel without touching or reaching across the sterile field.
20 Repeat step 16 or 17 for all sterile pieces needed to complete the dressing change. All sterile dressing materials can be opened up at one time.
21 When you put on sterile gloves, you can transfer the dressings to the sterile field.

22　If you are not going to use the sterile supplies immediately or if you are called out of the room, cover the sterile field with sterile towels. Place the towels on the sterile field in a way that prevents crossing over the sterile field.

INTERVENTION: Changing a Sterile Dressing

1　Gather the equipment from the supply room.
2　Check client's ID band.
3　Assemble equipment.
4　Explain procedure to client.
5　Wash your hands thoroughly.
6　Remove tape from client's skin by pulling *toward* the incision.
7　Put on clean gloves.
8　Remove soiled dressing.
9　Discard gloves and dressings into plastic bag. Observe wound closely for signs of infection/healing.
10　Open sterile barrier and prepare sterile field.
11　Prepare cleansing solution.
12　Put on sterile glove. If you are working alone, place sterile glove on dominant hand, leaving other hand free to work with nonsterile supplies.
13　Cleanse wound. When cleansing an area, always start at the cleanest area and work away from that area. Never return to an area you have previously cleaned.
14　If a drain is present, cleanse under the drain and around the site with a four- by four-inch tissue and cleansing solution.
15　Place several tissues under the drain.
16　Using sterile, disposable forceps from the dressing kit, place several four- by four-inch tissues over wound. Cover with ABD pad if necessary, and tape securely. (Montgomery straps may be used if desired.)
17　Remove glove.
18　Close plastic bag and dispose of bag as isolation material.
19　Wash your hands thoroughly.
20　Check with client to see that he or she is comfortable before leaving room.

▶ **Dressing Change**

- Frequent dressing changes are preferable to reinforcing the same dressing. Organisms often culture in blood and wound drainage, especially after bowel surgery.
- Avoid pooling of excessive drainage under saturated dressing. Pools of drainage increase the number of organisms that come in contact with the suture line.

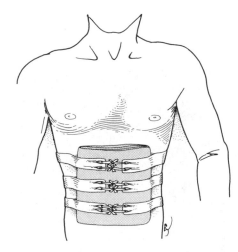

Montgomery straps are used when frequent dressing changes are needed.

INTERVENTION: Caring for a Draining Wound

1　Gather equipment from supply room.
2　Check client's ID band.
3　Assemble equipment.
4　Explain procedure to client. Ask client if he or she has any specific complaints that relate to wound care.
5　Wash your hands thoroughly.

131

History of smoking
Obesity
Old age
Anemia
Malnourishment
Low-serum protein level
Steroid therapy
Immunodeficiency
Chemotherapy
Radiation therapy
Diabetes
Shock
Acidosis
Hypoxemia
Infection
Wound dehiscence

6 Remove tape from client's skin by pulling *toward* the incision.
7 Put on clean gloves.
8 Remove soiled dressing.
9 Discard gloves and dressings into plastic bag.
10 Observe wound closely for signs of infection or healing.
11 If pin on the Penrose drain is crusted, replace it. Be careful not to dislodge drain or suction tubing.
12 Using cotton applicators or gauze pads, cleanse drain site with hydrogen peroxide and then saline.
13 Put on sterile gloves.
14 Apply gauze pad with a precut slit to drain, or apply or replace drainage bag.
15 Apply dry, sterile gauze pads over drain.
16 Apply ABD pads over sterile gauze.
17 Remove gloves and dispose of them in refuse bag.
18 Tape dressing or retie Montgomery straps.
19 Remove bag with soiled dressing from room.
20 Wash hands thoroughly.
21 Check with client to see if he or she is comfortable before leaving room.

INTERVENTION: Maintaining a Hemovac Suction

1 Check physician's orders and collect supplies.
2 Identify client and explain procedure, giving client time to ask questions.
3 Provide for comfort and privacy.
4 Wash your hands thoroughly.
5 Elevate bed to workable height.
6 Expose catheter insertion site while keeping client draped. Place Hemovac on bed protector.
7 Examine pump and catheter for patency, seal, and stability.
8 Remove Hemovac plug, which is labeled.
9 Pour collected drainage into graduate measure while compressing pump. Set collection aside.
10 Hold pump tightly compressed and reinsert plug to reestablish closed drainage system.
11 If catheter occludes, notify the physician.
12 Position catheter and evacuator on bed.
13 Read graduate measure and record amount.
14 Examine contents for color, consistency, and odor.
15 Discard contents, rinse container, and wash hands.
16 Send culture specimen to laboratory if ordered.
17 Make client comfortable and lower bed.
18 Compress evacuator at least every four hours to provide suction. To compress, take plug out and press evacuator together. Replace plug to reestablish suction.

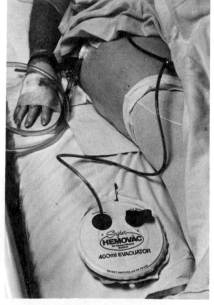

Empty drainage through Pouring Spout. Then compress evacuator and replace plug in Pouring Spout.

INTERVENTION: Obtaining Wound Drainage for Aerobic Culture and Sensitivity

1 Complete steps 1 to 5 for intervention "Caring for a Draining Wound."
2 Remove culture swab and wipe swab in wound. Avoid touching purulent exudate.
3 Swab area of inflamed wound. Avoid touching skin edges or other surfaces that will contaminate the swab.
4 Return swab to container.
5 Crush transport media vial, and push swab tip into contact with transport media.
6 Transport specimen to laboratory within 30 minutes so that organisms are still viable.

INTERVENTION: Obtaining Wound Drainage for Anaerobic Culture and Sensitivity

1 Complete steps 1 to 5 for intervention "Caring for a Draining Wound."
2 Remove culture swab and wipe in wound as you did with aerobic culturing. Be sure you do not tip anaerobic transport media tube because it contains carbon dioxide. Tipping will "spill" the gas out, making it useless to transport anaerobic organisms.
3 Return swab to container.
4 Transport specimen to laboratory *immediately*.
5 *Alternative method*
   a Draw up exudate in syringe with all air expelled or have a physician aspirate the wound.
   b Transport specimen to laboratory *immediately*.

INTERVENTION: Irrigating Wounds

1 Gather irrigation equipment and dressing material.
2 Check client's ID band.
3 Assemble equipment.
4 Explain procedure to client and answer any questions.
5 Wash hands thoroughly.
6 Set up sterile area or open equipment packages on overbed table.
7 Position client so that solution will flow from wound to basin.
8 Remove and discard used dressing.
9 Place chux under client. Place a bath blanket under chux when irrigating a large wound. The blanket will absorb any spilled irrigation solution.
10 Place bedside stand near working area with all packages open.
11 Put on sterile gloves following correct procedure.
12 Inspect area surrounding wound for redness, tissue integrity, and signs of granulating tissue.
13 Gently place Robinson catheter into uppermost area of wound to prevent tissue trauma. (For large wounds, position Robinson catheter in several areas of the wound.)

▶ **Wound Culture**

● Obtain wound culture for both aerobic and anaerobic organisms during scheduled dressing change before any medication or antimicrobial agents have been applied.
● Anaerobic organisms may appear on gram stain even though they are not grown in the culture. When anaerobes are suspected, use anaerobic culturing methods to obtain a specimen.

133

14 Attach barrel of asepto syringe to Robinson catheter.

15 Place sterile basin under wound area.

16 Pour room temperature irrigating solution from sterile graduate.

17 Allow irrigating solution to flow over wound so that all organisms, tissue debris, and drainage are washed into basin. Cleanse from cleanest to dirtiest area of wound if possible.

18 Repeat until all irrigation solution has been used.

19 After the irrigation, cleanse client's skin and dry surrounding area.

20 Apply sterile dressing.

21 Dispose of equipment according to isolation protocol, and obtain fresh supplies for next irrigation.

22 Check to see that client is comfortable before leaving room.

EVALUATION

EXPECTED OUTCOMES

1 Granulation takes place and healing occurs. *If not*, follow these alternative nursing actions:

ANA: Assess dressing to see if it is impairing the healing process. Wounds healing by second intention must not be allowed to "seal over," but must heal from the bottom upward.

ANA: Assess client's nutritional status. A high-protein diet may be indicated.

ANA: Culture wound to identify presence of microorganisms.

2 Sterility is maintained during dressing change. *If not*, follow these alternative nursing actions:

ANA: Remove and discard contaminated dressings and apply sterile dressings.

ANA: Review sterile dressing change procedure with staff.

3 A noncontaminated specimen is collected for culture. *If not*, follow these alternative nursing actions:

ANA: Discard contaminated specimen and container.

ANA: Obtain new specimen.

ANA: Review procedure for obtaining specimen with staff.

4 Adhesive-backed drainage bag works efficiently to contain drainage and skin integrity is maintained. *If not*, follow these alternative nursing actions:

ANA: If leakage appears under seal, clean skin with soap and water, and apply karaya ring or blanket with hole cut just large enough to cover drain site and drainage bag.

ANA: If skin appears moderately red with broken areas, clean area with soap and water. Apply aluminum paste or antacid from bottom of unshaken bottle. Dry, sprinkle with karaya powder, spray with skin prep, and apply new drainage bag.

ANA: If skin is weeping with ulcerated areas, prepare site as in previous ANA, but apply karaya powder until it no longer darkens from absorbed moisture. Cover ulcerated spots with small non-adherent dressing pieces before spraying with skin prep.

ANA: If massive drainage appears, connect drainage bag to suction system, using Sump suction or large thoracic catheter with a large gauge needle inserted as air vent.

ANA: If drainage is massive and skin is too irritated for bag application, consult physician about inserting suction catheter directly into wound.

ANA: If wound is too extensive for application of drainage bag or if ABD pads cannot contain drainage, make a doughnut-shaped ring out of peripads covered with stretch gauze. Place ring around wound and fill center with ABD pads wrapped together with stretch gauze. Hold dressing in place with abdominal binder or draw sheet.

ANA: If permanent large draining wound, consult physician about making a mold of silicone gel to fit inside wound, thus reducing size of drainage area.

UNEXPECTED OUTCOMES

1 Wound becomes infected with different microorganisms.
   ANA: Do culture and sensitivity to identify pathogen.
   ANA: Wash your hands thoroughly to prevent the spread of infection.
   ANA: Pay strict attention to changing dressings. Consult with physician for new orders.
2 Edges of wound split open (wound dehiscence).
   ANA: Place client in supine position. Apply butterfly tape to wound edges. Cover opening with sterile dressings. Apply binder for abdominal incisions.
   ANA: Culture incision if signs of infection are present.
   ANA: Observe client for signs of shock. If client in shock, notify physician immediately.
   ANA: Encourage high-protein diet.
3 Evisceration occurs (protrusion of bowel contents).
   ANA: Institute emergency measures: Place client in supine position. Cover bowel with sterile gauze moistened with sterile saline. Insert intravenous catheter and infuse normal saline. Reassure client. Obtain vital signs, and treat for shock if present.
   ANA: After above measures, notify physician and prepare client for return to surgery.
   ANA: After repair, increase protein and vitamin C in diet. Apply abdominal binder.
4 Wound hemorrhages.
   ANA: Outline area of blood on dressing with a pen and observe outline to see how quickly the bleeding spreads.
   ANA: If bleeding is excessive, notify physician immediately.
   ANA: Apply pressure to site if there is bleeding.

Charting
- Condition of wound
- Characteristics of drainage
- Type of dressing applied
- Cultures obtained
- Application
- Type and amount of irrigating solution used
- Method used for irrigating
- Observation of wound site, including amount, color, and odor of drainage, and appearance of suture site.
- Observation of granulating tissue and redness
- Pertinent observations concerning client's tolerance of procedure
- Observation of skin condition around incision site
- Changes in vital signs that indicate possible infection
- Type of dressing applied
- Observations on wound irrigation
- Type and amount of irrigating solutions used
- Unusual tension on sutures if present

ACTION: TREATING DECUBITUS ULCERS

Rationale for Action

- To identify the stage of the ulcer
- To provide appropriate treatment for specific ulcer stage
- To promote healing of established ulcer
- To prevent new ulcer formation
- To prevent spread of pathogens from ulcerated area

ASSESSMENT

1 Assess stage of ulcer.
2 Identify if infection is associated with decubitus ulcer.
3 Evaluate effectiveness of ulcer treatment.
4 Assess healing process of the ulcer.
5 Assess other bony prominences for potential formation of decubiti.

PLANNING

GOALS

- Staging of decubitus ulcer is accurately assessed.
- Decubitus ulcer is treated effectively according to stage of ulcer formation.
- Healing of decubitus ulcers takes place.

EQUIPMENT

- Soap and water
- Heat lamp
- Op-Site kit
  Alcohol soaks
  Sterile 10-cm × 10-cm gauze pads
  Betadine prep pad
  Scissors
  Paper tape
- Appropriate skin care tray for stage of ulcer

▶ **Stages of Decubitus Ulcers**

Stage 1: Erythematous skin not relieved by stimulation or relief of pressure.

Stage 2: Superficial tissue damage; involves excoriation, vesiculation, or skin breakdown.

Stage 3: Ulceration involves the dermis (full thickness loss of skin); may or may not include subcutaneous tissue level; produces serosanguineous drainage.

Stage 4: Ulceration deep into structures (full thickness loss of skin) with invasion of deep tissue and/or structures such as fascia, connective tissue, muscle or bone.

Use of Stage 2 skin care tray is explained as an example. The three other skin care trays utilize different materials and include instructions.

INTERVENTION: Applying Op-Site

1 Obtain Op-Site kit. Op-Site can be used for any stage of ulcer formation. Choose appropriate size of Op-Site.
2 Apply to flat surface for application. Coccyx area cannot be treated with Op-Site.
3 Wash your hands.
4 Explain procedure to client.
5 Provide privacy.
6 Wash decubitus ulcer area with soap and water.
7 Dry area thoroughly.
8 Apply Betadine prep pads over decubitus ulcer and surrounding tissue.
9 Wash area with sterile saline.
10 Apply plasticizing agent (skin prep, skin gel) over surrounding tissue. Do not apply on ulcer because the agent contains alcohol, which will burn ulcer area.
11 Allow area to dry thoroughly.
12 Loosen Op-Site from one side of backing paper.

13 "Walk on": start at one edge of site and gently lay the Op-Site down, keeping it free of wrinkles. Overlap wound at least 2.5 cm on all sides.
14 Cut off green tabs from Op-Site after wound is covered.
15 Observe ulcer area daily.
16 If large amount of secretions or serous fluid accumulate under Op-Site, aspirate with a number 26-gauge needle.
17 Change Op-Site only when loose.
18 "Work-off" Op-Site from one edge to the other.
19 Position client for comfort.
20 Remove and discard equipment.
21 Wash your hands.

INTERVENTION: Using Skin Care Tray

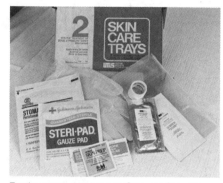

Equipment contained in Stage 2 Skin Care Tray.

1 Obtain appropriate tray for stage of ulcer. (Stage 2 kit is explained.)
2 Wash your hands.
3 Explain procedure to client.
4 Provide privacy.
5 Wash decubitus ulcer with povidone-iodine for three minutes.
6 Rinse area with water and dry thoroughly. (May use heat lamp for drying.)
7 Apply Maalox and allow to dry. If area is infected, an antibiotic ointment may be used instead of Maalox.
8 Dust Karaya powder over Maalox, removing the excess powder.
9 Apply protective skin prep to area surrounding the ulcer. Allow to dry.
10 Apply Stomahesive. Do not cut Stomahesive, but use entire sheet.
11 Secure edges of Stomahesive with nonallergic plastic tape. (Picture-frame the Stomahesive in a similar manner as with colostomy bag.)
12 Change Stomahesive every 24 hours. Do not tear off wound.
13 Position client for comfort.
14 Remove equipment from room.
15 Wash your hands.

EVALUATION

EXPECTED OUTCOMES

1 Stage of decubitus ulcer is accurately assessed. *If not,* follow these alternative nursing actions:
   ANA: Wash area carefully to ensure better observation of ulcer area.
   ANA: Consult with enterostomal therapist to assist in accurate identification of stage of ulcer.
2 Decubitus ulcer is treated effectively according to stage of ulcer formation. *If not,* follow these alternative nursing actions:
   ANA: Reassess for stage of ulcer to determine if appropriate treatment is being provided.

137

ANA: Determine if proper technique was used to apply protective covering.

ANA: Determine if protective covering is kept in place for stated length of time.

3 Healing of decubitus ulcer takes place. *If not*, follow these alternative nursing actions:

ANA: Obtain order for water bed or flotation pads to prevent additional pressure areas.

ANA: Obtain order for wound culture if drainage continues and healing is prevented.

ANA: Prepare client for possible skin graft.

UNEXPECTED OUTCOMES

1 Client does not have sufficient exercise and appetite decreases.

ANA: Encourage small frequent feedings.

ANA: Offer high-calorie drinks like eggnog or Isocal.

2 Client does not heal with traditional types of treatments.

ANA: Apply vitamin E to ulcer area. Open capsules and place liquid on affected area.

ANA: Sprinkle granulated sugar over ulcer.

ANA: Take fresh peelings from orange, place directly over wound, and tape down with nonallergic tape.

Charting

- Client's general skin condition
- Assessment of wound, i.e., drainage, evidence of tissue granulation
- Type of ulcer care given, i.e., kit used
- Stage of ulcer
- Location, size, color, odor, and possible cause of ulcer

TERMINOLOGY

antiseptics Agents that are applied to body tissues, such as skin or mucous membrane, to destroy or retard the growth of microorganisms.

autoinfections Infections that arise from an individual's own body flora.

barrier nursing Any technique that reduces the risk of cross contamination.

cell-mediated immunity Reaction to antigens by cells rather than antibody molecules present in body fluids.

chemotaxis Attraction and repulsion of living protoplasm to a chemical stimulus.

colonization Organisms present in body tissue, but not multiplying or invading the tissue.

depilatory Agent that removes hair from skin surfaces.

disinfectants Chemical agents that are used to destroy or reduce microorganisms on inanimate surfaces and objects.

disinfection A process that employs physical and chemical means to remove, control, or destroy most of the organisms that may be present on equipment or materials.

duration of the infectious challenge Sustained exposure to even a relatively small number of organisms that poses a significant risk to the client (e.g., intravenous catheters become colonized with microorganisms).

endogenous   Organisms natural to an individual's own body.

exogenous   Organisms external to an individual's own body.

humoral immunity   Acquired immunity where the circulating antibody is predominant.

infection   Establishment of a disease process that involves invasion of the body tissue by microorganisms and the reaction of the tissues to their presence and to the toxins generated by them.

nosocomial infection   An infection acquired while in the hospital that was not present or incubating at the time of admission.

opsonin   A substance in blood serum that acts upon microorganisms and other cells and facilitates phagocytosis.

outbreak   A critical incident where infections occur above an established level and are caused by the same etiological agent.

resident (normal) flora   Organisms natural to an individual's own body. Organisms multiply in the environment, not merely survive there.

sepsis   Condition resulting from the presence of pathogenic bacteria and their products.

sterile   Free from any living microorganisms.

susceptible sites   An area that is sensitive to or can be invaded by a bacterium or other infectious agent.

virulence   Recognized pathogenic organisms designated because of their ability to invade and propagate in normal, intact, uncompromised individuals. Some organisms that are avirulent for normal individuals become pathogenic when defense mechanisms are impaired.

LEVEL II
Maintenance of Homeostasis

CHAPTER 5
Assessing Vital Signs

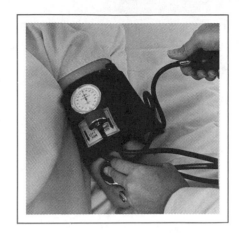

Vital signs, also called cardinal signs, reflect the body's physiological status and provide information critical to evaluating homeostatic balance. This chapter will discuss the important vital signs and the nurse's responsibility in assessing them to determine the client's state of health.

TEMPERATURE

Temperature control of the body is a homeostatic function, regulated by a complex mechanism involving the hypothalamus. The temperature of the body's interior (core temperature) is maintained within ±1° F except in the case of febrile illness. The surface temperature of the skin and tissues immediately underlying the skin rises and falls with a change in temperature of the surrounding environment. Core temperature is maintained when heat production equals heat loss. The temperature regulating center in the hypothalamus keeps the core temperature constant by a negative feedback mechanism. Temperature receptors, which determine if the body is too hot or too cold, feed into the hypothalamus. These receptors are heat sensitive neurons in the preoptic area of the anterior hypothalamus, skin temperature receptors for both hot and cold, and temperature receptors in the spinal cord, abdomen, and internal organs. When the body becomes overheated, heat sensitive neurons in the preoptic area stimulate sweat glands to secrete fluid. This

LEARNING OBJECTIVES

Identify the cardinal signs that reflect the body's physiological status.

List three mechanisms which increase heat production.

Describe how disease alters the "set point" of the temperature regulating center.

Compare and contrast autoregulation and the autonomic nervous system and how they control the circulatory system.

Describe alternative nursing actions that can be performed when temperature is not within normal range.

Define the pulse and indicate how it is an index of heart rate and rhythm.

Compare the respiratory rate and rhythm to pulse and blood pressure.

List and describe the nursing actions for alterations in respiratory patterns.

List six factors which affect blood pressure. Outline appropriate nursing actions for hypotension and hypertension.

enhances heat loss through evaporation. Blood vessels also vasodilate, as sympathetic centers in the posterior hypothalamus are inhibited. The vasoconstrictor mechanism of the skin vessels is reduced, thereby conducting heat from the core of the body to the body surface. Heat loss occurs through radiation, evaporation, and conduction.

Regulatory Mechanisms When the body core is cooled below 98.6° F (37° C), heat conservation is affected. Intense vasoconstriction of the skin vessels results from release of sympathetic centers from inhibition, and stimulation from skin and spinal cord cold receptors. There is also piloerection and a decrease in sweating to conserve heat.

Heat production is increased by three mechanisms: stimulation from the skin and spinal cord cold receptors drives the primary motor center for shivering; stimulation of the sympathetic nervous system and circulating epinephrine and norepinephrine increases cellular metabolism; and increased thyroxine output increases cellular metabolism.

The "set point" is the critical temperature level at which the regulatory mechanisms attempt to maintain the body's core temperature. Above the set point, heat losing mechanisms are brought into play and below that level heat conserving and producing mechanisms are set into action.

Disease can alter the set point of the temperature regulating center to cause fever, a body temperature above normal. Brain lesions, pyrogens from bacteria or viruses, or degenerating tissue (i.e., gangrenous areas or myocardial infarction) also increase the set point. Dehydration can cause fever due to lack of available fluid for perspiration and by increasing the set point, which brings more heat conserving and producing mechanisms into play. When the "thermostat" is suddenly set higher, the client complains of feeling cold, has cool extremities, shivers and has piloerection. Hypoxia can occur due to increased oxygen requirements with the increased metabolism of heat production. When the "thermostat" returns to normal, heat losing mechanisms again come into play. The client feels hot and starts perspiring.

When body temperature falls below the normal range, the client experiences hypothermia and complains of being cold, shivers, and has cool extremities. Hypothermia may be caused by accidental exposure, frostbite, or GI hemorrhage. Medically induced hypothermia is now used for some surgical interventions. The ability of the hypothalamus to regulate body temperature is greatly impaired when the body temperature falls below 94° F (34.4° C) and is lost below 85° F (29.4° C). Heat production by cells is also depressed by a low temperature.

Measuring Body Temperature An accurate oral or rectal temperature records the core temperature. The normal range of an oral temperature is 97° to 99.5° F, or 35° to 38.4° C. Rectal temperatures are approximately 1° F higher. Temperature may vary according to age, time of day (lower in the morning and higher in the afternoon and evening), amount of exercise, or extremes in the environmental temperature.

The thermometer is the instrument used to measure body heat. Oral and rectal (also used for axillary temperature) thermometers are glass tubes containing mercury. When exposed to heat, the mercury expands, moves up the glass, and records the body temperature. The thermometer is marked in degrees and tenths of degrees and the range is 93° to 108° F (34° to 42.2° C).

Electronic thermometers, now widely used in hospitals, are more accurate than glass thermometers. In addition, they have disposable covers, which promote infection control, and therefore should be used when available. The electronic thermometer plugs into a receptable and has a heat sensor that records the client's core temperature in only a few seconds.

Heat sensitive tapes are also used to record temperature. The tape is applied to the skin, and color changes indicate the temperature level. These tapes are both disposable and nonbreakable. They are most appropriate for use with normal newborns, small children, and in situations where proper cleaning of the thermometer is difficult.

PULSE

The pulse is an index of the heart's rate and rhythm. Pulse rate is the number of heart beats per minute. With each beat the heart's left ventricle contracts and forces blood into the aorta. This forceful ejection of blood produces a wave that is transmitted through the arteries to the periphery of the body. The pulse is a transient expansion of a vessel resulting from internal pressure changes.

The pulse wave is influenced by the elasticity of the larger vessels, blood viscosity, and arteriolar and capillary resistance. Other characteristics of the pulse wave are size or amplitude, its type or contour, and its elasticity. Old age, with its arteriosclerotic changes in the blood vessels, speeds up the pulse wave velocity. The pulse wave changes in shape as it moves toward the periphery.

Circulatory System Control   The circulatory system is under the dual control of autoregulation and the autonomic nervous system. This dual control allows the circulatory system to vary blood flow to meet the body's requirements.

Local control of blood flow is called autoregulation. Blood flow is adjusted to the changing metabolic activity of different tissues. At constant levels of tissue metabolism, the flow is adjusted in response to changing arterial pressure. Tissues vary in their degree of autoregulation.

The autonomic nervous system regulates circulation through the vasomotor center in the medulla oblongata. Stimulation of this area causes vasoconstriction of resistance vessels (primarily precapillary sphincters but also arterioles and veins). This condition results in increased arterial blood pressure. Stimulation also increases heart rate and cardiac contractility. On the other hand, sympathetic inhibition causes vasodilation.

The baroreceptor reflex is another important circulatory control mechanism. Baroreceptors (pressoreceptors) are located in the walls of the carotid sinus and aortic arch. Increased blood pressure causes the baroreceptors to transmit signals to the medulla, which inhibits sympathetic action. The result is vasodilation and decreased blood pressure and heart rate. With a drop in blood pressure, the opposite occurs. The baroreceptors transmit signals to stimulate the vasomotor center, which causes vasoconstriction, and increased blood pressure and heart rate.

Heart Rate and Rhythm   The normal heart rate is from 60 to 80 beats per minute (BPM) in the resting adult, slightly faster in women than in men, and more rapid in children and infants (90 to 140 BPM). Older people usually have a slight increase in rate (70 to 80 BPM). Tachycardia is a pulse rate over 100 beats per minute. Bradycardia is a pulse rate below 60 beats per minute.

Heart rhythm is the time interval between each heartbeat. Rhythm varies according to the status of the client. Normally, the heart rhythm is regular although slight irregularities do not necessarily indicate cardiac malfunction. An intermittent pulse occurs when the normal pattern of the pulse rate is broken; if recurrent, this irregular rhythm requires cardiac evaluation as it may be indicative of cardiac disease. A consistent irregular rhythm, or arrhythmia, is indicative of cardiac malfunction.

Variance in heart rate, either increased or decreased, may be attributed to many factors such as drug intake, lack of oxygen, loss of blood, exercise, and body temperature. When evaluating a pulse rate, it is important to ascertain the normal baseline for each client and then to determine variances from the normal for that particular client. The heart normally pumps about 5 liters of blood through the body each minute. This cardiac output is calculated by multiplying the heart rate per minute by the stroke volume, the amount of blood ejected with one contraction. Increasing the heart rate is one of the first compensatory mechanisms the body employs to maintain cardiac output.

Evaluating Pulse Rate   The quality of the pulse rate is determined by the amount of blood pumped through the arteries. Normally, the amount of pumped blood remains fairly constant; when it varies, it is also indicative of cardiac malfunction. A so-called bounding pulse occurs when the nurse is able to feel the pulse by exerting only a slight pressure over the artery. If, by exerting firm pressure, the nurse cannot clearly determine the flow, the pulse is called weak or thready.

Outside the body trunk, the arterial pulse can be felt over arteries that lie close to the body surface and over a bone or firm surface that can support the artery when pressure is applied. The radial artery is palpated most frequently since it is the most accessible. The femoral and carotid arteries are used in cases of cardiac arrest to determine the adequacy of perfusion. It is important to note characteristics of peripheral pulses: 0 = absent; 1+ = weak; 2+ = normal; and 3+ = full and bounding.

Remember, the pulse is not always an accurate indication of the force of cardiac contractions. If cardiac contractions are weak or ventricular filling is incomplete, the pulse will be weak; however, in the case of aortic stenosis, the pulse may be weak in spite of forceful cardiac contraction.

RESPIRATION

Respiration is the process of bringing oxygen to the body and removing carbon dioxide. The lungs play a major role in this process. Their function is to maintain arterial blood homeostasis by maintaining the pH of the blood. The lungs accomplish this by the process of breathing.

Breathing consists of two phases, inspiration and expiration. Inspiration is an active process in which the diaphragm descends, the external intercostal muscles contract, and the chest expands to allow air to move into the tracheobronchial tree. Expiration is a passive process in which air flows out of the respiratory tree.

The respiratory center in the medulla of the brain and the level of carbon dioxide in the blood both control the rate and depth of respiration. Peripheral receptors in the carotid body and the aortic arch also respond to the level of oxygen in the blood. To some extent, respiration can be voluntarily controlled by breath holding and hyperventilation. Talking, laughing, and crying also affect respiration.

The diaphragm and the intercostal muscles are the main muscles used for breathing. Other accessory muscles, such as the abdominal muscles, the sternocleidomastoid, the trapezius, and the scalene, can be used to assist with respiration if necessary.

Evaluating Respiratory Rate   The quality of breathing is important baseline information. Normal respiration is effortless, quiet, automatic, and regular. When the breathing pattern varies from normal, it needs to be evaluated thoroughly. For example, bronchial sounds heard over the large airways are fairly loud. There is normally a pause between inspiration and expiration. Softer sounds are heard over the other lung areas, and there are no pauses between inspiration and expiration. If breathing is noisy, labored, or strained, an obstruction may be affecting the breathing pattern that could lead to major alterations in homeostasis.

In addition to evaluating the breathing pattern, it is also necessary to evaluate the rate and depth of respiration. Normal respiratory rate for a resting adult is 12 to 20 breaths per minute. The respiratory rate for infants ranges from 24 to 30 breaths per minute and is often irregular. Older children average about 20 to 26 breaths per minute. The ratio of pulse to respiration is usually 5:1 and remains fairly constant.

The depth of a person's respiration is the volume of air that moves in and out with each breath. The tidal volume is 500 cc in the healthy adult. Alveolar air is only partially replenished by atmospheric air with each inspiratory phase. Approximately 350 cc (tidal volume minus dead space) of new air is exchanged with the functional residual capacity volume during each respiratory cycle. Accurate tidal volume can be measured by a spirometer, but a nurse can judge the approximate depth by placing the back of the hand next to the client's nose and mouth and feeling the expired air. Another method of estimating volume capacity is to observe chest expansion and to check both sides of the thorax for symmetrical movement.

After assessing the pattern, type, and depth of respirations, it is important to observe the physical characteristics of chest expansion. The chest normally expands symmetrically without rib flaring or retractions. In addition, observation of chest deformities should also be made, as all of these signs yield information about the respiratory process and the overall health status of the client.

BLOOD PRESSURE

The heart generates pressure during the cardiac cycle to perfuse the organs of the body with blood. Blood flows from the heart to the arteries, into the capillaries and veins, and then reverses the cycle as it flows back to the heart. Blood pressure in the arterial system varies with the cardiac cycle, reaching the highest level at the peak of systole and the lowest level at the end of diastole. The difference between the systolic and diastolic blood pressure is the pulse pressure, which is normally 30 to 50 mm Hg.

Factors That Affect Blood Pressure

Cardiac Output   The force of heart contractions and the amount of blood ejected by the heart in one minute influences blood pressure, especially systolic pressure.

Peripheral Vascular Resistance   Resistance to the flow of blood is due to resistant vessels under the influence of the autonomic nervous system. Peripheral vascular resistance is the most important factor in diastolic pressure.

Elasticity and Distensibility of the Arteries   Elasticity refers to ability of the blood vessel walls to spring back after blood is ejected into them. When blood is ejected into the aorta and large arteries, the arterial vessel walls distend. Recoil during diastole propels blood through the arterial tree and maintains diastolic pressure. Distensibility decreases with age, resulting in decreased diastolic pressure and increased systolic pressure. Arteriosclerosis is an example of a condition that will increase blood pressure.

Blood Volume   Increased blood volume causes an increase in both systolic and diastolic blood pressure, whereas decreased blood volume causes the reverse effect. Hemorrhage will decrease blood pressure while over hydration or excessive blood transfusions cause an increase in blood pressure.

Blood Viscosity   Blood viscosity influences blood flow velocity through the arterial tree. For example, increased viscosity, which occurs with polycythemia, increases resistance to blood flow, whereas decreased viscosity, resulting from anemia, decreases resistance.

Chemicals Chemicals or drugs also have an important influence in blood pressure. For example, epinephrine and norepinephrine produce a profound vasoconstrictor effect on peripheral blood vessels. Other substances, such as aldosterone, released by the adrenal cortex, renin, released by the juxtaglomerular apparatus of the kidney, and histamine all produce effects which raise or lower the blood pressure.

Chemoreceptors Chemoreceptors in the aortic arch and carotid sinus also exert control over the blood pressure. They are sensitive to changes in PaO_2, $PaCO_2$ and pH. Decreased PaO_2 stimulates the chemoreceptors, which stimulate the vasomotor center. Increased $PaCO_2$ and decreased pH directly stimulate the vasomotor center, causing increased peripheral vascular resistance.

Measuring Blood Pressure Measuring blood pressure provides important information about the overall health status of the client. For example, the systolic pressure provides a data base about the condition of the heart, arteries and the arterioles. The diastolic pressure indicates vessel resistance. The pulse pressure, the difference between the systolic and diastolic pressure, provides information about cardiac output. A single blood pressure reading, however, does not provide adequate data from which conclusions can be drawn about all of these factors. Rather, a series of blood pressure readings should be taken to establish a baseline for further evaluation.

Normal blood pressure in an adult varies between 100 to 140 mm Hg systolic and 60 to 90 mm Hg diastolic. As blood moves toward smaller arteries and into arterioles, where it enters the capillaries, pressure falls to 35 mm Hg. It continues to fall as blood goes through the capillaries, where the flow is steady and not pulsatile. As blood moves into the venous system, pressure falls until it is the lowest in the venae cavae.

Blood pressure varies widely. A blood pressure of 100/60 mm Hg may be normal for one person but may be hypotensive for another. Hypotension (90 to 100 mm Hg systolic) in a healthy adult without other clinical symptoms is little reason for concern.

VITAL SIGN CHART FOR CHILDREN

AGE	RANGE OF NORMAL PULSE	(AVERAGE)	AVERAGE BLOOD PRESSURE	AVERAGE RESPIRATION
Newborn	70 – 170	120	80/45	40 – 90
1 year	80 – 160	115	90/60	20 – 40
2 years	80 – 130	110	95/60	20 – 30
4 years	80 – 120	100	99/65	20 – 25
6 years	75 – 115	100	100/56	20 – 25
8 years	70 – 110	90	105/56	15 – 20
10 years	70 – 110	90	110/58	15 – 20

GUIDELINES FOR MANAGING CLIENTS

Vital signs include four critical assessment areas: temperature, pulse, respiration, and blood pressure. The term vital is used because the information gathered is the clearest indicator of overall client status.

- These four signs form baseline evaluation data necessary for an on-going evaluation of a client's condition. If the nurse has established the normal range for a client, deviations will be more easily recognized.
- Routine vital signs are important to assess on every client and should be accomplished by a staff member who is familiar with the client's health history so results can be evaluated against previous data.
- Vital signs should be taken at consistent intervals. The more critical the client's condition, the more often these signs need to be taken and evaluated.
- Vital signs are not only indicators of a client's present condition but also cues to a positive or negative change in a client's status.

Obtaining the total picture of a client's health status is a main objective of client care. Although vital signs yield important information in themselves, they gain even more relevance when compared to the client's diagnosis, laboratory tests, history, and records.

- Temperature represents the balance between heat gain and heat loss and is regulated in the hypothalamus of the brain. Variations in temperature indicate the health status of the body; if hyperthermia is present due to pyrogens, nervous system disease, or injury, the thermostatic function may be out of balance.
- The pulse is an index of the heart's action, and by evaluating its rate, rhythm, and volume, one can gain an overall view of the heart's action.
- Respiration, the act of bringing oxygen into the body and removing carbon dioxide, yields data on the entire breathing process of a client. When the pattern of respiration is altered, on-going evaluation will yield important cues to a client's changing condition.
- Blood pressure readings provide information about the condition of the heart, the arteries and arterioles, vessel resistance, and the cardiac output. Serial readings provide the best indication of a client's cardiac status.

ACTION: DETERMINING CORE TEMPERATURE

ASSESSMENT

1 Determine which method is appropriate for obtaining temperature.
   a Oral method.
- Accurate method of determining body temperature.
- Used only for alert and cooperative clients.
- Not appropriate for use with clients requiring nasogastric, nasal, or oral intubation.

Rationale for Action
- To determine if core temperature is within normal range
- To provide baseline data for further evaluation
- To determine alterations in disease conditions

b Rectal method.
- Appropriate for uncooperative, confused, or comatose clients or for clients on seizure precautions.
- Used for clients receiving oxygen, unless contraindicated by illness or with nasal or oral intubation.
- Appropriate for clients with wired jaws, facial fractures, or other abnormalities, or for clients with nasogastric intubation.
- Contraindicated for clients who have had abdominal peritoneal resection or hemorrhoidectomy.

c Axillary method.
- Either rectal or oral thermometer used depending on hospital policy.
- Not accurate for adults.
- Used with infants in a controlled environment.

d Electronic thermometer.
- Most accurate.
- Prevents infection.
- Use when available.

2 Determine number of times temperature needs to be taken daily.
3 Compare temperature with other vital signs to establish baseline data.

▶ Fever may be normal for first day or two after surgery, for second or third day after a myocardial infarction, and after a CVA.

PLANNING

GOALS

- Baseline data established with consistent recording of core temperatures.
- Body function is evaluated.
- Alterations in temperature are identified early.

EQUIPMENT

- Rectal or oral glass mercury thermometer
- Digital thermometer probe
- Tissues
- Lubricant on a paper wipe for rectal method

INTERVENTION: Taking an Oral Temperature

1 Wash your hands.
2 Rinse thermometer in cold water if kept in a chemical solution, and wipe dry with tissue.
3 Grasp thermometer with thumb and forefinger and shake vigorously by flicking wrist in downward motion to lower mercury level.
4 Check temperature reading on thermometer.
5 Explain procedure to client.
6 Place thermometer in client's mouth under tongue and ask client to hold lips closed.
7 Leave in place 3 to 5 minutes if using glass mercury thermometer.

Comparison of thermometers calibrated to Fahrenheit and Centigrade.

8　Remove thermometer and wipe it with tissue from fingers down to bulb. Discard tissue.

9　Read temperature by rotating thermometer until mercury level is clearly visible. Shake thermometer down and replace in container.

10　Wash hands.

11　Record client's temperature according to hospital procedure.

INTERVENTION: Taking a Rectal Temperature

1　Wash your hands.

2　Rinse thermometer in cold water if kept in a chemical solution, and wipe dry with tissue.

3　Grasp thermometer with thumb and forefinger and shake vigorously, flicking wrist in downward motion, to lower mercury level.

4　Check temperature reading on thermometer.

5　Explain to client what you intend to do.

6　Lubricate tip of thermometer with lubricant on a paper wipe.

7　Provide privacy; instruct and assist client to turn on side with knees slightly flexed.

8　Fold back bed linen to expose client's buttocks.

9　Separate buttocks with left hand so anal opening is visible.

10　Insert thermometer into rectum approximately 3.5 cm (1½ inches).

11　Leave in place about three minutes with client resting. Hold in place if client expels thermometer.

12　Remove thermometer and wipe it with tissue from fingers down to bulb. Discard tissue.

13　Read temperature by rotating thermometer until mercury level is clearly visible, shake thermometer down.

14　Assist client to a comfortable position.

15　Wash thermometer in warm, soapy water, rinse, and put away.

16　Wash your hands.

17　Record client's temperature according to hospital procedure.

INTERVENTION: Taking an Axillary Temperature

1　Wash your hands.

2　Rinse thermometer in cold water if kept in a chemical solution, and wipe dry with tissue.

3　Grasp thermometer with thumb and forefinger and shake vigorously, flicking wrist in downward motion, to lower mercury level.

4   Check temperature reading on thermometer.
5   Explain to client what you intend to do.
6   Assist client to a comfortable position and expose axilla.
7   Place thermometer (usually oral) in axilla and fold down client's arm across the chest.
8   Leave in place 5 to 8 minutes.
9   Remove thermometer and wipe it with tissue from fingers down to bulb. Discard tissue.
10 Read temperature by rotating thermometer until mercury level is clearly visible, shake down, and replace in container.
11 Assist client to a comfortable position.
12 Wash your hands.
13 Record client's temperature according to hospital procedure.

INTERVENTION: Using an Electronic Thermometer

1   Remove thermometer from charger unit.
2   Place carrying strap around your neck.
3   Grasp probe at the top of the stem using your thumb and forefinger. Do not put pressure on the top because it is the ejection button.
4   Firmly insert probe into disposable probe cover.
5   Slide probe under front of client's tongue and along the gum line to the sublingual pocket at the base of the tongue.
6   For oral temperature instruct client to close lips. Lips should close at the rise of the probe cover.
7   For rectal temperature, position client on side, separate buttocks and insert probe 1.2 cm. Tissue contact is ensured when probe is positioned to the side of the anus.
8   Remove probe when audible signal occurs. Client's temperature is now registered on the dial.
9   Discard probe cover into trash by pushing ejection button.
10 Record temperature and then return probe to storage well.
11 Return thermometer unit to charging base. Ensure charging base is plugged into electrical outlet.

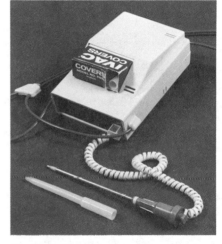

Electronic thermometer and carrying strap. When taking temperature place individual cover over probe.

EVALUATION

EXPECTED OUTCOME

Temperature is within normal range. *If not,* follow these alternative nursing actions:

ANA: Recheck temperature with new thermometer as occasionally thermometers are inaccurate.

ANA: Check intake and output for possible dehydration, and increase fluid intake unless contraindicated (i.e., in congestive heart failure, cardiogenic shock, or increased intracranial pressure).

ANA: Apply tepid sponges.

ANA: Decrease room temperature and remove excess covers.

ANA: If ASA or Acetaminophen ordered, give one dose as an antipyretic.

▶   For rectal temps—use red colored probe.

151

▶ Fever is any abnormal elevation of body temperature. The most common signs and symptoms are:
- Perspiration over body surface
- Body warm to the touch
- Chills and shivers
- Flushed face
- Client complains of feeling cold alternately with feeling hot
- Increased pulse and respirations
- Complaints of malaise and fatigue
- Parched lips and dry skin
- Convulsions, especially with children

Charting
- Record temperature, core and surface skin temperature
- Result of cooling measures for fever or warming measures for hypothermia
- Changes in pulse and respirations with fever or hypothermia and result of nursing measures
- Record skin discoloration with hypothermia

UNEXPECTED OUTCOMES

1 Fever develops.
   ANA: Check possible sources of infection, and take preventative measures.
   a Wounds: Adhere to strict aseptic technique in changing dressings.
   b Pulmonary: Encourage deep breathing and coughing; maintain a patent airway and adequate hydration of bedridden, inactive, or postoperative clients; encourage early ambulation after surgery.
   c Urinary: Avoid catheterization if possible. Use strict aseptic technique if catheterization is necessary.
   d Thrombophlebitis: Encourage active leg exercises, use of antiembolic stockings or Ace bandages, and early ambulation.
2 Despite initial cooling measure, temperature remains elevated because of destruction of hypothalamus from brain disease or injury.
   ANA: Request cooling blanket order from physician.
   ANA: Continue to administer antipyretic drugs.
3 Temperature remains elevated because of bacterial produced pyrogens.
   ANA: Request physician's order to culture possible sources of infection and the organism's sensitivity to antibiotic therapy.
   ANA: Request physician's order for tepid sponge bath.
4 Hypothermia occurs.
   a Medically induced to decrease oxygen requirements for surgery or GI hemorrhage or as a result of cold operating rooms.
   ANA: Apply warm blankets upon return from surgery.
   ANA: Maintain adequate hydration since blood vessels will dilate when body warms up and blood pressure could drop with vasodilation.
   b Accidental exposure to cold.
   ANA: Maintain patent airway as gag reflex may be weak or absent.
   ANA: Check skin for discoloration.
   ANA: Apply wet heat at 110° F (43.3° C) to warm client adequately since blood supply may not be adequate.
   c Ventricular fibrillation from hypothermia.
   ANA: Defibrillation as per order.
   d Frostbite.
   ANA: Thaw affected areas immediately with 110° F (43.3° C) water to prevent permanent damage.

ACTION: TAKING THE PULSE RATE

ASSESSMENT

1 Assess appropriate site to obtain pulse.
2 Check pulse whenever client's status changes.
3 Take an apical-radial pulse on clients with irregular rhythms or those on heart medications.

4 Obtain baseline peripheral pulses in any client going for cardiac or vascular surgery or medical clients with diabetes, arterial occlusive diseases such as Raynaud's or Buerger's disease, atherosclerosis, or aneurysm.

PLANNING

GOALS

- Heart rate or number of times the heart beats per minute is determined. The heart rhythm, volume, and quality is determined.
- Blood flow to all parts of the body is ascertained — all pulses are present.
- Pulse rate is evaluated in relation to other vital signs and interrelationship is consistent.

EQUIPMENT

- Watch with sweep second hand
- Felt pen
- Stethoscope
- Sphygmomanometer

Rationale for Action

- To determine if the pulse rate is within the normal range and if rhythm is regular
- To evaluate the equality of corresponding arterial pulses
- To monitor and evaluate the amplitude and contour of the pulse wave and the arteries' elasticity
- To monitor and evaluate changes in the client's status
- To reflect the function of vital organs

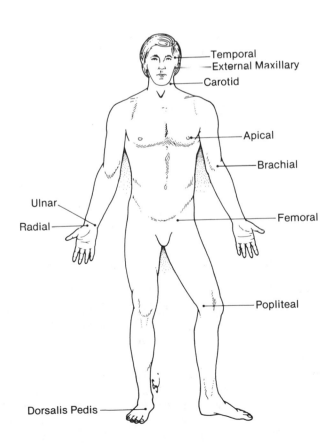

Temporal
External Maxillary
Carotid
Apical
Brachial
Ulnar
Radial
Femoral
Popliteal
Dorsalis Pedis

Radial artery most common site for palpating pulse. Other pulse sites are identified.

▶ Peripheral pulses may be absent or weak. The size (amplitude) of a pulse depends on the degree of filling of the artery during systole (ventricular contraction) and of emptying during diastole (ventricular relaxation). The size of a pulse is described as being large or small and measures the pulse pressure (the difference between systolic and diastolic pressure). The type (contour) of pulse felt by the fingers depends on how fast the pulse pressure changes and is described as being quick or prolonged.

▶ Mark location where peripheral pulses are found with a felt pen to assist other health care members in easily detecting pulses.

153

The pulse should be taken every one to two hours on an acutely ill hospitalized client and less frequently (every 4 to 8 hours) on more stable hospitalized clients. Once a day is adequate for clients in long term care facilities. Do not wait until the next routine schedule if the client develops unexpected symptoms.

Clinical Alert

When the carotid pulse is palpated, take care not to exert too much pressure as this could stimulate a vagal response and slow the heart rate. Palpate only one side at a time.

INTERVENTION: Taking the Pulse Rate

1 Gather equipment.
2 Wash your hands.
3 Check client's name and identification band.
4 Take pulse rate with routine vital signs.
5 Place client in a reclining position with the trunk of the body at a 30 degree angle.
6 Palpate arteries by using pads of the middle three fingers of your hand. Press the artery against the bone or underlying firm surface to occlude vessel and then gradually release pressure.
7 Count the pulse rate.
  a When taking a radial pulse, count the pulse rate for 30 seconds and multiply by two for a minute rate if the rhythm is regular.
  b When taking an apical pulse, or if the radial pulse rate is irregular, count the rate for one minute. Determine if there is a pattern to the irregularity or if it is chaotically irregular.
  c When the rhythm is irregular, auscultate the apical pulse and palpate the radial pulse simultaneously to note a pulse deficit. To auscultate the apical pulse, place a stethoscope over the apex of the heart. The apex is normally located in the fifth intercostal space left of the sternum in the midclavicular line.
  d Assess pulse volume by feeling the pressure of the beat.
8 Palpate the radial and pedal pulses simultaneously to determine if the pulses arrive without delay.
9 Check to see that client is comfortable.
10 Record pulse rate, rhythm, pattern, and volume.

EVALUATION

EXPECTED OUTCOMES

1 Pulse rate is within normal range, and rhythm is regular. *If not,* follow these alternative nursing actions:
  ANA: Repeat procedure and/or validate findings with R.N. before reporting to physician.
  ANA: Identify alteration in normal range and rhythm.
    a Presence of arrhythmias (tachycardia, bradycardia, etc.)
    b Absent or weak peripheral pulses.
    c Atrial fibrillation.
    d Sinus arrhythmias.
  ANA: Complete ANA's suggested in Unexpected Outcomes.
2 All peripheral pulses are equal in amplitude and contour when compared with the corresponding pulse on the other side and when compared to the next proximal site. *If not,* follow these alternative nursing actions:
  ANA: Vary site slightly and change the amount of finger pressure because pressure can obliterate the pulse. In the absence of other symptoms, a weak or absent pulse should not be considered a sign of vascular problems.

fluids, volume expanders, or blood as ordered by physician and assess response.

ANA: For hypotension take vital signs more frequently (every 15 minutes to 2 hours) until condition has stabilized.

ANA: If cardiac output is decreased due to myocardial infarction or cardiomyopathy, raise the legs, decrease peripheral resistance with vasodilators as ordered by physician, replace fluid as needed, and increase contractility with appropriate drugs as ordered. If accompanied by pain, relieve with reassurance, analgesia, oxygen, and rest. Assess response, vital signs, and mental status frequently.

ANA: Although vasodilation following surgery is normal, look for signs of hemorrhage, and notify physician if blood pressure continues to fall.

ANA: If fear or grief is the cause, allow client to ventilate his or her feelings. Spend enough quality time with client to enable him or her to "talk through" fears.

ANA: For clients with trigeminal pain, administer analgesia when necessary and assess response.

ANA: For clients with septic shock, maintain high suspicions for susceptible clients. Assess mental status and warmth of skin. Notify physician, and administer antibiotics and oxygen. Evaluate respiratory status and assess response to treatment.

ANA: For clients with cardiac tamponade, notify physician immediately. Reassure client and prepare for emergency pericardiocentesis.

ANA: For clients with cardiac arrhythmias, determine origin of arrhythmia and treat with proper drug, precordial thump, emergency cardioversion, or defibrillation.

2 Hypertension (blood pressure consistently over 140/90 mm Hg).

ANA: For clients with severe hypertension take vital signs more frequently (every 15 minutes to 2 hours) until condition has stabilized.

ANA: If client is anxious or excited, institute relaxation techniques to lower blood pressure.

ANA: Allow client to rest after strenuous exercise.

ANA: Relieve pain with reassurance, change of position, and analgesia as ordered by physician.

ANA: For clients with essential hypertension, administer antihypertensive and diuretic drugs as ordered by physician. Evaluate response by checking blood pressure in reclining, sitting, and standing position. Instruct client in diet therapy such as low-salt, low-fat and inclusion of vitamins and garlic.

ANA: For clients with hypoxia, relieve with oxygen administration in whichever mode is most effective.

ANA: For clients with kidney disease, assist client in adapting to long term dialysis or transplant. Give assistance with dietary restrictions. Assess response to medical treatment.

ANA: Check pulses in lower extremities. If reduced or delayed, check blood pressure in legs. Apply wider cuff around lower third of

▶ Routinely, the blood pressure for an acutely ill client should be taken every 1 to 2 hours, and the blood pressure of more stabilized clients should be taken every 4 to 8 hours. Clients with severe hypotension or hypertension, with low blood volume, or on vasoconstrictor or vasodilator drugs require checking every 5 to 15 minutes.

▶ In persons with hypertension, an auscultatory gap may be present. This gap is an absence of sounds after the first Korotkow's sounds appear and then the reappearance of the sounds at a lower level. This condition can be avoided if the brachial artery is palpated first and the cuff is inflated above the level where the pulsations disappear.

161

the thigh and apply stethoscope over popliteal artery. Normally pressure is higher in the legs but is lower with coarctation of the aorta. If thigh is too large, wrap cuff around calf and palpate dorsalis pedis or posterior tibial pulse.

ANA: For clients with polycythemia, treat cause as directed. Prepare for possible phlebotomy.

ANA: For clients with endocrine disorders, instruct client in possible diagnostic studies, and prepare for surgery.

ANA: For clients with anemia, administer medications and blood products as ordered by physician.

ANA: For clients with hyperthyroidism, provide rest from external stimuli, and administer medications as ordered by physician.

ANA: For clients with aortic insufficiency and atherosclerosis, follow medical treatment. Surgery may be a possibility so prepare for adequate preoperative instruction.

ANA: For clients with increased intracranial pressure, check for other signs such as changes in consciousness, movement (hemiparesis, positive Babinski reflex), change in pupillary response, inequality of pupils, or pupil size. Notify physician at once and follow orders.

ANA: For fluid overload, restrict fluids and administer diuretics as ordered. Observe rate of all IV fluids.

Charting

- Systolic blood pressure
- Diastolic blood pressure
- Level of muffled Korotkow's sounds and their disappearance (for example: 126/80/72 mm Hg)
- Response to alternative nursing actions
- Presence of pulsus paradoxus or pulsus alternans

TERMINOLOGY

Types of Respirations

apnea Absence of breathing.

Biot's Abrupt interruptions or pauses between a faster than normal and deeper respiratory rate.

bradypnea Slow, regular respirations. Rate is below 10 per minute.

Cheyne-Stokes Periods of apnea appear throughout cycle. Respirations become deeper and faster than normal followed by a slower rate and progressing to periods of apnea lasting up to 60 seconds.

hyperpnea Deep respirations at a normal rate.

tachypnea Respiratory rate increased above 20 breaths per minute. Rate remains regular in pattern.

Types of Pulses

normal pulse Pulse pressure is about 30 to 40 mm Hg. It is smooth and rounded and is felt as a sharp upstroke and gradual downstroke.

small, weak pulse Pulse pressure is diminished. It is smooth and rounded but is felt as a gradual upstroke and prolonged downstroke. It is commonly seen in conditions resulting in decreased cardiac output, such as heart failure and shock, and with obstruction to left ventricular ejection, such as aortic stenosis.

large, bounding pulse Pulse pressure is increased. It is felt as a slapping against the fingers because of the rapid upstroke and quick downstroke. It is seen in conditions of increased cardiac output, such as exercise, anxiety, alcoholic intake, and pregnancy. It is also noted in pathology with fever, anemia, hyperthyroidism, liver failure, complete heart block with bradycardia, and hypertension. When there is a rapid runoff of blood, such as with aortic insufficiency ("water-hammer" pulse) and patent ductus arteriosus, this type of pulse is characteristic. Increased rigidity in the aorta, which occurs with aging and arteriosclerosis, also causes this type of pulse.

bigeminal pulse Pulse occurs with premature beats and is a disturbance in rhythm. The premature beat decreases the stroke volume for that beat and so is weaker than the normal beat.

pulsus alternans Rhythm is regular but the amplitude alternates from beat to beat.

pulsus paradoxus Pulse diminishes in amplitude with inspiration because more blood remains in the lungs. The resulting increased negative thoracic pressure provides less return to the left ventricle and decreases stroke volume. This condition is really an exaggeration of what normally occurs during the respiratory cycle.

sinus arrhythmia Common in children and young adults. The heart rate accelerates with inspiration and slows with expiration.

premature beats A pacemaker outside the sinus node fires earlier than the sinus node, the normal pacemaker of the heart. Since the beat is early, the stroke volume is less because the ventricles do not have time to fill. This condition causes a pause in rhythm, which may result in a pulse deficit. A pulse deficit occurs when the heart rate counted at the apex by auscultation is greater than the heart rate counted by palpation of the radial pulse. The pulse wave is not transmitted to the periphery to produce a palpable radial pulse.

atrial fibrillation A chaotically irregular pulse rate with a pulse deficit.

CHAPTER 6
Completing Physical Assessment

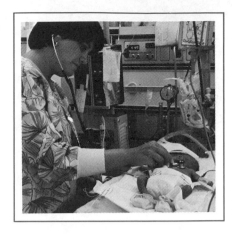

This chapter outlines the techniques of physical assessment, the first step in the nursing process. It also includes information about charting and obtaining a health history.

Because assessments are often conducted rapidly, in situations where many other activities are occurring, they need to be practical and methodical.

ASSESSMENT TECHNIQUES

An assessment technique is practical if it can be accomplished easily, with minimal equipment. The techniques discussed in this chapter can be performed in less than ten minutes, using a stethoscope, flashlight, your hands and observational skills. Although you may not be able to perform assessments rapidly at first, you will have many opportunities to practice your skills since every client needs to be assessed at least once during a shift.

The four phases of assessment are inspection, auscultation, palpation, and percussion. Inspection is an overview of the client. While interviewing the client, observe such characteristics as hair, skin, general posture and psychosocial behavior; in other words, the general appearance of the client. Auscultation is accomplished by using a stethoscope to listen to respiratory, heart, and bowel sounds. Palpation and percussion are performed using fingers and hands to assess abnormalities of sound such as vocal fremitus, enlarged organs, organ displacement, and expansion of the chest or abdomen.

LEARNING OBJECTIVES

Describe the client's clinical condition by performing a physical assessment.
List the four phases of physical assessment.
Outline the essential elements obtained from a health history.
Describe abnormal manifestations associated with each specific body system for one client you are caring for.
List at least five essential elements included in a mental status assessment.
Compare and contrast the commonalities and dissimilarities in at least three selected religious groups.
List the assessment modalities in each stage of pregnancy.
Identify client learning needs and outline prenatal class content.
List the characteristics observed in a newborn assessment which are pertinent to the newborn.
Identify major abnormalities in the pediatric client when an altered health status occurs.

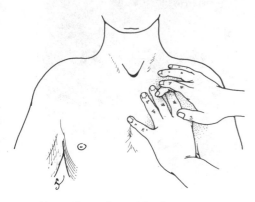

Use entire surface of five fingers when percussing for abnormalities.

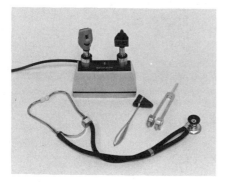

Instruments used to complete a physical assessment: stethoscope, ophthalmoscope, otoscope, percussion hammer, and tuning fork.

As you conduct the assessment, use your hands for palpation. Using the proper technique will provide you with more complete findings and cause minimal discomfort to the client. When palpating an area, use the entire surface of all five fingers. Apply pressure slowly but firmly. Sudden pressure or probing with one finger may cause discomfort or cause the client to tense the area you are palpating.

The two basic physical assessment formats are head-to-toe and body systems. This chapter recommends a modified systems approach. You start at the client's head and examine the client's body as you move from head to toe.

To ensure that your assessment is methodical, follow the same format each time. It is not important which of the several formats you choose, only that you follow the same one consistently.

Types of Equipment The primary instrument used during assessment is the stethoscope. As you use this instrument, remember that any movement, such as moving your fingers on the chest piece or tubing or moving the chest piece on the skin, can cause extraneous noise that obliterates the sounds you want to hear.

All stethoscopes consist of earpieces, tubing, and a head, which contains a bell chest piece and a diaphragm chest piece. Ear pieces should shut out extraneous noise without causing discomfort. The tubing should be no longer than 38 cm in length, or part of the sound will be lost during transmission. The diaphragm piece should be applied firmly to the skin. The bell piece should be placed on the skin very lightly to pick up low-pitched sounds such as heart murmurs. If the bell is pressed firmly, it stretches the skin and acts like a diaphragm.

Another instrument, the flashlight, is needed during the neurological examination and for viewing the oral cavity. The tuning fork, ophthalmoscope, and otoscope are needed when a more complete physical assessment is required.

HEALTH HISTORY

A total physical assessment should include a health history. The client's past health conditions, current problems, and present needs should be clearly identified in this process. Past experiences with the health care delivery system, perceptions of illness, and concepts regarding health in general can also be included.

Information obtained from the interview and the physical assessment comprises the basis for establishing the individualized nursing care plan. A complete health history includes the following elements:

- *Biographical information*: age, sex, whether client is a good historian.
- *Chief complaint*: condition that brought client to health care facility.
- *Present health status or illness*: onset of the problem; clinical manifestations, including severity of symptoms; pain characteristics if present; and factors that aggravate or improve the condition.
- *Health history*: general state of health, past illnesses, surgeries, hos-

pitalizations, allergies, current medications, general habits such as smoking or consuming alcohol.

- *Family history*: age and health status of parents, siblings, and children; cause of death for immediate family members; history of diseases found in family members.
- *Psychosocial factors, lifestyles*: cultural beliefs that influence health management; religious or spiritual beliefs.
- *Nutrition*: dietary habits, preferences, or restrictions.

A complete physical assessment follows the health interview and all the information is compiled into a written record. This becomes part of the client's chart, a legal document. The recorded data also serves as a baseline for determining, evaluating, and changing therapy for the client. Charting must be objective, concise, and specific in order to be an effective tool for client care.

NEUROLOGICAL ASSESSMENT

The neurological examination is begun with the initial contact with the client. Evaluation of verbal responses, movement, and sensation are carried out throughout the examination. In addition, a general assessment of the function of the cerebrum, cerebellum, cranial nerves, spinal cord, and peripheral nerves is done. The level of consciousness is the most sensitive and reliable index of cerebral function.

Glasgow Coma Scale

Eyes Open
4 opens eyes spontaneously
3 opens eyes in response to speech
2 opens eyes in response to pain
1 does not open eyes to painful stimuli

Verbal Response
5 oriented to person, place, and time
4 not oriented but is able to converse
3 words and phrases make little or no sense
2 responds with incomprehensible sounds
1 nonresponsive verbally

Motor Response
5 obeys commands appropriately
4 purposefully removes painful stimuli
3 flexes arm, nonpurposely, to pain
2 extends elbows and internally rotates wrists, nonpurposely, in response to pain
1 no motor response

Scoring
Normal response:	14 points
Comatose state:	7 or less
Indicative of brain death:	3 (lowest possible score)

ASSESSMENT	NORMAL	ABNORMAL
LEVEL OF CONSCIOUSNESS		
Evaluate **verbal responses** If client seems awake and alert but does not respond properly, check to see if client is blind, deaf, or speaks another language	Alert Restless Responds to verbal command Answers questions appropriately Speaks clearly Oriented to time, person, place	Lethargic Drowsy Hard to awaken Unable to give date, month, place Irritable Does not recognize family Does not respond to own name
Observe and test **motor responses** on both sides of body	Eyes open Ability to stick out tongue, squeeze fingers, move extremities	Eyes closed Does not follow directions to stick out tongue, squeeze fingers, or move extremities

ASSESSMENT	NORMAL	ABNORMAL
Exert pressure on nailbed with pen Apply pressure to supraorbital notch Pinch ear lobes or between big toe and second toe	Responds to painful stimuli by reaching out or trying to stop pressure	Does not respond to painful stimuli Assumes *decorticate posturing* (legs extended; feet extended with plantar flexion; arms internally rotated and flexed on chest): due to lesion of corticospinal tract near cerebral hemisphere Assumes *decerebrate posturing* (arms stiffly extended and hands turned outward and flexed; legs extended with plantar flexion): may be due to lesion in diencephalon, pons, or midbrain Assumes *flaccid posturing* (no motor response): may be due to extreme brain injury to motor area of brain

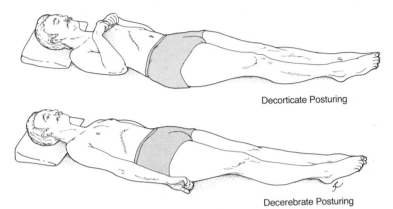

Decorticate Posturing

Decerebrate Posturing

Decorticate and Decerebrate posturing.

Involuntary movements

choreiform (jerky and quick): present in Sydenham's chorea
athetoid (twisting and slow): present in cerebral palsy
tremors: hyperthyroid, cerebellar ataxia, parkinsonism
spasms: cord injured clients
convulsions: epilepsy, heat stroke
asterixis: liver disease, uremia

PUPIL ASSESSMENT

Observe **appearance of pupils** by holding eyelids open and checking for:		
Size of pupils	Diameter: 1.5 to 6 mm	Unilateral dilation: sign of third cranial nerve involvement Bilateral dilation: sign of upper brainstem damage Dilated and nonreactive: sign of increased intracranial pressure or ipsilateral oculomotor nerve compression from tumor or injury
Shape of pupils	Round and midposition	Midposition and fixed: sign of midbrain involvement Pinpoint and fixed: sign of pontine involvement
Equality of pupils	Equal	Unequal: sign that parasympathetic and sympathetic nervous systems are not in synchronization
Observe **reaction to light** by using pen light in darkened room Open eyelid being tested; cover opposite eye Move light toward client's eye from side position	Pupil constricts promptly	Sluggish reaction: early warning of deteriorating condition Light reflex is the most important sign differentiating structural from metabolic coma

ASSESSMENT	NORMAL	ABNORMAL
Observe consensual **light reflex** Hold both eyelids open Shine light into one eye only Observe opposite eye	Pupil constricts	Pupil does not constrict: sign that connection between brainstem and pupils is not intact

MOTOR FUNCTION

ASSESSMENT	NORMAL	ABNORMAL
Assess **muscle strength** Test hand grip by asking client to squeeze your fingers		Absence of motor function: may be sign of hemiplegia (paralysis of one side of the body); paraplegia (paralysis of the legs and/or lower part of the body); quadriplegia (paralysis of arms and legs)
Test arm strength by asking client to close eyes and hold arms out in front with palms up	Maintain position for 20 to 30 seconds	Inability to maintain position with both arms: possible sign of hemiplegia
Assess **flexion** and **extension** strength in extremities Stand in front of client, place your hand in front of client, and ask client to push your hand away	Equal response in both arms	
Place your hand on client's forearm and ask client to pull his or her arm upward		
Position client's leg with knee flexed and foot resting on bed; as you try to extend leg, ask client to keep his or her foot down	Equal response in both legs	
Place one hand on client's knee and one hand on client's ankle; ask client to straighten his or her leg as you apply resistant force to knee and ankle		
Assess **muscle tone** Flex and extend client's upper extremities to assess how well client resists your movements	Client resistance is apparent	Increased resistance: sign of increased muscle tone from muscle rigidity or spasticity Increased in UMN lesions and parkinsonism Decreased resistance: sign of decreased muscle tone from flaccidity Decreased in LMN and cerebellar lesion
Flex and extend client's lower extremities to assess resistance		
Assess **coordination** *Hand coordination* Ask client to pat both thighs as rapidly as he or she can	Client able to perform coordinated movements upon request	Uncoordinated movements: may be due to cerebellum or basal ganglia involvement

ASSESSMENT	NORMAL	ABNORMAL
Ask client to turn his or her hands over and back in quick succession		
Ask client to touch each finger to his or her thumb in rapid succession — repeat with other hand		
Foot coordination		
Place your hands close to client's feet		
Ask client to tap your hands alternately with the balls of his or her feet		
Hand positioning coordination		
With client's eyes open, extend your hand in front of client's face		
Ask client to touch his or her nose with index finger several times in rapid succession		
Repeat test with client's eyes closed		Inability to perform task with eyes closed: may be due to loss of positioning sense
Leg positioning coordination		
Ask client to put heel on opposite knee and to slide heel down leg to foot		
Assess **reflexes**		
Blink reflex		
Hold client's eyelid open	Eyes close immediately	Absence of blink response; eyelid continuously in open position: due to fifth or seventh cranial nerve not being intact
Approach client's eye unexpectedly from side of head or brush client's eyelashes		
Gag and swallow reflex		
Open client's mouth and hold tongue down with tongue blade		Absense of gag and swallow reflex; inability to swallow food or liquid: due to ninth or tenth cranial nerve not intact
Touch back of pharynx on each side with applicator stick		
Plantar response (Babinski reflex)		
Run top of pen along outer lateral aspect from heel to little toe of client's foot	Flexion of toes	Great toe dorsiflexes; other toes fan: due to upper motor neuron lesion
Continue tracing a line across ball of foot toward great toe		

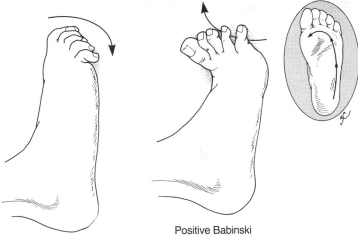

Negative Babinski

Positive Babinski

Negative and positive Babinski response.

ASSESSMENT	NORMAL	ABNORMAL
Deep tendon reflex		
Ask client to relax	Biceps reflex: flexion at elbow and contracting of biceps muscle	Absent or diminished: sign of C^5 or C^6 injury
Position limb to be assessed so that muscle is somewhat stretched		
Using reflex hammer, strike tendon quickly while applying additional tendon stretch	Triceps reflex: extension at elbow and contraction of triceps muscle	Absent or diminished: C^7 or C^8 injury
Assess according to scale	Knee reflex: extension of knee and contraction of quadriceps	Absent or diminished: C^2, C^3 or C^4 injury

Grading Scale

4+   Hyperactive (indicative of disease state)
3+   More brisk than usual but not indicative of disease state
2+   Average/normal
1+   Slightly diminished, low normal
0   No response

SENSORY FUNCTION

Assess **superficial sensations**

Pain

Ask client to close eyes	Ability to distinguish between sharp and dull sensations	Alterations in pain or temperature sensations: indicate lesion in posterior horn of spinal cord or spinothalamic tract of cord
Stroke skin with safety pin, alternating blunt end and sharp end of pin		
Ask client to distinguish sharp and dull pain		

ASSESSMENT	NORMAL	ABNORMAL
Temperature		
Fill two test tubes with water, one hot, one cold	Ability to distinguish between hot and cold	
Ask client to close eyes and touch client's skin with test tubes		
Touch		
Ask client to close eyes		
Stroke cotton wisp over client's skin	Ability to identify light touch	
Positioning		
Ask client to close eyes		
Grasp client's finger with your thumb and index finger	Ability to identify position	
Move client's finger up and down		
Ask client to identify direction finger is moving		Inability to determine direction of movement: may be due to loss or injury of position sense
VITAL SIGNS		
Assess rate and quality of **respirations**	Regular rate: 12 to 20	Cheyne-Stokes (rhythmic rising and falling of depth of respiration): may be due to deep cerebral or cerebellar lesion
		Central neurogenic hyperventilation
		Apneustic
		Cluster breathing
		Ataxis
Monitor **arterial blood gases** if signs of respiratory imbalances occur	pH: 7.35 to 7.45 pCO_2: 35 to 45 mm Hg HCO_3: 22 to 26 mEq/l	Alterations in pH and pCO_2 values: indicate respiratory imbalances
		pH below 7.35 and pCO_2 above 45: signs of acidosis
		pH above 7.45 and pCO_2 below 35: sign of alkalosis
		HCO_3 altered: indicates compensation
Assess **temperature**	Ability to maintain normal body temperature (approximately 98.6° F)	Inability to maintain normal temperature: may be due to damage to hypothalamus
If client is semi-comatose or comatose, take temperature rectally		No sweating below level of injury: due to spinal cord injury
If rectal temperature contra-indicated or if there are signs of increased intracranial pressure, take axillary temperature		Hypothermia

ASSESSMENT	NORMAL	ABNORMAL
Assess pulse Observe character of pulse Observe pulse rate	Regular rhythm (rate: 60 to 100)	Premature beats: may be due to hypoxia Slow pulse rate with accompanying widening pulse pressure and bradypnea: sign of increased intracranial pressure
Assess blood pressure Position neurological clients in low to semi-Fowler's position	Normal pressure (range 120/80 to 140/90)	Systolic blood pressure rises with diastolic pressure remaining same: sign of increased intracranial pressure Blood pressure over 140/90: sign of hypertension Blood pressure below 95/60: sign of hypotension

ASSESSMENT OF SKIN

The skin is the body's first line of defense against disease and injury. It is made up of three layers: the epidermis, the dermis, and the subcutaneous tissues.

The epidermis is divided into two avascular, or bloodless, layers: an outer layer that consists of dead keratinized cells and an inner layer that consists of live cells where keratin and melanin are formed. The dermis contains blood vessels, connective tissue, sebaceous glands and some of the hair follicles. The subcutaneous tissues contain the remainder of the hair follicles, fat, and the sweat glands.

Hair, nails, sweat glands, and sebaceous glands are appendages of the skin. There are two types of sweat glands: eccrine and apocrine. Eccrine glands are distributed over most of the body except for the palms and soles. These glands help control body temperature through their sweat production. The apocrine glands are found mainly in the axillary and genital areas and are stimulated by emotional stress. The decomposition of secretions in these glands causes body odor.

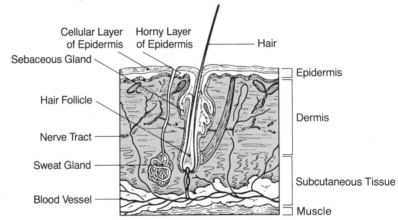

Skin is the first line of defense against disease and injury.

ASSESSMENT	NORMAL	ABNORMAL
Note **color** of the skin by assessing the oral mucous membranes, the conjunctiva, and the nail beds	Pink, tan, or brown, depending on the client's basic skin color	Decrease in color or pallor *Example*: anemia from acute blood loss (hemorrhage), renal failure, dietary deficiencies, or peripheral vascular disorders Vasoconstriction due to smoking, fear, or anger Jaundice (icterus): due to the presence of conjugated or unconjugated bilirubin in the blood and tissues; appears most frequently in the face and trunk; seen best under natural light

173

ASSESSMENT	NORMAL	ABNORMAL
		Cyanosis (blue, bluegray, or purple discoloration of the skin and mucous membranes): caused by hypoxia, a result of an increased amount of reduced hemoglobin
		Peripheral: seen in nail beds and earlobes
		Example: anxiety or hypothermia
		Central: seen in nail beds, lips (circumoral) and oral mucosa
		Erythema (redness of the skin): caused by capillary congestion; occurs with inflammation or infection; usually a local finding
Note **pigmentation**		Hyperpigmentation
		Example: use of oral contraceptives, pregnancy, Addison's disease, and hyperthyroidism
Note **turgor** and **mobility**	Smooth and elastic	Tight or stretched and difficult to move: due to local or generalized edema
Pinch skin on an extremity If the fold persists, skin turgor is poor	Resilient and supple	Wrinkled: due to dehydration caused by rapid weight loss; appears as folds of skin on upper arms or abdomen
		Thin and translucent (parchment)
		Example: chronic steroid use
		Thin, shiny, and smooth with alopecia on lower extremities
		Example: chronic arterial insufficiency
Press finger into skin on ankle bone; grade amount of fluid from 1 to 4+	Resilient and no evidence of fluid retention	Pitting edema: excess intracellular fluid
		Example: congestive heart failure, renal failure, cirrhosis of the liver
Note **moistness** and **temperature** of the skin	Warm and dry	Warm (hot) and moist due to hyperthermia
		Cool and moist (cold and clammy): may be due to shock states
		Abnormally dry: may be due to dehydration, decreased sebaceous gland secretions, or the excessive use of soap
Assess for **sensation** — response to external stimuli	Feels touch, sensitive to heat and cold and pressure	Absence of touch or pain sensation
		Example: spinal cord injury or nerve damage
		Diminished heat and cold sensation
		Example: peripheral vascular disease
		Itching and tingling
		Example: peripheral vascular disease, drug incompatibility, histamine reaction
Note **lesions** on the skin Physical characteristics include color, elevation, shape, mobility, and contents	No lesions present	Macules (localized changes in color without elevation)
		Example: petechiae, first degree burns, purpura
		Papules, plaques, nodules (solid, elevated, varying in size)
		Example: psoriasis, xanthomas

Wheals (elevated, circumscribed, transient)
  Example: urticaria, insect bites)
Vesicles and bullae (clear, fluid-filled pockets
  between skin layers)
  Example: second degree burns
Pustules (vesicles or bullae filled with exudate)
  Example: furuncles, acne

ASSESSMENT OF HEAD AND NECK

The names of the regions of the head are derived from the bones that form the skull. Knowing the names of the bones and regions of the skull can assist in describing the location of the physical findings.

An understanding of the function of each lobe of the brain allows the nurse to be able to identify potential client problems when an injury occurs to that portion of the brain.

The brain is comprised of three segments, the brainstem, cerebrum and the cerebellum. There are twelve cranial nerves, which will be discussed in this chapter, and 31 spinal nerves with the respective dorsal and ventral roots.

The brainstem is divided into four sections. The diencephalon is comprised of the thalamus, which screens and relays sensory impulses to the cortex, and the hypothalamus, which regulates the autonomic nervous system, stress response, sleep, appetite, body temperature, water balance, and emotions. The midbrain is responsible for motor coordination and conjugate eye movements. The pons controls involuntary respiratory reflexes and contains projection tracts between the spinal cord, medulla, and brain. The medulla contains cardiac, respiratory, vomiting, and vasomotor centers. In addition, all afferent and efferent tracts must pass between the spinal cord and brain through the medulla.

The cerebral hemispheres have an outer layer formed by cellular gray matter, called the cerebral cortex. The two cerebral hemispheres are divided

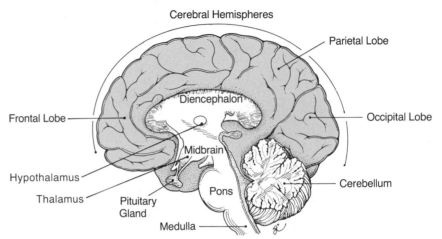

Three segments of brain: brainstem, cerebrum, cerebellum.

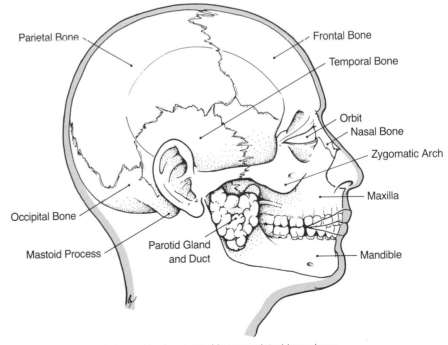

Lobes of brain covered by associated bone layer.

175

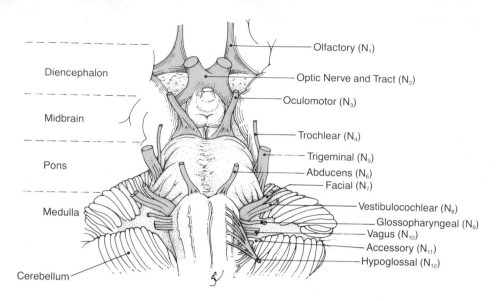

Diencephalon

Olfactory (N₁)

Optic Nerve and Tract (N₂)

Oculomotor (N₃)

Midbrain

Trochlear (N₄)

Trigeminal (N₅)

Pons

Abducens (N₆)

Facial (N₇)

Vestibulocochlear (N₈)

Medulla

Glossopharyngeal (N₉)

Vagus (N₁₀)

Accessory (N₁₁)

Hypoglossal (N₁₂)

Cerebellum

Brainstem and cranial nerves.

into four major lobes. The frontal lobe controls emotions, judgments, motor function and the motor speech area. The parietal lobe integrates general sensations, interprets pain, touch and temperature, and governs discrimination. The temporal lobe contains the auditory center and sensory speech center. The occipital lobe controls the visual area. The cerebellum coordinates muscle movement, posture, equilibrium and muscle tone.

The twelve cranial nerves are summarized below. The second through twelfth nerves arise from the brainstem.

The cranial nerves are 12 pairs of parasympathetic nerves with their nuclei along the brainstem.

First cranial nerve: olfactory. Sensory nerve

Second cranial nerve: optic. Sensory nerve; conducts sensory information from the retina

Third cranial nerve: oculomotor. Motor nerve; controls four of the six extraocular muscles; raises eyelid and controls the constrictor pupillae and ciliary muscles of the eyeball

Fourth cranial nerve: trochlear. Motor nerve; controls the superior oblique eye muscle

Fifth cranial nerve: trigeminal nerve. Mixed nerve with three sensory branches and one motor branch; the ophthalmic branch supplies the corneal reflex

Sixth cranial nerve: abducens. Controls the lateral rectus muscle of the eye

Seventh cranial nerve: facial. Mixed nerve; anterior tongue receives sensory supply; motor supply to glands of nose, palate lacrimal, submaxillary, and sublingual; motor branch supplies hyoid elevators and muscles of expression and closes eyelid

Eighth cranial nerve: acoustic. Sensory nerve with two divisions—hearing and semicircular canals

Ninth cranial nerve: glossopharyngeal. Mixed nerve; motor innervates parotid gland; sensory innervates auditory tube and posterior portion of taste buds

Tenth cranial nerve: vagus. Mixed nerve with motor branches to the pharyngeal and laryngeal muscles and to the viscera of the thorax and abdomen; sensory portion supplies the pinna of the ear, thoracic, and abdominal viscera

Eleventh cranial nerve: accessory. Motor nerve; innervates the sternocleidomastoid and trapezius muscles

Twelfth cranial nerve: hypoglossal. Motor nerve; controls tongue muscles

ASSESSMENT	NORMAL	ABNORMAL
EYE ASSESSMENT		
Note **visual acuity** by observing client performance of activities of daily living	Adequate performance of activities of daily living	Hyperopia (farsightedness) Myopia (nearsightedness)
Factors influencing visual acuity include client's previous status and age	Appropriate responses to environment	Cataract (opacification of the lens) Enucleation (loss of an eye): may have prosthesis in place
Note exact location, size, and color of any **external lesions**	No external lesions	Circumocular ecchymosis: may be sign of basal skull fracture
Palpate for mobility and firmness		Xanthalasma (small, yellowish, well-circumscribed plaques): may appear on eyelids of clients with lipid disorders *Example*: atherosclerosis
Note **equality of eyelid movement**	Eyelids are equal in movement	Ptosis (paralytic drooping of the upper eyelid)
Note color, consistency, amount, and origin of **discharge** from eyes	No discharge	Sty, or hordeolum Thick white discharge: may be due to conjunctivitis
Note **internal lesions**	No internal lesions	Conjunctival or ciliary injection (dilatation of the blood vessels)
Assess differences between **pupil size and reaction**	Both pupils are the same size	Anisocoria (indicates unequal pupil size): may be indicative of neurological trauma or deficit
Note presence of hemorrhage		Corneal edema (very soft, movable mass that looks like raw egg white): frequently occurs in clients who have increased intracranial pressure Arcus senilis (partial or complete whitish circle near the outer edge of the cornea): usually due to aging

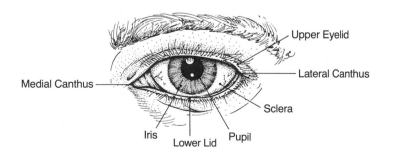

Normal eye anatomy

Medial Canthus — Upper Eyelid — Lateral Canthus — Sclera — Iris — Lower Lid — Pupil

ASSESSMENT	NORMAL	ABNORMAL
EAR ASSESSMENT		
Note **auditory acuity** by asking client to indicate if he or she hears normal sounds as you make them	Adequate responses to normal sounds Auditory changes due to aging	Deafness: may be caused by continued use of antibiotics Abnormal sounds in the ears *Example*: ringing or buzzing
Note exact size, color, and location of any **external lesions** Palpate lesions for mobility and firmness	No external lesions	Battle's sign (ecchymosis behind the ear): may be sign of basilar skull fracture
Note color, quantity, and consistency of any **discharge** from the ears Test clear fluid for glucose using a Labstix	No discharge	Cerebrospinal fluid leak: may be due to head injury. If drainage is blood and CSF, it will develop a "halo" with a reddish area in the center and a whitish circle if placed on white material Perforation of tympanic membrane: serosanguineous or purulent drainage

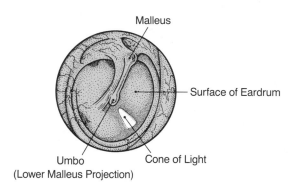

Normal Eardrum

Malleus

Surface of Eardrum

Umbo
(Lower Malleus Projection)

Cone of Light

NOSE ASSESSMENT		
Note any **structural changes** in the nose by observing client breathe Gently occlude one nostril at a time; ask client to breathe through the non-occluded nostril	Regular breathing with mouth closed Breathing through non-occluded nostril	Breathing through the mouth only: furuncles may occlude breathing Obstruction in the nose due to deviated nasal septum, or excessive mucus secretions
Note color, quantity, and consistency of any **discharge** from the nose	Minimal discharge	Cerebrospinal fluid leak (Fluid tests positive for glucose with Labstix.) Copious, watery-to-thick, mucopurulent discharge: may be due to acute rhinitis

ASSESSMENT	NORMAL	ABNORMAL
MOUTH AND LIP ASSESSMENT		
Note size, color, and location of any **external lesions** 　Palpate for mobility and 　　firmness	No external lesions	Excessive build-up of mucous secretions Dehydrated mouth or lips Fissures Pressure sores Necrosis
Note size, color, and location of any **internal lesions** 　Palpate for mobility and 　　firmness	No internal lesions	Moniliasis (a fungal infection indicated by white plaques similar to milk curd)
NECK ASSESSMENT		
Note any **lesion or swelling** in the neck 　Ask client to relax and flex neck 　　slightly 　Palpate the neck, using the 　　pads of your fingers to move 　　the skin and underlying 　　tissues	Occasional small, mobile discrete, nontender lymph nodes	Enlarged, tender immobile nodes

ASSESSMENT OF THE CHEST

The chest or thorax area extends from the base of the neck to the diaphragm. The overall shape of the thorax should be elliptical, although deformities such as barrel chest, pigeon chest or funnel chest do occur. Total assessment includes the external aspect: the nurse should observe for movement, posture, shape and symmetry, especially of the breast and axilla area; and the internal components of the lungs and the heart.

The lungs anteriorly extend from 2 – 4 cm above the inner third of the clavicle to the eighth rib at the mid-axillary line and the sixth rib at the midclavicular line.

Posteriorly, the lungs extend from the third thoracic spinous process and descend to the tenth process or, on deep inspiration, to the twelfth process.

Breath sounds of clients will be different due to the depth of breathing, underlying disease, obesity, etc. Be-

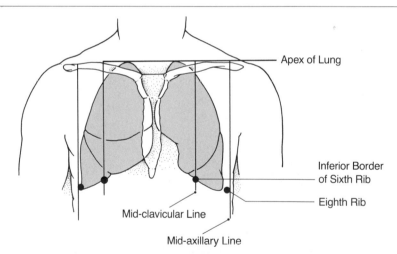

Anatomical relationship of lungs to skeletal structure.

cause of these differences, it is difficult to compare the breath sounds of one client with another. The basic principle to remember when auscultating the lungs is to do a comparison between the right and left lung. To make these comparisons, begin auscultating at the apices of one lung, alternating sides as you work down through both lungs. By comparing similar areas in both lungs, you will note changes and determine causes for these changes more easily.

Place the client in an upright sitting position with shoulders pulled forward. If the client is lying on his or her

179

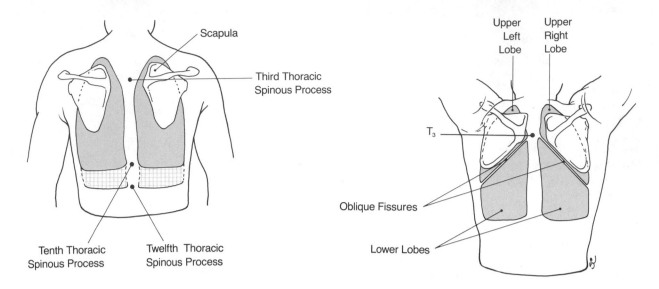

Posterior relationship of lung lobes to skeletal structure.

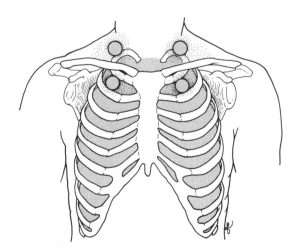

Stethoscope placement sites for anterior auscultation of breath sounds.

side, the lung closest to the bed will be mechanically compressed, and true lung sounds will not be heard.

Ask the client to breathe deeply, through the mouth. Breathing through the nose produces extra sounds that mask true lung sounds.

The heart is located directly behind the sternum, with the left ventricle projecting into the left chest. The heart is usually thought to be in the left chest for two reasons: the left ventricle produces the most movement (ventricular contraction), and three of the valve sound areas are located to the left of the sternum.

The action of the heart should be assessed both proximally and distally. Proximal assessment involves evaluating the heart sounds, the heart rate and the rhythm of the ventricular contractions to obtain information about the mechanical activity of the heart. Distal assessment involves evaluating the peripheral pulses to obtain information about the efficiency of the heart's circulatory effectiveness.

One method for assessing heart sounds is to start at the aortic area, moving slowly across to the pulmonic area, down to the tricuspid area, and over to the mitral area. This same general progression can also be used in reverse, starting at the mitral area and progressing up to the aortic area. Most clinicians begin the assessment at the mitral area, which is the point of maximum intensity and where the apical pulse is the loudest.

The most important point to re-member in heart assessments is to use the same method every time, repeating the same steps in the same sequence. By using one systematic approach, you will learn how to compare the different sounds more easily and not neglect to listen to all areas on the chest.

ASSESSMENT	NORMAL	ABNORMAL
THORAX ASSESSMENT		
Note the **general appearance** of the chest		
While client is standing or sitting	Straight spine, level shoulders	Breathing possible only when sitting forward with arms on pillows or overbed table
While client is in bed in high-Fowler's position	Relaxed breathing; rib cage moves symmetrically with respirations	Uses accessory muscles, i.e., scalene, trapezius, sternocleidomastoid, or pectoralis
	Estimate the anterior-posterior diameter (normally 5:7 ratio or as low as 1:2)	Intercostal or sternal retractions (present with obstruction and increased effort with atelectasis)
Note **shape of chest**		Deformities such as scoliosis, kyphosis or kyphoscoliosis
Note **shape of ribs**	Normal is downward	Horizontal is common in COPD
		Bulging of interspaces during exhalation (present with asthma and emphysema)
		Chest tilted to one side when client sits or stands: may be due to pain in ribs or chest wall or trauma, i.e., fractured ribs or surgery such as a thoracotomy

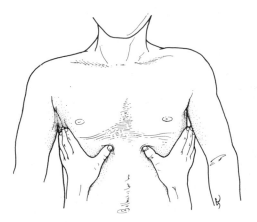
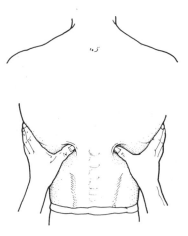

Measure chest excursion while client takes deep breath.

ASSESSMENT	NORMAL	ABNORMAL

Measure **chest excursion**, using your thumbs
  Place thumbs on posterior surface at level of and parallel to the tenth ribs
  Grasp lateral rib cage with hands
  Ask client to inhale
  Place thumbs on anterior surface with thumbs along each costal margin and hands along lateral rib cage
	On inhalation, the thumbs move equidistant away from spinal cord area	Flail chest: occurs when ribs are broken in two places; rib sections pulled abnormally inward during inhalations, rib sections pushed outward during exhalation
		Asymmetrical (unequal) chest excursion: occurs when client has a pneumothorax and cannot expand one side of chest; when client has fractured ribs; or when client's chest is splinted due to incisional pain
		Alteration in the thoracic movement indicates underlying disease of lung or pleura
		Barrel chest (increased anterior-posterior diameter): usually due to COPD
		Pigeon breast (congenital; sternum pushed away from spine): due to rickets
		Funnel breast (congenital; sternum retracted toward spine)

BREAST ASSESSMENT

ASSESSMENT	NORMAL	ABNORMAL

Inspect **size**, **symmetry** and **contour** of breasts
  Place client in sitting position
  Have client remove clothing from waist up
  Have client raise arms over her head
	Size varies with each client
	Breasts should be equal in size and symmetrical in position
		Masses, dimpling, or flattened areas: indicate possible cancer

Color, **edema**, and **venous pattern of skin**	Normal skin color with darker area surrounding nipples No edema or prominent vessels	Erythema: indicates infection or inflammatory carcinoma Edema or increased venous prominence: indicates carcinoma

Inspect **size and shape of nipples**
  Note direction in which they point, and any **rashes** or **discharge**
  To palpate breasts, position client supine or on side
  Using three fingers in a circular motion, compress breast tissue gently against chest wall
  Examine entire breast
  Make frequent checks to assess for changes
	Simple inversion of nipples is common
	
	Soft, elastic tissue with mobile nodules: indicates cystic disease
		Flattening, nipple pull, or axis deviation of nipple points: may be due to fibrosis associated with cancer
		Ulcerations of nipples and areola: may be due to Paget's disease
		Discharge: may not be malignant but should be observed closely
		Hard nodules fixed to skin or underlying tissue may indicate cancer
		When nodules are present
		  Describe location and quadrant of breast where found
		  Note size in centimeters
		  Describe consistency and shape
		  Note tenderness and mobility of nodule in relationship to underlying tissue

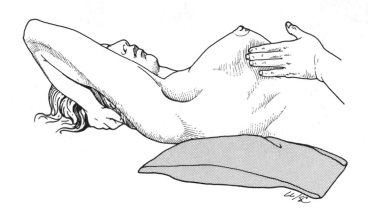

Examine breast systematically using a circular movement to compress breast tissue against chest wall.

ASSESSMENT	NORMAL	ABNORMAL
Palpate nipples Compress nipple between thumb and index finger to inspect for discharge	No discharge	Bloody discharge: may indicate papilloma
Note **elasticity** Observe for erection of nipple with pal ation	Elastic, no retraction of nipple	Loss of elasticity: indicates possible cancer Inversion, flattening, or retraction: may indicate cancer

LUNG ASSESSMENT

Complete a **general assessment** of the lungs

Respiratory rate	12 to 20 respirations/minute	Increased respiratory rate: may be due to increased metabolic needs (fever), mechanical injury, surgery, or trauma to chest wall
Respiratory depth or *volume*	Normal depth is equal to about 500 ml A normal or increased rate does not assume a normal tidal volume	Clients may have an increased rate to compensate for decreased tidal volume, but the resultant minute volume is still not sufficient. (Normal minute volume is 6 to 8 liters/minute.) Increased depth: due to neurological disease, ICP from trauma, drug overdose, exertion, fear, or anxiety Decreased depth: due to neurological disease, ICP from trauma, drug overdose, respiratory disease, or pneumothorax

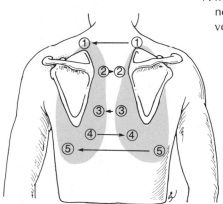

Auscultate breath sounds bilaterally.

ASSESSMENT	NORMAL	ABNORMAL
Note location and quality of **lung sounds**		
Vesicular breath sounds Heard over lung parenchyma (Heart will mask breath sounds on the left side) Lungs extended anteriorly to the sixth intercostal space Lungs extended posteriorly to T_{10} on expiration, to T_{12} on deep inspiration	Low to medium pitch, with low amplitude Soft, whooshing quality Inspiration two to three times longer than expiration	Rales: due to passage of air through fluid or mucus-filled airways; more frequently heard during inspiration Fine rales: high pitched, soft, and crackling Coarse rales: low pitched and bubbling
Bronchovesicular breath sounds Heard over the mainstem bronchi below the clavicles and adjacent to the sternum, between scapulae	Moderate to high pitch, with moderate amplitude Hollow, muffled quality Inspiration and expiration equal in duration	Rhonchi: produced by air passing through airways narrowed by edema, muscle spasms, or tenacious mucus; characterized as musical or sonorous according to pitch of sound (rhonchi in small airways are musical; those in larger airways are sonorous); more frequently heard during expiration
Bronchial breath sounds Heard over the trachea above the sternal notch Not true lung sounds, but important because they approximate the sounds heard in areas of atelectasis	High pitch and amplitude Harsh, loud, tubular quality Expiration twice as long as inspiration	Wheezes: produced by air passing through airways narrowed by smooth muscle contraction, secretions, or edema; characterized as high-pitched and musical; more frequently heard during expiration, especially in asthmatic clients Pleural friction rub: produced when irritated or inflamed pleura rub together in the absence of normal pleural fluid; characterized as high-pitched, jerky, and scratchy; frequently transient; may become louder if stethoscope pressed firmly to chest wall

HEART ASSESSMENT

Evaluate **atrioventricular heart sounds** (S_1 heart sound) *Mitral valve sounds*: located between the left atrium and left ventricle; heard best at left, fifth intercostal space at, or medial to, the midclavicular line *Tricuspid valve sounds*: located between the right atrium and the right ventricle; heard best at left, fifth intercostal space at the sternal border	S_1 (the first heart sound, a combination of the mitral and tricuspid sounds) heard best over the mitral and tricuspid areas Lubb sound	Heart sounds not heard in the area prescribed; e.g., with left ventricular hypertrophy, mitral sound moves laterally Relative strength of heart sounds in each area change, e.g., S_1 may be predominant at pulmonic area (left, second intercostal space at the sternal border), rather than S_2

ASSESSMENT	NORMAL	ABNORMAL
Evaluate **semilunar heart sounds** (S₂ heart sounds)		
Aortic valve sounds: located between the left ventricle and the aorta; heard best at right, second intercostal space at the sternal border	S₂ (the second heart sound, a combination of the aortic and pulmonic sounds): heard best over the aortic and pulmonic areas	Sounds altered with aortic stenosis (thrill) and hypertension (accentuated sound)
Pulmonic valve sounds: located between the right ventricle and the pulmonary artery; heard best at left, second intercostal space at the sternal border	Dubb sound	Pulsations with increased pressure, thrill with pulmonic stenosis and accentuated sound with pulmonary hypertension
Evaluate presence of **other heart sounds** Use bell of stethoscope		
S₃ (ventricular gallop): heard just after S₂, at the apex or at lower, left sternal border; occurs when blood flow changes from rapid to slow during ventricular diastole	Quiet and low pitched May be a physiological finding in some children and young adults	Sounds like ken-TUC-ky S₁ S₂ S₃ Almost always signifies cardiac decompensation when found in a client who has heart disease
S₄ (atrial gallop): heard just before S₁, at the apex or at lower, left sternal border; occurs when blood flow from atrial contraction meets increased resistance in ventricle	Not usually present	Sounds like TEN-nes-see S₄ S₁ S₂ Heard in clients with heart disease, especially coronary artery disease or myocardial infarction
Assess for **heart murmurs** Produced by atypical flow of blood through the heart, e.g., irregularity or partial obstruction, increased flow in normal area, flow into dilated chamber, flow through abnormal passage; regurgitant flow Occurs during systole (between S₁ and S₂) or during diastole (between S₂ and S₁)	Faint sound More common during systole Often found in children and young adults	Faint or loud enough to be heard without a stethoscope Occurs during systole or diastole (diastolic murmurs are almost always pathological) — found in older clients with heart disease or infants and children with congenital heart defects
Evaluate the **apical pulse** when assessing for general heart rate and rhythm of contractions Auscultate at the apex of the heart (left, fifth intercostal space at the midclavicular line) Palpate and view pulse, if client's chest wall is thin enough	Regular rhythm Heart rate: 60 to 100 beats/minute Moderate bradycardia common in well-trained athletes Mild tachycardia possible with stress, infection, or fever	Irregular rhythm, i.e., atrial fibrillation (no discernible rhythmic pattern) Abnormal rate Bradycardia (less than 60 beats/minute) Tachycardia (more than 100 beats/minute)

ASSESSMENT	NORMAL	ABNORMAL

Assess for **irregular apical pulse**
  With another nurse, take apical and radial pulses simultaneously
  Compare beats per minute for both pulses

Equal apical and radial pulses

Fewer beats at the radial area may indicate an irregular apical pulse

Palpate **peripheral pulses**: radial, brachial, femoral, popliteal, dorsalis pedis, posterior tibial
  (For special cases, after carotid surgery, palpate temporal pulse also)
  Follow these guidelines for palpating peripheral pulses:
  If pulse is not immediately palpable, examine adjacent area
  Pulse locations differ with clients
  Palpate weak pulses gently so that you do not obliterate pulse with too much pressure
  If you cannot differentiate your pulse from client's pulse, check your radial pulse or observe monitor pattern
  Repeat palpations of same area slowly
  Weak pulses may be difficult to feel

Easily palpated
Equally strong on both sides
Posterior tibial pulse usually weaker than femoral

Difficult to palpate
Unequal pulses
Weak pulses
Absent pulses

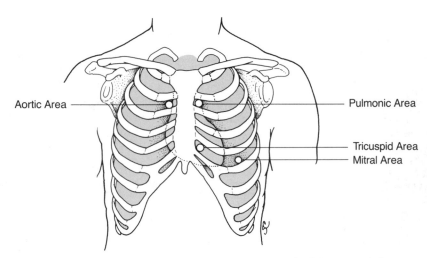

Use diaphragm of stethoscope to hear high-pitched (S_1, S_2) heart sounds.

ASSESSMENT OF THE ABDOMEN AND GENITOURINARY TRACT

The abdomen extends from the diaphragm to the pelvis. Generally speaking, there are two body systems present in this area: the gastrointestinal system and the genitourinary system.

The gastrointestinal system begins at the mouth and consists of the stomach, the small and large intestines and associated organs that include the liver, pancreas, and spleen.

The urinary tract consists of the kidneys, ureters, bladder, and the urethra. The urinary tract should be assessed frequently and accurately because changes in the status of the urinary organs can rapidly affect other body systems.

The most common way to assess the urinary tract is to note the quantity and quality of the urinary output. Some medications or foods produce unusual odors and

colors in urine, e.g., sulfasalazine (Azulfidine) turns urine a yellow-orange color; asparagus gives urine a musty odor.

External male genitalia include the penis, the scrotum, and the testicles. External female genitalia include the vulva, the urethral orifice, and the vagina.

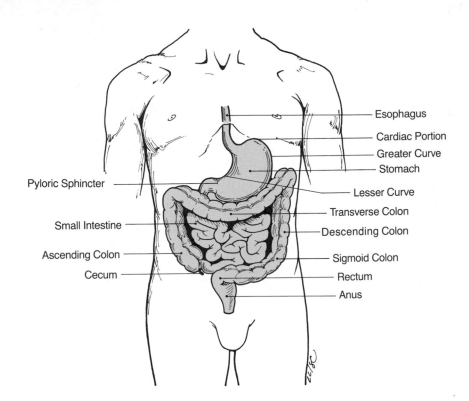

Esophagus
Cardiac Portion
Greater Curve
Stomach
Lesser Curve
Transverse Colon
Descending Colon
Sigmoid Colon
Rectum
Anus

Pyloric Sphincter
Small Intestine
Ascending Colon
Cecum

Abdominal organs.

ASSESSMENT	NORMAL	ABNORMAL
ABDOMEN		
Assess the **general contour** of the abdomen with client lying flat in bed	Abdomen flat between chest and pubis	Scaphoid (concave) abdominal contour: due to inadequate intake of food or IV calories, energy needs which exceed caloric intake, or to inadequate food absorption Protuberant abdomen: caused by hemorrhage after trauma, e.g., auto accident or surgery
Assess **circumference** for intra-abdominal hemorrhage by placing a tape measure around the largest circumference of the abdomen and drawing two lines around client's entire abdomen, one line at the top of the tape measure, one line at the bottom of the tape measure; perform measurement when client exhales	No increase in abdominal circumference	Abdominal circumference increases steadily within one to two hours

ASSESSMENT	NORMAL	ABNORMAL
Auscultate abdomen to assess presence and quality of **bowel sounds**		
Place diaphragm of stethoscope firmly on abdomen, lateral to and below umbilicus	Bowel sounds similar to fairly frequent gurgle	Increased bowel sounds: due to diarrhea or to partial bowel obstruction (sounds become high-pitched and tinkling or come in "rushes," followed by silence as obstruction progresses)
Listen for several minutes since bowel sounds are not continuous like pulses	Varying frequency of sounds with clients and time of day, i.e., more sounds right before and after eating	
	Decreased or absent bowel sounds after surgery	Decreased bowel sounds
	After general anesthesia, normal sounds in one to two days	Absent bowel sounds: may be due to complete bowel obstruction or systemic illness
	After abdominal surgery, normal sounds in three to five days	Bowel sounds hypoactive, quiet, and infrequent: may be due to paralytic ileus or no obvious cause
Palpate abdomen to determine condition of **abdominal muscles** and organs beneath muscles		
Tell client to relax, lie flat in bed, and flex knees		
Place your hand flat on client's abdomen, holding four of your fingers together and exerting pressure with the flat part of your fingers	Soft, pliant musculature when relaxed	Rigid, tender muscles: may be due to presence of inflammation or infection (peritonitis)
Never palpate with one finger or with finger tips		
Begin palpation at the pubis, moving upward. Palpate any problem areas last to minimize effects of discomfort		
Palpate all quadrants of abdomen to assess organs contained in each quadrant		
Superficial palpation: use slight pressure only		
Deep palpation: indent the abdominal wall 4 to 5 cm		

URINARY TRACT ASSESSMENT

Assess the **external urethra**	Orifice is pink and moist; clear, minimal discharge	Burning or pain at urethral orifice: may indicate urinary infection
Assess the quantity, color, odor, specific gravity, and pH of **urine output**	Output: 1200 to 1500 ml/24 hours, or 30 to 50 ml/hour	Increased output: may indicate potential diabetes or inappropriate ADH response
		Decreased output: may indicate dehydration, acute nephritis, cardiac disease, or renal failure

ASSESSMENT	NORMAL	ABNORMAL
	Clear, yellow-amber color (Vegetarians may have slightly cloudy urine)	Cloudy (turbid): may indicate possible urinary tract infection or early signs of hematuria Dark amber: may indicate very concentrated urine due to dehydration Dark amber to green: may indicate hepatitis or obstructive jaundice
	Slight odor (Ammonia-like odor indicates that specimen has been sitting for some time)	Foul-smelling: may indicate urinary tract infection, drug or specific food ingestion Sweet odor: may indicate acetone from keto-acidosis
	Specific gravity: 1.003 to 1.030	Specific gravity of more than 1.030: indicates dehydration Constant specific gravity of 1.010, regardless of fluid intake: indicates renal failure
	pH range from 4.5 to 7.5; average is 6-7	Acidic pH below 6.0: may indicate starvation or acidosis Alkaline pH greater than 7.0: indicates metabolic alkalosis
Assess for **blood** in urine using Hemastix or Labstix	No blood present	Mildly pink-tinged to grossly red-colored urine indicates blood in urine Sudden decrease or termination of urine output *Prerenal* causes affecting urine formation: inadequate intake, acute CHF, diabetes insipidus (large amounts of dilute urine output) *Renal* causes affecting quantity or makeup of urine: renal failure, acute tubular necrosis, glomerulonephritis *Postrenal* causes resulting in decreased urine output: BPH, blockage of ureters by kidney stones, or plugged catheter
Palpate for **bladder distension**	Not normally palpated	Distended bladder (firm, round mass) accompanied by discomfort and urge to void: indicates distention (common following surgery, where catheter is not used)
Assess for **pain**	No pain	Severe pain in the flank region (below ribcage posteriorly and lateral to spine): indicates kidney infection or stones
	Clear urine	Urine cloudy and odorous
GENITAL ASSESSMENT		
Visually examine the **male genitalia** 　Retract the foreskin of the penis to note cleanliness, any **lesions**, and **discharge**	Clean No odor No lesions No discharge Urethra opens midline of the tip of the glans	Unclean Odor Lesions and discharge: may indicate venereal disease Oval and round, dark erosion: may indicate syphilitic chancre Hypospadias: due to congenital displacement of the urethral meatus

189

ASSESSMENT	NORMAL	ABNORMAL
	Size of the penis and the scrotum vary	Indurated nodule or ulcer: may indicate carcinoma
	Two testicles in the scrotum	Mass in scrotum: indicates possible hernia, hydrocele, testicular tumor, or cyst
Visually examine **female genitalia**	Clean No odor	Unclean Odor
Assess for **lesions** or **discharge**	Minimal, clear discharge Menstrual flow Lochia (normal discharge after delivery) No lesions	Thick; thin, white, yellowish, or green discharge: may indicate Trichomonas Thick, white, and curdy discharge: may indicate Candida Lesions: could indicate syphilitic chancre, herpes infection, venereal wart, or carcinoma of vulva

MENTAL-SPIRITUAL ASSESSMENT

The mental assessment is completed throughout the physical assessment and history-taking time frame. It is not generally considered a separate entity. Mood, memory, orientation, and thought processes can be evaluated while obtaining the health history. A spiritual assessment can be obtained as a part of the health history, although specific socio-cultural beliefs may need to be ascertained separately. Nutritional preferences and restrictions can be accomplished as a part of a client care plan and may or may not be included in the general client assessment.

The purpose of a spiritual assessment is to facilitate the client adapting to the hospital environment and help the staff understand stressors the client may be experiencing as a result of belief systems.

The purpose of a mental status assessment is to evaluate the present state of psychological functioning. It is not designed to make a diagnosis; rather, it should yield data that will contribute to the total picture of the client as he or she is functioning at the time the assessment is made.

The specific rationale for completing a mental status assessment is:

- To collect baseline data to aid in establishing the etiology, diagnosis, and prognosis.
- To evaluate the present state of psychological functioning.
- To evaluate changes in the individual's emotional, intellectual, motor, and perceptual responses.
- To determine the guidelines of the treatment plan.
- To ascertain if some seemingly psychopathological response is, in fact, a disorder of a sensory organ (i.e., a deaf person appearing hostile, depressed, or suspicious).

- To document altered mental status for legal records.

The initial factors that the nurse must consider in completing a mental status assessment are to correctly identify the client, the reason for admission, record of previous mental illness, present complaint, any personal history that is relevant, (living arrangements, role in family, interactional experience), family history if appropriate, significant others and available support systems, assets, and interests.

The actual assessment process begins with an initial evaluation of the appropriateness of the client's behavior and orientation to reality. The assessment continues by noting any abnormal behavior and ascertaining the client's chief verbalized complaint. Finally, the evaluation determines if the client is in contact with reality enough to answer particular questions that will further assess the client's condition.

MENTAL STATUS ASSESSMENT

ASSESSMENT	NORMAL	ABNORMAL
GENERAL APPEARANCE, MANNER AND ATTITUDE		
Assess **physical appearance**	General body characteristics, energy level, sleep patterns	Inappropriate physical appearance, high or low extremes of energy, poor sleep patterns
Note **grooming**, mode of dress, and **personal hygiene**	Grooming and dress appropriate to situation, client's age, and social circumstance Clean	Poor grooming Inappropriate or bizarre dress or combination of clothes Unclean
Note **posture**	Upright, straight, and appropriate	Slumped, tipped, or stooped Tremors
Note speed, pressure, pace, quantity, volume, and diction of **speech**	Moderated speed, volume, and quantity Appropriate diction	Accelerated or retarded speech and high quantity Poor or inappropriate diction
Note relevance, content, and organization of **responses**	Questions answered directly, accurately, and with relevance	Inappropriate responses, unorganized pattern of speech Tangential, circumstantial or out-of-context replies
EXPRESSIVE ASPECTS OF BEHAVIOR		
Note **general motor activity**	Calm, ordered movement appropriate to situation	Overactive, e.g., restless, agitated, impulsive Underactive, e.g., slow to initiate or execute actions
Assess **purposeful movements** and **gestures**	Reasonably responsive with purposeful movements, appropriate gestures	Repetitious activities, e.g., rituals or compulsions Command automation Parkinsonian movements
Assess style of **gait**		Ataxic, shuffling, off-balance gait
CONSCIOUSNESS		
Assess **level of consciousness**	Alert, attentive, and responsive Knowledgeable about time, place, and person	Disordered attention; distracted, cloudy consciousness Delirious Stuporous Disoriented in time, place, and person

ASSESSMENT	NORMAL	ABNORMAL
THOUGHT PROCESSES AND PERCEPTION		
Assess **coherency**, **logic**, and **relevance** of thought processes by asking questions about personal history, e.g., "Where were you born?" "What kind of work do you do?"	Clear, understandable responses to questions Attentiveness	Disordered thought forms Autistic or dereistic (absorbed with self and withdrawn); abstract (absent-mindedness); concrete thinking (dogmatic, preaching)
Assess **reality orientation**: time, place, and person awareness	Orderly progression of thoughts based in reality Awareness of time, place, and person	Disorders of progression of thought: looseness, circumstantial, incoherent, irrelevant conversation, blocking Delusions of grandeur or persecution: neologisms, use of words whose meaning is known only to the client Echolalia (automatic repeating of questions) No awareness of day, time, place, or person
Assess **perceptions** and reactions to personal experiences by asking questions such as "How do you see yourself now that you are in the hospital?" "What do you think about when you're in a situation like this?"	Thoughtful, clear responses expressed with understanding of self	Altered, narrowed, or expanded perception Illusions Depersonalization
THOUGHT CONTENT AND MENTAL TREND		
Ask questions to determine general themes that identify **degree of anxiety**, e.g., "How are you feeling right now?" "What kinds of things make you afraid?"	Mild or 1+ level of anxiety in which individual is alert, motivated, and attentive	Moderate to severe (2+ to 4+) levels of anxiety
Assess **ideation** and **concentration**	Ideas based in reality Able to concentrate	Ideas of reference Hypochondria (abnormal concerns about health) Obsessional Phobias (irrational fears) Poor or shortened concentration
MOOD OR AFFECT		
Assess prevailing or **variability in mood** by observing behavior and asking questions such as "How are you feeling right now?" Check for presence of abnormal **euphoria**	Appropriate, even mood without wide variations high to low	Cyclothymic mood swings; euphoria, elation, ecstasy, depressed, withdrawn

ASSESSMENT	NORMAL	ABNORMAL
If you suspect **depression**, continue questioning to determine depth and significance of mood, e.g., "How badly do you feel?" "Have you ever thought of suicide?"	May be sad or grieving but mood does not persist indefinitely	Flat or dampened responses Inappropriate responses Ambivalence

MEMORY

Assess **past and present memory** and **retention** (ability to listen and respond with understanding or knowledge); ask client to repeat a phrase, e.g., an address	Alert, accurate responses Able to complete digit span Past and present memory appropriate	Hyperamnesia (excessive loss of memory); amnesia; paramnesia (belief in events that never occurred) Preoccupied Unable to follow directions
Assess **recall** (recent and remote) by asking questions such as "When is your birthday?" "What year were you born?" "How old are you?"	Good recall of immediate and past events	Poor recall of immediate or past events

JUDGMENT

Assess **judgment, decision-making ability** and interpretations by asking questions such as "What should you do if you hear a siren while you're driving?" "If you lost a library book, what would you do?"	Ability to make accurate decisions Realistic interpretation of events	Poor judgment, poor decision-making ability, poor choice Inappropriate interpretation of events or situations

AWARENESS

Assess **insight**, the ability to understand the inner nature of events or problems, by asking questions such as "If you saw someone dressed in a fur coat on a hot day, what would you think?"	Thoughtful responses indicating an understanding of the inner nature of an event or problem	Lack of insight or understanding of problems or situations Distorted view of situation

INTELLIGENCE

Assess **intelligence** by asking client to define or use words in sentences, e.g., recede, join, plural	Correct responses to majority of questions	Incorrect responses to majority of questions indicates possible severe psychiatric disorders

ASSESSMENT	NORMAL	ABNORMAL
Assess **fund of information** by asking questions such as ''Who is President of the United States?'' ''Who was the President before him?'' ''When is Memorial Day?'' ''What is a thermometer?'' (Consider client's cultural and educational background)	Correct responses to majority of questions	Deteriorated or impaired cognitive processes

SENSORY ABILITY

Assess the **five senses**, e.g., vision, hearing, tasting, feeling, and smelling abilities	Able to perceive, hear, feel, touch appropriate to stimulus	Lack of response Suspicious, hostile, depressed Kinesthetic imbalance

DEVELOPMENTAL LEVEL

Assess client's **developmental level** as compared to normal	Behavior and thought processes appropriate to age level	Wide span between chronological and developmental age Mentally retarded

LIFE-STYLE PATTERNS

Identify **addictive patterns** and effect on individual's overall health	Normal amount of alcohol ingested Smoking habits Prescriptive medications Adequate food intake for physical characteristics	High quantity of alcohol taken frequently Heavy smoker Addicted to illegal drugs Habituative medication; user of over-the-counter or legal medications Anorexic eating patterns Obese or overindulgence of food

COPING DEVICES

Identify **defense-coping mechanisms** and their effect on individual	Conscious coping mechanisms used appropriately such as compensation, fantasy, rationalization, suppression, sublimation or displacement Mechanisms effective, appropriate, and useful	Unconscious mechanisms used frequently such as repression, regression, projection, reaction-formation, insulation or denial Mechanisms inappropriate, ineffective, and not useful

SPIRITUAL ASSESSMENT

RELIGIOUS GROUP	BAPTISM	DEATH RITUALS	HEALTH CRISIS	DIET
Adventist	Opposed to infant baptism	No last rites	Communion or baptism may be desirable	No alcohol, coffee, tea, or any narcotic
Baptist	Opposed to infant baptism	Clergy support and counsels	Some believe in healing and laying on of hands Some sects resist medical help	Condemn alcohol Some do not allow coffee and tea
Black Muslim	No baptism	Prescribed procedures for washing body and shrouding	No faith healing	Prohibit alcohol and pork
Buddhist	Rites are given after child is mature	Send for Buddhist priest Last rite chanting	Family should request priest to be notified	Usually no restrictions although some are vegetarian
Christian Scientist	No baptism	No last rites No autopsy	Deny the existence of health crises Many refuse all medical help, blood transfusions, or drugs	Alcohol, coffee, and tobacco viewed as drugs and not allowed
Episcopalian	Infant baptism mandatory	Last rites not essential for all members	Medical treatment acceptable	Some do not eat meat on Fridays
Jehovah's Witness	No infant baptism	No last rites	Opposed to blood transfusions	Do not eat anything to which blood has been added
Judaism	No baptism but ritual circumcision on eighth day	Ritual washing of body	Medical treatment acceptable	Orthodox observe kosher dietary laws, which prohibit pork, shellfish, and the eating of meat and milk products at the same time
Methodist	Baptism encouraged	No last rites	Medical treatment acceptable	No restrictions
Mormon	Baptism eight years or older	Baptism of the dead very important	Do not prohibit medical treatment although they believe in divine healing	Do not allow alcohol, caffeine, tobacco, tea, and coffee
Roman Catholic	Infant baptism mandatory	Last rites are mandatory	No special requirements	Most ill people are exempt from fasting

This section outlines the essential assessment data that is required throughout pregnancy. Information obtained from this assessment assists the clinician in determining the progression of the pregnancy as well as identifying potential complications. When complications are identified early in the pregnancy, interventions may be planned that will preserve the fetus and protect the mother.

Initial physical findings will vary depending in what week of the pregnancy the examination is done. The information obtained from this assessment will provide baseline data in order to evaluate changes throughout the pregnancy. Clients are assessed monthly during the first seven months of gestation. In the seventh and eighth months assessments are done twice a month. In the ninth month weekly assessments are done.

A total assessment of the obstetrical client requires a complete health history. The health history includes personal medical history, family medical history, social history, menstrual history, contraceptive/sexual history, and previous obstetrical history.

The expected date of confinement (EDC) is determined during the first health care visit. The date of the last menstrual period (LMP) is needed to determine the EDC. Nägele's rule is generally used for determining the due date. To obtain the EDC, take the first day of the LMP, minus three months, and add seven days. If the date of the LMP is unknown, the EDC can be estimated when the first fetal heart tone (FHT) is audible using the doptone. This occurs about 11 to 12 weeks after conception. The fetoscope picks up the FHT at about 18-20 weeks gestation. When quickening (the first sign of life) occurs, the fetus is about 17 to 19 weeks gestation.

An important aspect of the maternal assessment involves identifying the client's knowledge of nutrition and physical care during pregnancy. A healthy client generally has fewer complications and a healthier infant. It is important that each obstetrical client be provided prenatal teaching.

A supplement containing nutritional aspects and recommendations for prenatal and postpartum clients is found at the end of this section to assist in providing the necessary information for client teaching. In addition, signs of pregnancy, major discomforts and relief measures, and the stages and phases of labor are outlined.

OBSTETRICAL ASSESSMENT

ASSESSMENT	NORMAL	ABNORMAL
INITIAL PHYSICAL ASSESSMENT		
Assess **breasts** and **nipples**		
Contour and size		
Presence of lumps	No lumps	Lumps
Secretions	Colostrum secretions in late first trimester or early second trimester	Secretions, other than colostrum
Assess **abdomen**		
Contour and size		
Changes in skin color	Linea nigra (black line of pregnancy along midline abdomen) Primiparas: coincidentally with growth of fundus Multiparas: after 13 to 15 weeks gestation	

ASSESSMENT	NORMAL	ABNORMAL
Striae (reddish-purple lines)	On breasts, hips, and thighs during pregnancy After pregnancy, faint silvery-grey	
Scars, rashes, or other skin disturbances	Usually none present	
Fundal height in centimeters (fingerbreadths less accurate): measure from symphysis pubis to top of fundus	Fundus palpable just above symphysis at 8 – 10 weeks Halfway between symphysis and umbilicus at 16 weeks Umbilicus at 20 – 22 weeks	Large measurements: EDC is incorrect; tumor; ascites; multiple pregnancy; and poly-hydramnios Less than normal enlargement: fetal abnormality, oligohydramnios, placental dysmaturity, missed abortion, fetal death
Perineum: scars, moles, rashes, warts, discharge		

BASELINE DATA

Evaluate **weight**		
Take **vital signs**, **blood pressure** (BP), **temperature**, **pulse**, and **respiration** (TPR)		
Evaluate **lab findings** Urine: sugar, protein, albumin	Negative for sugar, protein, and albumin throughout pregnancy	Positive for sugar, protein, and/or albumin
Human calcitonin (HCT) Hemoglobin (Hgb) Blood type and Rh factor	38% to 47% 12% to 16%	If Rh negative, father's blood should be typed If Rh positive, titers should be followed; possible RhoGAM at termination of pregnancy
Pap smear VD smears and screening		

ANTEPARTUM ASSESSMENT

Evaluate **weight** to assess maternal health and nutritional status and growth of fetus	1st trimester: 3 to 4 lbs 2nd trimester: 12 to 14 lbs 3rd trimester: 8 to 10 lbs Minimum weight gain during pregnancy: 24 lbs (2 lbs/week or 5 lbs/month)	Inadequate weight gain: possible maternal malnutrition Excessive weight gain: if sudden at onset, may indicate preeclampsia; if gradual and continual, may indicate overeating
Evaluate **blood pressure**	Fairly constant with baseline data throughout pregnancy	Increased: possible anxiety (Client should rest 20 to 30 minutes before you take BP again) Rise of 30/15 above baseline data: sign of pre-eclampsia Decreased: sign of supine hypotensive syndrome. If lying on back, turn client on left side and take BP again

ASSESSMENT	NORMAL	ABNORMAL
Evaluate **fundal height**	Drop around 38th week: sign of fetus engaging in birth canal Primipara: sudden drop Multipara: slower, sometimes not until onset of labor	Large fundal growth: may indicate wrong dates, multiple pregnancy, hydatidiform mole, polyhydramnios, tumors Small fundal growth: may indicate fetal demise, fetal anomaly, retarded fetal growth, abnormal presentation or lie, decreased amniotic fluid
Determine **fundal position**, using Leopold's maneuvers. Complete external palpations of the pregnant abdomen to determine fetal position, lie, presentation and engagement		
First maneuver: to determine part of fetus presenting into pelvis Second maneuver: to locate the back, arms, and legs; fetal heart heard best over fetal back Third maneuver: to determine part of fetus in fundus Fourth maneuver: to determine degree of cephalic flexion and engagement	Vertex presentation	Breech presentation or transverse lie

Steps of Leopold's maneuvers.

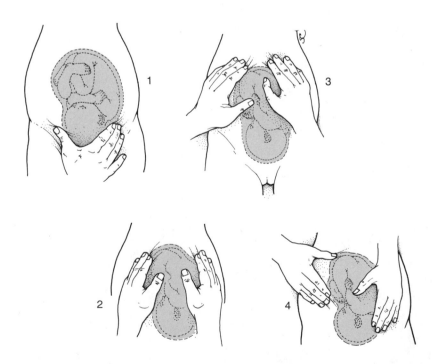

ASSESSMENT	NORMAL	ABNORMAL
Evaluate **fetal heart rate** by quadrant, location, and rate	120 to 160 beats/minute	More than 160 or less than 120: may indicate fetal distress. *Notify physician*
Check for presence of **edema**	In lower extremities towards end of pregnancy	In upper extremities and face: may indicate preeclampsia
Evaluate **urine** (clean catch mid-stream)	Negative for sugar, protein, and albumin	Positive for sugar: may indicate subclinical or gestational diabetes Positive for protein and/or albumin: may indicate preeclampsia
Evaluate **levels of discomfort** (See Obstetrical Supplement at end of this section)		

INTRAPARTUM ASSESSMENT

Assess for **lightening** and **dropping** (the descent of the presenting part into the pelvis)	Several days to two weeks before onset of labor Multipara: may not occur until onset of labor Relief of shortness of breath and increase in urinary frequency	No lightening or dropping: may indicate disproportion between fetal presenting part and maternal pelvis
Check if **mucous plug** has been expelled from cervix	Usually expelled prior to onset of labor	
Assess for **"bloody show"**	Clear, pinkish, or blood-tinged vaginal discharge that occurs as cervix begins to dilate and efface	
Assess for **ruptured membranes**		
Time water breaks	Before, during, or after onset of labor	Breech presentation: frank meconium or meconium staining
Color of **amniotic fluid**	Clear, straw color	Greenish-brown: indicates meconium has passed from fetus, possible fetal distress Yellow-stained: fetal hypoxia 36 hours or more prior to rupture of membrane or hemolytic disease
Quantity of amniotic fluid	500 to 1000 ml of amniotic fluid, rarely expelled at one time	Polyhydramnios: excessive fluid over 2000 cc Observe newborn for congenital anomalies: craniospinal malformation, orogastrointestinal anomalies, Down's syndrome and congenital heart defects Oligohydramnios: minimal fluid, less than 1000 cc Observe newborn for malformation of ear, genitourinary tract anomalies, and renal agenesis
Odor of fluid	No odor	Odor: may indicate infection; deliver within 24 hours

ASSESSMENT	NORMAL	ABNORMAL
Fetal heart rate	120 to 160 beats/minute Regular rhythm	Decreased: indicates fetal distress with possible cord prolapse or cord compression Accelerated heart rate: initial sign of fetal hypoxia Absent: may indicate fetal demise
Evaluate **contractions** *Frequency*: from start of one contraction to start of next	3 to 5 minutes between contractions	Irregular contractions with long intervals between: indicates false labor
Duration: from beginning of contraction to time uterus begins to relax	50 to 90 seconds	Over 90 seconds: uterine tetany; stop pitocin if running
Intensity (strength of contraction): measured with monitoring device	Peak 25 mm Hg End of labor may reach 50-75 mm Hg	Over 75 mm Hg: uterine tetany or uterine rupture

LABOR AND DELIVERY ASSESSMENT

First stage

Latent phase (0 to 10 cm dilatation)	0 to 5 cm over 6 to 10 hours	Prolonged time in any phase: may indicate poor fetal position, incomplete fetal flexion, CPD, or poor uterine contractions
Active phase (5 to 7 cm)		
Transition phase (8 to 10 cm)	Progresses from 8 to 10 cm in 1 to 2 hours	Labor less than 3 hours: indicates precipitous labor, increasing risk of fetal complications, or maternal lacerations and tears
Assess for **bloody show**		
Observe for presence of **nausea or vomiting**		
Assess **perineum**	Beginning to bulge	
Evaluate **urge to bear down**		Often uncontrolled Multipara: can cause precipitous delivery "Panting" (can be controlled until safe delivery area established)
Second stage (10 cm to delivery)	Primipara: up to 2 hours Multipara: several minutes to 2 hours	Over 2 hours: increased risk of fetal brain damage and maternal exhaustion
Assess for **presenting part**	Vertex with ROA or LOA presentation	Occiput posterior, breech, face or transverse lie
Assess **caput** (infant head) Multipara: move to delivery room when caput size of dime Primipara: move to delivery room when caput size of half dollar	Visible when bearing down during contraction	"Crowns" in room other than delivery room: delivery imminent (Do not move client)

ASSESSMENT	NORMAL	ABNORMAL
Assess **fetal heart rate**	120 to 160/minute	Decreased: may indicate supine hypotensive syndrome (Turn client on side and take again.) Hemorrhage (Check for other signs of bleeding; notify physician.) Increased or decreased: may indicate fetal distress secondary to cord progression or compression (Place client in Trendelenburg's or knee-chest position; give oxygen if necessary; inform physician.)
Evaluate **breathing**	Controlled with contractions	Heavy or excessive: may lead to hyperventilation and/or dehydration
Evaluate **pain** and **anxiety**	Medication required after dilated 4 to 5 cm unless using natural childbirth methods	Severe pain early in first stage of labor: inadequate prenatal teaching, backache due to position in bed, uterine tetany
Third stage (from delivery of baby to delivery of placenta)	Placental separation occurs within 30 minutes (usually 3-5 minutes)	Failure of placental separation Abnormality of uterus or cervix, weak, ineffectual uterine contraction, tetanic contractions causing closure of cervix Over 3 hours: indicates retained placenta
Fourth stage (first hour postpartum)		Mother in unstable condition (hemorrhage usual cause) Highest risk of hemorrhage in first postpartum hour
Temperature	36.5° to 37.5°C	Over 37.5°C: may indicate infection Slight elevation: due to dehydration from mouth breathing and NPO
Pulse	Pulse: 60 to 100	Increased: may indicate pain or hemorrhage
Respiration	Respirations: 12-22	
Blood pressure	Blood pressure: 140-120/80	Increased: may indicate anxiety, pain or posteclamptic condition Decreased: hemorrhage

POSTPARTUM ASSESSMENT

Assess **vital signs** every 15 minutes for 1 hour, every 30 minutes for 1 hour, every hour for 4 hours, every 8 hours, and as needed	Pulse may be 45-60/minute in stage 4 Pulse to normal range about third day	Decreased BP and increased P: probably postpartum hemorrhage; elevated temperature above 38°C: indicates possible infection Temperature elevates when lactation occurs
Assess **fundus** every 15 minutes for 1 hour, every 8 hours for 48 hours, then daily	Firm (Like a grapefruit) in midline and at or slightly above umbilicus Return to prepregnant size in 6 weeks: descending at rate of 1 fingerbreadth/day	Boggy fundus: immediately massage gently until firm; report to physician and observe closely; empty bladder; medicate with pitocin if ordered Fundus misplaced 1 to 2 fingerbreadths from midline: indicates full bladder (Client must void or be catheterized.)

ASSESSMENT	NORMAL	ABNORMAL
Assess **lochia** every 15 minutes for 1 hour, every 8 hours for 48 hours, then daily		
Color	3 days postpartum: dark red (rubra) 4 to 10 days postpartum: clear pink (serosa) 10 to 21 days postpartum: white, yellow brown (alba)	Heavy, bright-red: indicates hemorrhage (Massage fundus, give medication on order, notify physician.) Spurts: may indicate cervical tear No lochia: may indicate clot occluding cervical opening (Support fundus; express clot.)
Quantity	Moderate amount, steadily decreases	
Odor	Minimal	Foul: may indicate infection
Assess **breasts** and **nipples** daily	Day 1 to 2: soft, intact, secreting colostrum Day 2 to 3: engorged, tender, full, tight, painful Day 3+: secreting milk Increased pains as baby sucks: common in multiparas	Sore or cracked (Clean and dry nipples; decrease breast feeding time; apply breast shield between feeding.) Milk does not "let down": help client relax and decrease anxiety; give glass of wine or beer
Assess **perineum** daily	Episiotomy intact, no swelling, no discoloration	Swelling or bruising: may indicate hematoma
Assess **bladder** every four hours	Voiding regularly with no pain	Not voiding: bladder may be full and displaced to one side, leading to increased lochia (Catheterization may be necessary.)
Assess **bowels**	Spontaneous bowel movement 2 to 3 days after delivery	Fear associated with pain from hemorrhoids
Assess mother-infant **bonding**	Touching infant, talking to infant, talking about infant	Refuses to touch or hold infant
Evaluate **Rh-negative status**	Client does not require RhoGAM	RhoGAM administered

OBSTETRICAL GUIDELINES

This supplement contains pertinent information regarding recommendations for prenatal and postpartum clients; signs of pregnancy, major discomforts and relief measures; and the stages and phases of labor.

ASSESSMENT	NORMAL	ABNORMAL
RECOMMENDATIONS FOR PRENATAL CLIENTS		
Instruct about **nutrition**		
Instruct about intake of **sodium**, which is essential for maintaining increased body fluids needed for adequate placental flow, increased tissue requirements, and adequate renal blood flow		
Instruct about **exercise** Exercise is beneficial in moderation Continued exercise in familiar sports throughout pregnancy is recommended Participation in new or unfamiliar sports is not recommended	Fatigue in early pregnancy: may need to decrease exercise	Excessive fatigue: may indicate too much exercise
Instruct about **rest** Frequent rest periods are necessary to prevent fatigue Legs should be elevated to promote venous return Crossing legs at knees should be avoided to prevent pressure on veins	Venous stasis in legs and feet late in pregnancy: may occur due to weight of fetus on femoral plexus	
Instruct about **clothing** Bras should support with wide shoulder straps Client may need several sizes during pregnancy Shoes should be supportive, with low heels Clothing should be loose and comfortable. Client should avoid constrictive clothing, especially on legs		
Instruct about **bathing** Tub baths are acceptable if membranes intact and no bleeding Client should be helped when getting in and out of the tub		Tub baths avoided: client large and unstable on feet; signs of bleeding, onset of labor

ASSESSMENT	NORMAL	ABNORMAL
Instruct about **drugs** and **tobacco** Tobacco should be eliminated or decreased Alcohol should be eliminated		Alcohol use associated with small-for-gestational-age infants (SGA) If mother is allergic to alcohol: fetal alcohol syndrome
Instruct about **sexual relations**	Continuation if no bleeding, ruptured membranes, or premature contractions	
Instruct about **preparations for labor and delivery** at about 30th to 32nd week of gestation		
Instruct about **major discomforts** and **relief measures**		

RECOMMENDATIONS FOR POSTPARTUM CLIENTS

Instruct about **nutrition**		
Instruct about **exercise**	Return to previous level of activity slowly, progressively, with physician's approval	Early, strenuous exercise: may lead to fatigue and hemorrhage
Encourage adequate **rest**		
Inform about **care of baby** Bathing/skin care Diapering/dressing Feeding/burping Sleeping/positioning Temperature/signs of illness Medical check-ups/immunizations Safety Growth and development		
Instruct about **contraceptives** if necessary	Nursing: use condom, gel, foam for first 6 weeks then method of choice may be used Nonnursing: may use oral contraceptives after delivery	
Instruct about **sexual relations**	Resume when episiotomy healed and lochia stopped	Pain with intercourse: may need water-based jelly for lubrication for four to six months; episiotomy may not be healed

THEORIES OF CHILDBIRTH

Factors that influence pain in labor

1. Preconditioning by "old wives' tales," fantasies, and fears. Accurate information about the childbirth process can often alleviate effects of preconditioning.
2. Pain produces stress, which in turn affects the body's functioning. Interpretations of and reactions to pain can be altered by a refocusing of attention and by conditioning.
3. Feelings of isolation. Social expectations and tension may also increase feelings of pain.

Childbirth education

1. Each method varies somewhat but basic underlying concepts are similar. Birth is viewed as a natural occurrence. Knowledge about the birth experience dispels fears and tension, and distraction and concentration during labor and delivery modify the pain experience.
2. Purpose is to promote relaxation enabling the mother to work with the labor process. Allows parents to take an active part in the birth process, thereby increasing self-esteem and satisfaction.
3. Goals are accomplished by means of:
   Education: anatomy and physiology of reproductive system, and the labor and delivery process; replacement of misinformation and superstition with facts. May include classes on nutrition, discomforts of pregnancy, breast-feeding, infant care, etc.
   Training: controlled breathing and neuromuscular exercises.
   Presence of father, or significant other, in labor and delivery rooms to serve as coach and lend support.
4. Common methods presently available:
   Read method (Natural Childbirth) introduced by Grantly Dick-Read in England. Believed pain in childbirth was psychological rather than physiological. Pain brought about by fear and tension.
   Lamaze method.
   Bradley method.
   Scientific relaxation for childbirth.
5. *LeBoyer technique*: used in delivery room to reduce stress of birth upon infant.
   Includes increasing room temperature to one comfortable for infant, reducing external stimuli by dimming lights, keeping noise level to a minimum.
   Infant is placed in skin-to-skin contact on mother's abdomen and gently stroked; cord clamping is delayed until pulsation stops.
   Infant is submerged up to head in a bath of warm water until it appears relaxed, then is dried and wrapped snugly in a warm blanket.
6. Classes for parents expecting delivery by C-section are now being given.

MAJOR DISCOMFORTS AND RELIEF MEASURES

DISCOMFORT	TRIMESTER MOST PROMINENT	RELIEF MEASURES
Nausea and vomiting	1st	Eat five or six small, frequent meals. In between meals, have crackers without fluid Avoid foods high in carbohydrates, fried and greasy, or with a strong odor Take antinausea drug if prescribed
Frequency	1st and 3rd	Wear perineal pads if there is leakage
Heartburn	2nd and 3rd	Avoid fatty, fried, and highly spiced foods Have small frequent feedings Use an antacid; *avoid* sodium bicarbonate
Abdominal distress	1st, 2nd, and 3rd	Eat slowly, chew food thoroughly, take smaller helpings of food
Flatulence	2nd and 3rd	Maintain daily bowel movement Avoid gas-forming foods. Take antiflatulents as prescribed by physician

DISCOMFORT	TRIMESTER MOST PROMINENT	RELIEF MEASURES
Constipation	2nd and 3rd	Drink sufficient fluids. Eat fruit and foods high in roughage Exercise moderately Take stool softener if prescribed by physician. Do *not* use mineral oil
Hemorrhoids	3rd	Apply ointments, suppositories, warm compresses Avoid constipation and get adequate rest
Insomnia	3rd	Exercise moderately to promote relaxation and fatigue Change position while sleeping If severe, take medication as prescribed by physician
Backaches	3rd	Rest and improve posture — use a firm mattress Use a good abdominal support, wear comfortable shoes Do exercises such as squatting, sitting, and pelvic rock
Varicosities of legs and vulva	3rd	Avoid long periods of standing or sitting with legs crossed Sit or lie with feet and hips elevated Move about while standing to improve circulation Wear support hose; *avoid* tight garters
Edema of legs and feet	3rd	Elevate feet while sitting or lying down Avoid standing or sitting in one position for long periods
Cramps in legs	3rd	Extend cramped leg and flex ankles, pushing foot upward with toes pointed toward knee Increase calcium intake
Pain in thighs or aching of perineum	3rd	Alternate periods of sitting and standing Rest
Shortness of breath	3rd	Sit up Lie on back with arms extended above head
Breast soreness	1st, 2nd, and 3rd	Wear brassiere with wide adjustable straps that fits well
Supine hypotensive syndrome	3rd	Change position to left side to relieve pressure of uterus on inferior vena cava
Vaginal discharge	3rd	Practice proper cleansing and hygiene. Avoid douche unless recommended by physician Observe for signs of vaginal infection common in pregnancy

The basic methods of pediatric assessment are similar to those used for assessing adults. However, the pediatric nurse should be cognizant of some specific differences in techniques, observations, and findings. For example, physical examination findings must be placed within the context of the child's growth and development continuum. Normal and abnormal development of the child's body systems and the child's cognitive processes should also be considered.

Because children are generally not as compliant as adults during physical examinations, it is important to plan your approach before any examination. Knowledge of a child's growth and developmental level, as well as a child's fears and level of understanding, is essential for a successful examination.

Before touching an infant, make sure your hands are warm. Start with the nonintrusive portions of the examination, such as observing muscle tone and body symmetry. Progress to the more intrusive portions, such as adducting hips for dislocation. When a child is quiet, listen to the heart rate and rhythm and respirations. An active or crying child makes auscultation difficult.

When you are assessing toddlers allow the child to sit on his or her mother's lap for security. Use simple terms to explain what you are about to do. Before using a stethoscope or tongue blade, let the child examine it. Begin the examination with the least threatening procedures; gradually proceed to the more threatening ones. For example, observe the child's hands and feet, chest and abdomen; then auscultate and percuss these areas. Observe the child's genital area; examine the child's head, eyes, face, neck, mouth, ears, nose, and throat. (Toddlers do not like anyone holding their heads!)

When assessing school-age children you will be aware that the school-age child is generally more cooperative than a younger one. During the examination, let the client manipulate the instruments and listen to the stethoscope. Allow the child to keep on underwear until you assess the genitalia. Begin the examination by assessing the child's vital signs, moving from head to toe. Examine the genitalia last. When you conduct this part of the examination, allow the child adequate privacy. Also during the examination, talk with the child about his or her daily activities. This will serve two purposes: it distracts the child from the task at hand; and it gives you an opportunity to assess the child's activities and determine if they are appropriate to the child's age.

The assessment of the adolescent should proceed with the physical examination as with an adult. Use your discretion to determine whether the parent should be present. Respect the wishes of the young adult in this matter. As you conduct the examination, explain every procedure. Pay particular attention to the adjustment the young adult is making to physical and emotional changes in his or her life.

ASSESSMENT	NORMAL	ABNORMAL
NEWBORN ASSESSMENT		
SKIN ASSESSMENT		
Note skin **color** and **lesions**	Pink Mongolian spots Capillary hemangiomas on face or neck	Cyanosis, pallor, beefy red Petechiae, ecchymoses, or purpuric spots: signs of possible hematologic disorder Cafe au lait spots (patches of brown discoloration): possible sign of congenital neurological disorder Raised capillary hemangiomas on areas other than face or neck

ASSESSMENT	NORMAL	ABNORMAL
	Localized edema in presenting part	Edema of peritoneal wall
	Cheesy white vernix	Poor skin turgor: indicates dehydration
	Desquamation (peeling off)	Yellow discolored vernix (meconium stained)
	Milia (small white pustules over nose and chin)	Impetigo neonatorum (small pustules with surrounding red areas)
	Jaundice after 24 hours; gone by second week	Jaundice at birth or within 12 hours
		Dermal sinuses (opening to brain)
		Holes along spinal column
		Low hairline posteriorly: possible chromosomal abnormality
		Sparse or spotty hair: congenital goiter or chromosomal abnormality
Note color of **nails**	Pink	Yellowing of nail beds (meconium stained)
Note **skin tone**	Strong, tremulous	Flaccid, convulsions
		Muscular twitching, hypertonicity

HEAD AND NECK ASSESSMENT

Note **shape of head**	Fontanels: anterior open until 18 months; posterior closed shortly after birth	Depressed, tense, bulging, or absent fontanels: indicates hydrocephalus or dehydration
		Cephalohematoma that crosses the midline
		Microcephaly and macrocephaly
Assess **eyes**	Slight edema of lids	Purulent discharge
		Lateral upward slope of eye with an inner epicanthal fold in infants not of Oriental descent
		Exophthalmos (bulging of eyeball): may be congenital anomaly, sign of congenital glaucoma or thyroid abnormality
		Enophthalmos (recession of eyeball): may indicate damage to brain or cervical spine
	Pupils equal and reactive to light by three weeks of age	Constricted pupil, unilateral dilated fixed pupil, nystagmus (rhythmic nonpurposeful movement of eyeball): continuous strabismus
	Intermittent strabismus (occasional crossing of eyes)	
	Conjunctival or sclera hemorrhages	Haziness of cornea
	Symmetrical light reflex (light reflects off each eye in the same quadrant): sign of conjugate gaze	Absence of red reflex; asymmetrical light reflex
Note **placement of ears**, shape and position		Low set ears: may indicate Down's syndrome
Assess **nose**	Discharge, sneezing	Thick, bloody nasal discharge

ASSESSMENT	NORMAL	ABNORMAL
Assess **mouth**	Sucking, rooting reflexes Retention cysts (pears) Occasional vomiting	Cleft lip, palate Flat, white nonremovable spots (thrush) Frequent vomiting: may indicate pyloric stenosis Vomitus with bile: fecal vomiting Profuse salivation: may indicate tracheo-esophageal fistula
Assess **neck**	Tonic neck reflex (Fencer's position)	Distended neck veins Fractured clavicle Unusually short neck Excess posterior cervical skin Resistance to neck flexion
Assess **cry**	Lusty cry	Weak, groaning cry: possible neurological abnormality High-pitched cry; hoarse or crowing inspirations; cat-like cry: possible neurological or chromosomal abnormality

CHEST AND LUNG ASSESSMENT

Assess the **chest**	Circular Enlargement of breasts Milky discharge from breasts	Depressed sternum Retractions, asymmetry of chest movements: indicates respiratory distress and possible pneumothorax
Assess the **lungs**	Abdominal respirations Respiration rate: 30 to 50 Respiration movement irregular in rate and depth Resonant chest (hollow sound on percussion)	Thoracic breathing, unequal motion of chest, rapid grasping or grunting respirations, flaring nares Deep sighing respirations Grunt on expiration: possible respiratory distress Hyper-resonance of chest or decreased resonance

HEART ASSESSMENT

Assess the **rate**, **rhythm**, and **murmurs** of the heart	Rate: 100 to 180 at birth; stabilizes at 120 to 140 Regular rhythm Murmurs: significance cannot usually be determined in newborn	Heart rate above 200 or less than 100 Irregular rhythm Dextrocardia, enlarged heart

ABDOMEN AND GASTRO-INTESTINAL TRACT ASSESSMENT

Assess the **abdomen**	Prominent	Distention of abdominal veins: possible portal vein obstruction

ASSESSMENT	NORMAL	ABNORMAL
Assess the **gastrointestinal tract**	Bowel sounds present	Visible peristaltic waves
		Increased pitch or frequency: intestinal obstruction
		Decreased sounds: paralytic ileus
		Distention of abdomen
	Liver 2 to 3 cm below right costal margin	Enlarged liver or spleen
	Spleen tip palpable	Midline suprapubic mass: may indicate Hirschsprung's disease
	May be able to palpate kidneys	Enlarged kidney
	Bladder percussed 1 to 4 cm above symphysis pubis	Distended bladder; presence of any masses
	Umbilical cord with one vein and two arteries	One artery present in umbilical cord: may indicate other anomalies
	Soft granulation tissue at umbilicus	Wet umbilical stump or fetid odor from stump

GENITOURINARY TRACT ASSESSMENT

Assess the **genitalia**	Edema and bruising after delivery	Inguinal hernia
	Unusually large clitoris in females a short time after birth	
	Vaginal mucoid or bloody discharge may be present in the first week	
Urethra orifice	Urethra opens on ventral surface of penile shaft	Hypospadias (urethra opens on the inferior surface of the penis)
		Epispadias (urethra opens on the dorsal surface of the penis)
		Ulceration of urethral orifice
Testes	Testes in scrotal sac or inguinal canal	Hydroceles in males

SPINE AND EXTREMITIES ASSESSMENT

Assess the **spine**	Straight spine	Spina bifida, pilonidal sinus; scoliosis
Assess **extremities**		Asymmetry of movement
	Soft click with thigh rotation	Sharp click with thigh rotation: indicates possible congenital hip
		Uneven major gluteal folds: indicates possible congenital hip
		Polydactyly (extra digits on a hand or foot); syndactyly (webbing or fusion of fingers or toes)
Assess **anus and rectum**	Patent anus	Closed anus: no meconium

ASSESSMENT	NORMAL	ABNORMAL

PEDIATRIC ASSESSMENT

MEASUREMENTS

Measure **height** and **weight** and plot on a standardized growth chart	Height/weight proportional Sequential measurements: pattern follows normal growth curves	Height/weight below third percentile Sudden drop in percentile range of height and/or weight: possible sign of disease process or congenital problem
Assess **temperature** (axillary until six years of age)	Axillary 97° F; 36.4° C Elevations following eating or playing not unusual	Temperature of 104° to 105° F: corresponds roughly with 101° to 102° F in an adult Large daily temperature variations Hypothermia: usually result of chilling

Measure **circumference of head and chest**
  Examine or check circumferences when child is less than two years old
  Compare measurements with standardized charts
	Head at birth: about 2 cm greater than chest
	During first year: equalization of head and chest
	After two years: rapid growth of chest; slight increases in size of head
		Increase in head circumference greater than 2.5 cm per month: sign of hydrocephalus

VITAL SIGNS

Assess **pulse** apically	Birth to one year: 120 to 140 One year: 80 to 160 Two years: 80 to 130 Three years: 80 to 120 Over three years: 70 to 115	Pulse over 180 after first month of life: cardiac or respiratory condition Inability to palpate femoral pulses: possible coarctation of the aorta
Assess **respirations**	Birth: 30 to 50 Six years: 20 to 25 Puberty: 14 to 16 (Young children have abnormally high respiration rate with even slight excitement)	Consistent tachypnea: usually a sign of respiratory disease Respiratory rate over 100: lower respiratory tract obstruction Slow rate: may be sign of CNS depression
Assess **blood pressure**	Birth: 60 to 90 mm Hg systolic 20 to 60 mm Hg diastolic Rise in both pressures: 2 to 3 mm Hg per year of age Adult level reached at puberty	Elevated blood pressure in upper extremities: coarctation of aorta Narrowed pulse pressure (normal or elevated diastolic with lowered systolic; less than 30 mm Hg difference between systolic and diastolic readings): possible sign of aortic or subaortic stenosis or hypothyroidism Widened pulse pressure: possible sign of hyperthyroidism

211

ASSESSMENT	NORMAL	ABNORMAL
APPEARANCE		
Observe **general appearance**	Alert, well-nourished comfortable, responsive	Lethargic, uncomfortable, malnourished, gross anomalies, dull
Listen to **voice and cry**	Strong, lusty cry	Weak cry, low- or high-pitched cry: may indicate neurological problem or chromosomal abnormality
	Facial expression animated	Expressionless, unresponsive
	No indications of pain	Doubling over, rubbing a body part, general fretfulness
	No odor	Musty odor: sign of phenylketonuria, diphtheria
		Odor of maple syrup: may be maple syrup urine disease
		Odor of sweaty feet: one type of acidemia
		Fishy odor: may be metabolic disorder
		Acetone odor: acidosis, particularly diabetic ketoacidosis
SKIN ASSESSMENT		
Assess **pigmentation**	Usually even	Multiple cafe au lait spots: possible neurofibromatosis
	Pigmented nevi common	Cyanosis
	Large, flat, black and blue areas over sacrum, buttocks (Mongolian spots)	Jaundice
		Pallor
Assess **lesions**	Usually none	Erythematous lesions
	Adolescence: acne	Multiple macules, papules, or vesicles
		Petechiae and ecchymoses: may indicate coagulation disorder
		Hives
		Subcutaneous nodules: may indicate juvenile rheumatoid arthritis
Note **consistency of skin**	Good turgor	Poor turgor
	Smooth and firm	Dryness
		Edema
		Lack or excess of subcutaneous fat: sign of malnutrition or excess nutrition
Assess **nails**	Nail beds: normally pigmented	Cyanosis
	Good nail growth	Pallor
		Capillary pulsations
		Pitting of the nails: possible sign of fungal disease or psoriasis
		Broad nail beds: possible sign of Down's syndrome or other chromosomal abnormality

ASSESSMENT	NORMAL	ABNORMAL
Assess **hair** (consistency appropriate to ethnic group)	No excessive breaking	Dry, coarse, brittle hair: possible sign of hypothyroidism Alopecia (loss of hair): may be psychosomatic or due to drug therapy Unusual hairiness in places other than scalp, eyebrows, and lashes: may indicate hypothyroidism, vitamin A poisoning, chronic infections, reaction to Dilantin therapy Tufts of hair over spine or sacrum: may indicate site of spina bifida occulta or spina bifida Absence of the start of pubic hair during adolescence: possible hypothyroidism, hypopituitarism, gonadal deficiency, or Addison's disease
Assess **lymph nodes**	Nontender, movable, discrete nodes up to 3 mm in diameter in occipital, postauricular, parotid, submaxillary, sublingual, axillary, and epitrochlear nodes Up to 1 mm in diameter inguinal and cervical nodes	Tender or enlarged nodes: may be sign of systemic infection

HEAD AND NECK ASSESSMENT

ASSESSMENT	NORMAL	ABNORMAL
Assess **scalp**	Usually without lesions	Ringworm, lice
Assess frontal and maxillary **sinuses**	Nontender	Tenderness: indicative of inflammatory process
Assess **face**	Symmetrical movement	Signs of facial paralysis Twitching: could be due to psychosomatic causes
Evaluate the **eyes**		
Gross screening of vision with Snellen chart	With younger child, ability to follow movement and to see objects placed a few feet away	Inability to follow movement or to see objects placed a few feet away
Sclerae	Completely white	Yellow sclera: sign of jaundice Blue sclera: may be normal or indicative of osteogenesis imperfecta
Placement in eye socket	Normally placed	Exophthalmos (protrusion of eyeball) Enophthalmos (deeply placed eyeball)
Iris	At rest: upper and lower margins of iris visible between the lids	Setting sun sign (iris appears to be beneath lower lid): if marked, may be sign of increased intracranial pressure
Movement	In newborn, intermittent strabismus	Fixed strabismus or intermittent strabismus continuing after six months of age: indication of muscle paralysis or weakness Nystagmus (constant motion of eye): characteristic of cerebellar lesions and brain tumors

213

ASSESSMENT	NORMAL	ABNORMAL
Eyelids	Fully covers eye Fully raised on opening	Ptosis of eyelid: may be an early sign of a neuro-logical disorder Sty
Conjunctiva	Clear	Inflammation Conjunctivitis Hemorrhage Stimson's lines (small red transverse lines on conjunctiva)
Cornea	Clear	Opacity: sign of ulceration Inflammation Redness
Discharge	Tears	Purulent discharges: note amount, color, consistency
Pupils	Round, regular Clear, equal Brisk reaction to light Accommodation reflex (pupil contraction as object is brought near the eye)	Sluggish or asymmetrical reaction to light: indicates intracranial disease Lack of accommodation reflex
Lens	Clear	Opacities (cataracts)

Evaluate the **ears**

Sinuses	None present	Small holes or pits anterior to ear: may be super-ficial but could indicate the presence of a sinus leading into brain
Position	Top of ear above level of eye	Top of ear below level of eye: congenital defects
Discharge	None	Discharge: note color, odor, and amount
Hearing	In infant: turning to sound In older child: response to whis-pered command	Diminished hearing in one or both ears

Assess the **nose**

	No secretions	Secretions: note characteristics Any unusual shape or flaring of nostrils
	Breathing through nose	Breathing through mouth

Assess the **mouth**

		Circumoral pallor: possible sign of cyanotic heart disease, scarlet fever, rheumatic fever, hypo-glycemia; also seen in other febrile diseases Asymmetry of lips: seen in nerve paralysis
	Intact palate	Cleft palate
	Teeth in good condition In older child, presence of per-manent teeth	Delayed appearance of deciduous teeth: may indicate cretinism, rickets, congenital syphilis, or Down's syndrome; may be normal Poor tooth formation: may be seen with systemic diseases Green or black teeth: seen after iron ingestion or death of tooth Stained teeth: may be seen after prolonged use of tetracyclines

ASSESSMENT	NORMAL	ABNORMAL
Assess the **gums**	Retention cysts in newborn	Inflammation, abnormal color, drooling, pus, tenderness Black line along gums: may indicate lead poisoning
Assess the **tongue**	Moves freely	Tremors on protrusion: may indicate chorea, hyperthyroidism White spots (thrush) Tongue-tie
Assess the **throat**	Tonsils normally enlarged in childhood	White membrane over tonsils White pus on sacs, erythema
Assess the **larynx**	Normal vocal tones	Hoarseness or stridor: possible respiratory tract obstruction
Assess the **neck**	Short in infancy Lengthens at two to three years Trachea slightly right midline	Trachea deviated to left or right: may indicate shift with atelectasis
Thyroid	Not enlarged	Enlarged: may be due to hyperactive thyroid, malignancy, goiter
Motion	Full lateral and upward/downward motion	Limited movement with pain: may indicate meningeal irritation, lymph node enlargement, rheumatoid arthritis, or other diseases

LUNGS AND THORAX ASSESSMENT

ASSESSMENT	NORMAL	ABNORMAL
Assess the **lungs**	Normally clear breath sounds bilaterally	Presence of rhonchi, rales or wheezes Diminished breath sounds heard over parts of lung
	No retractions	Mild or severe intercostal or sternal retractions
	Symmetry of diaphragmatic movement	Asymmetry of movement
Assess the **sputum**	None or small amount of clear sputum in morning	Thick, tenacious sputum with foul odor Blood-tinged or green sputum
Assess the **breasts**	Slightly enlarged in infancy Generally slightly asymmetrical at puberty	Discharge or growth in male

HEART ASSESSMENT

ASSESSMENT	NORMAL	ABNORMAL
Assess **heart sounds**	S_1, S_2, S_3	S_4: indicates congestive heart failure
Assess **femoral pulses**	Strong	Weak
Note **edema**	None present	Edema: note location (initially periorbital) and duration

ASSESSMENT	NORMAL	ABNORMAL
Note **clubbing** of fingers	None present	Clubbing: note location and duration
Note **murmurs**		Murmur grade three or higher
Note **cyanosis**	None normally present	Circumoral or peripheral cyanosis: indicates respiratory or cardiac disease
		Abnormal pulse rate for age

ABDOMEN ASSESSMENT

Assess **skin condition**	Soft	Hard, rigid, tender
Assess for **peristaltic motion**	Not visible	Visible peristalsis: may indicate pyloric stenosis
Assess **shape**	Slightly protuberant in standing adolescent	Large protruding abdomen: may indicate pancreatic fibrosis, hypokalemia, rickets, hypothyroidism, bowel destruction, constipation
		Inguinal hernias, unilateral or bilateral: observe for reducibility
	Umbilical protrusion	Umbilical hernia

GENITOURINARY TRACT ASSESSMENT

Assess **female genitalia**		
Discharge	Mucoid	Foul or copious discharge; any bleeding prior to puberty
Assess **male genitalia**		
Presence of urethral orifice	Orifice on distal end of penis	Hypospadias or epispadias (urethral orifice along inferior or dorsal surface)
Urethral opening	Normal size	Stenosis of urethral opening
Foreskin	Covers glans completely	Foreskin incompletely formed ventrally when hypospadias present
Placement of testes	Descended testes	Undescended testes
		Enlarged scrotum
Assess **urine output**	Full, steady stream of urine	Urine with pus, blood, or odor
		Excessive urination or nocturia: possible sign of diabetes
Check **anus and rectum**	No masses or fissures present	Hemorrhoids, fissures, prolapse, pinworms
		Dark ring around rectal mucosa: may be sign of lead poisoning

MUSCULOSKELETAL ASSESSMENT

Assess **extremities**	Coloration of fingers and toes consistent with rest of body	Cyanosis: can indicate hypothermia, respiratory, or cardiac disease
		Clubbing of fingers and toes: indicates cardiac or respiratory disease

ASSESSMENT	NORMAL	ABNORMAL
	Quick capillary refill on blanching	Sluggish blood return on blanching: indicates poor circulation
	Temperature same as rest of body	Temperature variation between extremities and rest of body: indicates neurological or vascular anomalies
	Presence of pedal pulses	Absence of pedal pulses indicates circulatory difficulties
	No pain or tenderness	Presence of localized or generalized pain
	Straight legs after two years of age	Any bowing after two years of age: may be hereditary or indicate rickets
	Broad-based gait until four years of age; feet straight ahead afterwards	Scissoring gait: indicates spastic cerebral palsy
		Persistence of broad-based gait after four years of age: possible abnormalities of legs and feet or balance disturbance
		Any limp or ataxia
Assess **spine**	No dimples	Presence of dimple or tufts of hair: possible spina bifida
	Flexible	Limited flexion: indicates central nervous system infections
		Hyperextension (opisthotonos): indicates brainstem irritation, hemorrhage, or intracranial infection
	No lateral curvature or excessive anterior posterior curvature	Presence of lordosis, kyphosis, or scoliosis
Assess **joints**	Full range of motion without pain, edema, or tenderness	Pain, edema, or tenderness: indicates tissue injury
Assess **muscles**	Good tone and purposeful movement	Decreased or increased tone
	Ability to perform motor skills approximate to developmental level	Spasm or tremors: may indicate cerebral palsy
		Atrophy or contractures

NEUROLOGICAL ASSESSMENT

Refer to adult section on neurological assessment for complete overview

Assess **fine motor movements**	Presence of fine motor activity approximate to age	Continued presence of primitive reflexes after fading of reflex should normally occur: may indicate brain damage
Assess presence of **reflexes**		Any asymmetry of movement

CHAPTER 7
Managing Stress and Pain

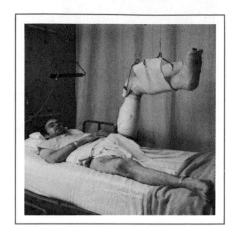

COPING WITH STRESS

Stress is a universal phenomenon that all human beings in all cultures experience. The concept of stress has been with man since the beginning of time, but it was not until William Osler and Walter Cannon began their investigation that stress was actually linked to illness. By 1950 Dr. Hans Selye, an endocrinologist and biologist and the world expert on stress, scientifically demonstrated that stress played a major role in certain diseases such as gastric ulcers and high blood pressure. Since Dr. Selye's early research, authorities from medicine, biology, physiology, sociology, psychology, and anthropology have studied and written thousands of articles on the subject of stress. With the undeniable fact that stress affects an individual's total life, it is imperative that the nurse have a basic understanding of stress, its effect on humans, how humans cope and adapt to stress, and how the nurse can deal with his or her own stress and help clients deal with theirs. The stress of life is life itself according to Dr. Barbara Brown. To examine stress and its impact on human beings in this culture, we have to examine one's total life experience.

Western medicine is entering an era of transformation. The whole context of the medical profession is changing. Clients and professionals alike are examining alternatives to traditional patterns of treatment and are devising new modes of health care delivery. These changes are

LEARNING OBJECTIVES

Define stress and discuss the impact of stress on the body.

Describe Selye's general adaptation syndrome.

List at least three different categories of stressors.

Identify five major signals of stress.

Outline the factors that alter resistance to stress.

Discuss three specific methods to control stress.

Explain what is meant by the Holistic Model of Stress Reduction.

Define what is meant by pain.

Discuss the Gate Control Theory.

Outline the main points of one noninvasive method of relieving pain.

State the main parameters of pain assessment.

Summarize at least two methods of relieving pain.

219

occurring at a time when the structure of the health care system in this country (and indeed the world) desperately needs new ways of dealing with health and illness. And, as we change our focus from illness to health, we need new perspectives for health care.

Perhaps the greatest impetus for these changes has come about in response to new knowledge about the role of stress in our lives. Dr. Selye believes that efforts to manage and find cures for diseases is an ineffective approach to creating wellness. He and other prominent scientists think that the only viable approach is to examine man's ability to cope and adapt to stress. At the second international conference on stress held in Monte Carlo eminent physician Dr. Arnold Fox stated that stress is either the main cause or a strong contributing factor in all diseases of mankind. Most of these scientists now attribute 70 to 80 percent of all diseases to stress.

Dr. Brown, however, believes that 100 percent of diseases have stress factors at the root. The view that disease is caused by invading micro-organisms or that ill people are merely victims or even that all disease can be cured by modern science is erroneous. New definition of existing problems necessitates finding new solutions. The current emphasis on stress and stress reduction methods may be a new solution to old problems. The current emphasis on stress is relevant to our times, and as nurses, we need to recognize and understand stress and the impact of stress on us as individuals, on our profession, and, most particularly, on our clients.

Stress is a difficult term to define precisely, for there is not one specific source or one definite response. Dr. Selye states that stress may be viewed as the common denominator of all the body's adaptive reactions. Stress may be grief as well as joy, pleasure as well as unhappiness, cold as well as heat, fear as well as elation. In fact, stress covers the total range of mental, emotional, and physical demands on the body that will respond with predictable biochemical and general adaptation changes. Health is determined by the body's being in a state of balance in which the whole organism functions in harmony. Stress can be defined as a state of arousal or agitation which throws the body out of balance. While a certain amount of stress is necessary for survival, when it becomes prolonged and intense, our adaptive responses weary and the negative aspects begin to take their toll on our bodies and our minds.

The Impact of Stress   Psychologically, stress may be viewed as the experience an individual has when the demands placed on the body exceed the ability to cope; thus, the body is thrown out of balance. Physiologically, stress initiates certain bodily processes, such as the "fight or flight" mechanism, which result in a threat to homeostasis. Early in the 1900s Dr. Cannon, a Harvard physiologist, coined the term "homeostasis." As a result of his work, certain adjustment mechanisms of the body, such as blood sugar level, temperature, hydration, etc., were identified. According to Dr. Cannon, the stress response resulted in these mechanisms being activated, which in turn threw the body out of balance.

Rather than a specific response, Dr. Selye focuses on a general adaption process as a response to stress. This process is the body's attempt to adapt and maintain homeostasis. Dr. Selye further defines stress as the rate of wear and tear on the body and states that the only freedom from stress is death.

Dr. Selye's general adaptation syndrome occurs in three stages. The first stage, *the alarm stage*, occurs when a generalized response throughout the body responds to stressors such as trauma, infection, pain, cold, heat, fear. The purpose of the alarm reaction is to mobilize the body's defenses to meet the stressor. Biochemically, during alarm, the hormonal levels of the adrenal cortex and lymph glands increase. The anti-inflammatory hormones, the adrenocorticotropin hormones, cortisone, and cortisol are produced along with pro-inflammatory hormones, aldosterone, and desoxycorticosterone. This is the shock phase when the autonomic nervous system comes into full play. The second stage, *the resistance stage*, occurs when the body's defenses are mobilized to produce hormones to cope with the alarm stage. The body chemistry either repels or adapts to the stressor. During this phase the organism is successful in adapting to the stressor, and the biochemical changes resulting from the alarm phase return to the pre-alarm stage. Any life change causes alarm and resistance and the stress accrued through life reduces the body's adaptive abilities. Continuous high degrees of stress will deplete the organism's adaptive abilities at a much greater rate than normal stress levels. *The final stage* occurs when the stress is prolonged and the body can no longer cope effectively. The result is exhaustion and the body may become ill with disease. The organism's adaptive abilities are depleted and the organism loses its ability to deal with the stress. The organism goes into shock, and if the stress is not alleviated, the result may be the death of the organism.

The general adaptation syndrome varies widely in intensity. A reaction to positive stimuli, such as getting married or learning you are going to have a baby, will activate stress response but it may result in less damage than a negative stressor even though it does temporarily throw the body out of balance. Moreover, a person does not respond with the same intensity to all negative stressors. For example, you would not respond with the same degree of intensity to jumping in a cold pool as you would to turning a corner and seeing a man pointing a gun at you.

The local adaptation syndrome is the manifestation of stress in a limited part of the body. The body responds locally to the stressor, such as a burn or a cut to a finger. The local response may also trigger a general response if the ability of the body to respond to the specific area is greatly affected by the condition of the whole organism. An upper respiratory infection causes much different response within a healthy child than in a child with cystic fibrosis. The better the organism as a whole is at adapting to stress, the more effective the local adaptive response.

Response to Stress Responses to stress then can be categorized into several different patterns: the physiological response, where there is loss or gain in weight, increase in hormone levels, increase in blood pressure, or a psychosomatic symptom; the psychological response, which may also result in a psychosomatic illness or psychiatric manifestations, such as depression, mania, withdrawal from reality, or neurosis; the behavioral response, where one hits out, becomes aggressive (fights) or withdraws, becomes immobilized or turns inward (physical or emotional flight); interpersonal mode, where communication effectiveness decreases, relationships deteriorate, trust in others diminishes, the ability to form and maintain close, intimate, loving ties with another person decreases; and, finally, the affective response, where one's emotions are affected so that anxiety is high and emotions are unstable, labile, unpredictable, and inappropriate to the situation. All of the above modes of response relate the negative elements of response patterns. Of course, these modes can be used in a positive way so that stress becomes nondetrimental. All life is basically stress-producing as it demands the organism to adapt to continual internal and external changes. There is no way to eliminate the stressors, but individuals can learn to minimize the harmful effects and utilize response modes in a positive way.

SELYE'S STRESS ADAPTATION SYNDROME

STAGE	GENERAL FUNCTION	INTERPERSONAL	BEHAVIORAL	AFFECTIVE	COGNITIVE	PHYSIOLOGICAL
1 Alarm reaction	Mobilization of body defenses	Interpersonal communication effectiveness decreases	Task oriented Increased restlessness Apathy, regression Crying	Feelings of anger, suspiciousness, helplessness Anxiety level increases	Alert Thinking becomes narrow and concrete Symptoms of thought blocking, forgetfulness, and decreased productivity	Muscle tension Increase in epinephrine and cortisone Stimulation of adrenal cortex and lymph glands Increase in blood pressure, heart rate, blood glucose
2 Stage of resistance	Adaptation to stresses Resistance increases	Interpersonal communication self-oriented Uses interpersonal relationships to meet own needs	Automatic behaviors Self-oriented behaviors Fight or flight behavior apparent	Increased use of defense mechanisms Emotional responses may be automatic or exaggerated	Thought processes more habitual than problem solving oriented	Hormonal levels return to pre-alarm stage All physiological responses return to normal or are channeled into psychosomatic symptoms
3 Stage of exhaustion	Depletion or exhaustion of organs and resources Loss of ability to resist stress	Disintegration of personal interactions Communication skills ineffective and disorganized Self-oriented	Restless, withdrawn, agitated; may become violent or self-destructive Diminished productivity	Depressed, flat, or inappropriate Exaggerated or inappropriate use of defense mechanisms Decreased ability to cope	Thought disorganization, hallucinations, preoccupation Reduced intellectual processes	Exhaustion, with increased demands on organism Adrenal cortex hormone depletion Death, if stress is continuous and excessive

Stressors may be chemical, physical, developmental, and emotional. Graduating from nursing school, being promoted, failing to be promoted, having arguments, and playing a tough game of racketball are all stressful events and require adaptation and change at some level. By understanding stress, we can more easily identify stress factors and their effects on clients who need and/or seek health care. Whether a client is having a baby, undergoing open heart surgery, or seeking counseling for emotional problems, each of these individuals is experiencing stress in his or her own particular manner. How the individual adapts or fails to adapt depends on several factors: personality and emotional makeup and past experiences in dealing with stress (response repertoire).

People are able to create many different forms of disease as well as emotional and spiritual scars. And the more we use our reserves of adaptation energy, the more likely we are to age and hasten our death. In fact, Dr. Selye warns that there is no evidence that the basic reserves of energy for adaptation can be restored. These may be genetically programmed. The more reserves you use handling everyday stress, the less you have for major crises or for growing older. The latest research indicates that there is a direct relationship between the amount of stress encountered in everyday life and aging.

It is important to remember that the stress syndrome can be both positive and negative. Any change or alteration in the balance of life can create stress. The Holmes and Rahe stress scale is an excellent example of the varying conditions in life that result in stress. We are all unique individuals and we respond differently to various stressors. Thus, it does not matter whether the stress is positive or negative, light or severe. What matters is how we develop adaptive mechanisms to cope with these stressors. The ability to cope or solve a problem can be translated as the ability to withstand stress and create life experiences that do not work against you. The implications of stress theory — that by being able to withstand stress, by coping with it, diluting it when it occurs, or eliminating it you can actually affect your life — are tremendously exciting. It means that you are not doomed to inevitable illness later in life. You are not preprogrammed for premature aging. The fact is you control your own health. To quote the *Journal* of American Medical Association, "Nature did not intend us to grow old and ill; we were designed to die young in old age but free of disease."

Along with coping with his or her own stress, it is the responsibility of the nurse to be aware that clients suffer from the stress phenomena and that part of the nurse's role is to assist clients to adapt and cope with stress. How can this behavioral objective be implemented?

First, the nurse must have an understanding of the role of stress.
- Understand and accept the theory of stress — what it is and what it does to the body.
- Be cognizant of the manifestations of stress: tiredness, apathy, frequent illness, lack of interest or aliveness, unwillingness to seek out new challenges, inability to cope with change, and many other symptoms.

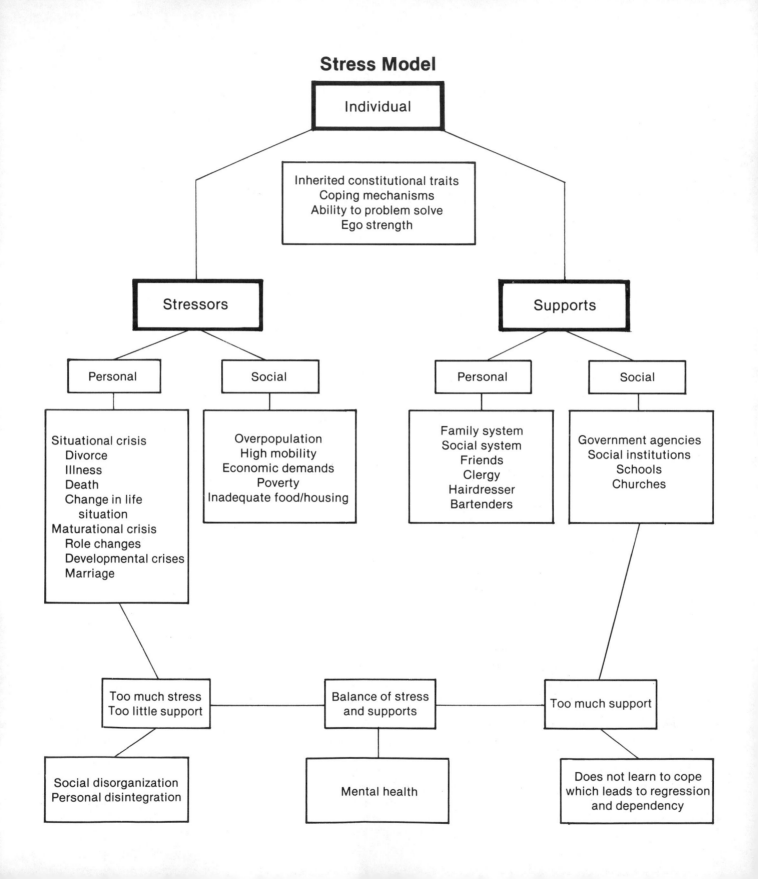

Stress Model

- Elicit the factors that alter resistance to stress (illness, hospitalization, pain, medication, family pressures, etc.).
- Make a plan and implement it, designing specific actions to reduce stress, such as relaxation methods.
- Educate the individual about how to control his or her own stressors.

Secondly, the nurse may carry out specific behaviors in the hospital setting.

- Counsel the client and family on the theory of stress; together, examine how the client's particular stressors impact his or her lifestyle.
- Reinforce the adaptive process of the client by meeting his or her needs, listening to concerns, administering care, and providing emotional support.
- Assist in the reduction of negative aspects of stress by assisting the client to alter adaptive behaviors.

GUIDELINES FOR MANAGING CLIENTS

Human beings move naturally toward wellness and away from illness.

- Human beings have a capacity to be aware of self and of others in relation to self.
- Human beings are capable of taking responsibility for healing themselves.
- Human beings have the ability to regulate the status of their own health and wellness.

Stress is a universal phenomenon that all human beings experience.

- Current research indicates that 80 percent of diseases are stress induced.
- There is no one specific source of stress nor one definitive response.
- Stress may come from environmental, physical, emotional, mental, and even social sources. Responses also range from physiological to behavioral to emotional.
- A certain amount of stress is necessary for survival but when it becomes prolonged and intense, the individual experiences negative effects.

Dr. Selye's theory, general adaptation syndrome, focuses on a general adaptation process as a response to stress.

- This process occurs in three stages — the alarm stage, the resistance stage, and, finally, the stage of exhaustion.
- This syndrome varies in intensity and a person does not respond with the same intensity to all negative stressors.

Clients suffer from stress and part of the nurse's role is to assist clients to adapt and cope with the stress.

- Nurses must understand the role of stress and how it may be manifested in each individual.
- Nurses must be able to examine with the client the factors that alter the resistance to stress.
- Finally, nurses must be able to introduce and implement measures to reduce stress.

ACTION: IDENTIFYING STRESS—IMPACT AND RESPONSE

ASSESSMENT

Rationale for Action
- To identify presence of stress in client
- To identify how stress impacts on the body
- To determine the client's responses to stress
- To evaluate stress interventions that will have a positive effect on stressed client

1 Identify the client who demonstrates stressed behavior.
2 Evaluate, with the client, the past and present stressors that the client has experienced.
3 Evaluate the stressors' effect on the client's body and for signs of distress in the body. Examples of stress impact are:
   a Cardiovascular system: increased pulse and blood pressure, evidence of angina, arrhythmias, migraine headaches, disturbance of heat and cold mechanisms.
   b Gastrointestinal system: ulcers, ulcerative colitis, constipation or diarrhea, imbalance in sugar absorption.
   c Musculoskeletal system: backache, tension headaches, arthritis, proneness to accidents.
   d Autoimmune system: infections, flu, allergies, rheumatoid arthritis, cancer.
4 Assess client's level of energy and the degree to which it is depleted.
5 Evaluate client's awareness of thoughts, attitudes, values, and beliefs that influence stress response and adaptation.
6 Assess present level of distress in the client's body.
7 Assess possible causes of stress that are affecting client.
   a Environmental stressors: input overload such as sights, sounds, smells; actions and demands of others in the environment; or monotony.
   b Physical stressors: hunger, heat or cold, dangerous environment, injury, or pain.
   c Emotional stressors: loss of something of value, frustrations of needs and drives, and/or threats to self-concept.
   d Psychosocial stressors:
   Conflicting cultural values (i.e., the American values of competition and assertiveness vs. the need to be dependent).
   Future shock — physiological and psychological stress resulting from an overload of the organism's adaptive systems and decision-making processes brought about by too rapidly changing values and technology.
   Cultural shock — stress developing in response to the transition from a familiar environment to unfamiliar one; involves unfamil-

iarity with communication, technology, customs, attitudes and beliefs (i.e., immigrating, being confined in a hospital or prison); crowding and urban life.

Job choice and the work environment (about 80 percent of the workers in our country are estimated to be unhappy in their jobs).

8 Assess the factors that influence how the client responds to stress.

  a Characteristics of the stressful event: magnitude, intensity, duration.

  b Client's biological and psychological inclinations.

  c Soundness of support system.

PLANNING

GOALS

* Client who is severely stressed is identified.
* Client is able to evaluate the general stressors that impact on his or her life.
* Client identifies the current sources that result in stressed behavior.
* Client is aware of response patterns to stressors and is able to alter them appropriately.

INTERVENTION: Determining Impact of Stress on Client

1 Discuss the concept of stress with client to elicit his or her understanding of the impact on body.

  a Stress is a physical, chemical, or emotional factor that causes bodily or mental tension and that may be a factor in disease causation; it is a state resulting from factors that tend to alter an existing equilibrium.

  b Dr. Selye's definition of stress.

    A state manifested by a specific syndrome that consists of all the nonspecifically induced changes within the biologic system. The body is the common denominator of all adaptive responses.

    Stress is manifested by the measurable changes in the body.

    Stress causes a multiplicity of changes in the body.

2 Provide a relationship where client feels free to discuss his or her life patterns that relate to stress.

3 Discuss the impact of stress on client. Cover physical, emotional, mental, and social areas of life that are affected by stress.

4 Formulate a plan with the client to reduce or eliminate at least some of the sources of stress.

INTERVENTION: Determining the Response Patterns to Stress

1 Discuss the client's body response to stress in his or her life.

  a The body's response to stress is a self-preserving mechanism that automatically and immediately becomes activated in times of danger.

Caused by physical or psychological stress: disease, injury, anger, or frustration.

Caused by changes in internal and/or external environment.

  b There are a limited number of ways an organism can respond to stress (a cornered amoeba cannot fly).

2 Assist client to understand his or her response patterns.

3 Provide problem-solving assistance so client can examine new, more appropriate response patterns.

4 Refer client to resources (therapy classes, books, relaxation tapes) that will assist him or her to develop new responses.

EVALUATION

EXPECTED OUTCOMES

1 Client is able to evaluate the general stressors and identify sources of stress in his or her life. *If not*, follow these alternative nursing actions:

ANA: Start at the beginning and reexplain the theory of stress and what is meant by stressor.

ANA: Administer a stress scale, such as the Holmes and Rahe stress test, which rates various life situations to determine the amount of stress one is experiencing.

ANA: Suggest that client ask family and friends to help identify stressors.

2 Client is aware of response patterns to stress and is able to alter patterns appropriately. *If not*, follow these alternative nursing actions:

ANA: Examine client's behavior in all five modes — interpersonal, behavioral, affective, cognitive, and physiological — to identify specific responses.

ANA: Evaluate adaptation modes to determine whether they are adaptive or maladaptive. (See Selye's Stress Adaptation Syndrome chart.)

ANA: Suggest ways to alter response patterns, i.e., relaxation methods, visualization, exercise, consultation.

UNEXPECTED OUTCOMES

1 Client moves into the stage of exhaustion and stress becomes dangerous to health.

ANA: Immediately take measures to remove stressors through medication, complete rest, etc.

ANA: Implement specific stress reducing measures such as relaxation processes, visualization, biofeedback, etc.

2 Client refuses to acknowledge stress is impacting on his life.

ANA: Attempt to elicit feelings of client before giving information about the role of stress and effect on one's body.

ANA: Refer client to resources, articles and knowledgeable persons who can discuss the impact of stress and the importance of eliminating stressors.

Charting
- Identify stressed behavior observed in client
- Separate physical from emotional and environmental stressors
- Relate how client is responding to stress
- Pertinent verbalizations of client related to stress

ACTION: MANAGING STRESS

ASSESSMENT

1 Identify potential stressors (see previous action).
2 Assess adaptation factors that influence stress management.
  a Age: adaptation is greatest in youth and young middle life and least at the extremes of life.
  b Environment: adequate supply of required materials is necessary.
  c Adaptation involves the entire organism.
  d The organism can more easily adapt to stress over a period of time than suddenly.
  e Flexibility of organism influences survival.
  f Expenditure of energy: the organism usually uses the adaptation mechanism that is most economical in terms of energy.
  g Presence of illness that decreases the organism's capacity to adapt to stress.
  h The adequacy or deficiency of the adaptation responses.
3 Assess the effects of stress on the client.
  a Increased anxiety, anger, helplessness, hopelessness, guilt, shame, disgust, fear, frustration, or depression.
  b Behaviors resulting from stress:
     Apathy, regression, withdrawal.
     Crying, demanding.
     Physical illness.
     Hostility, manipulation.
     Senseless violence, lashing out.
4 Identify the major signals of stress.
  a Irritability, hyperactive behavior, or depression.
  b Impulsive, unpredictable behavior.
  c Crying jags.
  d Inability to concentrate or complete a task.
  e Feelings of unreality, withdrawal.
  f Loss of energy or absence of joy in living.
  g High anxiety level — "free-floating anxiety."
  h Emotional instability, inappropriate laughter.
  i Dizziness or weakness.
  j Tremors or nervous tics.
  k Pounding heart, abnormal beats.
  l Teeth-grinding at night.
  m Insomnia, nightmares.
  n Increased perspiration.
  o Diarrhea, nausea, indigestion, or vomiting.
  p Headaches, migraine.
  q Over or undereating; loss or gain of weight.
  r Increased smoking.
  s Increased dependence on alcohol, drugs.
  t Accident proneness.
  u Illness and disease.

Rationale for Action
- To maintain stability of organism during stress
- To repair damage caused by high stress level
- To restore body to normal composition and activity
- To cope with stress in an adaptive rather than a maladaptive mode

229

► **Danger Signals of Stress**

Depression
Uncontrolled hyperactive behavior
Lack of concentration
Feelings of unreality
Loss of control
Pervasive high anxiety level
Physical manifestations of
  Irregular heartbeats
  Tremors, tics
  Gastrointestinal disturbance
  Skin disturbance
Insomnia
Disease

► **Suggestions for Coping**

- Prioritize tasks to be completed, and identify activities that need to be accomplished
- Forget unimportant details; do not try to remember too many things. Concentrate on the essential issues and details.
- Eliminate past unpleasant events from the mind and focus on present.
- Do not cling to unpleasant experiences and emotions that clog emotional ability to respond to here and now.
- Discard habit of anticipating negative outcomes, which is often worse than the actual event.
- Do not yearn for things relating to the past or the future; focus attention on present desires.

PLANNING

GOALS

- The client is aware of the impact of stress on his or her body and life.
- Client works toward reducing environmental stressors.
- Body stressors are identified and removed as far as possible.
- Mind stress is identified and alleviated.
- Client learns to exchange chronic stressful patterns of thought and behavior for positive coping mechanisms.

INTERVENTION: Manipulating the Environment to Reduce Stress

1 Modify external environment of the client so that adaptation responses are within his or her capacity.
2 Support the efforts of the client to adapt or to respond.
3 Provide client with the materials required to maintain constancy of his or her environment.
4 Understand the body's mechanisms for accommodating stress.
5 Prevent additional stress.
6 Reduce external stimuli and input through senses.
7 Reduce or increase physical activity depending on the cause of and response to stress.

INTERVENTION: Monitoring Stress Level

1 Teach client to be aware of stress sensations in his or her body — recognize physical symptoms.
2 Suggest that client frequently monitor thought patterns to identify those thoughts that cause automatic tensing responses (tight muscles, increase in heartbeat, butterflies in stomach).
3 Assist client to make decisions whether these thoughts are essential to survival or if they can be changed, eliminated, or replaced.
4 Assist client in planning to set aside periods each day for self-stress evaluation.

INTERVENTION: Coping with Stress

1 Identify client's stress tolerance level.
  a Recognize the body's alarm signals (see major signals in assessment).
  b Assess signal correctly as signifying high level of stress.
2 Analyze stress status.
  a Estimate total amount of stress client is experiencing — too much indicates need for a rest.
  b Recognize where in body or mind the stress is manifesting — uneven stress indicates need for a diversion.
3 Suggest client utilize diversion methods of coping.
  a Physical diversion: jogging, swimming, cooking, cleaning, etc.

b Mental diversion: reading, painting, going to a movie, or simply thinking about a pleasant memory.
4 Plan with client how to use rest as a way to cope with stress.
   a Vacation, leave of absence from job, frequent naps, etc.
   b Eliminate major stressors so result is rest from stress input.
5 Teach client how to use concentration or meditation techniques to relieve mind stress.
6 Remind client that laughter is a great tranquilizer and healer as well as a stress reducer.
7 Plan with client how to manage time so that input can be reduced and goals limited.

INTERVENTION: Managing Stress from a Holistic Model

1 Manage stress through exercise.
   a Poor physical condition becomes a stressor.
   b State contributes to lethargy, a constant fatigue level, low resistance for illness, and lessens adaptive responses.
   c Good physical condition results in stamina, reserves necessary to withstand stress, and protection against unpredictable stress periods.
   d Exercise prepares body physically for stress caused by cold or heat conditions.
   e Consistent exercise prepares body to handle stress emotionally.
2 Manage stress through diet.
   a Certain foods and drug substances (caffeine, alcohol, sugar, junk foods, preservatives, smoking) are potent stressors to our bodies.
   b Consuming high-stress foods results in negative body changes such as hypertension, high cholesterol, labile blood sugar levels, and a rapid, bounding pulse rate.
   c Consuming a low-stress diet results in more energy and stamina to cope with stress.
   d A low-stress diet includes fat and protein intake to equal 10 to 15 percent of consumed calories. Remainder of intake should be raw or barely cooked vegetables, fruits, whole grains, nuts, low-fat dairy products, and plenty of liquids. Eliminate sodas, caffeine products, and most alcohol. Exclude refined sugars and carbohydrates and convenience or processed foods.
   e Vitamin supplements: vitamin C, B-complex, mineral supplements. Examine diet and experiment with different vitamin-mineral supplements letting your body report on positive results.
3 Manage stress by altering lifestyle patterns.
   a Eliminate unnecessary stressors in your life.
   b Change those parts of your life that are particularly stressful.
   c Develop personal methods for coping with stress: walking in the woods, painting, listening to music, reading, practicing yoga, etc.
   d Assess your lifestyle periodically and alter habits as necessary to reduce stress.

▶ The term holistic implies wholeness; a harmonious individual that integrates mind, body, and spirit into a functioning unit. A holistic stress model implies modifying all parts of one's life so that stress is both encountered and alleviated from an integrated perspective.

Did you know that you can test the stress effect of certain foods on your body by taking your pulse? It will be higher after ingesting high stress foods (sugar). A pulse rate of 90 means your heart beats over 9 million more times a year than a heart beat of 72. Save your heart—eat low-stress foods.

Did you know that fried chicken and french-fried potatoes will increase the pulse rate while broiled chicken and baked potatoes will not?

Did you know that ingesting sugar stresses the pancreas, disrupts blood sugar levels, leads to vitamin B complex deficiency, and disturbs calcium levels in the body?

231

INTERVENTION: Alleviating Stress Through Controlled Breathing

1 Have client sit so that his or her back is well supported, with spine straight but not rigid.
2 Have client place feet flat on floor and place hands on legs.
3 If client is lying down, have him or her place hands at side.
4 Have client find a comfortable position, close eyes, and take a deep slow breath through nostrils.
5 Continue giving the client the following instructions.
   a Extend your abdominal muscles.
   b Hold your breath for the count of four. Then very slowly release the air through slightly parted lips, making a whoosh sound.
   c When you think that all the air is out, hold your stomach in to push out even more air.
   d Repeat this breathing pattern several times so that your body will relax.
   e Breathe in through your nostrils to the count of four — one-two-three-four. Hold it — one-two-three-four — and expel the breath all the way out slowly, slowly releasing the air through your mouth.
   f As the air goes out, feel all of the tension drain out with it.
   g Now double the count, and breathe in slowly, filling your lungs all the way to the top to the count of eight. 1-2-3-4-5-6-7-8. Hold it — 1-2-3-4 — and now slowly release the breath — 5-6-7-8.
   h Again breathe in slowly to the count of twelve. 1-2-3-4-5-6-7-8-9-10-11-12. Hold it to the count of eight — 1-2-3-4-5-6-7-8 — and slowly release the air through your mouth to the count of 12 — 1-2-3-4-5-6-7-8-9-10-11-12.
   i Continue with your regular breathing pattern, letting the air breathe for you.
6 Stop the process by having the client open his or her eyes.

INTERVENTION: Utilizing a Relaxation Process
As a Method for Reducing Stress

1 Place client in a comfortable position.
   a Have client sit so that back is well supported and spine is straight. Have client put both feet on the floor and hold hands comfortably in lap.
   b If sitting is uncomfortable, have client lie on a bed and support areas of the body so that he or she is comfortable.
2 Have client concentrate on each key muscle of the body, tensing and relaxing each muscle until it is totally relaxed.
3 Have the client tense and release the muscles in the left toes, left foot, left calf, left thigh, and left leg.
4 Now have the client continue the process on the right leg, trunk, upper torso, arms, shoulders, neck, and face. Then have the client check to see that every muscle is relaxed.
5 Have client practice being totally relaxed.
6 Have client check for tight areas, any tension, any uncomfortable areas of sensations and let it all go. Have client describe the area and ask if he is willing to let the tension go.

INTERVENTION: Utilizing Meditation As a Method to Reduce Stress

1 Meditation is the process of relaxing the body and focusing and quieting the mind. The essence of this method depends on the ability to concentrate on an object, a word, or nothing.
2 The process of meditation begins with slow quiet breathing and deep muscle relaxation.
3 During meditation, there is a decrease in oxygen consumption, blood pressure, pulse rate, respiration, brain wave activity, and blood lactate level (high in anxious people).
4 Research indicates that meditation has a measurable effect on stress related conditions.

INTERVENTION: Utilizing Psychogenics As a Method to Reduce Stress

1 First, have client practice correct breathing procedures: inhale through nose, filling lungs from bottom to top. Have abdomen pouch out first, then draw the air in and up so that the entire lungs are filled. Hold the breath a few moments; then exhale through mouth.
2 Give client the following instructions for the "Windmill" exercise, adapted from Arica training. This exercise is particularly useful under high stress conditions.
   a Stand relaxed, with feet parallel about one foot apart, and with arms hanging loosely at your sides.
   b Bend knees slightly, and remain loose at the hip level.
   c Inhaling evenly, make six backward circles by swinging the left arm backward and then the right arm as the left reaches the top of its swing, similar to the crawl in swimming.
   d Holding your breath, make sixteen backward circles, eight with each arm.
   e Now exhale evenly, making six forward circles, three with each arm.
3 Have the client repeat the exercise three times and then relax.
4 The physiological effect of this exercise is a return to acid-base balance and recovery from stress. As the client completes the technique, he or she will again be able to cope.

EVALUATION

EXPECTED OUTCOMES

1 The client is aware of body-mind stress and the impact on his or her body. *If not*, follow these alternative nursing actions:
   ANA: Introduce the concept of stress, its impact on the body, and the result. Discuss theory as well as practical aspects.
   ANA: Refer client to resources, articles, and persons who can relate from experience the importance of understanding stress.
2 Client reduces environmental stressors. *If not*, follow these alternative nursing actions:

ANA: Introduce body cleansing measures, such as jogging or running in an unpolluted area.

ANA: Have client take additional vitamins, especially high B-complex and C, which assist in cleansing the blood.

ANA: Discuss with client the possibility of changing work or home location.

3 Client is able to identify and alleviate stress caused from mental concerns. *If not*, follow these alternative nursing actions:

ANA: Utilize autogenic tapes that instruct the client via relaxation and visualization how to reduce mental stress.

ANA: Assist client to try meditation techniques or refer to an expert to master this stress-reduction method.

UNEXPECTED OUTCOMES

1 Known relief measures for stress are ineffective.

ANA: Refer client to an expert in stress reduction, i.e., psychiatrist, hypnotherapist.

ANA: Refer client to a holistic health practitioner who will be able to integrate a variety of relief measures.

2 Client does not have adequate coping mechanisms for stress.

ANA: Explore additional coping mechanisms with client, for example, community resources, physicians, holistic practitioners, etc.

ANA: Assist client to integrate new coping mechanisms. Remain with client when under severe stress until coping is effective.

Charting

- Effects of stress on client-stress level
- Adaptation or coping modes of client
- Danger signals of stress observed in client
- Methods used for stress relief
- Result of stress reduction methods
- Referrals suggested for stress reduction

COPING WITH PAIN

The experience of pain is direct and personal. In this culture we tend to view pain as a negative condition and often will go to any lengths to avoid the sensation. The positive aspect of pain is that it is an early warning system; its presence triggers an awareness that something is wrong in our body. Without the sensation of pain we could not survive, for we would have no cues with which to modify our reactions and direct our behavior. One perspective of pain is that it is a message to our conscious self to check out any pain sensation before it gets worse, for that is the nature of pain. Without intervention it may well get worse.

McCaffery defines pain as "whatever the patient experiencing pain says it is, existing whenever he says it does." The nurse is totally dependent on the client to describe the sensation of pain, identify the location, and tell about what kind of pain is being experienced.

The most important information in pain assessment, then, is the client's report. The pain experience is totally subjective. The onset of acute pain stimulates the sympathetic nervous system "fight or flight" response that results in certain signs or symptoms. While observation of these symptoms provides objective data, it cannot be considered conclusive evidence to the identification of pain—that must come from the client.

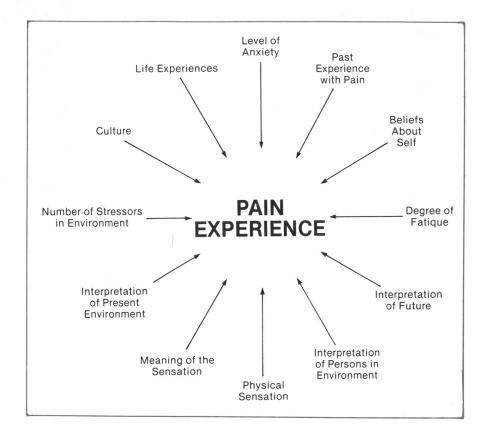

The diagram shows "PAIN EXPERIENCE" at the center with arrows pointing toward it from the following factors:

- Level of Anxiety
- Life Experiences
- Past Experience with Pain
- Beliefs About Self
- Culture
- Degree of Fatique
- Number of Stressors in Environment
- Interpretation of Present Environment
- Interpretation of Future
- Meaning of the Sensation
- Interpretation of Persons in Environment
- Physical Sensation

The pain experience is a mixture of physical sensations, physiologic changes, and psychosocial factors. The client's interpretation of the physical sensation is influenced by the client's culture, previous experiences with and without pain, beliefs about self, interpretation of the future, present environment, and the persons in that environment. The intensity of pain is influenced by what the sensation means to the client, the client's level of anxiety, degree of fatigue, and the number of stressors in the client's environment.

Pain Pathways The pathway to pain is a complicated, wondrous expression of how our amazing bodies work. First there is the source of pain, a direct causative factor. Stimulation of a pain receptor may be mechanical, chemical, thermal, electrical, or ischemic. The sensation travels along the sensory pathways through the dorsal root ending at the second order neuron in the posterior horn. Afferent fibers cross over to the anterolateral pathway and ascend in the lateral spinothalamic tract to the thalamus. The autonomic nervous system is activated, and the fibers then travel to the postcentral gyrus in the parietal lobe, the sensory area of the cerebral cortex. Pain reception occurs in the thalamus, where awareness and integration take place, and pain interpretation occurs in the cerebral cortex. Once awareness of the pain takes place and it has been interpreted by the cerebral cortex, the person becomes aware and

Types of Pain

Superficial: localized, short duration, sharp sensation.

Deep pain: long duration, diffuse, dull aching quality, associated autonomic responses, musculoskeletal tension, nausea.

- Visceral: internal organs.
- Somatic: neuromuscular, segmental distribution.
- Referred: area stimulated (deep) and area pain referred to (superficial) are innervated by nerve fibers arising from same segment of spinal cord.
- Secondary to skeletal muscle.

Central pain: autonomic reflex pain syndrome.

- Causalgia: lesion of peripheral nerve.
- Phantom: after amputation.
- Central: lesion in CNS, affecting pain pathway.

Psychogenic: due to emotional factors without anatomic or physiological explanation.

the response patterns are activated. Delayed, enhanced, or distorted responses to pain are influenced by a client's previous experiences, culture, existing physiological or psychological state, or degree of trust in the treatment team.

The sensation of physical pain arouses some specific responses in the client. The sympathetic nervous system response is usually stimulated by superficial pain, and the parasympathetic nervous system response is usually stimulated by deeper pain and results in the slowing down of all the systems to conserve energy.

Gate Control Theory   The neurophysiological basis of pain can be explained by several theories, none of which is mutually exclusive nor totally comprehensive. One of the most popular and credible concepts is the gate control theory. The first premise of the gate control theory states that the actual existence and intensity of the pain experience is dependent upon the particular transmission of neurological impulses. Secondly, gate mechanisms along the nervous system control the transmission of pain. Finally, this theory speculates that if the gate is open, the impulses that result in the sensation of pain are able to reach the conscious level. If the gate is closed, the impulses do not reach the level of consciousness and the sensation of pain is not experienced.

Three primary types of neurological involvement affect whether the gate is open or closed. The first type involves activities in the large and small nerve fibers that affect the sensation of pain. Pain impulses travel along small diameter fibers. The large diameter nerve fibers close the gate to the impulses that travel along the small fibers. The technique of using cutaneous stimulation on the skin, which has many large diameter fibers, may help to close the gate to the transmission of painful impulses, thereby relieving the sensation of pain.

Interventions that apply this theory to practice include massage, hot and cold applications, touch, acupressure, and transcutaneous electric nerve stimulation. These interventions are described in detail later in this chapter.

The second form of neurological involvement is the impulses from the brainstem that affect the sensation of pain. The reticular formation monitors in the brainstem regulate sensory input. If the person receives adequate or excessive amounts of sensory stimulation, the brainstem transmits impulses that close the gate and inhibit pain impulses from being transmitted. If on the other hand, the client experiences a lack of sensory input, the brainstem would not inhibit the pain impulses, the gate would be open, and the pain impulses would be transmitted. Interventions that apply to this part of the gate control theory are those related in some way to sensory input, such as techniques of distraction, guided imagery, and visualization.

The third type of neurological involvement is the neurological activities or impulses in the cerebral cortex and thalamus. A person's thoughts, emotions, and memories may activate certain impulses in the cortex that trigger pain impulses, which are transmitted to the conscious level.

Past experiences relating to pain affect how the client responds to current pain. For this reason, it is important to explore the client's previous experiences and teach the client what to expect from the present situation.

Interventions that apply to this part of the gate control theory include utilizing and teaching various relaxation techniques, teaching the client what expectations to have about pain as related to a specific illness, allowing the client to feel he or she has some control over the taking of medication for pain relief, and giving medications properly (i.e., preventively) before the pain is so severe that the client fears he or she will receive no relief.

The Discovery of Endorphins A recent and exciting theory of pain relief was developed when Avron Goldstein, looking for morphine and heroin receptors, discovered that receptors in the brain fit only morphine or morphine-like molecules. He asked himself why these receptors were located in the brain, when MSO_4 is not naturally found in this area. The answer, learned through diligent research, is that the brain produces natural brain opiates. These substances are hormones, chemicals produced by different parts of the body to regulate certain biological processes.

At the present time, five of these natural opiates have been found. Three are called endorphins, one dynorphin, and one enkephalin. Endorphins fit into special cells, called receptors, in order to activate their regulating powers. In addition to endorphin "keys" and receptor "locks," researchers have found antilocks, called antagonists, that keep endorphins from working. Endorphin receptors and anti-locks have been found throughout the body—in the stomach, intestines, pancreas, spinal cord, and bloodstream as well as the brain.

A beta-endorphin is 50 times stronger than morphine, and a dynorphin is 190 times stronger than morphine. In one test, fourteen men and women suffering from extreme pain from cancer were given tiny injections of an endorphin. *All* felt relief within minutes, and the relief lasted from one to three days.

Endorphins are now being produced synthetically, but they are very expensive and at this time used only for research. Researchers must discover how the body makes and releases endorphins before a method is developed to encourage the body to produce more of its own endorphins to control pain.

Noninvasive Pain Relief Measures Transcutaneous electric nerve stimulation (TENS) is a noninvasive method to relieve pain that has gained credibility and popularity in the past few years. The procedure involves stimulation to the skin via a mild electrical current. The stimulator is a solid-state battery-powered unit that has two to four electrodes attached by lead wires. These electrodes are placed on the skin, and the client experiences a buzzing, tingling, or vibrating sensation. This method relieves pain but just exactly how this phenomena occurs is not clear. What is apparent through clinical research is that this method offers

There are several theories that explain how TENS works:
  Increased production of endorphins.
  Fatigue of peripheral nerve fibers by high frequency electrical stimulation.
  Blockade of primary afferent fibers.
  Stimulation of afferent nerve fibers, which masks or modifies perception of pain.
  Gate theory (large cutaneous nerve fibers close the gate to the transmission of pain impulses).

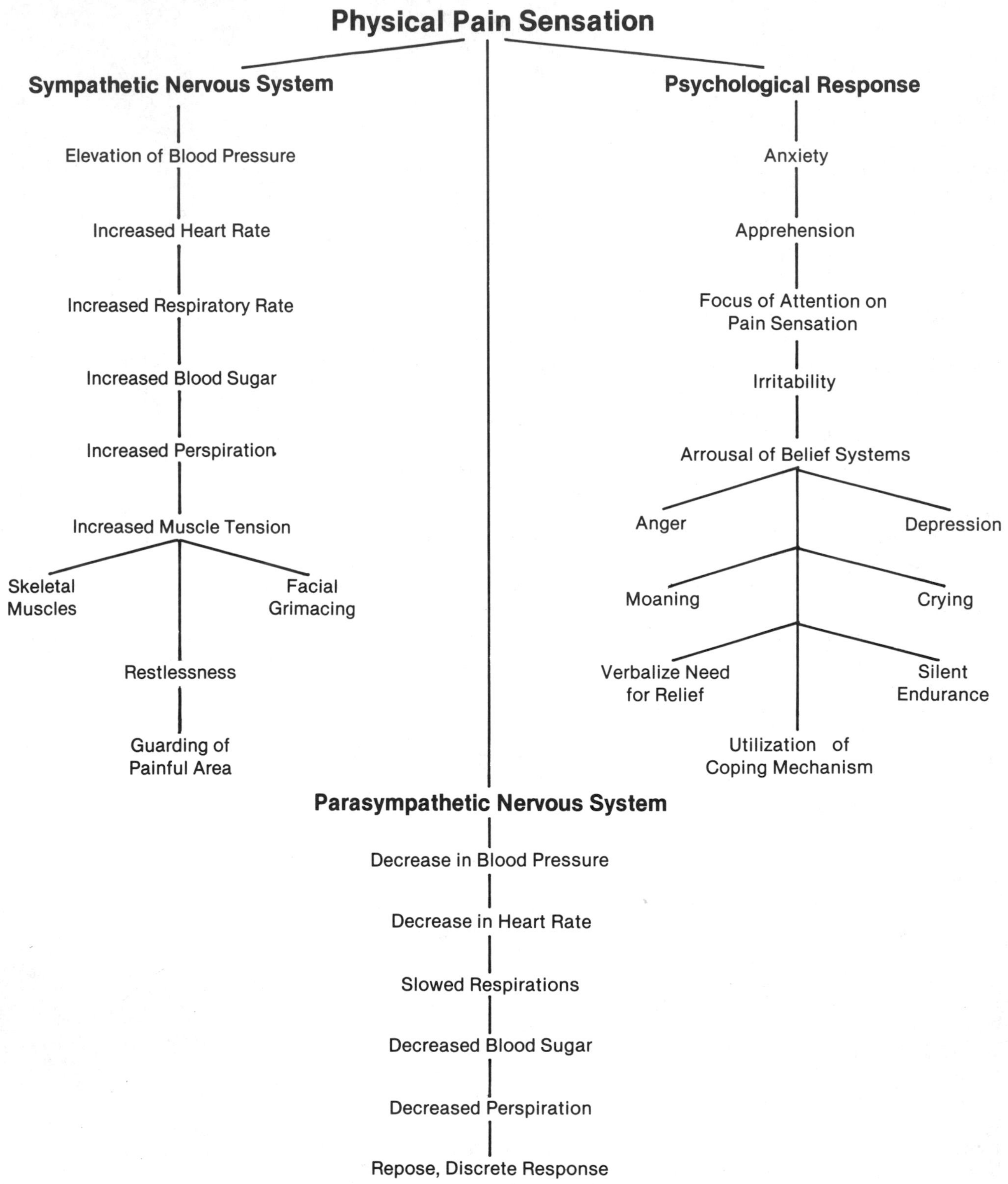

Physical Pain Sensation

Sympathetic Nervous System

Elevation of Blood Pressure

Increased Heart Rate

Increased Respiratory Rate

Increased Blood Sugar

Increased Perspiration

Increased Muscle Tension

Skeletal Muscles — Facial Grimacing

Restlessness

Guarding of Painful Area

Psychological Response

Anxiety

Apprehension

Focus of Attention on Pain Sensation

Irritability

Arrousal of Belief Systems

Anger — Depression

Moaning — Crying

Verbalize Need for Relief — Silent Endurance

Utilization of Coping Mechanism

Parasympathetic Nervous System

Decrease in Blood Pressure

Decrease in Heart Rate

Slowed Respirations

Decreased Blood Sugar

Decreased Perspiration

Repose, Discrete Response

relief from chronic and acute pain. In fact, the most common use today is for relief of chronic pain in adults.

Biofeedback is a second noninvasive method to relieve pain. It is also used to reduce stress. The biofeedback system is based on three principles: individuals can be taught to regulate any biological function that can be monitored by electrical instruments; changes in physiology in the body will be accompanied by changes in one's mental-emotional state and vice-versa; and biofeedback training can assist people to enter a relaxed state that is fundamental to consciously controlling internal functions.

The first phase of biofeedback training involves having the learner, who is hooked up to an electrical monitoring instrument (EEG, ECG, EMG, GSR), experience how behavior affects internal processes. The second phase involves imagining or visualization. The trainee experiences that thinking pleasant or happy thoughts slows down heart rate while unhappy thoughts speed up the heart rate. The third and last phase teaches the trainee to imagine heaviness and warmth in his or her arms and hands or around the heart. At the same time the trainee is instructed to notice that the heart beat decelerates. Conversely, when constriction is felt, the heart beat increases. This last phase establishes a link between internal sensations (warmth around the heart) and the effect on a body system (slowing of heart rate).

When the trainee understands that he or she can duplicate the sensation through visualization and affect his or her body processes, an important principle has been learned; once these connections have been made, the biofeedback equipment is no longer necessary and the trainee can manipulate certain internal functions on demand.

There are many pain-reduction techniques and medications. The physical sensation of pain itself is usually a small factor in the pain experience. Indeed, the physiologic response of muscle tension alone may increase pain. Rarely is pain relief successfully achieved with only one method. Two or more methods have an additive effect. Also, massive doses of narcotics do not always control pain because pain has been allowed to escalate. Relief of pain by prescribing small, frequent doses of medication and preventing escalation of pain can provide the client with a comfortable and speedy recovery.

The most significant aspect of pain relief is the relationship that exists between the nurse and the client. The client knows that the nurse has the power to relieve pain or to withhold pain relief. This knowledge creates anticipatory anxiety. The client who has a nurse who is supportive and caring and who will assist the client with pain management will need and ask for less medication. On the other hand, the clock watcher craves pain relief. This client's anxiety and pain escalate with each moment that the client realizes his or her needs are of little concern to the nurse.

Nursing interventions that provide the best pain relief are those that elicit behaviors incompatible with the behaviors of pain. For example, when the client is talking about something of great interest or pleasure,

▶ To understand more about how our minds control our bodies and how to exert control over our bodies, read Kenneth Pelletier's *Mind as Healer, Mind as Slayer.* New York, Delta Books (1977).

he or she is not talking about pain. If distracted, the client is not focusing on pain. Relaxation is as incompatible with muscle tension and anxiety as breathing slowly and deeply is incompatible with rapid, shallow respirations. The nurse should teach pain-relief techniques when there is no experience of pain, preferably before surgery so that the client can practice. The nurse should also encourage the client to use techniques that the client has already found effective, no matter how ''unscientific'' they may be.

GUIDELINES FOR MANAGING CLIENTS

The experience of pain is direct, personal, and subjective.

- The most important information in pain assessment is the client's report.
- The client's interpretation of pain is influenced by perception, culture, previous experiences with pain, beliefs about self, and environment.
- At any one time the pain experience can be intensified by psychophysiological factors. The intensity of each factor will vary.

There are several neurophysiological theories that attempt to explain the phenomenon of pain and pain relief.

- The gate control theory proposes that the actual existence and intensity of pain is dependent upon the particular transmission of neurological impulses.
- The theory of endorphins — receptor keys and locks — is an explanation of pain relief and how it occurs.
- Transcutaneous electric nerve stimulation and biofeedback are noninvasive measures employed to relieve pain.

ACTION: ACHIEVING PAIN RELIEF

ASSESSMENT

1 Assess type of pain.
  a Acute pain: short duration of a few seconds to six months.
  b Chronic pain: longer duration of six months to years.
  c Intractable pain: severe and constant and resistant to relief measures.
2 Assess location.
  a Ask client to point to area of the body or verbalize.
  b Ask if pain is superficial or deep.
  c Ask if pain is diffuse or localized.
  d Ask if pain radiates and where it goes.
3 Assess quality.
  a Stabbing, knife-like.   d Vise-like, suffocating.
  b Throbbing.   e Searing, burning.
  c Cramping.   f Other.

Rationale for Action
- To prevent pain from retarding recovery
- To prevent pain from causing nausea and vomiting which could result in fluid and electrolyte imbalance
- To prevent pain from causing undue fatigue
- To prevent pain from inhibiting moving, ambulating, turning and coughing, and thereby increasing possibilities of secondary problems from inactivity (pneumonia, emboli)
- To relieve pain or prevent pain from escalating by relaxing muscles (muscle tension increases with pain)
- To decrease client's anxiety that present and future pain relief will not be achieved
- To bring pain relief to a level acceptable to the client

4   Assess intensity.
   a   Ask client to indicate intensity of pain on a scale of zero to ten, zero being no pain and ten being the most pain ever experienced.
   b   Use this scale to assess relief of pain after intervention.
5   Assess onset and precipitating factors.
   a   How movement affects pain.
   b   If coughing affects pain.
   c   Impact of emotion on pain, i.e., arguing with spouse or receiving disturbing news.
6   Assess aggravating factors.
   a   How position affects pain.
   b   Environmental stressors.
   c   Fatigue.
7   Assess associated factors.
   a   Nausea.
   b   Vomiting.
   c   Bradycardia/tachycardia.
   d   Hypotension/hypertension.
   e   Profuse perspiration.
   f   Apprehension or anxiety.
8   Assess alleviating factors.
   a   Position.
   b   Elevation of inflamed extremity.
   c   Techniques used at home for pain relief.
9   Assess client's behavioral responses to pain.
   a   Depression, withdrawal, or crying.
   b   Stoicism or expressiveness.

▶ Carefully assess the client's "pain." Never assume it is "just incisional." For example, it may be caused by an impending M.I., kidney stone or bruise from operating table.

PLANNING

GOALS

- Pain is controlled to the client's satisfaction.
- The client is not resistant to turning, coughing and deep breathing, ambulating, or sitting in a chair due to presence of pain.
- The client is free from nausea and vomiting due to pain.
- The client's anxiety is decreased.

EQUIPMENT

For touch
- Cream or talcum powder
- Massage oil
For relaxation
- A printed relaxation technique (the nurse can read slowly to client until client learns technique)
- A cassette recorder and tape
For TENS
- Cutaneous stimulator with lead wires and leads
- Cream for lead placement

For heat or cold
- Aquathermic pad
- Gel pack
- Ice bag or collar

INTERVENTION: Achieving Pain Relief Using Medication

1 Check physician's orders.
2 Use a preventive approach to pain management. Give medication before pain becomes severe.
3 Follow steps outlined in Assessment to determine nature, quality, and extent of pain.
4 Start with p.o. medications. If ineffective or only mildly effective, give IM medications, or combine p.o. and IM medications.
5 Evaluate result of pain medication. Was it effective? How long did effect last? What was the extent of relief?
6 Evaluate client for possible side effects of the medication.
7 Discuss with physician effects of medication and whether a change of prescription is needed.

Clinical Alert

If client is receiving radiation therapy, no creams, ointments or lotions are to be used on his or her skin during treatment and post-treatment periods.

INTERVENTION: Alleviating Pain Through Touch

1 Determine whether client achieves more relief from pain with massage over painful area, near painful area, or from foot rub, back rub, or hand rub.
2 Warm your hands by rubbing them together or rinsing in warm water.
3 Warm lotion to be used by holding closed bottle under warm running water.
4 Massage area of choice with slow and steady motion.
5 Use deep pressure or light stroking motion, whichever is more comfortable for the client.

INTERVENTION: Alleviating Pain Using Heat or Cold

1 Determine whether heat, which increases circulation, or cold, which impairs circulation, brings more relief to client.
2 Obtain order from physician for heat application. Obtain a temperature regulated device. (Example: aquathermic pad.) Apply as described in Chapter 11.
3 For cold application, obtain a gel pack or ice bag. Apply as described in Chapter 11.

INTERVENTION: Achieving Pain Relief Using Relaxation Techniques

1 Help client assume a comfortable position.
   a If lying, place support under knees, lower legs, and under head. Be sure body is in good alignment.

b If sitting, sit comfortably positioned with both feet on the floor, hands on knees, back straight, and head balanced comfortably straight.

2 Instruct client to inhale deeply, hold breath for a moment, then exhale deeply. Repeat several times.

3 Give the following instructions to client, using a slow soothing voice.

a Continue to breathe in and out slowly. Concentrate on my voice and follow my words.

b Find a point of tension in your body.

c As you identify the tension, tense the area up even more.

d Then relax the area, letting all the tension drain out.

4 Continue with these instructions until the client has had time to relax all points of tension.

5 To end the process, instruct client to open eyes slowly and say, ''I feel relaxed and awake.''

6 For further examples of the relaxation process, see Managing Stress in this chapter.

▶ A commercially available relaxation cassette tape may also be used to teach this technique. Several tapes are available where the voice of an experienced therapist is accompanied by a soothing musical background. (See bibliography at the end of this book)

INTERVENTION: Relieving Pain Through Visualization

1 Follow steps 1-4 of previous intervention.

2 Then continue to instruct client in steps of visualization as follows:

a After achieving a state of relaxation, imagine a ball of healing white light forming around the area of pain.

b With each breath it becomes bigger and bigger, surrounding the entire painful area.

c See the ball of white light surrounding the pain begin to move out of your body.

d Watch it float away like a large white balloon.

e Now take a few moments and visualize your body free of pain.

f When you are ready, open your eyes, feeling relaxed and refreshed.

INTERVENTION: Achieving Pain Relief Using TENS
(Transcutaneous Electric Nerve Stimulation)

1 Obtain physician's order (may be intermittent or continuous).

2 Choose the area for application of electrodes. (Check electrode placement chart by manufacturer of TENS unit.)

a Place electrode on skin over or near the area of pain.

b Identify trigger points (specific points which are extremely sensitive when stimulated) and place electrode.

c Identify acupressure point, and place electrode.

d Place electrode on peripheral nerves, enervating area of pain. (Client adjusts each pair of electrodes to produce a sensation that is pleasant and to relieve pain.)

▶ Studies indicate success with certain conditions
- Chronic pain in adults
- Chronic pain in children
- Postoperative pain
- Increased hyperactivity in gastrointestinal tract postoperatively
- Acute trauma pain

Contraindicated in certain conditions
- Pacemakers
- Myocardial ischemia
- Arrhythmias
- Pregnancy

3 Apply electrodes.
   a Some electrodes are water conductive: moisten with water.
   b Some electrodes require a conductive gel: place gel on electrode before attaching to skin.
4 Instruct client to adjust intensity of skin stimulation until it creates a pleasant sensation that relieves the pain.

EVALUATION

EXPECTED OUTCOMES

▶ Caution the client to report any changes in characteristics of pain or level of discomfort. A change may reflect alteration in condition, another disorder or a potential complication.

1 Pain is controlled to the client's satisfaction. *If not*, follow these alternative nursing actions:
   ANA: Try an alternative method of pain control. Begin with back care and position change and work up the scale of pain relief to more intensive techniques.
   ANA: Teach client a variety of methods to alleviate pain so he or she can feel in control and be able to choose method appropriate to circumstances.
   ANA: Suggest that client use medication or pain control method early, before pain becomes too severe.
2 The client's pain is relieved and does not interfere with ambulation or sitting in a chair. *If not*, follow these alternative nursing actions:
   ANA: Administer pain medication before assisting client to perform these activities.
   ANA: Assist the client to reduce fears through discussion as a lessening of fear may reduce his or her pain.
   ANA: Encourage client to take responsibility and plan his or her own schedule for pain medications and activity.
3 The client is free from nausea and vomiting due to pain. *If not*, follow these alternative nursing actions:
   ANA: Obtain order for and administer antiemetic along with narcotic.
   ANA: Report side effect and request order to change narcotic.
   ANA: Utilize deep breathing and relaxation exercises.
4 Client's anxiety level is low. *If not*, follow these alternative nursing actions:
   ANA: Since anxiety is often fear of the unknown, prepare client giving him or her adequate information and discuss fears and concerns.
   ANA: Assist client to use coping mechanisms that have worked in the past.
   ANA: Have client practice relaxation techniques to reduce anxiety.
   ANA: Reevaluate medications and obtain order for and administer anti-anxiety drug.

UNEXPECTED OUTCOMES

1 Client achieves no relief from relaxation, visualization, or massage.
   ANA: Try combining methods with use of medications, i.e., use these methods while waiting for medication to take effect.

ANA: Be sure client's environment is conducive to learning and practicing techniques.

ANA: Client has to trust technique before it will be effective. Have client talk to another person who has found technique helpful.

2 Client achieves little or no relief from TENS.

ANA: Use another brand or type of stimulator.

ANA: If using continuous cutaneous stimulation, try using intermittent stimulation and vice versa.

3 Client achieves no pain relief from electrode placement sites used according to manufacturer's directions.

ANA: Check with physical therapist for suggestions of alternative placement.

ANA: Experiment with placing electrodes in other areas to determine if pain is relieved.

ANA: Check other manufacturers' placements charts.

4 Client develops skin irritation at electrode sites.

ANA: Use hypoallergic tape to secure electrodes.

ANA: Discontinue tape. Use velcro or elastic bandage to hold electrodes in place.

ANA: If rash appears to be caused by gel:

Mix cortisone gel with the electrode cream.

Change gel. Cleanse skin and electrodes with soap and water frequently.

5 Client develops constipation from regularly administered narcotic preparations.

ANA: Obtain order for and administer stool softener and peristaltic stimulant.

ANA: Encourage intake of high-fiber diet, if not contraindicated.

ANA: Encourage adequate fluid intake.

Charting

- Describe the client's pain, including location, quality, intensity, precipitating factors, associated factors, and aggravating factors
- Describe alleviating factors, including what the client does to relieve pain as well as nursing assistance
- Describe behavioral changes due to pain relief or the absence of objective changes in response to the medication and/or nursing interventions
- If there is a poor response to therapy, state what other measures will be attempted and chart results
- Continue to document attempts to relieve pain until relief occurs and the client is satisfied

TERMINOLOGY

adaptive reaction A response in which the person attempts to improve or alter his or her condition in relation to the environment.

autogenic training A method of deep muscle relaxation that enables one to reduce the stress response, regain homeostasis, and prepare to handle additional stress.

autonomic nervous system The part of the nervous system that regulates the functioning of internal organs and glands; it controls such functions as digestion, respiration, and cardiovascular activity.

biofeedback A training technique that utilizes monitoring instruments to assist people to control stress-related disorders through self-regulation of internal functions.

dynamics of homeostasis Danger or its symbols, whether internal or external, resulting in the activation of the sympathetic nervous system and the adrenal medulla. The organism prepares for flight or fight.

fight or flight   One's immediate response to stress that is, although archaic and often inappropriate, part of our central nervous system biological heritage.

general adaptation syndrome   A general theory of stress response formulated by Dr. Hans Selye; describes the action of stress response in three stages — the alarm reaction, the stage of resistance, and the stage of exhaustion.

homeostasis   The maintenance of a constant state in the internal environment through self-regulatory techniques that preserve an organism's ability to adapt to stress.

parasympathetic nervous system   A division of the autonomic nervous system that regulates acetylcholine and conserves energy expenditure; it slows down the systems.

stress   A nonspecific response of the body to any internal or external event or change that impinges on a person's system and creates a demand.

stressor   A specific demand that gives rise to a coping response.

sympathetic nervous system   A division of the autonomic nervous system that controls energy expenditure and mobilizes for action when confronted with a threat.

CHAPTER 8
Therapeutic Agents

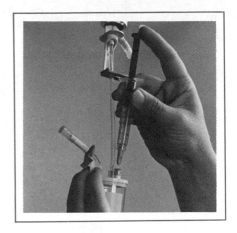

This chapter presents the conceptual basis for administering therapeutic agents. It includes basic information about drugs, drug metabolism, and the nursing actions involved in their administration.

Therapeutic agents are drugs or medications which, when introduced into a living organism, modify the physiological functions of that organism. The term "therapeutic agent" usually refers to a chemical compound. If this substance has an effect on body functions, it can also be a vitamin, mineral, herb, or even a natural food. In this chapter, the term "therapeutic agents" refers to drugs and their actions.

DRUG METABOLISM

Drug metabolism in the human body is accomplished in four basic stages: absorption, transportation, biotransformation, and excretion. In order for a drug to be completely metabolized, it must first be given in sufficient concentration to produce the desired effect on body tissues. When this "critical drug concentration" level is achieved, body tissues change.

Absorption The first stage of metabolism refers to the route a drug takes from the time it enters the body until it is absorbed in the circulating fluids. Drugs are absorbed by the mucous membranes, the gastrointestinal tract, the respiratory tract, and the skin. The mucous membranes are one of the most rapid and effective routes of absorption because they are highly vascular. Drugs are absorbed through these membranes by diffusion, infiltration, and osmosis.

Drugs that are given by mouth are absorbed in the gastrointestinal tract. Portions of these drugs dissolve and are absorbed in the stomach. The rate of absorption depends on the pH of the stomach's contents, the food content in the stomach at the time of ingestion, and the presence of disease conditions. Most of the drug concentrate dissolves in the small intestine where the large vascular surface and moderate pH level enhance the process of dissolution.

Parenteral methods are the most direct, reliable, and rapid route of absorption. Methods of administration include intradermal, subcutaneous, intramuscular, intravenous, and intra-arterial injections. The actual administration site will depend on the type of drug, its action, and the client. For example, a client with an anaphylactic reaction will receive epinephrine intravenously since this is the fastest route for drug absorption in an emergency situation.

Another route of administration that is faster than the gastrointestinal tract but not as rapid as parenteral injections is inhalation or nebulization of medications through the respiratory system. Drugs administered through the respiratory tract must be made up of small particles that can pass through to the alveoli in the lungs.

The final mode of absorption is the skin. Most drugs, when applied to the skin, produce a local, rather than a systemic effect. The degree of absorption will depend on the strength of the drug as well as where it is applied on the body surface.

Transportation The second stage of metabolism refers to the way in which a drug is transported from the site of introduction to the site of action. When a drug enters or is absorbed by the body, it binds to plasma protein in the blood and is transported through circulation to all parts of the body. As a drug moves from the circulatory system, it crosses cell membranes and enters the body tissues. Some of the drug is also distributed to and stored in fat and muscle, where greater masses of tissue attract the drug.

The amount of the drug that is distributed to body tissues depends on the permeability of the membranes and the blood supply to the absorption area. A drug that first accumulates in the brain may move into fat and muscle tissue and then back to the brain because the drug is still chemically active. As the drug is released in small quantities from the tissues and travels back to the brain, equal drug and blood concentration levels in the body are maintained.

Biotransformation The third stage of metabolism takes place as the drug, which is a foreign substance in the body, is converted by enzymes into a less active and harmless agent that can be easily excreted. Most of this conversion occurs in the liver through synthetic and biochemical reactions, although some conversion does take place in the kidney, plasma, and intestinal mucosa. In synthetic reactions, liver enzymes conjugate the drug with other substances to make it less harmful for the body. In biochemical reactions, drugs are oxidized, reduced, hydrolyzed, and synthesized so that they become less active and more easily eliminated from the body.

Excretion   The final stage in metabolism takes place when the drug is changed into an inactive form or excreted from the body. The kidneys are the most important route of excretion because they eliminate both the pure drug and the metabolites of the parent drug. During excretion, these two substances are filtered through the glomeruli, secreted by the tubules, and either reabsorbed through the tubules or directly excreted. Other routes of excretion include the lungs (which exhale gaseous drugs), feces, saliva, tears, and mother's milk.

Factors That Affect Drug Metabolism   There are many factors that affect drug metabolism. They include personal attributes, such as body weight, age, and sex; physiological factors, such as state of health or disease processes; acid-base and fluid and electrolyte balance; permeability; diurnal rhythm and circulatory capability. Genetic and immunologic factors play a role in drug metabolism, as do psychological, emotional and environmental influences, drug tolerance, and cumulation of drugs. Responses to drugs vary, depending on the speed with which the drug is absorbed into the blood or tissues and the effectiveness of the body's circulatory system.

DRUG ADMINISTRATION

The method of drug administration influences the action of that drug on the body. To obtain a systemic effect, a drug must be absorbed and transported to the cells or tissues that respond to it. How a drug is administered will depend on the chemical nature and quantity of the drug, as well as the desired speed of effect and the overall condition of the client. Common routes of administration to obtain systemic effects include the following: oral, sublingual, rectal, inhalation, and parenteral. Parenteral injections are made in these sites: intradermal, subcutaneous, intramuscular, intraosseous, and occasionally intracardiac, intrapericardial, and intraspinal.

Source and Naming of Drugs   The primary sources from which drugs are compounded are roots, bark, sap, leaves, flowers, and seeds of plants. Other natural sources include animal organs or organ cells and secretions and mineral sources. Synthetic drugs, such as sulfonamides, are made in a laboratory from chemical substances.

Most drugs are given chemical, generic, and trademark names. A chemical name which refers to the chemical derivation of the drug is ethyl, 1-methyl-4-phenylisonipecotate hydrochloride. A generic name, meperidine hydrochloride, reflects the chemical family to which the drug belongs but is shorter and simpler. Demerol is a trademark name; this is the most common way in which a drug is known. Once a drug is registered with a brand name (Demerol ®) that drug can be manufactured only by its legal owner.

Safety Procedures When you administer drugs, you must follow certain safety rules, which are also known as "The Five Rights." These rules should be carried out each time you give a drug to a client.

The Five Rights

1 Right medication:
   Compare drug card medication sheet or drug Kardex with drug container three times.
   Know action, dosage, and method of administration.
   Know side effects of the drug.
2 Right client—check client's ID band and door number.
3 Right time
4 Right method of administration
5 Right amount:
   Check all calculations of divided doses with another nurse.
   Check heparin, insulin, and intravenous digitalis doses with another nurse.

Documenting the Medication A medication administered to a client must have a physician's order or prescription before it can be legally administered. The physician's order is a verbal or written order, which is recorded in a book or file or in the client's chart. If an order is given verbally over the telephone, you must write a verbal order in the client's chart for the physician to sign at a later date. Written orders are safer because they leave less room for potential misunderstanding or error. A drug order should consist of seven parts:
1 The name of the client
2 The date the drug was ordered
3 The name of the drug
4 The dosage
5 The route of administration and any special rules of administration
6 The time and frequency the drug should be given
7 The signature of the individual who ordered the drug

There are two basic types of drug orders: routine and one time only drug orders. A routine medication is administered according to instructions until it is cancelled by another order. Routine medication orders can also be used for prn drugs. These drugs are administered when the client needs the medication, not necessarily on a routine time schedule. Medication for bowel elimination is a type of prn drug which is not necessarily administered every day. When you administer medications, you should assess the continued validity of any routine order. Physicians occasionally forget to cancel an order when it is no longer appropriate for a client's condition. One time only orders are administered as stated, only one time. These orders may be given at a specified time or "stat," which means immediately.

If you prepare a medication, you must also give it to the client and chart it after the client has taken the required dosage. If a client refuses a medication, you should chart that the medication was refused and report this information to the physician. When you chart medications, be sure to use the correct abbreviations and symbols.

If you find an error in a drug order, such as inaccurate dose or method of administration, it is your responsibility to question the order. If you cannot understand or read the order, verify it with the physician. Do not guess at the order as this constitutes gross negligence. In many hospitals it is the pharmacist's responsibility to contact physicians when medication orders are unclear.

Always report medication errors to the physican immediately so that potential danger to the client is minimized. While no nurse or doctor would intentionally commit an error, errors do occur. When they do, it is important that measures be taken immediately to assess and evaluate the client's status and to institute a plan of action to reverse the effects of the medication.

Errors in medication should also be documented in a medication incident report and on the client's record. This documentation is necessary for both legal reasons and nursing audits. Nursing audits are conducted to determine if an error in medication indicates one primary problem, a particular source of problems, or a range of problems that seem to have no connection.

Each hospital has its own policies and protocols for administering medications. Before administering any drugs, you must find out what these policies are and perform them accordingly.

GUIDELINES FOR MANAGING CLIENTS

The primary purpose for performing nursing interventions associated with drug administration is to safely administer drugs **with an appropriate knowledge base. As you perform these interventions, refer to the following guidelines:**

• Determine the correct dosage, actions, side effects, and contra-indications of any medication before you administer the medication to a client.

• Determine if medications ordered by the physician are appropriate for the client's condition. This is part of your professional responsibility.

• Question the physician about any medication orders that are incomplete, illegible, or inappropriate for the client's condition. Remember, you may be liable if you make a medication error. Report every medication error to the physician and nursing administrator and complete a medication incident report.

• Check to determine if the medication ordered is compatible with the client's condition and with other medications prescribed.

Clinical Alert

Before administering any medication, check client's Identaband and ask client to state name.

251

- Ascertain what the client has been eating or drinking before administering a medication so that you can determine what effect the client's diet will have on the medication. For example, you would not give an MAO inhibitor to a client who had just ingested cheddar cheese or wine.
- Check to see that the calculated drug dosage for young children and elderly people is appropriate, as they usually require smaller doses of medications.
- Adjust drug dosages for very thin or obese clients according to their weight. For example, a thin client may require less morphine than an obese client to obtain the same therapeutic effect.
- Consider the diagnosis of the client when administering drugs. If, for example, a client has kidney failure, he or she will not be able to excrete certain drugs.

ACTION: APPLYING MEDICATIONS TO THE SKIN

Rationale for Action

- To absorb medication more rapidly through use of certain topical medications, i.e., Nitro-Bid paste
- To treat skin disorders or lesions caused by burns or abnormal growths
- To dilute effects of a drug (local action may be less than systemic)
- To apply an agent that stops, slows, or prevents the growth of microorganisms
- To provide a local anesthesia to specified parts of the body

ASSESSMENT

1 Observe for open lesions, rashes, or areas of erythema and skin breakdown. If any are present, you may need to select another route for drug administration.
2 Assess for known allergies as related by the client and/or as noted in the chart. Note any allergies that may cause abnormal skin problems.
3 Observe local changes in the skin occurring from the use of the drug.
4 Assess for proper medication administration by following safety procedures.

PLANNING

GOALS

- Skin returned to normal state
- Alleviation of symptoms for which medication was administered
- Decreased pain
- Control of microorganisms

EQUIPMENT

- Medication container
- Application tube (if needed)
- 2 × 2 pads for cleansing
- Tongue blade
- Gloves
- Sterile gauze (for burn dressing)
- Commercially prepared burn dressings.

INTERVENTION: Preparing Skin Medications

1. Obtain client's medication record. Medication record may be a drug card, medication sheet, or drug Kardex, depending on the method of dispensing medications in your facility.
2. Compare the medication record with the most *recent* physician's order.
3. Wash your hands.
4. Gather necessary equipment including gloves or tongue blade as needed.
5. Remove the medication from the drug box or tray on medication cart.
6. Compare the label on the medication tube or jar to the medication record.
7. Place medication tube or jar (include a tongue blade with jar) on a tray, if not using medication cart.

INTERVENTION: Applying Ointments and Salves

1. Take medication to client's room; check room number and client's identaband against medication card or sheet.
2. Wash your hands.
3. Provide client privacy.
4. Squeeze medication from a tube or, using a tongue blade, take ointment out of jar.
5. Spread a small, smooth, thin quantity of medication evenly over client's skin surface using your fingers or a tongue blade.
6. Protect skin surface with a dressing, if needed, so that medication cannot rub off.
7. Cleanse skin surface with soap and water between medication applications, unless contraindicated by client's condition.
8. Check to see that client is comfortable before leaving room.
9. Return medication to appropriate storage area.

INTERVENTION: Applying Topical Vasodilator Medications

1. Take medication to client's room; check room number and client's identaband against medication card or sheet.
2. Wash your hands.
3. Provide client privacy.
4. Put on gloves to prevent absorbing any medication yourself.
5. Obtain premeasured paper, which accompanies medication tube.
6. Place prescribed medication directly on paper (usually one-half to one-inch strip).
7. Apply medicated paper to anterior surface of chest. You may apply medicated paper to any area of the body; however, most clients feel the medication works better if applied to the chest surface.
8. Alternate areas of the chest with each dose of medication.
9. Check to see that client is comfortable before leaving room.
10. Return medication to appropriate storage area.

INTERVENTION: Applying Antibacterial Ointment to Burns

1 Take medication to client's room; check room number and identa-band against medication card or sheet.
2 Wash your hands.
3 Provide client privacy.
4 Squeeze medication from a tube or, using a tongue blade, take ointment out of jar.
5 If *no dressing is ordered*, apply drug directly to burn area; using sterile gloves and tongue blade, cover entire burn area with medication to provide an occlusive effect.
6 If *dressing is ordered*, use sterile gloves to rub drug directly into sterile gauze. Then apply medicated gauze to burn area. (Commercially prepared premedicated gauze dressings can be applied directly to burn area, using sterile technique.) Cover medicated dressings with sterile Kerlix.
7 Check to see that client is comfortable before leaving room.
8 Return drug and/or equipment to appropriate storage area.

EVALUATION

EXPECTED OUTCOMES

1 Skin returned to normal state. *If not*, follow these alternative nursing actions:
ANA: Assess effectiveness of medication for condition. Obtain order for medication replacement if skin not returned to normal state.
ANA: Assess for signs of skin irritation due to medication.
ANA: Discontinue medication when skin irritation occurs and notify physician.
2 Alleviation of symptoms for which medication was administered. *If not*, follow these alternative nursing actions:
ANA: For allergic responses (hives, increased itching, or rash), hold medication and notify physician.
ANA: Obtain order for antihistamine if indicated.
3 Decreased pain. *If not*, follow these alternative nursing actions:
ANA: Burning sensation is felt on skin: Notify physician and obtain order to discontinue drug. Treat burned areas symptomatically with lotion such as zinc oxide.
ANA: Pain continues or is intensified when medication is applied to burn area: Ensure that all burn areas are covered completely. Sterile dressings may need to be applied, in addition to medications, over the burn area.
4 Control of microorganisms. *If not*, follow these alternative nursing actions:
ANA: Obtain order for culture and sensitivity to identify if causative organism is altered.
ANA: Reevaluate medication type and strength in relation to identified microorganism.
ANA: Obtain order for systemic-acting medication.

Charting
- Appropriate medication form for facility
- Name of drug
- Dosage
- Times ordered
- Time administered
- Method of administration
- Initials of nurse administering drug
- In nurses notes make comments on skin condition, any areas of irritation, erythema, etc.

ACTION: APPLYING MEDICATIONS TO MUCOUS MEMBRANES

ASSESSMENT

1 Observe for open lesions, rashes, or areas of erythema and breakdown. If any are present, you may need to select another route for drug administration.
2 Assess for known allergies as related by the client and/or as noted in the chart.
3 Observe local changes in the mucous membranes (remember that mucous membranes are essential to assess in the dark-skinned client).
4 Assess for proper medication administration by following safety procedures.

PLANNING

GOALS

- Mucous membrane returned to normal state
- Alleviation of symptoms for which medication was administered
- Decreased pain
- Control of infection or inflammation

EQUIPMENT

- Medication container
- Application tube (if needed)
- Medication dropper for nasal drops
- 2 × 2 pads for cleansing
- Tongue blade
- Gloves

INTERVENTION: Preparing Mucous Membrane Medications

1 Obtain client's medication record. Medication record may be a drug card, medication sheet, or drug Kardex, depending on the method of dispensing medications in your facility.
2 Compare the medication record with the most *recent* physician's order.
3 Wash your hands.
4 Gather necessary equipment including eye dropper, gloves or tongue blade as needed.
5 Remove the medication from the drug box or tray on medication cart.
6 Compare the label on the medication bottle, tube or jar to the medication record.
7 Place medication bottle, tube or jar (include a tongue blade with jar) on a tray, if not using medication cart.

Rationale for Action

- To dilute effects of a drug (local action may be less than systemic)
- To apply an agent that stops, slows, or prevents infection or inflammation
- To provide local anesthesia to specified parts of the body to relieve pain or discomfort
- To provide relief of nasal congestion
- To provide more appropriate surface for absorption, i.e., mucous membrane

INTERVENTION: Applying Drugs to Mucous Membranes

1 Check drug information to determine if appropriate for application to mucous membranes.
2 Verify which method is most appropriate for application: instillation, swabbing, spraying, irrigation, or douching.
3 Take medication to client's room; check room number and identa-band against medication card or sheet.
4 Wash your hands.
5 Provide client privacy.
6 Complete application according to specific method of application.
7 For specific information on application methods, review drug information pamphlets which accompany medications.

INTERVENTION: Instilling Nose Drops

1 Take medication to client's room; check room number and identa-band against medication card or sheet.
2 Wash your hands.
3 Place client in sitting position with head tilted back, or in supine position with head tilted back over a pillow.
4 Fill dropper with prescribed amount of medication.
5 Place dropper 1 cm inside the nares and instill correct number of drops. Repeat procedure in both nares.
6 Instruct client not to sneeze and to keep head tilted back for five minutes to prevent medication from escaping.
7 Check to see that client is comfortable before leaving room.
8 Return medication to appropriate storage area.

Clinical Alert

Only use nebulizer or spray that emits fine particles of suspended drugs into the upper respiratory tract. Substances containing oil cause lipoid pneumonia if the substance reaches the lower respiratory structures.

Instruct client to tilt head backwards when instilling nose drops.

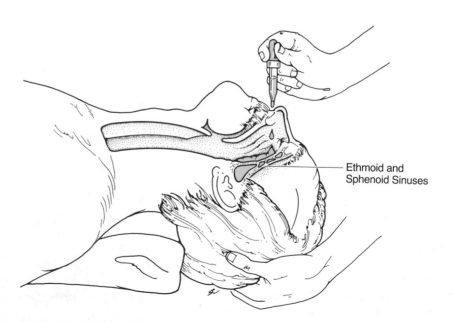

Ethmoid and Sphenoid Sinuses

EVALUATION

EXPECTED OUTCOMES

1 Mucous membrane returned to normal state. *If not*, follow these alternative nursing actions:
ANA: Assess effectiveness of medication for condition. Obtain order for medication replacement if needed.
ANA: Discontinue medication when irritation occurs and notify physician.
2 Alleviation of symptoms for which medication was administered. *If not*, follow these alternative nursing actions:
ANA: For allergic responses (hives, increased itching, or rash), hold medication and notify physician.
ANA: Obtain order for antihistamine if indicated.
3 Increased comfort and relief. *If not*, follow these alternative nursing actions:
ANA: Burning or itching sensation felt on mucous membrane (if not a usual side effect of drug): Notify physician and obtain order to discontinue drug.
4 Control of infection or inflammation. *If not*, follow these alternative nursing actions:
ANA: Obtain order for culture and sensitivity to identify if causative organism is altered.
ANA: Reevaluate medication type and strength in relation to identified microorganism.
ANA: Obtain order for systemic-acting medication.

Charting
- Use appropriate medication form for facility
- Name of drug
- Dosage
- Method of administration
- Times ordered
- Time administered
- Initials of nurse administering drug
- In nurses notes discuss status of mucous membrane, client tolerance of medication and observed effects of medication

ACTION: ADMINISTERING ORAL MEDICATIONS

ASSESSMENT

1 Assess that oral route is the most efficient means of medication administration.
2 Check medication orders for completeness and accuracy.
3 Assess client's physical ability to take medication as ordered:
   a Swallow reflex present
   b State of consciousness
   c Signs of nausea and vomiting
   d Uncooperative behavior
4 Check to make sure you have the correct medication for the client.
5 Assess correct dosage when calculation is needed.

PLANNING

GOALS

- Client is able to ingest and metabolize medication without feelings of nausea or vomiting.

Rationale for Action
- To offer the most common, easiest, and least expensive route of administering medications
- To provide a sustained drug action and increased absorption time via waves of peristalsis, which bring the drug into contact with the mucosal lining of the gastrointestinal tract

▶ With advent of unit dose system, prepackaged medications are placed in individual trays in a medication cart, which is taken to the client's room. Even though medications are prepackaged, you are still responsible for ensuring that the correct drug is administered to the correct client.

▶ Medication Cart

- Generally used with unit dose medication system.
- This system allows medications to be dispensed directly from cart outside client's room.
- Cart remains locked at all times while nurse is dispensing medications to client.
- Cart may be left unattended in hallway but must remain locked.

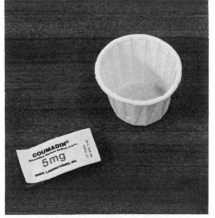

When using a unit dose medication system, keep the drug in the wrapper until you reach the client's bedside. Read the medication label as a check.

- Client emotionally accepts medication.
- Client experiences a sustained action of drug and a positive effect on his or her body.

EQUIPMENT

- Medication: tablet, capsule, or liquid
- Water (none if liquid preparation), juice, or milk (if not contraindicated by drug absorption) to prevent gastric irritation
- Mortar and pestle for crushing pills (if needed)
- Drug card, medication sheet, drug Kardex
- Drug cart, if unit dose system is used

INTERVENTION: Using Equivalent Tables to Calculate Drug Dosages

1 To convert milligrams to grains, use the following formula:

Example: Convert 180 milligrams to grains.

$$\frac{1 \text{ gr}}{\text{Mg in gr}} = \frac{\text{Dose desired}}{\text{Dose on hand}}$$

$$\frac{1}{60} = \frac{X}{180}$$
$$60X = 180$$
$$X = 3 \text{ grains}$$

2 You may also make this conversion as a ratio:

1 gr:60 mg::X gr:180 mg   60X = 180
                                              X = 3 grains

3 Check equivalency tables in the drug supplement.

INTERVENTION: Calculating Oral Dosages of Drugs

1 To calculate oral dosages, use the following formula:

$$\frac{D}{H} = X$$

where D = dose desired
          H = dose on hand
          X = dose to be administered

Example: Give 500 mg of Ampicillin when the dose on hand is in capsules containing 250 mg.

$$\frac{500 \text{ mg}}{250 \text{ mg}} = 2 \text{ capsules}$$

2 To calculate oral dosages of liquids, use the following formula:

$$\frac{D}{H} \times Q = X$$

where Q = quantity

Example: Give 375 mg of Ampicillin when it is supplied as 250 mg/ 5 ml.

$$\frac{375 \text{ mg}}{250 \text{ mg}} \times 5$$
$$1.5 \times 5 = 7.5 \text{ ml}$$

You can also set up a direct proportion and following the algebraic principle, cross multiply:

$$\frac{375 \text{ mg}}{X} = \frac{250 \text{ mg}}{5 \text{ ml}}$$
$$250X = 1875$$
$$X = 7.5 \text{ ml (of strength 250 mg/5 ml)}$$

INTERVENTION: Preparing Oral Medications

1   Obtain client's medication record. Medication record may be a drug card, medication sheet, or drug Kardex, depending on the method of dispensing medications in your facility.
2   Compare the medication record with the most *recent* physician's order.
3   Wash your hands.
4   Gather necessary equipment.
5   Remove the medication from the drug box or tray on medication cart.
6   Compare the label on the bottle or drug package to the medication record.
7   Correctly calculate dosage if necessary and check the dosage to be administered.
8   Pour the medication from the bottle into the lid of the container and then into the medicine cup. With unit dosage, take drug package from medication cart tray and place in medication cup. Do not remove drug from drug package.
9   Check medication label again to ensure correct drug and dosages if drug is not prepackaged.
10 Place medication cup on a tray, if not using medication cart.
11 Return the multidose vial bottle to the storage area. If medication to be given is a narcotic, sign out the narcotic record sheet with your name.

INTERVENTION: Administering Oral Medications to Adults

1   Take medication tray or cart to client's room; check room number against medication card or sheet.
2   Check the client's identaband and ask client to state name so that you are sure you have correctly identified him or her.
3   Place client in sitting position, if not contraindicated by his or her condition.

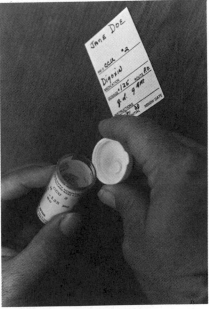

Drop tablet into lid before placing in medication cup and check against card or medication sheet.

▶ Check medication three times before taking to client
● when taking medication from storage area
● before placing medication into medicine cup
● before placing medicine bottle back into storage area (unless you are using the unit dose system)

▶ When pouring a liquid, set medicine cup on firm surface and read fluid level at the lowest point of the meniscus.
● Tablets and capsules are given with water to prevent antagonism of chemical properties of the drug.
● Cough syrups and antacids are not followed by water because they dilute the topical effect.
● Crushed pills or liquids may be mixed with a small quantity of bland food, if not contraindicated by the client's diet.

4 Tell the client what type of medication you are going to give and explain the actions this medication will produce.

5 If prepackaged medication is used, read label, take medication out of package, and put into medication cup.

6 Give the medication cup to the client.

7 Offer a fresh glass of water, or other liquid, to aid swallowing and give assistance with taking medications.

8 Make sure the client swallows the medication.

9 Discard used medicine cup.

10 Position client for comfort.

11 Record the medication on the appropriate forms.

INTERVENTION: Administering Oral Medications to Children

1 Follow the procedures for the previous intervention, keeping the following guidelines in mind:

  a Play techniques may help to elicit a young child's cooperation.

  b Remember: the smaller the quantity of diluent (food or liquid), the greater the ease in eliciting the child's cooperation.

  c Never use a child's favorite food or drink as an enticement when administering medication because the result may be the child's refusal to eat or drink anything.

  d Be honest and tell the child that you have medicine, not candy.

2 Assess child for drug action and possible side effects.

3 Explain medication action and side effects to parents.

EVALUATION

EXPECTED OUTCOMES

1 Client is able to ingest and metabolize medication without feeling nauseated or vomiting. *If not*, follow these alternative nursing actions:

  ANA: Repeat administration in one-half to one hour.

  ANA: Obtain order for antiemetic if nausea continues.

  ANA: If vomiting recurs, notify physician so that administration route can be altered or drug changed.

2 Client emotionally accepts medication. *If not*, follow these alternative nursing actions:

  ANA: Ask client to tell you why he or she refuses medication and help client to work through negative feelings.

  ANA: Offer explanation of medication's action and purpose for written order.

  ANA: Offer medication again.

  ANA: Notify physician if client continues to refuse medications.

3 Client experiences a sustained action of drug and a positive effect on the body. *If not*, follow these alternative nursing actions:

  ANA: Assess response to drug by evaluating vital signs, signs of allergic reaction, etc.

  ANA: Report drug response to physician.

UNEXPECTED OUTCOME

Client has an allergic or anaphylactic response to the medication.

ANA: Immediately stop or hold medication.

ANA: Notify physician at once; prepare to administer antihistamine.

ANA: If reaction is severe:
Keep client flat in bed with head elevated.
Take vital signs every 10–15 minutes.
Assess for hypotension or respiratory distress—if latter present administer oxygen via nasal prongs at 6 l/minute.
Have emergency equipment available.
Provide psychological support to client to alleviate fears.
Record type and progression of allergic reaction.

Charting

- Use appropriate medication form for facility
- Name of drug
- Dosage
- Times ordered
- Time administered
- Method of administration
- Initials of nurse administering drug
- In nurses' notes make comments on client tolerance, concerns or other appropriate information

ACTION: ADMINISTERING SUBLINGUAL MEDICATIONS

ASSESSMENT

1 Be certain that the drug can be administered sublingually, as only a few drugs are given via this route: nitroglycerin, glucagon.
2 Assess client's ability to understand and follow verbal directions.
3 Check to see if the area underneath the client's tongue is excoriated and/or painful. If so, do not give medication.

PLANNING

GOALS

- Therapeutic effects obtained within minutes, if drug is totally absorbed.
- Tablet dissolves and client experiences therapeutic effect.

EQUIPMENT

- Medication (kept in dark bottle as nitroglycerin is light-sensitive and loses its potency when exposed to light)
- Medication card or appropriate method for correctly identifying client and medication

Rationale for Action

- To provide the most appropriate route for fast absorption of drugs such as nitroglycerin and glucose
- To provide the most efficient method of absorption. Absorption is enhanced by the thin layer of epithelium underneath the tongue, as well as by the vast network of capillaries in that area.

INTERVENTION: Administering Sublingual Medications

1 Follow the procedures for preparing and administering oral medications, with these exceptions:
   a Explain that client must not swallow drug or drink any liquid until the drug is completely absorbed.
   b Ask client to place drug under his or her tongue, or to hold tongue up so that you can place medication under the tongue. Do not give water to client.
2 Assess client for drug action and possible side effects.

▶ Sublingual medications, such as nitroglycerin or fast-acting glucose, can be administered to nonresponsive clients because these medications dissolve rapidly and quickly with no chance of aspiration.

EVALUATION

EXPECTED OUTCOMES

1 Therapeutic effect is achieved as chest pain is relieved following administration of nitroglycerin given sublingually. *If not*, follow these alternative nursing actions:

ANA: Check nitroglycerin bottle for expiration date as potency of drug decreases after six months.

ANA: Administer another nitroglycerin tablet in five minutes. You may give client two more tablets over 15 minute time period.

ANA: If chest pain has not subsided, seek medical attention for possible myocardial infarction.

2 Therapeutic effect is experienced within minutes with administration of quick-acting glucose. *If not*, follow these alternative nursing actions:

ANA: Assess for signs of diabetic ketoacidosis.

ANA: Obtain order for blood sugar and urine S/A.

ANA: Obtain order, if needed, to start intravenous infusion of normal saline for ketoacidosis or IV glucose for insulin reaction.

UNEXPECTED OUTCOME

Comatose condition is unaltered with the administration of glucagon sublingually.

ANA: Give glucagon sublingually or intravenously to determine if glucose dose increases blood glucose level and reverses insulin reaction.

ANA: Assess for conditions other than hypoglycemia or insulin reaction that may be eliciting comatose response.

Charting
- Use appropriate medication form for facility
- Name of drug
- Dosage
- Times ordered
- Time administered
- Method of administration
- Initials of nurse administering drug
- In nurses' notes make comments on client tolerance, concerns or other appropriate information

ACTION: ADMINISTERING PARENTERAL MEDICATIONS

ASSESSMENT

1 Determine appropriate method for administration of drug:
  a Intradermal (intracutaneous): injection is made below surface of the skin.
  b Subcutaneous: small amount of fluid is injected beneath the skin in the loose connective tissues.
  c Intramuscular: larger amount of fluid is injected into large muscle masses in the body.
  d Intravenous: medication is injected or infused directly into a vein — route used when immediate drug effect is desired.
2 Evaluate condition of administration site for presence of lesions, rash, inflammation, lipid dystrophy, ecchymosis, etc.
3 Assess for tissue damage from previous injections.
4 Assess client's level of consciousness.
  a For client in shock: certain methods (subcutaneous) will not be used.

Rationale for Action
- To rapidly deliver medication to maintain high-blood titers of the medication
- To ensure adequate absorption and more predictable results

b For presence of anxiety: make sure client is allowed to express his or her fear of injections and offer explanations of ways in which injections will be less frightening.

5 Check client's written and verbal history for past allergic reactions. Do *not* rely solely on client's chart.

6 Review client's chart noting previous injection sites, especially insulin and heparin administration sites.

7 Check label on medication bottle to determine if medication can be administered via route ordered.

PLANNING

GOALS

● Injection process is completed without technical complications.
● Injection is as painless as possible.
● Medication enters bloodstream promptly and is effectively utilized by the tissues.

EQUIPMENT

● Alcohol wipes
● Vials or ampoules of medications
● Bottle of diluent (when necessary)
● Intravenous catheters or needles
● IV solutions and IV tubing
● Bandaid or tape and dressing for IV insertions
● Syringe with appropriate needles
  Intradermal injections: short bevel 26-gauge, ⅜-inch needle
  Subcutaneous injections: 25-gauge, ½- to ⅝-inch needle

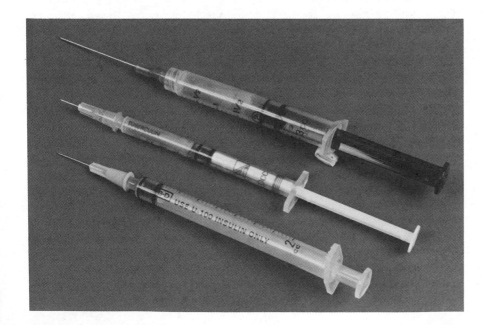

Syringes used for parenteral medication administration.

Intramuscular injections: deltoid muscle requires 23–25-gauge, ⅝ needle; needle size for thigh and buttock area varies 1 to 3 inches; oil base medications require 20-gauge needle; water base medications require 22-gauge needle; 18–23-gauge needles can be used in varying lengths from 1 to 1½ inches. 18-gauge needles are rarely used.

· *Intravenous injections*: See chapter on Fluid and Electrolytes for equipment.

INTERVENTION: Calculating Parenteral Dosages of Drugs

1 To calculate parenteral dosages, use the following formula:

$$\frac{D}{H} \times Q = X$$

Example: Give client 40 mg Gentamicin. On hand is a multidose vial with a strength of 80 mg/2 ml.

$$\frac{40}{80} \times 2 = 1 \text{ ml}$$

2 Check your calculations before drawing up medication.
3 See Calculations of Solutions in Drug Supplement.

INTERVENTION: Preparing Injections

1 Wash hands
2 Obtain equipment for injection: Needle and syringe, alcohol wipes, medication tray (medication container if needed).
3 Assemble the needle and syringe. Select the appropriate size needle, considering the size of the client's muscle mass and the viscosity of the medication.
4 Open the alcohol wipe and cleanse the top of the vial or break top of ampoule.
5 Remove the needle guard and place on alcohol wipe or medication tray.
6 Pull back on barrel of syringe to markings where medication will be inserted.
7 Pick up vial, insert needle into vial and inject air in an amount equal to the solution to be withdrawn by pushing barrel of syringe down. If using an ampoule, break off top at colored line, insert needle, but do not inject air into ampoule as it causes displacement and possible loss of medication through leakage.
8 Extract the desired amount of fluid. Remove needle from container and cover needle with guard. Needle should be changed to prevent tracking medication on skin and subcutaneous tissue.
9 Double check drug and dosage against drug card or medication sheet and vial or ampoule.
10 Place syringe on tray if tray available.

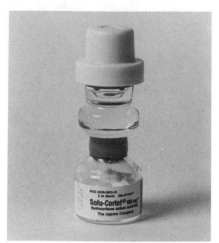

Mix-o-Vial is a convenient package for certain drugs, containing solute and solvent in one vial. To mix, push on stopper to force solvent into solute, shake well, wipe with alcohol, and withdraw medication into syringe.

Invert ampoule after breaking off top, then insert needle without injecting air. Medication will not drip out and this method enables all liquid to be withdrawn without contamination.

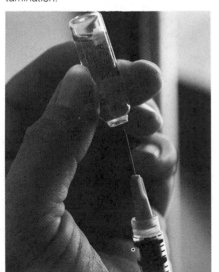

11 Check label and drug card or medication sheet for accuracy before returning multidose vial to correct storage area.

12 Return multidose vial to correct storage area or discard used vial or ampoule.

INTERVENTION: Administering Intradermal Injections

1 Take medication to client's room. Check room number against medication card or sheet.

2 Check client's identaband and ask client to state name.

3 Explain the medication's action and the procedure for administration to client.

4 Wash hands.

5 Select the site of injection.

6 Cleanse the area with an alcohol wipe, wiping in circular area from inside to outside.

7 Take off needle guard and place on tray.

8 Grasp client's forearm from underneath and gently pull the skin taut.

9 Insert the needle at a 10 to 15 degree angle with the bevel of needle facing up.

10 Inject medication slowly. Observe for wheals and blanching at the site (normal finding).

11 Withdraw the needle, wiping the area gently with a dry 2 × 2 pad to prevent dispersing medication into the subcutaneous tissue.

12 Return the client to a comfortable position.

13 Discard supplies in appropriate area.

14 Chart the medication and site used.

Intradermal or Intracutaneous Injections

- Injection sites: inner aspect of forearm or scapular area of back
- Purpose: for antigens for skin or for tuberculin tests
- Amount injected: ranges from 0.01 to 0.1 cc
- Absorption rate: slow

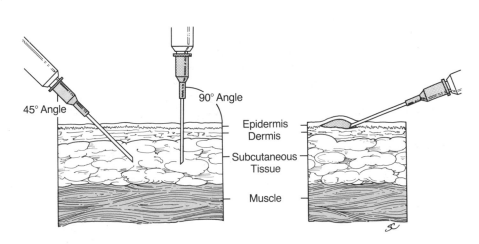

45° Angle

90° Angle

Epidermis
Dermis

Subcutaneous Tissue

Muscle

(a) Insert needle at 45 or 90 degree angle for subcutaneous injection. (b) Insert needle at 15 degree angle under the epidermis for intradermal injection.

Subcutaneous Injections

- Injection site: abdomen, lateral aspects of upper arm or thigh
- Purpose: for medications that are absorbed slowly, to produce a sustained effect
- Amount injected: variable—small amount of fluid. If repeated doses are necessary, as with insulin for a diabetic, rotate injection sites

When drugs are absorbed into the venous circulation from the upper GI tract, they must traverse the liver before entering the systemic circulation. Parenteral drugs are, therefore, more potent.

▶ Do not inject air directly into insulin solution as this causes bubbles in the solution which can alter the actual dosage being administered.

INSULIN TYPES AND ACTION

TYPES	ONSET	PEAK	DURATION
Rapid Acting			
Regular	½ to 1	2 to 4	6 to 8
Semilente	½ to 1	2 to 8	12 to 16
Intermediate Acting			
NPH	1 to 1½	8 to 12	24
Lente	1 to 1½	8 to 12	24
Long Acting			
Protamine zinc (PZI)	4 to 8	14 to 20	24 to 36
Ultralente	4 to 8	16 to 24	36

INTERVENTION: Administering Subcutaneous (Sub q) Injections

1. Take medication to client's room.
2. Set tray on a clean surface, not the bed.
3. Check client's identaband and ask client to state name.
4. Explain action of medication and procedure of administration.
5. Provide privacy when injection site is other than on the arm.
6. Wash hands.
7. Select site for injection by identifying anatomical landmarks. Remember to alternate sites each time injections are given.
8. Cleanse area with alcohol wipe. Using a circular motion cleanse from inside outward.
9. Take off needle guard.
10. Express any air bubbles from syringe.
11. Insert the needle at a 45-degree angle.
12. Pull back on the plunger.
13. Inject the medication slowly.
14. Withdraw needle quickly, and massage area with alcohol wipe to aid absorption and lessen bleeding. Put on bandaid if needed.
15. Return client to a position of comfort.
16. Discard used supplies in proper areas. Remember to break needle from syringe and discard needle in safety container.
17. Chart the medication and site used.
18. For injecting insulin, see following Intervention, "Administering Insulin Injections."

INTERVENTION: Administering Insulin Injections

1. Gather equipment, check medication orders, injection site, and rotation chart. Insulin does not need to be refrigerated.
2. Wash hands.
3. Obtain specific insulin syringe for strength of insulin being administered (U40, U80, U100).
4. Rotate insulin bottle between hands to bring solution into suspension if needed.
5. Wipe top of insulin bottle with alcohol.
6. Take off needle guard.
7. Pull plunger of syringe down to desired amount of medication and inject that amount of air into the insulin bottle.
8. Draw up ordered amount of insulin into syringe.
9. Expel air from syringe.
10. Replace needle guard.
11. Check medication card, bottle, and syringe with another RN for accuracy.
12. Take medications to client's room.
13. Double check site of last injection with client.
14. Provide privacy.
15. Wash hands.
16. Follow protocol for administration of medications by subcutaneous injections.

INTERVENTION: Administering Two Insulin Solutions

1 Follow steps 1–5 Administering Insulin Injections.
2 Inject prescribed amount of air into intermediate acting (NPH, Lente) or long acting (PZI, Ultralente) bottle.
3 Pull needle out of insulin bottle and withdraw plunger to prescribed short acting (Regular, Semilente) insulin dosage.
4 Inject air into short acting insulin bottle and withdraw medication.
5 Expel all air bubbles.
6 Insert needle into second insulin bottle taking care not to push any short acting insulin into bottle. This can be avoided by putting pressure on plunger with your small finger when inserting into bottle.
7 Invert bottle and pull back on plunger to obtain prescribed amount of insulin. Remember the total insulin dose will include the amount of short acting insulin already drawn up into syringe.
8 Follow steps 8–15 Administering Sub q Injections to complete procedure.

NEW INSULIN PREPARATIONS PURIFIED PORK INSULIN, U100

Actrapid
   Short acting
   Rapid effect
   Duration: 6 to 8 hours
   Method: IV and sub q

Semitard
   Prompt purified pork insulin
   Short acting
   Duration 12 to 16 hours
   Zinc suspension
   Method: sub q

Monotard
   Purified pork insulin
   Intermediate acting
   Duration: 24 hours
   Zinc suspension
   Method: sub q

Lentard
   Purified pork and beef insulin
   Intermediate acting
   Duration: 24 hours
   Zinc suspension
   Method: sub q administration only

Ultratard
   Extended purified beef insulin
   Long acting
   Duration: 36 hours
   Zinc suspension
   Method: sub q

The term "purified" means that the insulin has undergone additional purification. These medications must be stored in the refrigerator. Produced by Novo Labs, Inc.

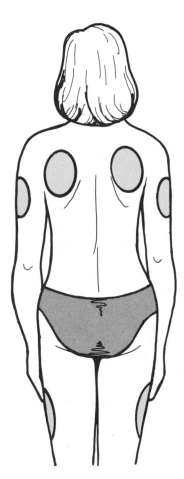
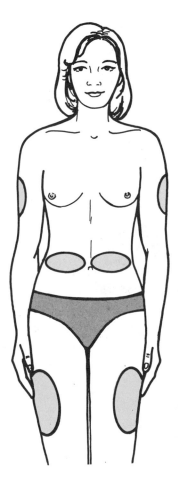

Rotate sites for subcutaneous injections given on a continuing basis.

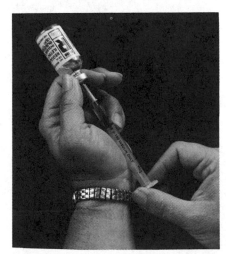

Use specific insulin syringe for strength of insulin being administered.

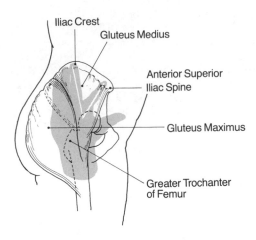

Iliac Crest

Gluteus Medius

Anterior Superior
Iliac Spine

Gluteus Maximus

Greater Trochanter
of Femur

(a) Insert needle in "V" area after placing
heel of hand over greater trochanter of
femur, spreading index and middle fingers
and forming "V".

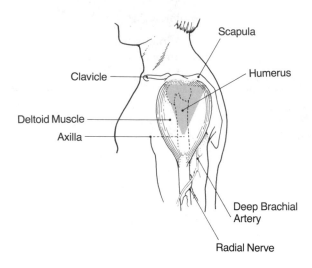

Scapula

Clavicle

Humerus

Deltoid Muscle

Axilla

Deep Brachial
Artery

Radial Nerve

(b) Administer IM or subcutaneous injection
in deltoid area. Identify lower edge of
acromium process and point on lateral arm
in line with axilla.

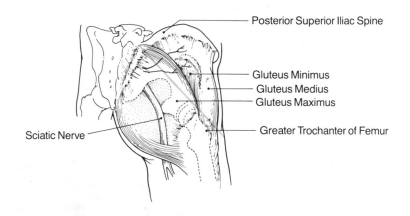

Posterior Superior Iliac Spine

Gluteus Minimus
Gluteus Medius
Gluteus Maximus

Greater Trochanter of Femur

Sciatic Nerve

(a) Place injection in gluteus medius above
and outside diagonal line for IM injections.

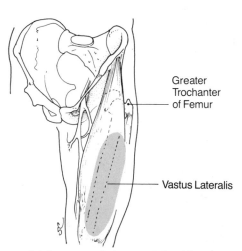

Greater
Trochanter
of Femur

Vastus Lateralis

(b) Insert needle in area defined from
one hand breadth above knee and one
hand breadth below greater trochanter in
vastus lateralis.

INTERVENTION: Administering Intramuscular (IM) Injections

1 Take medication to client's room. Check room number against medication card or sheet.
2 Check client's identaband and have client state name.
3 Set tray on a clean surface, not the bed.
4 Explain the procedure to client.
5 Provide privacy for client.
6 Wash your hands.
7 Select the site of injection by identifying anatomical landmarks. Remember to alternate sites each time injections are given.
8 Cleanse the area with alcohol wipe. Using a circular motion cleanse from inside outward.
9 Hold the syringe; take off needle cover.
10 Express air bubbles from syringe. Some clinicians suggest leaving a small air bubble at the tip so that all medicine will be expelled.
11 Insert the needle at 90-degree angle.
12 Pull back on plunger. If blood returns, you know you have entered a blood vessel and need to reposition the needle and aspirate again.
13 Inject the medication slowly.
14 Withdraw the needle and massage the area with an alcohol wipe. Put on a bandaid, if needed.
15 Return client to a comfortable position.
16 Discard supplies in appropriate area.
17 Chart the medication and site used.

(a) Insert needle at 90 degree angle and deep into muscle tissue for intramuscular injections.
(b) Pull skin tight and to one side before inserting needle to prevent tracking of medications. This method allows medication to be retained in muscle layer rather than seeping along needle track.

Intramuscular Injections

- Injection site: lateral aspect of thigh (vastus lateralis), buttocks (gluteus maximus), ventral gluteal area, upper arm (deltoid)
- Purpose: to promote rapid absorption of the drug; to provide an alternate route when drug is irritating to subcutaneous tissues; to provide a less painful route for parenteral medications
- Amount injected: variable—may be large amount of fluid
- Absorption rate: depends on circulatory state of client

All needles and syringes must be broken before discarding in refuse box.

Using Z-Track Method
- Used for iron injections
- Draw up prescribed medication into syringe
- Draw up 0.3 to 0.5 cc of air into syringe
- Replace needle with 3″ needle to penetrate deep into muscle
- Pull skin laterally away from injection site
- Cleanse site with alcohol
- Insert needle
- Inject medication slowly—and wait ten seconds
- Withdraw needle
- Allow retracted skin to go back into place
- Do not massage site
- Increase absorption rate through ambulation
- Skin discoloration can occur if Z-track method is not used

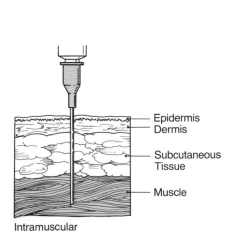

Epidermis
Dermis

Subcutaneous Tissue

Muscle

Intramuscular

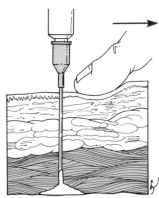

Z-Track Injection

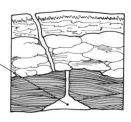

Medication

EXPECTED OUTCOMES

1   Injection process is completed without technical complications. *If not*, follow these alternative nursing actions:

ANA: If needle fails to pierce the underlying tissues remove needle and, using new site and clean needle, repeat procedure. Explain what you are doing and reassure client, making sure he or she is relaxed.

ANA: If a lump appears after administration, massage area to aid absorption. Verify with physician whether dose should be repeated.

ANA: If aspiration of blood occurs, withdraw, use clean needle and inject medicine into new site.

2   Injection is as painless as possible. *If not*, follow these alternative nursing actions:

ANA: Assess area thoroughly for lipid dystrophy or ecchymosis to prevent pain from injections.

ANA: Distract client before injection is administered.

ANA: Put pressure on injection site with hand not being used for inserting syringe. This pressure takes mind off actual needle insertion.

ANA: Review techniques for alleviating pain during injections.

ANA: Place topical anesthetic on injection site before inserting needle. This method is used for IV or intradermal injections.

ANA: Infuse xylocaine intradermally into site where IV catheter is to be inserted.

3   Medication enters bloodstream promptly and is effectively utilized by the tissues. *If not*, follow these alternative nursing actions:

ANA: Reassess needle length used. If not appropriate for site, use different needle. You may feel a ⅝" needle is sufficient for IM injections for thin people but in fact, the medication will be given Sub q rather than IM as ordered.

ANA: If medication infiltrates subcutaneous tissues, apply warm compresses and notify physician so that medication can be given via another route.

ANA: Assess that drug concentration is adequate for particular client.

ANA: Assess level of hydration: client dehydrated – drug will not absorb efficiently; client over-hydrated – drug will not disseminate.

UNEXPECTED OUTCOMES

1   Sciatic nerve is touched with needle.

ANA: Notify physician. Fill out incident report. Take greater care to identify anatomical landmarks.

ANA: Obtain order for warm, moist packs.

ANA: Medicate for pain.

2   Client has an anaphylactic allergic response.

ANA: Position client for optimal cerebral perfusion – flat or 30-degree elevation if dyspneic.

▶ **Techniques for Alleviating Pain During Injections**

- Encourage client to relax area to be injected: place client on side with flexed knee or out flat on abdomen, if giving injection in buttock.
- Reduce puncture pain by "darting" needle.
- Prevent antiseptic from clinging to needle during insertion by waiting until skin antiseptic is dry.
- If you must draw needle through rubber stopper, use a new needle for injection of medication.
- Avoid injecting sensitive or hardened body areas.
- After needle is under skin, aspirate to be certain that needle is not in a blood vessel.
- Inject medication slowly.
- Maintain grasp on syringe.
- Withdraw needle quickly after injection.
- Massage relaxed muscle gently to increase circulation and to distribute medication.

ANA: Maintain patent airway.

ANA: Obtain order from physician for antihistamine (or epinephrine if severe reaction).

ANA: Administer oxygen at 6 l/min via nasal prongs after bronchodilation has occurred.

3 Intermediate acting insulin contaminates regular insulin bottle when drawing up two insulins.

ANA: Regular insulin bottle must be discarded as regular insulin is used for emergency treatment and now would not have rapid onset of action.

ANA: Repeat procedure for drawing up two insulin solutions.

Charting

- Use appropriate medication form for facility
- Name of drug
- Dosage
- Method of administration
- Times ordered
- Time administered
- Initials of nurse administering drug
- In nurses notes make appropriate comments concerning client's condition, concerns, feelings, etc

ACTION: ADMINISTERING SUPPOSITORY MEDICATIONS

ASSESSMENT

1 Check to make sure that administration route is appropriate for ordered medication.
2 Observe for signs of rectal irritation and/or bleeding.
3 Observe for hemorrhoids.
4 Check sphincter control.

PLANNING

GOALS

- Medication is inserted without technical complications
- Medication is absorbed and is effectively utilized

EQUIPMENT

- Suppository as ordered
- Disposable glove or fingercot
- K-Y jelly

Rationale for Action

- To provide alternate route when upper GI tract is malfunctioning, i.e., vomiting
- To offer alternate route when drug has offensive taste or odor
- To maintain chemical integrity of drug when digestive enzymes change the chemical properties of the drug
- To obtain high blood concentration of the drug

INTERVENTION: Inserting Rectal Suppositories

1 Follow safety procedures for administering drugs.
2 Place medication on a tray, if not using medication cart.
3 Take medication to room, check room number and identaband against medication card or sheet.
4 Explain procedure to client.
5 Provide privacy by closing door and/or pulling curtain.
6 Wash your hands.
7 Place client in the Sim's (left lateral) position.
8 Remove the foil wrapper from the suppository.
9 Put K-Y jelly on tip of suppository to facilitate insertion.
10 Using a fingercot or disposable glove, insert the suppository into the rectal canal beyond the anal sphincter.

271

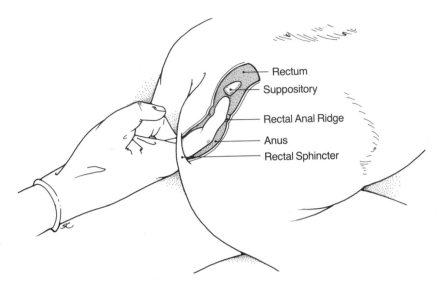

Insert rectal suppository beyond the rectal-anal ridge to ensure it is retained.

11 Instruct the client to lie quietly for fifteen minutes until the medicine is absorbed.
12 Return after fifteen minutes to check on client and make him or her comfortable.
13 Chart medication and results obtained.

INTERVENTION: Inserting Vaginal Suppositories

1 Follow safety procedures for administering drugs.
2 Take medication to client's room.
3 Check number and identaband against medication card or sheet.
4 Explain procedure to client.
5 Provide privacy by closing door and/or pulling curtain.
6 Wash your hands.

Insert vaginal suppositories at least two inches using glove or applicator as shown in this drawing.

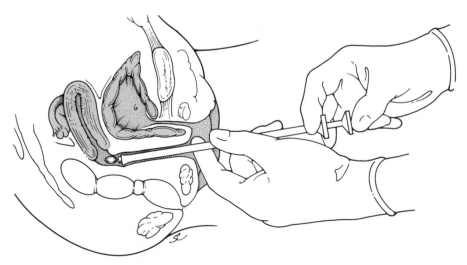

7   Place client in the dorsal recumbent or Sim's position.

8   Remove the foil wrapper from the suppository.

9   Using a disposable glove, insert the suppository into the vaginal canal at least two inches.

10 Instruct the client to lie quietly for fifteen minutes until the suppository is absorbed.

11 Return to client after fifteen minutes to check on client.

12 Chart medication and any evidence of discharge or odor from vagina.

EVALUATION

EXPECTED OUTCOMES

1   Medication is inserted without technical complications. *If not,* follow these alternative nursing actions:

ANA: If fecal impaction is present, obtain order for cleansing enema and repeat procedure.

ANA: If hemorrhoids are present and/or painful upon insertion, lubricate suppository well, have client take deep breath and insert gently.

ANA: If rectal bleeding from hemorrhoids or fissures occurs, do not insert suppository, and notify physician.

2   Medication enters bloodstream and is effectively utilized. *If not,* follow these alternative nursing actions:

ANA: Check to see if medication was immediately expelled.

ANA: If suppository fails to dissolve, check expiration date and obtain new supply.

ANA: Instruct client to maintain appropriate position so that drug is absorbed.

UNEXPECTED OUTCOME

Client unable to retain suppositories.

ANA: Observe if sphincter is competent.

ANA: Instruct client to maintain position for at least 15 minutes in order to allow any absorption.

ANA: Suggest to physician that an alternate route or a different medication be tried.

Charting
- Use appropriate medication form for facility
- Name of drug
- Dosage
- Times ordered
- Time administered
- Method of administration
- Initials of nurse administering drug
- In nurses notes make comments on skin condition, mucous membranes, burn area

ACTION: ADMINISTERING EYE MEDICATIONS

ASSESSMENT

1   Check to make sure that medication is appropriate for route ordered.

2   Assess client's level of consciousness to ensure cooperation during administration since medications are instilled into the lower conjunctival sac.

3   Check medication expiration date.

Rationale for Action
- To provide direct route for local effect
- To decrease intraocular pressure
- To provide means for eye evaluation

273

PLANNING

GOALS

- Client cooperates with instillation of eye medication
- Desired therapeutic effect is obtained

EQUIPMENT

- Eye drops or ointment
- Cotton ball or swab

INTERVENTION: Administering Eye Drops

1 Wash your hands.
2 Follow safety procedures for administering drugs.
3 Place medication on a tray, if not using medication cart.
4 Take medication to client's room, check room number against medication card or sheet.
5 Check client's identaband and ask client to state name.
6 Wash your hands.
7 Explain procedure to client.
8 Tilt client's head slightly backward.
9 Squeeze prescribed amount of medication into eye dropper. Hold dropper with bulb in uppermost position.
10 Give tissue to client for wiping off excess medication.
11 Expose lower conjunctival sac.
12 Drop prescribed medication into center of sac. (Do *not* place medication directly on cornea, since medication can cause injury to cornea.)
13 Ask client to close eyelids and move eyes to distribute solution over conjunctival surface and anterior eyeball.
14 Remove excess medication from surrounding tissue.

Drop eye medication in center of conjunctival sac.

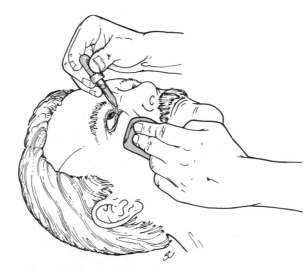

INTERVENTION: Administering Eye Ointments to Upper Lid

1 Follow steps 1 through 7 on page 274.
2 Instruct client to look down.
3 Grasp client's lashes near center of upper lid with your thumb and index finger. Draw lid down and away from eyeball.
4 With your opposite hand, place applicator horizontally along upper part of eyelid.
5 While pressing down on applicator, quickly turn eyelid up over the applicator.
6 Squeeze ointment over entire lid starting at the inner canthus.
7 Instruct client to close lid and move eye to assist in spreading medication, if not contraindicated.
8 Remove excess medication from surrounding tissue.

INTERVENTION: Administering Eye Ointments to Lower Lid

1 Follow steps 1 through 7 on page 274.
2 Take protective guard off medication tip.
3 Gently separate client's eyelids with your thumb or two fingers, and grasp lower lid near the margin of the lower lid immediately below the lashes. Exert pressure downward over the bony prominence of the cheek.
4 Instruct the client to look upward.
5 Place eye medication on the entire lower lid. Squeeze 2 cm of ointment from tube starting at the inner canthus.
6 Ask client to close eyelids and move eyes to assist in spreading ointment under the lids and over the surface of the eyeball.
7 With a cotton ball or soft tissue, remove the excess medication from client's eye and cheek.

EVALUATION

EXPECTED OUTCOMES

1 Client cooperates with instillation of eye medication. *If not*, follow these alternative nursing actions:
ANA: If client is unable to hold eyes open and blink, help client into a comfortable position, explain the procedure, encourage client to cooperate, and repeat the medication.
ANA: Use techniques of distraction for clients who are unable to keep eyes open during instillation of medication.
2 Desired therapeutic effect is obtained. *If not*, follow these alternative nursing actions:
ANA: If no relief is obtained or if eye is reddened, notify physician for new orders.
ANA: If severe irritation occurs obtain order for and apply sterile eye soaks to ease pain and discomfort.

Charting

- Use appropriate medication form for facility
- Name of drug
- Dosage
- Method of administration
- Times ordered
- Time administered
- Initials of nurse administering drug

Rationale for Action

- To soften ear wax
- To relieve pain
- To apply anesthetic agent
- To provide route for antibacterial medications

UNEXPECTED OUTCOME

Infection is introduced because of break in aseptic technique.

ANA: Medication dropper contaminated. Discard dropper and obtain new one.

ANA: Review the recommended procedures for administering the medication and have another nurse observe until you perfect the skill of administering eye medications.

ACTION: ADMINISTERING EAR MEDICATIONS

ASSESSMENT

1 Assess client's ability to cooperate with instillation.
2 Assess client's ability to be positioned on side.

PLANNING

GOALS

- Client cooperates with instillation
- Desired therapeutic effect obtained

EQUIPMENT

- Medication, warmed to body temperature
- Dropper for instilling medication
- Cotton wick

INTERVENTION: Administering Ear Medications

1 Before preparing medication for administration, warm medication bottle to body temperature (98.6° F).
2 Follow steps 1 through 7 on page 274.
3 Fill medication dropper with prescribed amount of medication.
4 Position client on side, with ear to be treated in uppermost position.
5 Prepare client for instillation of ear medications as follows:
  a *Infant*: Draw the auricle gently downward and backward to separate the drum membrane from the floor of the cartilaginous canal.
  b *Adult*: Lift the pinna upward and backward.
6 Insert a loose cotton wick into the canal to maintain a continuous application of the solution (optional).
7 Instruct client to remain on his or her side for 15 minutes following instillation to prevent medication from escaping.

EVALUATION

EXPECTED OUTCOMES

1 Client cooperates with instillation. *If not*, follow these alternative nursing actions:
ANA: Obtain assistance to hold client on his or her side in a supine position.

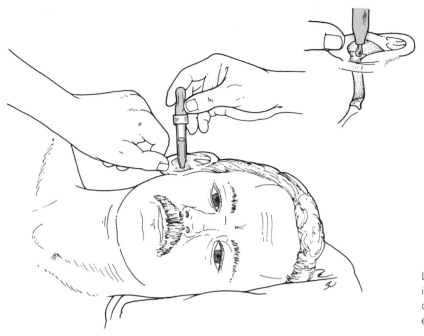

Lift auricle upward and backward for instilling ear medications for adults. Pull auricle downward and backward for instilling ear medications for children.

ANA: Have someone stay with client after instillation to ensure client remains on his or her side.

2   Desired therapeutic effect is obtained. *If not*, follow these alternative nursing actions:

ANA: Inform physician that client is still experiencing the same symptoms.

ANA: Ask physician for new medication orders.

UNEXPECTED OUTCOMES

1   Client moves unexpectedly, causing medication to run down client's neck.

ANA: Repeat explanation of procedure to client.

ANA: Readminister medication while holding client in correct position. Keep client positioned on side for 15 minutes after instillation.

2   Client complains medication is too warm.

ANA: Check to ensure medication is only heated to 98.6°F.

ANA: Observe client for any untoward effects.

Charting
- Use appropriate medication form for facility
- Name of drug
- Dosage
- Method of administration
- Times ordered
- Time administered
- Initials of nurse administering drug

Drug Supplement

This section is a supplement to the conceptual base of therapeutic agents. It contains information on systems of measurements, mathematic conversion tables, calculation of solutions, drug classification by action and by body system and basic laws governing drug dispensation.

APOTHECARY SYSTEM

A Older system, based on unrelated, arbitrary units of measure; gradually being replaced by metric system.
   1 Portions of a unit of measurement designated by common fractions, e.g., one-fourth grain, written as gr ¼.
   2 Symbols for ounces and drams are similar in form and must be written clearly (e.g., ꝫ is dram; ℥ is ounce).
   3 Symbols and abbreviations are placed before Roman numerals (5 grains written as gr v).

B Common apothecary measures and symbols
   drop   gtt
   minim   m
   dram   ꝫ
   ounce   ℥
   grain   gr

C Equivalents
   1 drop   = 1 minim
   15 drops   = 1 grain
   60 minims   = 1 fluid dram
   8 fluid drams   = 1 fluid ounce
   16 fluid ounces = 1 pint

METRIC SYSTEM

A French-invented system, based on rationally and related derived units; developed in the eighteenth century.
  1 Basic units of measure used in drug administration are the gram and liter.
  2 Other units are decimals, fractions, and Arabic numerals.
  3 Numbers and fractions are placed before symbols.

B Common metric measures and symbols

gram	gm
kilogram	kg
milligram	mg
milliliter	ml
liter	l

C Weight and volume equivalents with corresponding symbols

1 gram = 1,000 milligrams   1 gm = 1,000 mg
1 liter = 1,000 milliliters   1 l = 1,000 ml

HOUSEHOLD SYSTEM

A System based on familiar measures used in the home.
  1 Most measures are not sufficiently accurate for measure of medicines.
  2 Pints and quarts are also used in apothecary system.

B Common household measures and their abbreviations

pint	pt
teaspoon	t
tablespoon	T
quart	qt

MATHEMATIC CONVERSION

Approximate Equivalents

A The metric system is the universal system of weights and measures.
B Apothecary and metric systems do not use same size units; denominations of one system are not compatible with the other.
C Equivalency tables are established to list measurement denominations of one system in terms of another. (See Appendix 2, Tables A, B, and C.)
  1 Conversion from one system to another can be computed, but measurements are not equivalent in absolute terms.
  2 If there is occasion to compute, have computations checked by another licensed nurse.
    a Do not compute unless allowed to do so by your state Nurse Practice Act.
    b Check hospital policy for further guidelines.

CONVERSION TABLES

TABLE A HOUSEHOLD EQUIVALENTS (VOLUME)

METRIC	APOTHECARY	HOUSEHOLD
0.06 ml	1 minim	1 drop
5 (4) ml	1 fluid dram	1 teaspoonful
15 ml	4 fluid drams	1 tablespoonful
30 ml	1 fluid ounce	2 tablespoonfuls
180 ml	6 fluid ounces	1 teacupful
240 ml	8 fluid ounces	1 glassful

TABLE B APOTHECARY EQUIVALENTS (VOLUME)

METRIC		APOTHECARY
1 ml	=	15 minims
1 cc	=	15 minims
0.06 ml	=	1 minim
4 ml	=	1 fluid dram
30 ml	=	1 fluid ounce
500 ml	=	1 pint
1000 ml (1 l)	=	1 quart

TABLE C APOTHECARY EQUIVALENTS (WEIGHT)

METRIC						APOTHECARY
1.0	gm	or	1000 mg	=	gr xv	
0.6	gm	or	600 mg	=	gr x	
0.5	gm	or	500 mg	=	gr viiss	
0.3	gm	or	300 mg	=	gr v	
0.2	gm	or	200 mg	=	gr iii	
0.1	gm	or	100 mg	=	gr 1½	
0.06	gm	or	60 mg	=	gr 1	
0.05	gm	or	50 mg	=	gr ¾	
0.03	gm	or	30 mg	=	gr ½	
0.015	gm	or	15 mg	=	gr ¼	
0.010	gm	or	10 mg	=	gr ⅙	
0.008	gm	or	8 mg	=	gr ⅛	
4 g				=	1 dr	
30 g				=	1 oz	
1 kg				=	2.2 lbs	

Computation

A Drugs are not always labeled clearly as to number of tablets to administer, so computation may be necessary. Always have your computation checked by another licensed nurse.

B Method

    1 Both desired (ordered) dose and dose on hand must be in same unit of measurement, e.g., grains, grams, milligrams.

2　If not, convert so that unit of measure is the same.
   a　Refer to conversion tables.
   b　To convert one measure unit to another, basic equivalencies must be memorized.
3　After converting, divide desired dose by dose on hand to find amount to administer.

CALCULATION OF SOLUTIONS

Types of Solutions

A　Volume to volume (v/v): a given volume of solute is added to a given volume of solvent.
B　Weight to weight (w/w): a stated weight of solute is dissolved in a stated weight of solvent.
C　Weight to volume (w/v): a given weight of solute is dissolved in a given volume of solvent which results in the proper amount of solution.

Preparing Solutions

A　Liquid to drug solutions
   1　Determine the strength of the solution, the strength of the drug on hand, and the quantity of solution required.
   2　Use this formula for preparing solutions:

$$\frac{D}{H} \times Q = X$$

where D = desired strength
      H = strength on hand
      Q = quantity of solution desired
      X = amount of solute

Example: You have a 100% solution of hydrogen peroxide on hand. You need a liter of 50% solution.

$$\frac{50}{100} \times 1000 \text{ ml} = 500 \text{ ml}$$

If the strength desired and strength on hand are not in like terms, you need to change one of the terms.
Example: You have 1 liter of 50% solution on hand. You need a liter of 1:10 solution. 1:10 solution is the same as 10%.

$$\frac{10\%}{50\%} \times 1000 \text{ ml} = 200 \text{ ml}$$

Add 200 ml of the drug to 800 ml of the solvent to make a liter of 10% solution.

B Volume to volume solutions

   1 Use the formula:

$$\frac{D}{H} \times Q = X$$

where X = amount of stock solution used

Example: Prepare a liter of 5% solution from a stock solution of 50%.

$$\frac{5\%}{50\%} \times 1000 \text{ ml} = 100 \text{ ml}$$

Add 100 ml to 900 ml of diluent to make 1 liter of 5% solution.

DRUG CLASSIFICATION

Classification by Action

A Anti-infectives
   1 Antiseptics
      a Inhibit growth of microorganisms (bacteriostatic)
      b Cleanse wounds and skin infections, sterilize equipment, promote hygiene
   2 Disinfectants
      a Destroy microorganisms (bactericidal)
      b Destroy bacteria on inanimate objects (not appropriate for living tissue)

B Antimicrobials
   1 Sulfonamides
      a Inhibit the growth of microorganisms
      b Reduce or prevent infectious process, especially urinary tract infections
   2 Antibiotics (e.g., penicillin)
      a Interfere with microorganism metabolism
      b Reduce or prevent infectious process
      c Specific drug and dosage: based on culture and sensitivity of organism

C Metabolic drugs
   1 Hormones obtained from animal sources; found naturally in foods and plants
   2 Synthetic hormones

D Diagnostic materials
   1 Dyes and opaque materials: ingested or injected to allow visualization of internal organs
   2 Analyze organ status and function

E Vitamins and minerals
   1 Necessary to obtain healthy body function
   2 Found naturally in food or through synthetic food supplements

F Vaccines and serums
 1 Prevent disease and detect presence of disease
 2 Types
  a Antigenics: for active immunity
   - Vaccines: attenuated suspensions of microorganisms
   - Toxoids: products of microorganisms
  b Antibodies: stimulated by microorganisms or their products
   - Antitoxins
   - Immune serum globulin
  c Allergens: agents for skin immunity tests
   - Extracts of materials known to be allergenic
   - Used to relieve allergies
  d Antivenins: substances that neutralize venom of certain snakes and spiders

G Antifungals: check growth of fungi

H Antihistaminics
 1 Prevent histamine action
 2 Relieve symptoms of allergic reaction

I Antineoplastics: prevent growth and spread of malignant cells

Classification by Body Systems

Central Nervous System   Drugs affect CNS by either inhibiting or promoting the actions of neural pathways and centers.

A Action promoting drug groups (stimulants)
 1 Antidepressants: psychic energizers used to treat depression
 2 Caffeine: increases mental activity and lessens drowsiness
 3 Ammonia: used as stimulant to counteract fainting.

B Action inhibiting drug groups (depressants)
 1 Analgesics: reduce pain by interfering with conduction of nerve impulses
  a Narcotic analgesics: opium derivatives (morphine); may depress respiratory centers; must be used with caution and respiratory rate above 12
   - A narcotic antagonist drug counteracts depressant drugs
   - Such antagonist drugs are Lorfan, Narcan, and Nalline
  b Nonnarcotic antipyretics: reduce fever and relieve pain (ASA and Tylenol)
  c Antirheumatics: analgesics given to relieve arthritis pain; may reduce joint inflammation
 2 Alcohol: stimulates appetite when given in small doses; classified as a depressant
 3 Hypnotics: sedatives that induce sleep; barbiturates (phenobarbital) and nonbarbiturates (chloral hydrate)

    4   Antispasmodics: relieve skeletal muscle spasms; anticonvulsants prevent muscle spasms or convulsions

    5   Sedatives; produce relaxed, calming effect

    6   Tranquilizers

        a   Relieve tension and anxiety, preoperative and postoperative apprehension, headaches, menstrual tension, chronic alcoholism, skeletal muscle spasticity, and other neuromuscular disorders

        b   Tranquilizers and analgesics frequently given together (in reduced dosage); one drug enhances action of the other (synergy)

    7   Anesthetics: produce state of unconsciousness (general), blocks pain (local)

C   Precautions to be taken with CNS drugs:

    1   Drugs that act on CNS may potentiate other CNS drugs.

    2   Client may be receiving other medications; find out drug name and dosage.

    3   Dependence on CNS drugs may occur.

Autonomic Nervous System   This system governs several body functions. Drugs that affect the ANS will also affect other system functions.

A   The ANS is made up of two nerve systems: the sympathetic and parasympathetic.

    1   Parasympathetic: the stabilizing system

    2   Sympathetic: the protective emergency system

B   Basic drug groups

    1   Adrenergics: mimic the actions of sympathetic system

        a   Vasoconstrictors: stimulants such as Adrenalin

- Constrict peripheral blood vessels
- Increase blood pressure
- Dilate bronchial passages
- Relax gastrointestinal tract

        b   Vasodilators: depressants such as nicotinic acid

- Antagonists of epinephrine and similar drugs
- Vasodilate blood vessels
- Increase tone of GI tract
- Reduce blood pressure
- Relax smooth muscles

        Caution: If drug is to be stopped, reduce dosage gradually over a period of a week; do not stop dosage suddenly.

    2   Cholinergics: mimic actions of parasympathetic system

        a   Cholinergic stimulants (e.g., Prostigmin or Neostigmine)

- Decrease heart rate
- Contract smooth muscle
- Constrict pupil in eye
- Increase peristalsis
- Increase gland secretions

    b Cholinergic inhibitors (anticholinergics)
- Decrease gland secretion
- Relax smooth muscle
- Dilate pupil in eye
- Increase heart action

Gastrointestinal System   Drugs affecting GI system act upon muscular and glandular tissues.

A Antacids: counteract excess stomach acidity (Maalox)
1. Have alkaline base
2. Used in treatment of ulcers
3. Neutralize hydrochloric acid in the stomach
4. Given frequently (two-hour intervals or more often)
5. May be given with water
6. May cause constipation, depending on type of medication
7. Baking soda is a systemic antacid, which disturbs the pH balance in the body. Most other antacids coat the mucous membrane and neutralize HCl.

B Emetics: produce vomiting (emesis)

C Antiemetics: prevent vomiting or nausea; cause drowsiness (Emetrol)

D Digestants: relieve enzyme deficiency by replacing secretions in digestive tract

E Antidiarrheals: prevent diarrhea

F Cathartics: affect intestine and produce defecation
1. Provide temporary relief for constipation
2. Rid bowel of contents before surgery; prepare viscera for diagnostic studies
3. Counteract edema
4. Treat diseases of GI tract
5. Classifications
    a By degree of action
- Laxative: mild action
- Cathartic: moderate action
- Purgative: severe action

    b By method of action
- Increase bulk
- Lubricate mechanically
- Irritate chemically
- Increase or decrease water content with saline
- Disperse detergent or wetting agent
- Cathartics are contraindicated when abdominal pain is present

Respiratory System Drugs act on respiratory tract, tissues, and cough center; suppress, relax, liquefy, and stimulate.

A Respiratory stimulants: stimulate depth and rate of respiration

B Bronchodilators: relax smooth muscle of trachea

C Drug groups that provide cough relief:
   1 Antitussive agents (narcotic, nonnarcotic)
      • Sedatives: prevent cough
      • Not to be accompanied by water
   2 Demulcents: soothe respiratory tract
   3 Expectorants: liquefy bronchial secretions; increase amount of excretions in respiratory tract

Urinary System Drugs act on kidneys and urinary tract; increase urine flow, destroy bacteria, perform other important body functions.

A Diuretics
   1 Rid body of excess fluid and relieve edema.
   2 Some drugs that act on the GI tract and circulatory system are also diuretic in action

B Urinary antiseptics

C Acidifiers and alkalinizers: certain foods increase body acids or alkalies

Circulatory System Drugs act on heart, blood, and blood vessels; change heart rhythm, rate, and force and dilate or constrict vessels.

A Cardiotonics: used for heart-strengthening
   1 Direct heart stimulants: speed heart rate, e.g., caffeine, Adrenalin
   2 Indirect heart stimulants: e.g., digitalis
     a Stimulate vagus nerve
     b Slow heart rate and strengthen it
     c Improve heart action, thereby improving circulation
     d Do not administer if apical pulse is below 60

B Antiarrhythmic drugs: used clinically to convert irregularities to a normal sinus rhythm; monitor constantly with ECG when administering these drugs.
   1 Quinidine: used for its vasodepressor action
     a Slows impulse of sinoauricular node
     b Slows heart rate
     c Side effects: ringing in ears

C Drugs that alter blood flow
   1 Anticoagulants: inhibit blood-clotting action (heparin)
   2 Vasodilators: maintain blood fluidity

D Blood replacement

Miscellaneous Drug Classifications

A Anticonvulsant or antiepileptic drugs: drugs that control seizures, i.e., Dilantin (Hyperplasia of the gingiva, which is a side effect, requires frequent teeth brushing and dental checks.)

B Anti-inflammatories: drugs that reduce tissue inflammation, i.e., prednisolone (Observe client for gastric ulcers, Cushing's syndrome, and mood swings.)

C Antineoplastics: drugs that stop cell division, i.e., vincristine

D Antiparasitics: drugs used to rid the body of parasitic worms, amoebas, and protozoans, i.e., Antepar (Treat entire family.)

E Antiparkinsonism agents: drugs used to control symptoms of Parkinsonism, i.e., L-dopa

F Antituberculosis agents: drugs used to destroy tuberculosis bacteria, i.e., PAS, INH

G Hallucinogenics: drugs that induce hallucinations, i.e., LSD

H Hormones: substances secreted by the pituitary gland and the adrenal cortex (two organs needed for, among other things, sexual function) i.e., testosterone, estrogen

I Insulin and oral hypoglycemics: animal insulin or drugs that stimulate insulin production necessary for carbohydrate utilization (Site rotation prevents lipoid dystrophy and hypertrophy.)

J Narcotic antagonists: drugs that abolish the effect of opiates and opiate-like narcotics, i.e., Narcan

K Thyroid and antithyroid agents: drugs used either to stimulate or to suppress thyroid gland functions, i.e., hypothyroid (euthroid), hyperthyroid (iodine)

GOVERNING LAWS

Federal Food, Drug, and Cosmetic Act of 1938

A The Act is an update of the Food and Drug Act, first passed in 1906.

B It designates *United States Pharmacopeia* and *National Formulary* as official standards; gives the federal government the power to enforce standards.

C Provisions of the Act
  1 Drug manufacturer must provide adequate evidence of drug's safety.
  2 Drug manufacturer is responsible for the correct labeling and packaging of drugs.

D The Act was amended in 1952 to include control of barbiturates by restricting prescription refills.

E The Act was amended in 1962 to require substantial investigation of drugs and evidence that drugs are effective in terms of labeling claims.

Harrison Narcotic Act of 1914

A Provisions of the Act
1 Regulates manufacture, importation, and sale of opium, cocaine, and their derivatives.
2 Amendments have added addictive synthetic drugs to the regulated drug listing.

B Applications of the Act
1 Individuals who produce, sell, dispense (pharmacists), and prescribe (dentist, physicians) these drugs must be licensed and registered; prescriptions must be in triplicate.
2 Hospitals order drugs on special blanks that bear hospital registry number. The following information is recorded for each dose:
   a name of drug
   b amount of drug
   c date and time drug obtained
   d name of physician prescribing drug
   e name of client receiving drug

The Controlled Substance Act of 1970

A Provisions of the Act
1 Regulates potentially addictive drugs as to prescription, use, and possession.
   a Regulations refer to use in hospital, office, research, and emergency situations.
   b Regulations cover narcotics, cocaine, amphetamines, hallucinogens, barbiturates, and other sedatives.
2 Controlled drugs are placed in five different schedules or categorical listings, each governed by different regulations.
   a The regulations govern the manufacture, transport, and storage of the controlled drugs.
   b The use of the drugs is controlled as to prescription, authorization, the mode of dispensation, and administration.

B Application of the act for use of controlled drugs in hospital
1 The nurse is to keep the stock supply of controlled drugs under lock and key.
   a Nurse must sign for each dose (tablet, cc) of drug.
   b Key is held by the nurse responsible for administration of medication.
   c At the end of each shift, nurse must account for all controlled drugs in the stock supply.

2 Violations of the Controlled Substance Act
   a Violations punishable by fine, imprisonment, or both.
   b Nurses, upon conviction of violation, are subject to losing their licenses to practice nursing.

ABBREVIATIONS AND SYMBOLS FOR ORDERS, PRESCRIPTIONS, AND LABELS

aa	of each	os	mouth
a.c.	before meals	oz or $\mathfrak{z}$	ounce
ad lib.	freely, as desired	p.c.	after meals
Ba	barium	per	by, through
b.i.d.	twice each day	p.r.n.	whenever necessary
$\bar{c}$	with	q.h.	every hour
C	carbon	q.i.d.	four times each day
Ca	calcium	q.s.	as much as required
Cl	chlorine	q2h	every two hours
dr or $\mathfrak{z}$	dram	q3h	every three hours
et	and	q4h	every four hours
GI	gastrointestinal	R_x	treatment, "take thou"
gt or gtt	drop(s)	$\bar{s}$	without
H_2O	water	$\overline{ss}$	one-half (½)
H_2O_2	hydrogen peroxide	stat	immediately
IM	intramuscular	t.i.d.	three times a day
in.	inch	tsp	teaspoon
K	potassium	WBC	white blood cell
lb or #	pound	°	degree
m	minimum (a minim)	−	minus, negative, alkaline reaction
Mg	magnesium	+	plus, positive, acid reaction
N	nitrogen, normal	%	percent
Na	sodium	v	Roman numeral five
n.p.o.	nothing by mouth	vii	Roman numeral seven
q.d.	everyday	ix	Roman numeral nine
oob	out of bed	xiii	Roman numeral thirteen

CHAPTER 9
Assisting with Diagnostic Procedures

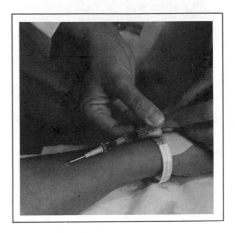

This chapter provides a fundamental overview of the more common diagnostic procedures with which you will come in contact during your clinical experience. The procedures are by no means inclusive and cannot possibly cover the variety of preprocedure and postprocedure interventions that accompany tests of this nature. It is recommended that students have a manual of laboratory and diagnostic tests available as a ready resource during their clinical experience.

The chapter is divided into five sections. Four of the sections are written according to the type of study being done, for example, dye injection studies and air contrast studies. The fifth section describes ways in which the nurse assists with the tests.

PREPARATION FOR DIAGNOSTIC TESTS

The nurse's responsibility begins with the initial scheduling of the test and continues after the results of the test are explained to the client. The physician explains the results of the test, but the nurse answers questions, interprets terminology, and listens to the client express his or her feelings or apprehensions.

The preparation of clients for diagnostic tests must be done on an individual basis. Some clients are well informed about the test they are scheduled to take. They know about diet and fluid restrictions, what to expect during the procedure, whether or not there is any discomfort with the test, and how long the procedure will take. Other clients need a great deal of interpretation and reinforcement of teaching. There are also clients who prefer not to have any explanation about the test. Nurses need to respect the client's preferences and provide only information requested unless it in some way is a danger to the client.

Many clients who are frightened are unable to communicate. Communicating with the client involves an active, verbal interchange of ideas as well as listening to the client's nonverbal cues. One effective way to allow clients time to think about questions is to provide a printed form explaining the diagnostic test. The form may cover such information as how long a test takes, equipment used for the test, and any sensations experienced during the test. Leaving the form at the bedside can stimulate interest on the part of the client and prompt the shy, reserved client to ask questions when you return later.

Another important aspect of client teaching involves the way in which you approach the client. Avoid giving the impression that you are in a hurry and that your job is so time-consuming that you have no time to answer any questions. On the other hand, be aware of the client's ability to hear what you have to say. If the client seems distracted, the client may be worried about finances, about who is watching the children, or whether or not the job will be waiting when he or she is discharged from the hospital. This preoccupation may prevent assimilation of knowledge and the client will be unprepared for the events that follow.

Remember, the client probably does not know medical jargon; therefore, explain procedures in terms the client can understand. If the client looks puzzled and does not ask any questions, evaluate how you presented the information.

Feedback is the only way in which you can evaluate the learner's knowledge. Feedback can be in the form of direct questioning about certain aspects of the test. Feedback can also be determined through direct observation of facial expressions, posturing, and activities.

This chapter will not confront the issue of client teaching, as that is reserved for another chapter in the book. Just remember the principles of good client-teaching when caring for clients undergoing diagnostic tests.

Dye Injection Studies Many x-rays utilize the normal contrasts of the body, such as air, water in soft tissues, and bone; however, for some tests a contrast media is required. Several types of contrast media are used routinely. Barium sulfate, helium, carbon dioxide, and organic iodides are some substances that are commonly used.

One of the major problems with the use of some contrast media is the adverse reaction or sensitivity that can occur. This is more common when iodine preparations are used. The degree of reaction varies from mild, such as nausea, to severe, such as cardiovascular collapse.

Barium can cause some uncomfortable feelings and problems with the gastrointestinal tract, but with proper postprocedure care this condition can be greatly reduced.

▶ Symptoms of dye reactions
Urticaria, hives
Nausea, vomiting
Respiratory distress
Decreased blood pressure

Radioactive Material Studies Radioisotopes consist of radionuclides, which distribute uniformly through normal tissue but unevenly in pathologically involved tissue. The radioisotopes emit radiation, gamma rays, and can be picked up by scanning devices.

Radioisotopes tend to concentrate in specific organ tissues and thus are more effective when administered for scanning a particular organ. For example, $_{131}$I (hippuran) is specifically used for kidney scanning while thallium 201 ($_{201}$Tl) is used for scanning heart tissue. Scanning allows visualization of organs that are unobservable by x-ray alone. Tumors present as areas of reduced radioisotopic activity. Radioisotope studies are contraindicated with pregnancy, breast-feeding mothers, or persons who are allergic to the radioisotopes.

The radioactive isotopes are administered intravenously or orally to the client. A specified time elapses before the scanning is done. This allows time for the radioactive material to reach the specific tissue under study. Then, a scanning device is used to record the concentration of radiation that emerges from the radioisotope.

Some clients are given blocking agents before the administration of the radioisotope. This prevents the radioactive material from entering other organs than those being studied. A common blocking agent is Lugol's solution. This is given to a client who is having a study done on any organ but the thyroid gland.

Air Contrast Studies The most common air contrast studies are the pneumoencephalogram, the ventriculogram, and air contrast studies of the colon.

Visualization of the cerebral ventricular system is accomplished by injecting small increments of sterile gas through a lumbar or cisternal puncture. The different densities of the gas and cerebral spinal fluid provide the necessary contrast for the x-ray films.

These studies are very difficult for clients because they are positioned in a somersaulting chair and rotated 360 degrees throughout the procedure, which can lead to severe nausea and vomiting. The client often takes this test knowing that an immediate craniotomy may be necessary. This knowledge therefore compounds the client's anxiety and fear. In addition, the client experiences an excruciating headache along with nausea during the test. The headache will decrease in intensity following the test and will not be completely eradicated for several days.

ASSISTING THE PHYSICIAN DURING TESTS

In this section, information about positioning clients during examination and preprocedure and postprocedure care will be outlined for several procedures. Nurses are frequently called upon to assist the physician with procedures at the bedside as well as in the treatment room. The procedures presented in this chapter are the most common ones performed in the hospital unit. It is important that the nurse be aware of the correct client positioning in order to facilitate the procedure, decrease complications, and decrease the time it takes to complete the procedure.

GUIDELINES FOR MANAGING CLIENTS

Clients undergoing diagnostic tests are usually frightened and often unable to communicate their fears.

- Nurses need to use both active teaching and active listening to identify cues in the client's ability to understand the procedure.
- Teaching about the diagnostic test needs to be done on an individual basis determined by the client's needs.
- Delivery of the content must be in a way that allows the client to understand the terminology.
- The time chosen for the client teaching should be unhurried and at a time when the client is not preoccupied.

Preparations for diagnostic tests must be carried out correctly to ensure good test results.

- Clients undergoing colon examinations with barium must be adequately cleansed of stool prior to the test to allow the barium to act as a contrast media.
- When several tests are being done within a short time, be sure the contrast media used in one test does not interfere with the results of another test.
- An n.p.o. status for clients undergoing dye injection tests should be maintained in order not to dilute the dye.
- Clients undergoing tests that can cause nausea and vomiting must be kept n.p.o.

Allergic reactions to dye and radioisotopes can occur.

- Always question clients about allergies to shellfish, iodine, or other contrast media when dye injection studies are scheduled.
- Alert the radiologist to clients who have allergies to food and drugs even though they are not allergic to shellfish.
- Instruct the client on the signs and symptoms most often experienced with allergic responses.
- Shortness of breath can accompany an allergic response. Have client take slow, deep breaths. Oxygen may need to be administered.

▶ Radiopaque substances and iodine dyes can affect the results of other studies.

▶ Clients allergic to food or drugs generally are allergic to some dyes used for diagnostic studies.

Rationale for Action
- To detect abnormal findings of body organs, i.e., kidney, gall bladder, liver, etc.
- To assist in diagnosis of disease states
- To determine if specific treatments have been successful in treating disease states

ACTION: CARING FOR THE CLIENT UNDERGOING DYE INJECTION STUDIES

ASSESSMENT

1 Assess client's knowledge of procedure to be done.
2 Identify any history of drug or food allergies.
3 Evaluate ability to follow directions before and during the test.
4 Assess vital signs and document for baseline data.

PLANNING

GOALS

- Client is able to complete test without untoward effects.
- Client understands procedure and anxiety level is under control.
- Client is properly prepared for diagnostic test.

EQUIPMENT

- Signed permit
- Pajama bottoms and hospital gown
- Dye injection material
- Patent IV or needle and syringe, tourniquet, and alcohol swab
- X-ray or fluroscopy equipment

PREPARATION

- Identify the specific diagnostic test that will be performed.
- Determine if any tests must precede others in order to schedule test appropriately.
- Obtain client's history to determine allergies to food or drugs and note these on the chart. Notify physician of findings.
- Identify specific preparations that need to be carried out before the studies.
- Monitor food and fluid restrictions that need to be altered for the studies.
- Obtain special consent forms for all invasive diagnostic studies after the physician has explained the study to the client.
- Provide client teaching regarding the study, including any special preparation required and restrictions imposed by the study.
- Provide psychological support and reassurance to the client.
- Obtain orders regarding medications or nutrition for clients with special problems, such as diabetes or seizure disorders.
- Carry out safety precautions immediately prior to the study:

Check identaband for accuracy.
Have client void if necessary.
Remove hairpins, jewelry, and dentures if necessary.
Chart premedication given.
Monitor safe transfer from bed to guerney or wheelchair.
Accompany client to x-ray department if needed. (Usually RNs accompany critically ill clients.)

Client Teaching

1. Assess client's and/or family's level of comprehension.
2. Describe the diagnostic study in terms that are understandable. Include the following data in your discussion:
   a. Description of procedure.
   b. Equipment used during test.
   c. Any discomfort or unusual sensations that might occur (i.e., hot, flushed skin or shortness of breath).
   d. Special preparations for the diagnostic study (enema, dye ingestion).
   e. Postprocedure nursing interventions.

INTERVENTION: Caring for the Client Having an Oral Cholecystogram

1. Explain purpose for procedure to client.
2. Identify allergies to shellfish or iodine.
3. Administer radiopaque medication after dinner.
   a. Number of tablets administered is based on weight of client.
   b. Tablets are given five minutes apart with one glass of water for each tablet.

4 Client is n.p.o. after midnight.
5 Client is taken to x-ray department.
6 Explain details of procedure to client.
   a Client will be x-rayed in standing and lying positions for good visualization of gallbladder and common bile duct.
   b If visualization does not occur, additional medications may be given and the test repeated the following day, or an IV cholangio-gram may be done.
7 Client is returned to room. Generally, the procedure takes a short time.

INTERVENTION: Caring for the Client Having an Intravenous Cholangiogram

1 Follow steps as appropriate in Preparing for Diagnostic Studies Utilizing Dye.
   a Procedure will involve dye injection given over 15 to 30 minutes.
   b Identify allergies to shellfish or iodine.
   c Client is taken to x-ray department.
2 Explain procedure to client.
   a Procedure will involve dye injection given over a 15 to 30-minute period.
   b X-rays will be taken every 15 to 30 minutes until the common bile duct tree is visualized.
   c The procedure may take one to three hours.
3 Client is returned to room.
4 Encourage fluids and offer diet.
5 Have client resume previous activity orders.
6 Monitor client for allergic response to dye.

INTERVENTION: Caring for the Client Having an Intravenous Pyelogram

1 Follow steps as appropriate in Preparing for Diagnostic Studies Utilizing Dye.
   a Give client clear liquids the evening before the IVP. Usual order is four to six glasses of fluid from 6 P.M. to midnight, then place client on n.p.o.
   b Give laxative or enema as ordered.
   c Identify allergies to shellfish or iodine.
   d Obtain permit.
   e Take client to x-ray department when notified.
2 Explain details of procedure to client.
   a Dye will be injected as a bolus.
   b X-rays are taken over period of one hour to determine extent to which dye is filtered through kidneys.
3 Warn client that dye can cause feelings of nausea, shortness of breath, and a hot, flushed effect.
4 Return client to room and have client resume ordered activity level.
5 Encourage fluids and offer diet.
6 Observe signs and symptoms for reactions to dye such as oliguria, nausea, and vomiting.

INTERVENTION: Caring for the Client Having a Myelogram

1 Follow steps as appropriate for Preparing for Diagnostic Studies Utilizing Dye.
   a Identify allergies to shellfish, iodine, or other contrast media.
   b Keep client n.p.o. for four to six hours.
   c Obtain baseline motor and sensory function.
   d Obtain permit.
   e Take client on guerney to x-ray department.
2 Explain details of procedure to client.
   a Client is placed in prone position with pillow under abdomen to allow visualization of ruptured disc or neoplasms.
   b A lumbar puncture needle is inserted between the vertebrae into the subarachnoid space.
   c A small amount of cerebral spinal fluid is sent to lab for study.
   d Contrast media is injected, and client is tilted on table to allow flow of dye to designated areas of spine to allow visualization by x-rays.
   e Contrast media (Pantopaque) is removed through aspiration. Explain to client that sudden, very painful radicular pain in legs may occur.
   f Procedure lasts about one hour.
   g Client is returned on guerney to room.
3 Keep client in supine position 8 to 12 hours without a pillow. Position client in Sim's position if ordered.
4 Monitor vital signs and motor and sensory function.
   a Cervical myelogram: check upper and lower extremities and bladder function.
   b Lumbar myelogram: check lower extremities and bladder function.
5 Medicate for pain as ordered.
6 Increase fluids to at least 2500 cc per day. Offer diet.
7 Monitor output and observe for distention.
8 Utilize comfort measures and relaxation techniques when needed.

INTERVENTION: Caring for the Client Having an Arteriogram

1 Explain purpose of procedure to client.
2 Identify allergies to shellfish, iodine, or any contrast media.
3 Obtain permit.
4 Shave and scrub puncture site when ordered.
5 Place client on n.p.o. if ordered.
6 Have client void before procedure.
7 Administer preprocedure medications if ordered and transport client to x-ray department.
8 Explain details of procedure to client.
   a Puncture site will be scrubbed and a local anesthetic administered.
   b Contrast media will be injected to visualize abnormalities or obstruction to specific vessels.

> **c** Client may be instructed to hold breath for x-rays. Procedure takes about one hour if an automatic film changer is used.
9 Client is returned on guerney to room.
10 Monitor vital signs, pulses, and puncture site, as with surgical clients.
11 Observe for signs of shock and presence of pain, which indicate hemorrhage or thrombosis.
12 Apply ice pack to puncture site if ordered. Do not flex extremity.
13 Maintain bedrest with head elevated slightly for 12 hours.
14 Offer fluids and diet as ordered and tolerated.
15 Provide comfort measures as needed.

INTERVENTION: Caring for the Client Having a Computerized Axial Tomography (CAT scan)

1 Explain purpose for procedure to client.
2 Identify allergies to shellfish or iodine.
3 Obtain permit.
4 Place client on n.p.o. as dye can cause nausea.
5 Administer preprocedure medication if ordered.
6 Client is taken on guerney to x-ray department.
7 Explain equipment and need for head to be placed in rubber cap. Face will not be covered.
8 Client will have IV injection of contrast material if enhanced study is to be done. Explain that a warm, flushed feeling or nausea can occur.
9 Instruct client to lie very still during procedure. Length of procedure, usually 30 to 60 minutes, depends on number of radiographs taken.
10 Return client to room.
11 Provide diet and force fluids to 3000 cc unless contraindicated.
12 Medicate for headache if needed.

INTERVENTION: Caring for the Client Having a Cardiac Catheterization

1 Explain purpose for procedure to client.
2 Obtain permit.
3 Identify allergies to drugs, iodine, shellfish, or any other contrast media.
4 Complete prep and shave of groin and/or brachial area.
5 Establish baseline data for vital signs, peripheral pulses, coagulation studies (PTT, Protime), ECG pattern.
6 Place client on n.p.o. after midnight.
7 In morning, obtain vital signs, take weight, have client void, and administer preprocedure medications.
8 Take client on guerney to cardiac catheterization lab.
9 Explain equipment and details of procedure to client.
> **a** Client is strapped onto a table. ECG leads and blood pressure equipment are applied.

b Groin or brachial area is scrubbed and injected with Xylocaine.

c Arterial and venous catheters are placed in femoral or brachial sites.

d When dye is injected for coronary artery visualization, explain to client that a warm, flushed feeling, shortness of breath, or nausea can occur.

e Client is asked to hold breath about ten seconds during dye injection.

f Reinforce that client will not fall off table as client may be turned on side for cineangiography. Total procedure takes one to one-and-a-half hours.

g Following catheterization, pressure is applied to puncture site for 10 to 15 minutes.

10 Transport client on guerney to room.

11 Provide post-cardiac-catheterization care.

a Monitor vital signs, puncture site, heart and lung sounds, and peripheral pulses as with a surgical client.

b Elevate extremity used for catheterization site. Keep extremity extended.

c Apply pressure dressing or sandbags to puncture site if bleeding continues.

d Encourage fluids and diet when vital signs are stable and no evidence of nausea or drowsiness is present.

12 Position client for comfort. Place on back for several hours post-procedure, then turn from side-to-side.

EVALUATION

EXPECTED OUTCOMES

1 Client is able to complete test without untoward effects. *If not*, follow these alternative nursing actions:

ANA: If client is allergic to shellfish or iodine, notify physician so contrast media can be changed or client can be treated with specific medications such as Benadryl.

ANA: Be observant for signs or symptoms of allergic responses and treat immediately.

2 Client understands procedure and client's anxiety level is under control. *If not*, follow these alternative nursing actions:

ANA: Repeat information about the test in terminology and in a manner the client can understand.

ANA: Utilize a different approach in teaching, such as using written material or utilizing filmstrip and audio-cassette.

ANA: Identify and eliminate any blocks present that can interfere with client's ability to listen to the information.

ANA: Ask another client to talk with client about the test.

3 Client is properly prepared for diagnostic test. *If not*, follow these alternative nursing actions:

ANA: Notify x-ray department and physician relating what action was not completed.

ANA: If n.p.o. status is not maintained, notify physician for orders. Sometimes the procedures are carried out anyway.

ANA: If preprocedure medication was not given at prescribed time, notify physician so he or she can determine if additional medication is needed.

ANA: Notify lab of change in type of procedure.

UNEXPECTED OUTCOMES

1 Client has allergic reaction.

ANA: If shortness of breath occurs, have client take slow, deep breaths. Oxygen may need to be administered. Place in low-Fowler's position unless contraindicated.

ANA: If nausea or vomiting occur, obtain orders and medicate with Compazine.

ANA: Administer Benadryl as ordered for treatment of hives or urticaria.

2 Client very apprehensive and refuses test at last minute.

ANA: Identify reasons for anxiety and attempt to allay fears.

ANA: Notify physician to cancel or postpone test to later time. Do not attempt to "talk client into it."

3 Client is given meal when on n.p.o. status.

ANA: Notify x-ray to change time of test. If possible, arrange for test to be done later in the day to avoid additional hospitalization.

ANA: Notify physician of delay in test.

ANA: Instruct client on what n.p.o. means.

ANA: Ensure that diet Rand has appropriate information on n.p.o. status.

4 Client is unable to take Telepaque tablets for oral cholecystogram because of nausea.

ANA: Notify physician so IV cholangiogram can be ordered.

5 Bleeding or hemorrhage occurs from arteriogram puncture site.

ANA: Apply direct pressure until pressure dressing can be applied.

ANA: Monitor amount of blood loss and possible signs and symptoms of shock.

ANA: Elevate and keep extremity in extension position.

ANA: Notify physician.

6 Client develops arrhythmias following cardiac catheterization.

ANA: Notify physician immediately.

ANA: Place client on cardiac monitor if not already on one.

ANA: Prepare for possible Code.

ANA: Start an IV with D_5W for drug administration if IV not present.

ANA: Monitor vital signs frequently.

7 Bleeding occurs at catheter insertion site following cardiac catheterization.

ANA: Apply pressure dressing.

ANA: Elevate extremity.

ANA: Monitor peripheral pulses.

ANA: Monitor vital signs.

ANA: If bleeding does not subside, notify physician.

Charting

- Preparation completed i.e., n.p.o., clear liquid dinner
- Client teaching completed
- Medication administered
- Allergies noted
- Unusual anxiety or fears of client
- How client transported to test
- Postprocedure care
- Appearance of dressing or puncture sites

ACTION: PREPARING THE CLIENT FOR DIAGNOSTIC STUDIES USING RADIOACTIVE MATERIAL

ASSESSMENT

1 Assess client's understanding of diagnostic test.
2 Evaluate client's ability to tolerate procedure.
3 Identify need for staff to accompany client to procedure.
4 Identify allergies to radioactive materials.
5 Assess vital signs and document for baseline data.

PLANNING

GOALS

- Client is physically prepared for diagnostic study.
- Client is psychologically prepared for diagnostic study.
- Client expresses understanding of diagnostic test.

EQUIPMENT

- Signed permit
- IV equipment (optional)
- Hospital gown and pajama bottoms

INTERVENTION: Preparing the Client for a Bone Scan

1 Explain purpose for procedure to client. If client is of child-bearing age, determine whether she is pregnant.
2 Have client ready for injection of tracer amount of radioactive material two hours before scan.
3 Force fluids for one hour.
4 Take client to nuclear medicine department.
5 Explain equipment to client. Client is positioned under scintillation camera.
6 Instruct client to remain very still for 20 minutes to ensure observation of bone abnormalities.
7 Return client to room and instruct to resume preprocedure activities.

INTERVENTION: Preparing the Client for a Lung Scan

1 Explain purpose for procedure to client.
2 Transport client to nuclear medicine department.
3 Explain equipment to client.
  a Closed-breathing system.
  b Scintillation camera.
4 Client is injected intravenously with a tracer amount of radioactive material.
5 Client is positioned in several ways to obtain clear images.
6 Instruct client to breathe through a closed system until all radioactive gas is cleared from the system.

Rationale for Action

- To prepare client physically to ensure that diagnostic test results in visualization of appropriate organ and regions within the organ
- To prepare client psychologically to prevent undue stress
- To complete client teaching to ensure client has an understanding of the procedure

▶ Pregnant personnel should avoid caring for clients who have undergone radioactive diagnostic studies for at least 24 hours after completion of studies.

301

7 Instruct client to lie quietly for 30 minutes as radiography is completed.
8 Transport client on guerney to room and instruct to resume prescan activities.

INTERVENTION: Preparing the Client for a Brain Scan

1 Explain purpose for procedure to client.
2 Obtain permit.
3 Take client to nuclear medicine department.
4 Explain equipment to client.
5 Place client's head under scintillation camera and instruct client to hold still for five minutes.
6 Client will have IV injection of radioactive materials.
7 Keep client comfortable and watch carefully for 90 minutes.
8 Client is next placed in several different positions to assist in distribution of radioisotopes.
9 Instruct client to hold still for 20 minutes to assist in radiography to determine presence of cerebral infarction, abscess, neoplasm, or contusions.
10 Return client to room, and have client resume prestudy activities.

EVALUATION

EXPECTED OUTCOMES

1 Client is physically prepared for diagnostic study. *If not*, follow these alternative nursing actions:
ANA: Notify nuclear medicine department to determine if test can be done later in the day. Usually preparations include enema for bone scan clients if lesion is suspected near abdomen or pelvis. Client may take radioactive iodine capsule or injection before going to nuclear medicine department.
ANA: Instruct staff on policy for preparing clients for study to prevent the recurrence.
2 Client is psychologically prepared for diagnostic study. *If not*, follow these alternative nursing actions:
ANA: Spend additional time with client to assess fears and answer questions.
ANA: Utilize relaxation techniques for clients with unusually high anxiety levels.
3 Client expresses understanding of diagnostic test. *If not*, follow these alternative nursing actions:
ANA: Observe for nonverbal cues of misunderstanding. These cues can be facial grimaces, posturing changes, staring into space.
ANA: Provide alternative teaching aids, such as audio-visual materials, to help client understand test.
ANA: Show and explain to client the equipment that will be used.
ANA: Ask client to explain the test to you in his or her own words. Correct any misinformation.

UNEXPECTED OUTCOMES

1 Client is unable to cooperate during the procedure.
   ANA   If not contraindicated by condition, client may be sedated.
   ANA   Nursing staff members may be asked to help client remain quiet. If so, nursing staff will need to wear lead apron shield.
2 Client is uncomfortable during procedure.
   ANA: Reposition client for comfort if possible. It may not be possible depending on area of body to be scanned.
   ANA: Provide support by propping client in position needed for scanning.

ACTION: PREPARING THE CLIENT FOR DIAGNOSTIC STUDIES USING AIR CONTRAST

ASSESSMENT

1 Assess ability of client to tolerate procedure.
2 Assess client's knowledge of procedure.
3 Assess vital signs and neurological signs, and document for baseline data.

Rationale for Action
- To prepare client psychologically and physically for the test
- To provide adequate baseline data to determine posttest complications
- To determine if client is able to understand and follow directions during the test

PLANNING

GOALS

- Client is able to cooperate during test.
- Client's headache is controlled.
- Client does not experience hypotension during and following test.
- Client's motor and sensory status remains unchanged.

▶ Clients will experience a very severe headache during the air contrast study.

EQUIPMENT

- Signed permit
- Pajama bottoms and gown
- IV equipment (optional)
- Lumbar or cisternal puncture tray
- Somersaulting chair
- Fluoroscopy unit

INTERVENTION: Preparing the Client for Pneumoencephalogram or Ventriculogram

1 Explain purpose for procedure to client.
2 Obtain permit. A possible craniotomy may need to be included on permit.
3 Place client on n.p.o. after midnight.
4 Obtain baseline vital signs, neurological signs, and motor and sensory function.
5 Have client void.

303

6 Remove dentures.
7 Administer preprocedure medication.
8 Transport to special procedures department, or operating room.
9 Explain equipment to client.
10 Position client in lateral or seated position (check position with physician).
11 Explain to client that during a pneumoencephalogram a small amount of cerebral spinal fluid will be obtained and then a small amount of air will be injected through the lumbar puncture needle.
   a X-rays will be taken to check placement of air.
   b Injection of additional air.
   c Positioning of client prone, supine, and upright during radiography.
12 Instruct client that when air is injected he or she might experience a severe headache, vertigo, nausea, diaphoresis, and chills.
13 Explain that the procedure visualizes a patency of the ventricular system and identifies any abnormalities. The procedure takes about one hour.
14 During a ventriculogram, air is injected directly into the ventricles through a small scalp incision in the frontal region. Explain to client that a hole is drilled in the skull and a spinal needle is inserted in the ventricle.
15 Explain to client that a ventriculogram takes about one hour and serves same purpose as a pneumoencephalogram. A ventriculogram is done if client has increased intracranial pressure.
16 Following the procedure, apply dressing to puncture site.
17 Transport client on guerney to room.
18 Monitor vital signs, neurological signs, and motor and sensory function as with a surgical client.
19 Provide comfort measures for headache, nausea, and generalized discomfort.
20 Keep client flat until headache has dissipated or decreased in intensity.
21 Provide quiet environment.
22 Encourage fluids unless contraindicated.
23 Offer diet.

EVALUATION

EXPECTED OUTCOMES

1 Client is able to cooperate during test. *If not*, follow these alternative nursing actions:
   ANA: Ensure that client is immobilized safely in somersaulting chair, especially the head.
   ANA: Medicate client to provide for maximum relaxation but still allow client to be able to follow directions.
2 Client's headache is controlled. *If not*, follow these alternative nursing actions:
   ANA: Increase fluid intake unless contraindicated.

ANA: Maintain supine position until headache is greatly decreased in intensity, about 48 hours.

ANA: Medicate every four hours to maintain blood level of drug.

ANA: Utilize relaxation techniques.

3 Client does not experience hypotension during or following test. *If this occurs*, follow these alternative nursing actions:

ANA: Obtain order for IV and IV fluids.

ANA: Start IV before beginning test and continue for 24 to 48 hours or until nausea subsides and client is taking fluids.

ANA: Apply elastic stockings pretest to decrease pooling of blood in lower extremities.

4 Client's motor and sensory status remains unchanged. *If not*, follow these alternative nursing actions:

ANA: Monitor neurological checks and complete sensory and motor exams frequently following test.

ANA: Immediately report any unusual or altered findings to physician.

UNEXPECTED OUTCOMES

1 Client's temperature increases and he or she complains of nausea and severe headaches.

ANA: Notify physician immediately. Client has experienced the most common complications following this procedure.

ANA: Obtain orders for and administer antiemetics.

ANA: Obtain blood cultures if ordered to determine if client has infection.

2 Client experiences respiratory distress.

ANA: Use relaxation techniques with client.

ANA: Administer oxygen if ordered.

Charting
- Pretest client teaching
- Baseline vital signs, neurological checks motor and sensory findings
- IVs
- Client's emotional status
- Premedication
- Posttest vital signs, neurological signs, motor and sensory findings
- Any evidence of severe headaches, nausea, vomiting, increased temperature

ACTION: PREPARING THE CLIENT FOR BARIUM STUDIES

ASSESSMENT

1 Assess results of laxative and enema administration to ensure a clean colon for the study.
2 Evaluate client's ability to cooperate with test. Notify physician if unable to "hold" enema solution.
3 Evaluate client's knowledge of test.

PLANNING

GOALS

- Client is able to cooperate with test.
- Client's colon is clear of stool.
- Barium is expelled following test.

Rationale for Action
- To confirm the diagnosis of bowel lesion, polyp, or obstruction
- To identify specific area to be resected during colon surgery
- To assess healing process of colon following inflammation or injury

▶ Barium studies should follow IVPs, ultrasound exams, and arteriograms as barium interferes with visualization of other structures.

► Obtain specific orders for enemas when client has severe abdominal pain, ulcerative colitis, or history of megacolon. Do not follow general preprocedural orders.

EQUIPMENT

- Enema tube
- Ordered solution for enema
- Barium sulfate
- Laxative
- Foley catheter
- Foley catheter with 30-cc bag (optional)

INTERVENTION: Preparing the Client for Barium Enema

1 Explain purpose for procedure to client.
2 Give clear liquid meal evening before procedure.
3 Place on n.p.o. after midnight.
4 Administer laxative in early evening before procedure.
5 Administer tap water enema morning of study.
6 Transport client to x-ray.
7 Explain details of procedure to client.
   a An enema tube is inserted and barium solution is administered into the large bowel in order to detect lesions, obstructions, or abnormalities.
   b X-rays are taken as the client is positioned several ways.
   c Client is asked to retain barium while x-ray is processed.
   d Client is allowed to expel barium in x-ray department.
   e Entire procedure takes one hour.
8 Transport client to room.
9 Force fluids unless contraindicated.
10 Administer laxative and/or enema as ordered.
11 Ensure client has bowel movement within two to three days.

INTERVENTION: Preparing the Client for Upper Gastrointestinal Study

1 Explain purpose of procedure to client.
2 Place client on n.p.o. after midnight.
3 Administer laxative and/or enema particularly if this test follows barium enema study.
4 Instruct client not to smoke to prevent an increase in flow of digestive juices.
5 Transport to x-ray department.
6 Explain details of procedure to client.
   a Client will be instructed to drink a cup of flavored barium.
   b Client is instructed to turn to several positions while x-rays are obtained.
   c X-rays will be taken every 30 minutes until barium advances through small bowel. This usually takes about two hours.
7 Transport client to room.
8 Force fluids unless contraindicated.
9 Administer laxative.
10 Ensure bowel movement within two to three days. Enema may need to be administered.

EVALUATION

1 Client is able to cooperate with test. *If not,* follow these alternative nursing actions:

ANA: Nursing staff may have to accompany client to x-ray to assist with procedure.

ANA: Foley catheter with 30-cc bag may need to be inserted and balloon inflated to hold barium in colon if client has poor sphincter control.

ANA: May need to sedate restless clients in order to assist them in remaining still during x-ray.

2 Client's colon is clear of stool. *If not,* follow these alternative nursing actions:

ANA: Notify x-ray department and reschedule procedure. Stool in colon prevents adequate visualization of polyps or obstructions.

ANA: Administer another enema unless contraindicated.

ANA: If after three enemas colon is not clear, notify physician for additional laxative order and reschedule test for next day.

3 Barium is expelled following test. *If not,* follow these alternative nursing actions:

ANA: Observe stool for at least two days. Stools will be light in color until barium is expelled.

ANA: Administer laxative for at least two days following test.

ANA: Administer enema if client has retention of barium after 24 hours.

UNEXPECTED OUTCOMES

1 Barium is unable to be expelled even following administrations of laxatives and enemas.

ANA: Administer oil retention enema.

ANA: Administer tap water enema following oil retention enema.

ANA: Continue to administer laxatives until barium is expelled.

2 Laxative and/or enemas are ordered for clients with ulcerative colitis or severe abdominal pain.

ANA: Do not administer either the laxative or enema without checking with the physician.

ANA: If physician confirms order, administer small amount of enema fluid carefully and observe and document effects on client.

ANA: Chart the type of pain if any, characteristics of stool, and any symptoms noted while enema is administered.

ANA: If client complains of excruciating pain, stop procedure and notify the physician.

3 Client's medications are administered in error.

ANA: Notify x-ray department and ask for specific orders as to what action needs to be taken regarding the test.

ANA: Complete a medication error form and send to nursing office.

Charting
- Laxative administered
- Type, amount of fluid, number of enemas administered
- Enema results, consistency of stool, color of returning enema solution
- Unusual symptoms such as pain, bleeding, or nausea associated with enemas
- Color of stool following test

ANA: If this is a frequent problem on the unit or in the hospital, an in-service education program should be given on which tests requiring medications can be withheld and which medications can be administered.

ACTION: ASSISTING PHYSICIANS WITH DIAGNOSTIC PROCEDURES

Rationale for Action
- To provide reassurance for clients undergoing diagnostic tests
- To position the client in a manner that facilitates the introduction of a needle through the skin surface to obtain a tissue sample
- To position client in a manner for ease in passing an instrument in order to visualize a body cavity

ASSESSMENT

1 Assess vital signs prior to, during, and following the procedure.
2 Assess client's ability to maintain position necessary for procedure.
3 Assess client's knowledge of procedure to be performed.
4 Review pertinent laboratory tests prior to procedure.

PLANNING

GOALS

- Diagnostic tests performed with minimal discomfort to client.
- Client positioned to ensure facilitation of needle insertion.
- Specimen obtained or fluids withdrawn for testing.
- Vital signs remain within normal range.

EQUIPMENT

▶ Check all diagnostic trays for contents to ensure that supplies necessary to complete the test are included. Many trays do not contain sterile gloves or antiseptic solution.

- Diagnostic tray or equipment specific for procedure
- Bath blanket
- Sterile collection bottles if indicated
- Sterile gloves
- Xylocaine injection, if not on tray

ADDITIONAL EQUIPMENT

For Papanicolaou Smear
- Two slides
- Cytology container

INTERVENTION: Assisting with a Lumbar Puncture

▶ A lumbar puncture should never be done on a client with head trauma or potential increased intracranial pressure. Removal of fluid from the spinal tract may cause the brain, because of edema, to herniate down through the tentorium. The CAT scan is now used more frequently to determine intracranial bleeding.

1 Explain procedure to client.
2 Obtain permit for procedure.
3 Obtain tray and any additional equipment needed, such as sterile gloves, bath blanket.
4 Open sterile tray if requested by physician. Pour antiseptic solution into sterile medicine cup if needed.
5 Position client in lateral recumbent position with his or her back at the edge of the examining table. Cover with bath blanket, exposing only client's back.
6 Pull up knees to abdomen and flex head on chest. This position widens the space between the spinous processes of the lower lumbar vertebrae for ease of needle insertion.

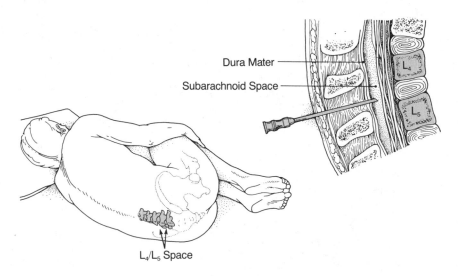

Dura Mater

Subarachnoid Space

L₄

L₅

L₄/L₅ Space

Place client in lateral Sim's position to facilitate needle insertion for lumbar puncture.

7   Assist client in relaxation exercises or instruct in deep, slow breathing through the mouth.
8   Assist physician with the Queckenstedt's test when requested. After opening pressure is obtained, apply compression to neck veins with your fingers.
9   Label cerebral spinal fluid samples with number on each specimen container.
10 After removal of needle, apply bandaid to puncture site.
11 Fill out lab slips for appropriate test, i.e., cell count, serology.
12 Instruct client to lie flat for 4 to 24 hours, depending on hospital policy. Head is to remain flat and even with position of body.
13 Encourage fluids if not contraindicated by client's condition.
14 Observe for spinal fluid leak from puncture site.
15 Assess for headaches or alterations in neurological status.

▶ Queckenstedt's test is used to identify blockage of CSF flow in the spinal subarachnoid space. Generally when neck pressure is applied, there is a rapid rise in pressure level on the manometer with a return to normal within seconds when pressure is released.

INTERVENTION: Assisting with a Liver Biopsy

1   Explain procedure to client.
2   Obtain permit for procedure.
3   Obtain lab values such as prothrombin time, bleeding time, and platelet count if ordered.
4   Obtain tray and any additional equipment needed such as sterile gloves, sandbag, bath blanket.
5   Open sterile tray.
6   Place client in supine position at the right edge of the bed. Raise right arm and extend it over the left shoulder behind the head. Turn head to left. This position provides maximal exposure of right intercostal space.
7   After the local anesthetic has been given, the client is instructed to take a deep breath and hold it on expiration. After the specimen is obtained, client can breathe normally.
8   Place bandaid over puncture site.

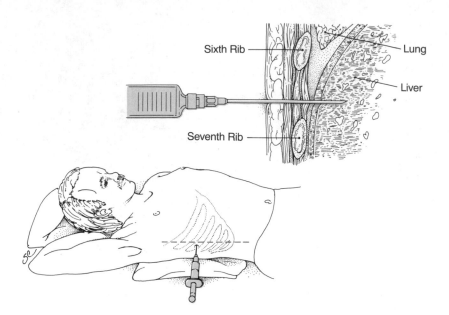

Sixth Rib — Lung

— Liver

Seventh Rib —

Instruct client to raise arm over head to facilitate needle insertion for liver biopsy.

9 Position client on right side for one hour. Sandbags may be placed under client's right side to provide hemostasis.
10 Instruct client to remain on bedrest for 24 hours.
11 Assess for signs of hemorrhage at least every hour for 12 hours.
12 Monitor vital signs as you would for a surgical client, every fifteen minutes for one hour, etc.

INTERVENTION: Assisting with a Thoracentesis

1 Explain procedure to client.
2 Obtain permit for procedure.
3 Position client on edge of bed with arms crossed and resting on the overbed table. This position provides good access to the intercostal spaces.
4 Provide adequate warmth and covering for client.
5 Obtain baseline vital signs and breath sounds.
6 Place unwrapped sterile tray on bedside stand. Open sterile gloves as indicated.
7 Assist physician as needed with skin prep.
8 Instruct client not to cough during placement of needle as pleural perforations can occur.
9 Following insertion of needle, observe client for pallor, dyspnea, tachycardia, chest pain, or vertigo. Report these findings immediately to the physician.
10 Apply bandaid or pressure dressing (as determined by policy) after fluid is removed.
11 Observe client for pulmonary edema (blood-tinged sputum) or cardiac distress (changes in respirations, pulse or color) as a shift in the mediastinum can occur with large fluid losses.

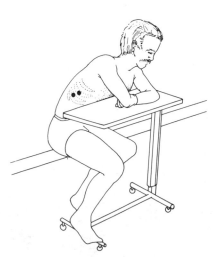

Position client leaning forward to expose intercostal space for thoracentesis.

12 Place client on unaffected side with head elevated 30 degrees for at least one hour.
13 Monitor vital signs and breath sounds as with postoperative clients for two hours.
14 Obtain chest x-ray following procedure to check for pneumothorax.
15 Record color, amount, consistency, and samples of fluid obtained.

INTERVENTION: Assisting with a Paracentesis

1 Explain procedure to client.
2 Obtain permit for procedure.
3 Have client empty bladder.
4 Position client in chair or on edge of bed with legs spread apart.
5 Provide adequate warmth and covering for client.
6 Obtain baseline vital signs.
7 Position and open tray on overbed table.
8 Open sterile gloves if needed.
9 Assist physician as needed.
10 Obtain vital signs and observe client for pallor and vertigo during procedures.
11 Apply pressure dressing following removal of needle.
12 Position client in bed. Semi-Fowler's to high-Fowler's position is usually most comfortable for client.
13 Monitor vital signs, urine output, and dressing for at least two hours.
14 Reinforce or change dressings as needed.
15 Record color, amount, consistency, and samples obtained for paracentesis.

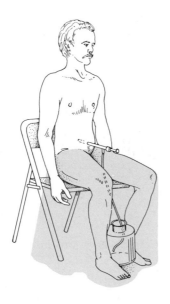

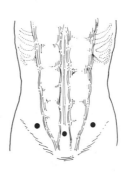

Place client in chair (preferred position) for trocar insertion and drainage during paracentesis.

INTERVENTION: Assisting with a Bone Marrow Aspiration

1   Explain procedure to client. Client will experience discomfort or pressure when needle is inserted.
2   Obtain permit for procedure.
3   Obtain tray and provide any additional equipment needed such as specimen container or gloves.
4   Premedicate with prescribed drugs.
5   Position client in supine position if sternum or anterior iliac crest is the biopsy site, or on abdomen if posterior iliac crest is the biopsy site. Usually place a sandbag under iliac crest area.
6   Open tray on overbed table.
7   Assist physician as needed. Apply direct pressure for 5 to 15 minutes following removal of needle to prevent bleeding.
8   Cover puncture site with small dressing or bandaid.
9   Monitor vital signs and observe puncture site for drainage, edema, or pain, as with surgical client.
10   Position the client for comfort.
11   Properly label specimens and send to laboratory.

INTERVENTION: Assisting with a Proctoscopy

1   Explain purpose for procedure to client.
2   Obtain permit.
3   Give clear liquid diet 24 hours before exam.
4   Administer laxative and enema as ordered the evening before exam.
5   Allow clear liquids after midnight as ordered.
6   Give tap water enema morning of examination.
7   Have client void before exam.
8   Transport client in wheelchair or on guerney to treatment room.
9   Position client on proctoscopy table or in a knee-chest position on regular examining table.
10   Position light for good exposure. Open tray and gloves and place lubricant on tray.
11   Explain equipment and details of procedure to client.
   a   Physician will digitally examine the rectum.
   b   Proctoscope is lubricated and passed through anus into the rectum to visualize any abnormality of rectum, sigmoid colon, and large bowel.
   c   Air may be introduced to increase visualization of bowel wall.
   d   Biopsy may be obtained by passing a snare through scope.
12   Return client in wheelchair or on guerney to room, and instruct to resume preexam activities.
13   Monitor stools for bleeding.
14   Encourage fluids, offer diet.

INTERVENTION: Assisting with a Vaginal Examination and Papanicolaou Smear

1   Explain procedure to client.

2 Instruct client not to douche before exam.
3 Assist client to examination room. Client may walk if not contra-indicated.
4 Position client in lithotomy position using stirrups.
5 Provide adequate coverings to preserve modesty and prevent chilling.
6 Open speculum package, gloves, and lubricant. Place on tray. Place cytology slides and container on tray.
7 Label two slides with client's name and area where smear obtained.
8 Position light for good exposure.
9 Stay with client if client is a child or physician is a male.
10 Assist physician as needed.
11 Place slides in cytology container and send to lab. Complete all cytology forms.
12 Assist client in perineal care.
13 Assist client to room.

INTERVENTION: Assisting with a Gastroscopy

1 Explain purpose for procedure to client.
2 Obtain permit.
3 Place client on n.p.o. after midnight.
4 Administer preprocedure medication if ordered.
5 Transport client to treatment room.
6 Explain equipment and details of procedure to client:
   a Client is given topical anesthetic to anesthetize the throat. An IV sedative is administered if necessary.
   b Place client on left side.
   c A scope is passed through mouth to stomach or duodenum (depending on exact procedure being done) to detect any lesions or abnormality of the gastrointestinal tract.
7 Transport client on guerney if sedated to room.
8 Maintain n.p.o. until gag reflex returns.
9 Observe for respiratory distress, bleeding, or alterations in vital signs.
10 Provide ice chips or throat lozenges for sore throat.

INTERVENTION: Assisting with a Cystoscopy

1 Explain purpose of procedure to client.
2 Obtain permit.
3 Transport client on guerney to cystoscopy room.
4 Place client in lithotomy position. Provide covering to preserve modesty and prevent chilling.
5 Prep external genitalia with povidone-iodine solution.
6 Explain equipment and details of procedure to client.
   a Cystoscope is inserted through the urethra to inspect bladder and urethral wall and facilitate a biopsy.
   b Bladder is filled with sterile water to assist in visualization of bladder wall.

    c Biopsy forcep may be passed through cystoscope to obtain tissue.
    d Bladder is emptied and scope removed.
7 Return client on guerney to room.
8 Observe closely for signs of septicemia, i.e., chills, fever, flushed feeling.
9 Force fluids unless contraindicated.
10 Monitor urine for persistent bright red color.
11 Assess client for severe pain (colicky pain is normal with uretheral catherization), continual burning, and frequency.

INTERVENTION: Assisting with an Amniocentesis

1 Explain purpose for procedure to client.
2 Obtain permit.
3 Have client void prior to test.
4 Transport client to treatment room.
5 Instruct client to lie quietly in supine position for 30 minutes.
6 Obtain fetal heart tones.
7 Open amniocentesis tray and gloves. Place Xylocaine nearby if not included on tray.
8 Explain details of procedure to client.
    a Physician preps abdomen with Betadine and/or alcohol.
    b Xylocaine injection will provide local anesthesia for needle insertion area.
    c Needle is inserted and amniotic fluid is withdrawn.
    d Amniotic fluid is placed in specimen container and labeled with client's name. Appropriate lab slips are completed.
9 Place small dressing or bandaid over needle site.
10 Monitor fetal heart tones and observe for signs of labor.
11 Instruct client to notify physician of any unusual occurrences or signs of labor.

EVALUATION

EXPECTED OUTCOMES

1 Diagnostic tests performed with minimal discomfort. *If not*, follow these alternative nursing actions:
ANA: Position client in a manner that facilitates ease of introduction of instrument or needle.
ANA: Supply physician with topical anesthesia medications, needles, and syringes.
ANA: Premedicate client if procedure is painful, i.e., gastroscopy or cystoscopy.
2 Vital signs remain within normal range. *If not*, follow these alternative nursing actions:
ANA: Notify physician immediately if client has increased temperature, chills, or flushed appearance following cystoscopy. These symptoms are indicative of sepsis.

ANA: Monitor vital signs, especially temperature. If temperature increases, notify physician. Be prepared to take blood cultures.

ANA: Monitor for signs of bleeding following biopsies, paracentesis, thoracentesis, and gastroscopy. Notify physician if bleeding or signs of shock occur following any of these procedures.

UNEXPECTED OUTCOMES

1 Client has spinal fluid leak following lumbar puncture.

ANA: Keep client in supine position.

ANA: Notify physician.

ANA: Keep sterile dressing over puncture site. Do not allow dressing to become wet.

ANA: If leak persists, physician may place client in Trendelenburg's position to prevent headache. This position is contraindicated in clients with increased intracranial pressure or following a craniotomy.

2 Client complains of shortness of breath or expectorates blood-tinged sputum following a thoracentesis.

ANA: Place client in Fowler's position.

ANA: Assess vital signs and lung sounds.

ANA: Administer oxygen if needed.

ANA: Obtain order for chest x-ray.

ANA: Have chest tube insertion tray available.

ANA: Allay client's fears and provide emotional support.

3 Urine output is blood-tinged following paracentesis.

ANA: Notify physician at once, bladder may have been punctured during procedure.

ANA: Monitor vital signs for shock.

ANA: Maintain client on bedrest.

Charting

- Preparation completed for test
- Client teaching completed
- How client tolerated procedure
- Fluid or specimens sent to lab for analysis
- Preprocedure and postprocedure vital signs
- Record color and amount of fluid withdrawn from paracentesis or thoracentesis
- Type of dressing applied
- Specific position assumed postprocedure

LEVEL III
Alterations in Homeostasis

CHAPTER 10
Alterations in Mobility

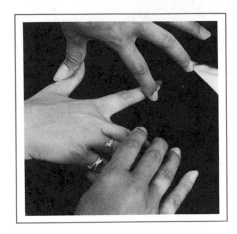

This chapter presents the conceptual basis for alterations in mobility. It includes nursing interventions and skills necessary to retain and achieve maximal movement.

ANATOMY AND PHYSIOLOGY OF THE MUSCULOSKELETAL SYSTEM

The musculoskeletal system protects the body, provides a structural framework, and allows the body to move. The primary structures in this system are muscles, bones, and joints.

Skeletal Muscles　Skeletal muscles move the bones around the joints by contracting and relaxing so that locomotion can take place. Each muscle consists of a body, or belly, and tendons, which connect the muscle to another muscle or to bone.

When skeletal muscles contract, they cause two bones to move around the joint between them. One of these bones tends to remain stationary while the other bone moves. The end of the muscle that attaches to the stationary bone is called the origin. The end of the muscle that attaches to the movable bone is called the insertion.

Muscles are designated flexors or extensors according to whether they flex the joint (decrease the angle between the bones) or extend the joint (increase the angle between the bones). For example, when the deltoid muscle contracts, it abducts the arm and raises it laterally to the horizontal position. The anterior fibers aid in flexion of the arm, and the posterior fibers aid in extension of the arm.

Joints Joints are the places where bones meet. Their primary function is to provide motion and flexibility. Although the internal structure of joints varies, most joints are composed of ligaments, which bind the bones together, and cartilage, or tissue, which covers and cushions the ends of the bones.

Bones Bones provide the major support for all the body organs. Bone is composed of an organic matrix, deposits of calcium salts, and bone cells. The organic matrix provides the framework and tensile strength for the bone. The calcium salts, which are about 75% of the bone, provide compressional strength by filling in the matrix. As a result, it is very difficult to damage a bone by twisting it or by applying direct pressure.

Bone cells include osteoblasts, osteocytes, and osteoclasts. Osteoblasts deposit the organic matrix; osteocytes and osteoclasts reabsorb this matrix. Because this process is usually in equilibrium, bone is deposited where it is needed in the skeletal system. If increased stress is placed on a bone, such as the stress of continued athletic activity, more bone will be deposited. If there is no stress on a bone, as is often the case with clients on prolonged bedrest, part of the bone mass will be reabsorbed or lost.

ALTERATIONS IN THE MUSCULOSKELETAL SYSTEM

Alterations in mobility can result from problems in the musculoskeletal system, the nervous system, and the skin. A primary cause for alterations in muscles is inactivity. With forceful activity muscles increase in size. With inactivity muscles decrease in size and strength. When clients are in casts or in traction, on prolonged bedrest, or unable to exercise, their muscles become weak and atrophied.

When a bone is fractured, a specific repair process takes place. This process begins with the formation of a blood clot at the site of the fracture. Once this clot is formed, osteoblasts and fibroblasts converge on the site and start laying down the organic matrix. Together, the fibrin net in the blood clot, the osteoblasts, and the organic matrix form a callus into which calcium salts are deposited. This callus evolves into regular bone tissue, which connects the pieces of original bone. In the final stage of the repair process, osteoblasts and osteoclasts remodel the callus area into a permanent and strong bone.

Alterations in joints result when mobility is limited by changes in the adjacent tissues. When muscle movement decreases, the connective tissue in the joints, tendons, and ligaments becomes thickened and fibrotic.

Chronic flexion and hyperextension can also cause alterations in the joints. Chronic flexion can cause joints to become "frozen" in one position so that they cannot be moved. Hyperextension occurs when joints are extended beyond their normal limits, which is usually 180 degrees. The results of hyperextension are pain and discomfort to the client and abnormal stress on the ligaments and tendons of the joints.

Alterations in bone are caused by disease processes, decalcification, and breaks caused from trauma, or twisting. Encouraging clients to stand and to walk is important because our bodies function best when they are in vertical positions. The lungs, for example, function best when the diaphragm is free to contract down into the abdominal cavity. When a person is horizontal, the abdominal organs press on the diaphragm and inhibit its movement, thus decreasing respiratory efficiency. Physical activity forces muscles to move and increase blood flow, which improves metabolism and facilitates such body functions as gastrointestinal peristalsis.

RESTORING MUSCULOSKELETAL FUNCTION

Orthopedic nursing involves the correction and prevention of alterations in the musculoskeletal system. To help clients achieve and maintain optimal mobility, nurses use preservative, restorative, and rehabilitative methods. Preservative methods, such as exercises and assisted ambulation, include those interventions that are needed to help clients maintain their normal mobility. Because the changes that occur in the human body when a person is hospitalized are varied and subtle, preservative methods are used with every client. Restorative methods, such as crutch walking and splinting, are used with clients who have decreased mobility caused by such factors as debilitating illness or major surgery. The purpose for applying restorative methods is to assist the client in achieving the level of mobility the client enjoyed before becoming ill. Rehabilitative methods, such as traction or amputee care, are used with clients after amputation, transection of the spinal cord, or a cardiovascular or cerebrovascular accident. The purpose for using these methods is to assist the client in attaining a higher level of mobility so that the client can function as independently as possible.

BODY MECHANICS

Knowledge of a client's body and how it moves is important. Knowledge of your own body and what happens to it when you care for clients with altered mobility is also important. Before you lift or move a client, study the medical history to determine the causes and consequences of the client's illness. This knowledge will enable you to move the client without causing him or her additional discomfort. Also, before you begin, thoroughly explain the procedures you will be completing so that you obtain the client's cooperation.

Trying to lift or move too much weight forces you to use your body incorrectly and frequently causes injuries. Incorrect lifting puts most pressure on the muscles of your lower back. Because these muscles are not strong enough to handle the stress, you can sustain severe injuries. If you do not follow the guidelines for body mechanics, you are putting yourself in jeopardy.

GUIDELINES FOR MANAGING CLIENTS

The primary purpose for performing nursing interventions associated with mobility is to improve the client's ability to move independently. As you perform interventions in this chapter, refer to these guidelines:

Muscles that are not used become weak and shortened.

- During prolonged bedrest, strength and endurance decrease rapidly.
- Clients can regain their muscle strength and mobility by practicing range-of-motion exercises daily.
- Clients with amputated extremities can increase their muscle strength and improve their mobility through range-of-motion exercises.

The human body functions best when it is frequently in a vertical position.

- Ambulation improves physical and mental well-being.
- Ambulation increases muscle strength and joint mobility. It also increases respiratory exchange, gastrointestinal muscle tone, and circulation.
- Without stress on bones calcium is liberated from bones and renal problems increase which can develop from calcium-based calculi.

Alterations in the alignment or loss of bone tissue can lead to major complications without appropriate nursing interventions.

- The ends of a fractured bone can damage adjacent soft tissues.
- Normal muscle tone will cause the ends of a fractured bone to overlap.
- A bone will heal in the position it is maintained.
- Before moving a client with a fracture, always immobilize the injured bone. Immobilization is complete when the joints above and below the fracture are immobilized.

Rationale for Action
- To prevent injury to yourself
- To prevent injury and falls to clients
- To evaluate client's musculoskeletal needs
- To teach by example how to use proper body mechanics

ACTION: UTILIZING PROPER BODY MECHANICS

ASSESSMENT

1 Evaluate personnel's knowledge of the principles of body mechanics.
2 Evaluate personnel's knowledge of how to use correct muscle groups for specific activities.

3 Assess knowledge and correct any misinformation about body alignment and how to maintain it with each position.
4 Assess knowledge of physical science and application to balance and body alignment.
5 Assess the competency of spinal cord and associated musculature.
6 Assess the muscle mass of the long, thick, and strong muscles of the shoulders and thighs.

PLANNING

GOALS

- Proper body mechanics are utilized in caring for clients.
- Injuries are prevented.
- Good posture promotes optimum musculoskeletal balance.
- Proper body mechanics facilitate caring for clients.
- Knowledge of musculoskeletal system, body alignment, and balance assists the nurse in caring for clients.
- Correct body mechanics promote health, enhance appearance, and assist body function.

INTERVENTION: Establishing Body Alignment Stance

1 Establish a firm base of support by placing both feet flat on the floor, with one foot slightly in front of the other.
2 Distribute weight evenly on both feet.
3 Slightly bend both knees.
4 Hold abdomen firm and tuck buttocks in so that rib cage is in alignment with spine.
5 Hold head erect and secure firm stance.
6 Use this stance as the basis for all actions in moving, turning, and lifting clients.

INTERVENTION: Maintaining Proper Body Alignment

1 Begin with the proper stance established in the previous intervention.
2 Evaluate working height necessary to achieve objective.
   a Test parameters of possible heights, i.e., bed moves within an approximate range of 45 cm from floor.
   b Establish a comfortable height in which to work; usual height is between waist and lower level of hip joint.
3 Test that this level minimizes muscle strain by extending your arms and checking that your body maintains proper alignment.
4 If you need to work at a lower level, flex your knees. Do not bend over at the waist as this results in back strain.
5 Make accommodations for working at high surface levels because reaching up may result in injury to the back through hyperextension of muscles.

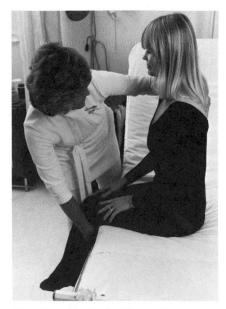

Maintain proper body alignment when assisting clients to move; for example, dangling from the bedside.

321

6 Work close to your body so that your center of gravity is not mis-aligned and your muscles are not hyperextended.
7 Use your longest and strongest muscles (biceps, quadriceps, and gluteal) when moving and turning clients.
8 Whenever possible, roll, push, and pull objects instead of lifting.

INTERVENTION: Utilizing Coordinated Muscle Movements in Body Alignment

1 Plan muscle movements to distribute workload before you actually begin turning, moving or lifting clients.
  a Establish a clear plan of action before you begin to move.
  b Take a deep breath so oxygen is available for energy expenditure.
  c Tense antagonistic muscles (abdomen) to those you will be using (diaphragm) in preparation for the movement.
  d Release breath and mobilize major muscle groups (abdominal and gluteal) to do the work.
2 Move muscles in a smooth coordinated manner to avoid putting strain on one muscle and to be more efficient.
3 Do not make jerky uncoordinated movements as this may cause injury and/or even frighten the client.
4 When you are working with another staff member, coordinate plans and movements before implementing them.

INTERVENTION: Utilizing Basic Principles for Correct Body Mechanics

1 Move an object by pushing and/or pulling to expend minimal energy.
  a Stand close to the object.
  b Place yourself in proper body alignment stance.
  c Tense muscles and prepare for movement.
  d Pull toward you by leaning away from the object and letting arms, hips, and thighs (*not back*) do the work.
  e Push away from you by leaning toward object utilizing body weight to add force.
2 When changing direction, use pivotal movement-moving muscles as a unit and in alignment, rather than rotating or twisting upper part of body.
3 When working at lower surface levels, do not stoop by bending over. Flex body at knees, and keeping back straight, use thigh and gluteal muscles to accomplish task.
4 Use the muscles of arms and upper torso in an extended, coordinated movement parallel to body stance when reaching to prevent twisting or hyperextension of muscles.
5 Lift or carry clients or objects with the maximum use of body alignment principles:
  a Determine that the movement is within your capability to perform without injury.
  b Place yourself in proper body alignment stance.
  c Stand close to and grasp the object or person near the center of gravity.

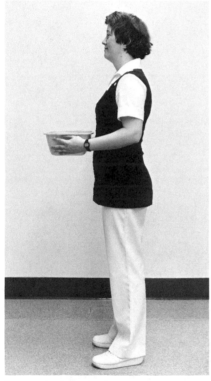

Proper stance: place both feet flat on floor, distribute weight evenly, and hold head erect with spine straight.

d Cognitively prepare muscles, take a deep breath, and set muscles.

e Lift object with arms or by stooping and using leg and thigh muscles.

f Carry the object or person close to your body to prevent strain on back.

g Take frequent rest periods to prevent additional strain.

EVALUATION

EXPECTED OUTCOMES

1 Correct body mechanics are utilized in caring for clients. *If not*, follow these alternative nursing actions:

ANA: Identify areas of your body where you feel stress and strain.

ANA: Evaluate the way you use body mechanics.

ANA: Attend an in-service program on using body mechanics appropriately.

ANA: Concentrate on how you are using your body when moving and turning clients.

ANA: Position bed and equipment at a comfortable height and proximity to working area.

ANA: Use your longest and strongest muscles to prevent injury.

2 Injuries are prevented. *If not*, follow these alternative nursing actions:

ANA: Report any back strain immediately to supervisor.

ANA: Complete incident report.

ANA: Go to health service or emergency room for evaluation and immediate care.

ANA: Evaluate any activities that lead to injury to determine incorrect use of body mechanics.

ANA: Prevent additional injury by obtaining assistance when needed.

ANA: Use devices such as turning sheets to assist in turning difficult clients.

Proper alignment: to maintain proper body alignment bend knees before lifting objects.

The Hoyer lift is a mechanical device used to move immobilized or difficult clients without staff strain.

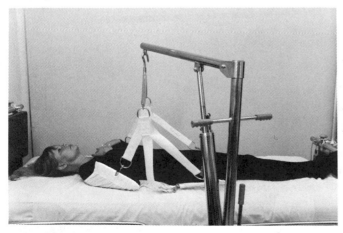

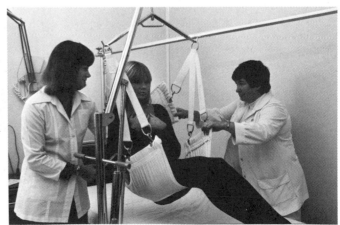

3 Proper body mechanics facilitate caring for clients. *If not,* follow these alternative nursing actions:

ANA: Evaluate client's condition and body weight to determine if mechanical devices such as Hoyer lift need to be used in moving client.

ANA: Clients with braces or heavy casts generally require additional personnel for moving and turning.

ANA: Clients with spinal cord injuries require two to three personnel for moving and turning.

UNEXPECTED OUTCOMES

1 Nurse uses poor body mechanics and injures client.

ANA: Assess the client's extent of injury.

ANA: Notify physician.

ANA: Complete incident report.

ANA: Carry out physician's orders for follow-up treatment.

2 Due to staffing shortage, nurse is unable to obtain sufficient assistance with turning and moving clients.

ANA: Place turning sheets on all clients who are difficult to move.

ANA: Use principles of leverage in moving clients.

ANA: Until adequate staff is available, turn and position client from side to side at least every two hours.

ACTION: MOVING AND TURNING CLIENTS

ASSESSMENT

1 Observe the client and identify ways to improve the client's position.
2 Determine the client's physical ability to assist you with positioning.
3 Note the presence of tubes, incisions, etc., that will alter the movement procedure.

PLANNING

GOALS

- Increased comfort
- Maintenance of intact skin
- Optimal ventilatory capacity
- Complete joint movement

EQUIPMENT

- Pillows for positioning
- Drawsheets for trochanter rolls
- Turning sheet (pull sheet)
- Chair

Charting

- Injury to client resulting from poor body mechanics
- Devices needed for turning and moving
- Number of personnel required for turning and moving
- Ways in which client assists in turning and moving
- Special requirements of client for proper body alignment
- Special turning and moving requirements

Rationale for Action

- To provide increased comfort
- To provide optimal lung excursion and ventilation
- To help maintain intact skin
- To prevent injury due to improper movement
- To prevent contractures due to constant joint flexion

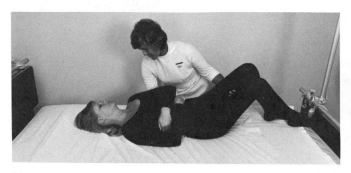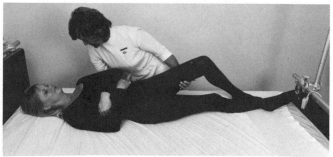

Move client up in bed by assuming proper body alignment stance, holding client securely and using leverage.

INTERVENTION: Moving the Client up in Bed by Yourself

1 Explain the rationale for the procedure to the client.
2 Lower the head of the bed so that it is flat or as low as the client can tolerate.
3 Raise the bed to a comfortable working height.
4 Remove the pillow and place it at the head of the bed to prevent striking the client's head against the bed.
5 Place one arm under the client's shoulders and the other arm under the client's thighs.
6 Instruct the client to put the arm that is closest to you under your arm and around your shoulder. Tell the client to put the other arm across the chest.
7 Instruct the client to bend legs and to put feet flat on the bed.
8 Lift and pull the client as he or she pulls with arms and pushes with feet.
9 Position the client comfortably, replacing the pillow and arranging bedding as necessary.

INTERVENTION: Moving the Client up in Bed with Assistance

1 Explain the rationale for the procedure to the client.
2 Lower the head of the bed so that it is flat or as low as the client can tolerate it.
3 Raise the bed to a comfortable working height.
4 Remove the pillow and place it at the head of the bed.
5 Position all nurses who are assisting you.
   a *Two nurses.* Position one nurse on each side of the client. Each nurse should have one arm under the client's shoulders and one arm under the client's thighs.
   b *Two nurses.* Position one nurse at the client's upper body. The nurse's arm nearest the head of bed should be under the client's head and opposite shoulder. The other arm should be under the client's closest arm and shoulder. Position the other nurse at the

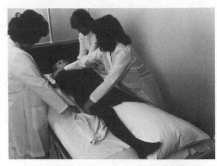

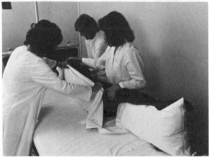

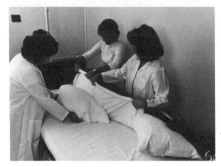

When client is immobile, use a three step process with assistance. Maintain proper alignment while positioning on side.

client's lower torso. The nurse's arms should be under the client's lower back and thighs.

c *Three nurses.* Position two nurses so that each one is supporting the client's shoulders as described above. Position the third nurse at the client's lower torso.

d *Four nurses.* Position two nurses so that each one is supporting the client's shoulders. Position the other two nurses on both sides of the client's hips or legs.

6 Coordinate the movements of all nurses.
7 Place pillow as shown to maintain proper alignment.

INTERVENTION: Turning the Client on the Side and Positioning the Client in Bed

1 Explain the rationale for the procedure to the client.
2 Lower the head of the bed completely or to a position that is as low as the client can tolerate.
3 Elevate the bed to a comfortable working height.
4 Move the client to the side of the bed away from the side where the client will finally be positioned.
5 Flex the client's knees.
6 Pull or push the client onto his or her side using the client's hips and shoulders as points of leverage.
7 Place pillow as shown in the illustration to maintain proper alignment.
8 Be sure to position the client's arms so that they are not under his or her body.

INTERVENTION: Turning the Client to a Prone Position

1 Explain the rationale for the procedure to the client.
2 Lower the head of the bed completely or to a position that is as low as the client can tolerate.
3 Elevate the bed to a comfortable working height.
4 Move the client to the side of the bed away from the side where the client will finally be positioned.
5 Position pillows on the side of the bed for the client's head, thorax, and feet.
6 Roll the client onto the pillows, making sure that the client's arms are not under his or her body.
7 Reposition pillows as necessary for the client's comfort.

INTERVENTION: Dangling the Client at the Side of the Bed

1 Lower the bed to the lowest position.
2 Raise the head of the bed until the client is sitting upright.
3 Stand at the client's waist with one of your arms under the client's arm and around upper back. Put your other arm over the client's legs.

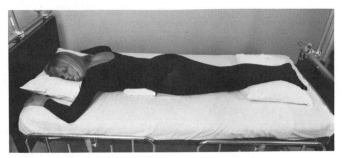
(a) Prone position

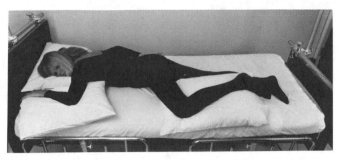
(b) Sim's (semi-prone) position

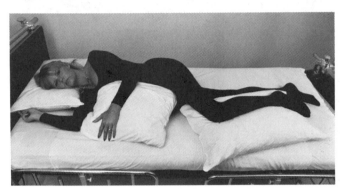
(c) Lateral (side-lying) position

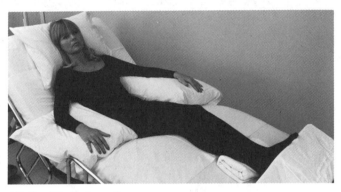
(d) Semi-Fowler's position

Maintain proper body alignment, support of extremities and comfort of the client when changing positions.

4 Bend the client's legs and grasp them at the knees.
5 In one motion, swing the legs over the side of the bed and pull the client's torso upright.
6 Stabilize the client by pushing your knees against the client's knees and grasping the torso under the client's arms.
7 Assess the client for dizziness or lightheadedness.

INTERVENTION: Moving the Client from Bed to Chair

1 Lock the bed in place.
2 Place a chair at the head of the bed. Be sure to lock chair wheels or have someone hold the chair as you move the client.
3 Dangle the client until he or she is stable.
4 Give the client nonslip shoes or slippers.
5 Stand directly in front of the client and place your arms under the client's arms.
6 Brace the client's knees with your knees and slide client to the edge of the bed.
7 Help the client straighten his or her legs by pulling with your arms and pushing with your knees.
8 Stabilize the client in a standing position.

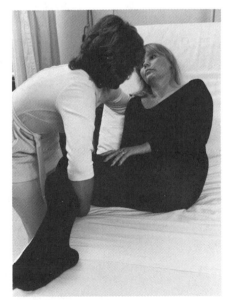
The first position in assisting a client to dangle on the side of the bed.

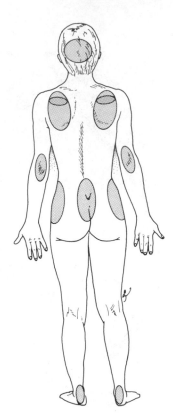

Prominent bony areas of the body may break down without adequate nursing care (see ANA's).

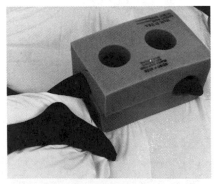

Utilize special devices to protect vulnerable areas.

9 Pivot the client 90 degrees until he or she is standing in front of the chair.
10 Help the client sit down, using your knees to brace his or her knees.

INTERVENTION: Logrolling the Client

1 Determine exactly why the client needs to be logrolled.
2 Obtain sufficient assistance to complete the procedure with ease.
3 Before moving the client, place pillows as follows:
   a at the client's head so that neck will not bend.
   b between the client's knees.
4 Position all assistants on the same side of the bed. (The person at the head will be in charge of moving the client.)
5 Move all parts of the client in one coordinated movement, i.e., head, shoulders, chest, abdomen, hips, thighs, and lower legs.
6 Maintain client's position with pillows, towels, or folded blankets.

EVALUATION

EXPECTED OUTCOMES

1 Increased comfort. *If not*, follow these alternative nursing actions:
   ANA: Reposition client, and if possible, get client up in chair.
   ANA: Provide back care and use of heating pad.
   ANA: Change to therapeutic mattress.
2 Maintenance of intact skin. *If not*, follow these alternative nursing actions:
   ANA: Reposition more frequently.
   ANA: Request modular water bed, flotation mattress, sheepskin, or eggcrate mattress.
   ANA: Rub pressure points with vitamin E four times a day.
   ANA: For severe decubiti, use Karaya or special decubiti care kit.
3 Optimal ventilatory capacity. *If not*, follow these alternative nursing actions:
   ANA: As much as possible, keep client in upright position to assist in lung expansion.
   ANA: Institute deep breathing and coughing, together with frequent moving and turning.
   ANA: Obtain order for incentive spirometer to increase client's ventilatory capacity.
4 Complete joint movement. *If not*, follow these alternative nursing actions:
   ANA: Alter positioning pattern to increase joint mobility to the affected joint.
   ANA: Institute or follow orders for ROM exercises.

UNEXPECTED OUTCOMES

1 Client unwilling to move due to fear of pain or discomfort.
   ANA: Explain rationale and need for procedure more thoroughly.
   ANA: If possible, medicate before the procedure.
   ANA: Obtain additional assistance to decrease client's apprehension.

2   Client unable to assist with movement.
   ANA: Use a turn sheet to provide more support for the client.
   ANA: Obtain additional assistance to help with moving ''dead'' weight.
3   Client unable to maintain any type of position without assistance.
   ANA: Use trochanter roll to prevent external rotation of client's hip.
   ANA: Use foam bolsters to maintain side-lying positions.
   ANA: Using folded towels, blankets, or small pillows, position client's hands and arms to prevent dependent edema.

Charting
- How often client turned or moved
- Condition of skin and joint movement
- Unexpected problems with moving or positioning client and solutions to problems
- Client's acceptance of and feelings about the procedure
- Number of staff needed to complete the procedure

ACTION: EXERCISING MUSCLES AND JOINTS

ASSESSMENT

1   Determine client's physical ability to perform exercises, i.e., level of consciousness, presence of casts, traction.
2   Ascertain present level of joint movement and/or muscle strength.
3   Note amount of spontaneous movement shown by the client.

Rationale for Action
- To improve or maintain joint function
- To improve or maintain muscle tone and strength
- To counteract effects of prolonged bedrest or immobilization
- To prevent contractures

PLANNING

GOALS

- Improved range of motion and muscle tone
- Increased comfort
- Prevention of deformities
- Preparation for ambulation

EQUIPMENT

- Hospital bed in a position as flat as the client can tolerate
- Sturdy nonslip shoes or slippers

Nursing Protocols
Muscle Exercise Sequence
1   Passive range of motion
2   Active assisted range of motion
3   Active range of motion

INTERVENTION: Performing Passive Range of Motion

1   Explain the rationale for the procedure to the client.
2   Position the client on the back with the bed as flat as possible.
3   Put all joints through range of motion. See illustrations on following page.

▶ *Passive Range-of-Motion Exercises*: All activity is carried out by the nurse so that the client has no muscle contraction. Passive ROM does not maintain or change the muscles but helps to maintain full joint motion and to prevent contractures.

INTERVENTION: Promoting Active Range of Motion

1   Explain the rationale for the procedure to the client.
2   Demonstrate the exercises that the client should perform.
3   Watch as the client does the exercises.
4   Correct any problems you notice in the client's performance.

▶ *Active Range-of-Motion Exercises*: The client produces the movement through muscle contraction and joint movement. These exercises may be used to maintain and increase muscle strength as well as to maintain full joint motion.

INTERVENTION: Providing Assisted Active Range of Motion

1   Explain the rationale for the procedure to the client.
2   Demonstrate the exercises that the client should perform.
3   Assist as the client performs the exercises.

▶ *Active Assisted Range-of-Motion Exercises*: The client does as much active exercise as is possible. If the client is very weak, the nurse should assist as necessary.

All of the following illustrations are examples of passive range of motion.

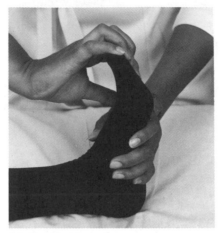

(a) Dorsiflexion.

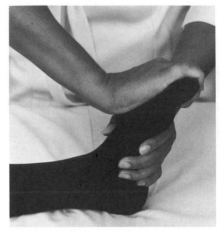

(b) Plantarflexion.

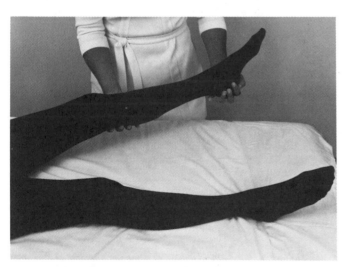

(a) Abduction (moving away from body).

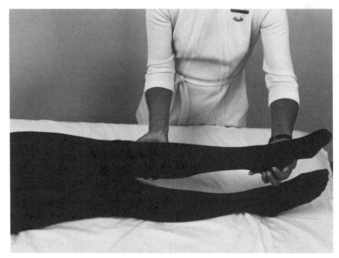

(b) Adduction (moving toward the body).

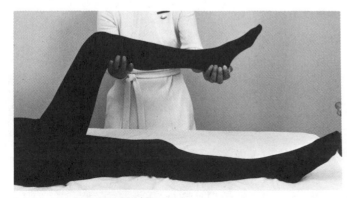

(c) Flexion of the knee and hip joints.

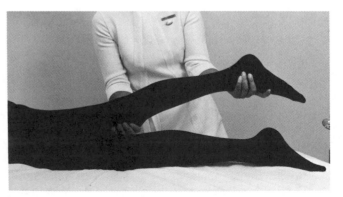

(d) Range of motion from prone position.

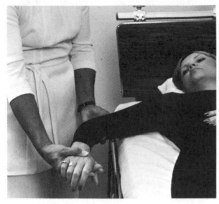
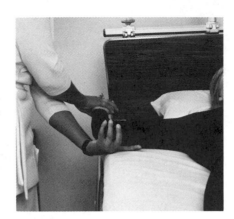
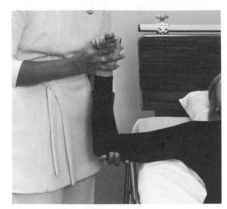

Internal and external rotation of shoulder.

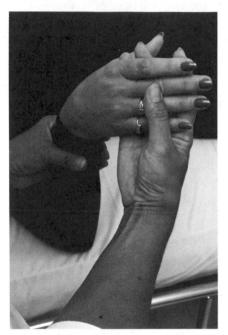
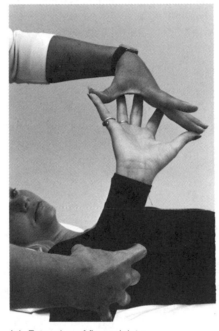
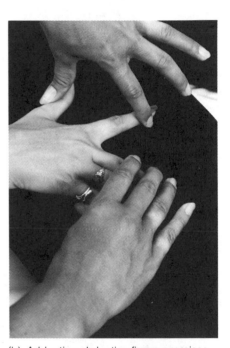

Rotation of the wrist.

(a) Extension of finger joints.

(b) Adduction-abduction finger exercises.

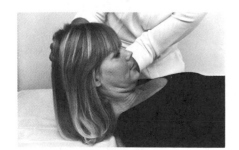
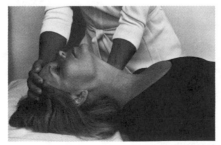
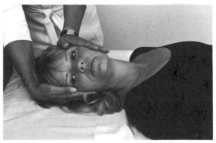

(a) Flexion of the neck.

(b) Extension of the neck.

(c) Rotation of the neck.

331

EVALUATION

EXPECTED OUTCOMES

Nurse-Client Teaching

1 Explain the importance of maintaining range of motion and muscle tone.
2 Demonstrate the exercises and answer the client's questions.
3 Encourage the client to do as many of the exercises as he or she can without help.
4 Encourage the client to increase the level of exercises as his or her strength increases.

1 Improved range of motion and muscle tone. *If not,* follow these alternative nursing actions:
ANA: Document the specific changes you observe in the client.
ANA: Notify the physician of any unanticipated change.
ANA: Institute more frequent exercise regimen.
ANA: Consult the physical therapist for more personalized exercises.
2 Increased comfort. *If not, or if movements cause pain,* follow these alternative nursing actions:
ANA: Evaluate reason for pain and change protocol if necessary.
ANA: Notify the physician if client experiences unusual pain or limitation in motion.
ANA: If pain is expected, medicate before doing range-of-motion exercises.

UNEXPECTED OUTCOME

Client continues to lose mobility and strength despite nursing intervention.
ANA: Discuss the need for additional physical therapy with the physician.
ANA: Assess the client for the need to use splints and braces to maintain the best physiologic position between exercise periods.

Charting

- Amount of time needed to complete exercises
- Any changes in condition of joint or joint mobility
- Movements that caused unusual pain or discomfort
- Amount of client participation

ACTION: ASSISTING WITH AMBULATION

ASSESSMENT

1 Assess client for dizziness when moved into an upright sitting position.
2 Determine if client feels pain from operative site.
3 Note weakness in client's legs.
4 Observe client's balance.

Rationale for Action

- To regain independence of action by regaining ability to walk
- To prevent paralytic ileus by increasing abdominal wall and gastrointestinal tract muscle tone
- To prevent thrombophlebitis by increasing circulation in the legs
- To promote healing by increasing circulation and muscle contraction

PLANNING

GOALS

- Increased feeling of physical and mental well-being
- Increased tolerance for exercise
- Better balance and muscle tone
- Decreased hospitalization

EQUIPMENT

- Robe or second hospital gown (Put on backwards so that client is not exposed.)

- Shoes or slippers that fit well and have nonslip soles
- Walker (if client is using one)

INTERVENTION: Ambulating with Two Assistants

1 Explain the rationale for the procedure to the client.
2 Help the client sit on the side of the bed.
3 Assess the client for dizziness or faintness. Keep the client in this position until the client is steady.
4 Position one nurse on each side of the client.
5 Have each nurse grasp the client's upper arm with the hand that is closest to the client.
6 Have each nurse grasp the client's hand with the other hand.
7 Encourage the client to maintain good posture and to look straight ahead, not down.
8 Ask the client to lift each foot to take a step. The client should not shuffle. Walk the client only as far as he or she is capable of walking and returning without exhaustion.

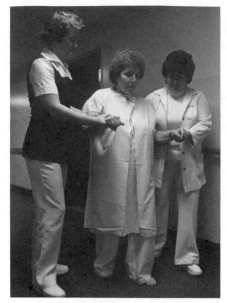

Each assistant grasps the client's upper arm and hand when ambulating.

Assist client to ambulate with a walker.

INTERVENTION: Ambulating with One Assistant

1 Explain the rationale for the procedure to the client.
2 Help the client sit on the side of the bed.
3 Assess the client for dizziness or faintness. Keep the client in this position until the client is steady.
4 Help the client to stand.
5 Grasp the client's upper arm with the hand that is closest to the client.
6 Grasp the client's hand with the other hand. If the client has a weaker side, stand on that side. For clients with CVA, stand on unaffected side.
7 Encourage the client to maintain good posture and to look straight ahead, not down.
8 Ask the client to lift each foot to take a step. The client should not shuffle. Walk the client only as far as the client is capable of walking and returning without exhausting him or herself.

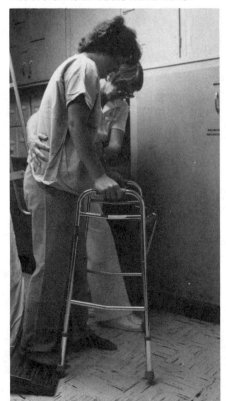

INTERVENTION: Ambulating with a Walker

1 Explain the rationale for the procedure to the client.
2 Help the client stand.
3 Tell the client to grasp the upper handles of the walker.
4 Have the client move the walker forward, keeping all four feet of the walker on the floor.
5 When the walker is stable, tell the client to walk into it.
6 Make sure the client lifts his or her feet to walk. The client should not shuffle.

EVALUATION

EXPECTED OUTCOMES

1 Increased feeling of physical and mental well-being. *If not*, follow these alternative nursing actions:
ANA: Ambulate more frequently for shorter periods and with more assistance to increase confidence.
ANA: Medicate at least one hour before ambulation to decrease pain.
ANA: With abdominal surgery, you may request order for binder to decrease fear of dehiscence.
ANA: Establish a nurse-client relationship so you can discuss altered self-image and fears.
2 Improved balance and muscle tone. *If not*, follow these alternative nursing actions:
ANA: Remind the client that he or she will not have to walk too far.
ANA: Ask other people to help you ambulate the client until the client is confident enough to walk on his or her own.
ANA: If necessary, enlist the aid of a stronger assistant whose presence may give the client additional psychological as well as physical support.
ANA: Gradually increase ambulation as muscle tone improves.

UNEXPECTED OUTCOMES

1 Client becomes dizzy or feels faint.
ANA: If in the client's room, help the client return to the chair or bed.
ANA: If in the hall, ease the client down the wall to the floor. Do not attempt to hold the client.
ANA: Summon help if possible.
2 Client is too weak to ambulate.
ANA: Provide active and passive ROM.
ANA: Begin ambulation protocol as soon as possible.

Charting
- Client's ability to balance
- Time and distance of ambulation
- Use of correct procedure for walker
- Client's perceptions of ambulation

Rationale for Action
- To increase client's level of activity after injury, such as fracture, or disease such as arthritis
- To improve muscle tone and joint flexibility
- To strengthen muscles weakened by immobility, trauma, or surgery
- To increase client's psychological sense of freedom

ACTION: TEACHING CRUTCH WALKING

ASSESSMENT

1 Assess the strength of the client's arms, back, and leg muscles.
2 Observe client's ability to balance him or herself.
3 Note any unilateral or unusual weakness.
4 Check client's medical history to find out exactly why the client needs crutches.

PLANNING

GOALS

- Improved ability to ambulate
- Increased muscle strength, especially in the arms and legs
- Increased feeling of well-being
- Better joint mobility

EQUIPMENT

- Properly fitted crutches
- Regular, hardsoled street shoes

INTERVENTION: Performing Muscle Strengthening

1 Explain the rationale for the exercises to the client.
2 Demonstrate the exercises that the client will practice.
   Quadriceps setting exercises
   a Try to hyperextend the client's leg by pushing the popliteal area (the area behind knee) into the bed and lifting heel off the bed.
   b Instruct client to contract muscles for a count of 5, then relax for a count of 5.
   c Have client repeat exercise two to three times, gradually working up to 10 to 15 times an hour.
   Gluteal setting exercises
   a Tell client to pinch his or her buttocks together for a count of 5 and to relax for a count of 5.
   b Client should repeat exercise 10 to 15 times an hour.
   Push-ups in sitting position
   a Tell client to sit up in bed with arms at sides.
   b Put books, boards, or something firm under the client's hands and have the client push down, raising hips off the bed. (This exercise may also be practiced while sitting in a chair.)
   c Client should repeat exercise until he or she can do 10 to 15 push-ups an hour.
   Push-ups in prone position
   a Tell client to lie prone in bed.
   b Ask client to place hands on the bed, close to the shoulders.
   c Tell client to extend arms and to push the upper part of the body into a upright position.
   d Client should repeat exercise until he or she can do 10 to 15 push-ups an hour.
3 Monitor as the client performs the exercises and correct any problems that may occur.
4 Assess the client for increasing strength as he or she continues to practice the exercises.

Nursing Protocol for Crutch Walking
1 Muscle strengthening exercises
2 Measuring for correct crutch size
3 Four-point crutch gait
4 Three-point crutch gait
5 Two-point crutch gait
6 Swing-to crutch gait
7 Swing-through crutch gait
8 Going upstairs and downstairs with crutches

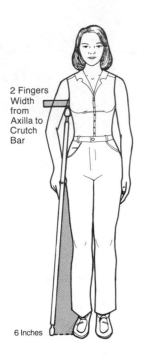

2 Fingers
Width
from
Axilla to
Crutch
Bar

6 Inches

Determine correct crutch length by proper measurement.

INTERVENTION: Measuring Client for Crutches

1. Explain the rationale for the procedure to the client.
2. Tell client to put on the shoes he or she will be wearing when using the crutches.
3. Ask client to lie flat in bed with arms at sides.
4. Measure the distance from the client's axilla (armpit) to a point six to eight inches out from heel.
5. Adjust hand bars on the crutches so that the client's elbows will always be slightly flexed.
6. Tell the client to stand with the crutches under arms.
7. Measure the distance between the client's axilla and the arm pieces on the crutches. You should be able to put two of your fingers in this space.

INTERVENTION: Teaching Crutch Walking—Four-Point Gait

1. Explain the rationale for the procedure to the client.
   a. The gait is rather slow but very stable.
   b. The gait can be performed when the client can move and bear weight on each leg.
2. Demonstrate the crutch-foot sequence to the client.
   a. Move the right crutch.
   b. Move your left foot.
   c. Move the left crutch.
   d. Move your right foot.

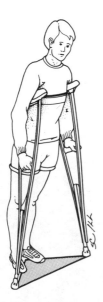

Tripod crutch stance.

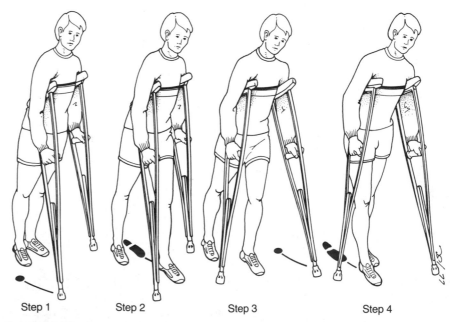

Step 1   Step 2   Step 3   Step 4

Four-point gait.

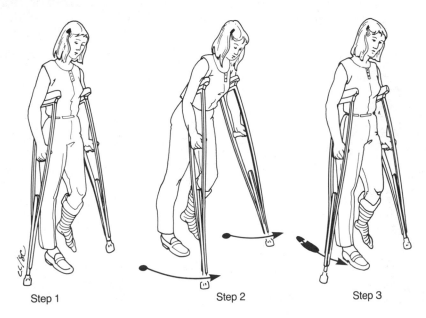

| Step 1 | Step 2 | Step 3 | Three-point gait. |

3 Help the client practice the gait. Be ready to help with balance if necessary.

4 Assess client's progress and correct mistakes as they occur.

INTERVENTION: Teaching Crutch Walking—Three-Point Gait

1 Explain the rationale for the procedure to the client.
 a The gait can be performed when the client can bear little or no weight on one leg or when the client has only one leg.
 b This gait is fairly rapid and requires fairly strong upper extremities and good balance.
2 Demonstrate the crutch-foot sequence to the client.
 a Two crutches will support weaker extremity.
 b Balance your weight on the crutches.
 c Advance forward on the foot that can bear your weight.
3 Help the client practice the gait.
4 Assess the client's progress and correct any mistakes as they occur.

INTERVENTION: Teaching Crutch Walking—Two-Point Gait

1 Explain the rationale for the procedure to the client.
 a This procedure is a rapid version of the four-point gait.
 b This gait requires more balance than the four-point gait.
2 Demonstrate the crutch-foot sequence to the client.
 a Advance your right foot and the left crutch simultaneously.
 b Advance your left foot and the right crutch simultaneously.
3 Help the client practice the gait.
4 Assess the client's progress and correct any mistakes as they occur.

Nurse-Client Teaching

1 Explain the procedure to the client before asking the client to practice.
2 Stress that learning how to use crutches will take time and may involve much practice.
3 Demonstrate tripod stance.
4 Explain why the client should not lean on the crutches at the axillae for long periods of time.

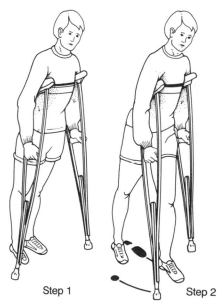

| Step 1 | Step 2 |

Two-point gait.

Swing-to Gait   Swing-through Gait

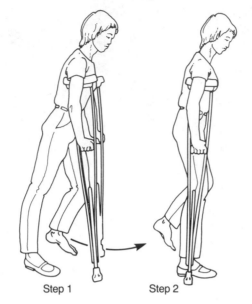

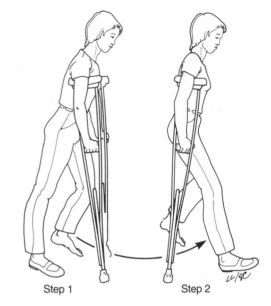

Step 1   Step 2   Step 1   Step 2

INTERVENTION: Teaching Swing-To Gait and Swing-Through Gait

1   Explain the rationale for the procedure to the client.
   a   These gaits are usually performed when the client's lower extremities are paralyzed.
   b   The client may use braces.
2   Demonstrate the crutch-foot sequence to the client.
   a   Move both crutches forward.
   b   Swing-to gait: Lift and swing your body onto the crutches.
   c   Swing-through gait: Lift and swing your body past the crutches.
   d   Bring crutches in front of your body and repeat.
3   Help the client practice the gaits.
4   Assess the client's progress and correct any mistakes as they occur.

INTERVENTION: Teaching Upstairs and Downstairs Ambulation with Crutches

1   Explain the rationale for the procedure to the client.
2   Demonstrate the procedure using a three-point gait.
   Going downstairs
   a   Start with your weight on the uninjured leg and crutches on the same level.
   b   Put the crutches on the first step of the stairs.
   c   Put your weight on the crutch handles and transfer your uninjured extremity to the step where you placed the crutches.
   d   Repeat until the client understands the procedure.
   Going upstairs
   a   Start with the crutches and your uninjured extremity on the same level.

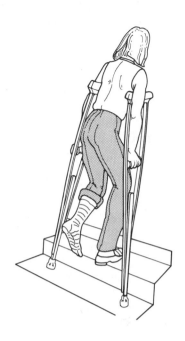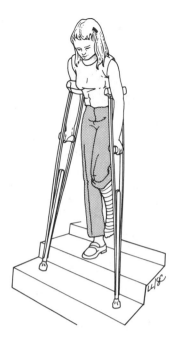

Manipulating stairs—up and down.

    b Put your weight on the crutch handles and lift the uninjured extremity onto the first step of the stairs.

    c Put your weight on the uninjured extremity and lift your other extremity and crutches to step.

    d Repeat until the client understands the procedure.

3 Help the client practice.

4 Make sure that the client has adequate balance. Be ready to assist if necessary.

5 Assess the client's progress and correct any mistakes as they occur.

EVALUATION

EXPECTED OUTCOMES

1 Improved ability to ambulate. *If not*, follow these alternative nursing actions:

ANA: Observe as the client practices the procedures to make sure that the client is completing the steps correctly for each gait.

ANA: Explain that it will take time to become proficient. Reassure the client that he or she will improve with continued practice.

2 Increased muscle strength, especially in the arms. *If not*, follow these alternative nursing actions:

ANA: Institute specific exercises (check with physical therapist) to increase muscle strength in arms.

ANA: Use crutches more frequently for shorter periods of time to build stamina.

3 Increased feeling of well-being. *If not*, follow these alternative nursing actions:

ANA: Assess fit of client's crutches. Measure fit again and adjust the crutches as needed.

ANA: Assess the client's ability to use the crutches and evaluate level of confidence.

UNEXPECTED OUTCOMES

1   Shoulder girdle is too weak to bear client's weight for crutch support
    ANA: Increase exercise of shoulder (biceps and triceps setting) to gain strength.
    ANA: Request order for overhead frame with trapeze for shoulder exercise sets.
2   Fear of falling while dependent on crutches.
    ANA: Slow down crutch protocol until client gains confidence at every level of mastery (e.g., four-point gait to two-point gait).
    ANA: Remain with client and give verbal reassurance and feedback for improvement.

ACTION: CARING FOR AND HANDLING CASTS

ASSESSMENT

1   Identify type of cast client is wearing.
2   Note condition for which the cast was applied.
3   Observe condition of the casted extremity.

PLANNING

GOALS

- Dry cast without cracks or indented areas
- Minimal discomfort from heat or edema
- Normal sensation, movement, and circulation

EQUIPMENT

- Bedboard
- Pillows covered with plastic

INTERVENTION: Caring for a Wet Cast (Plaster of Paris)

1   If client is wearing a spica or body cast, place a bedboard under the mattress to provide firm support.
2   Explain to the client that the cast will feel warm as the plaster dries.
3   Use ONLY the palms of your hands on the cast for the first 24 hours. (Fingers can cause dents in the cast which create pressure areas on the inside of the cast.)
4   Support the cast with pillows as necessary.
    a   Keep the casted extremity above the heart to decrease edema.
    b   Maintain the angles that were built into the cast.

Charting

- Time and distance of ambulation on crutches
- Balance
- Problems noted with technique
- Remedial teaching
- Client's perceptions of ambulation with crutches

Rationale for Action

Casting

- To immobilize extremity so that bone particles can be held together in reduction
- To correct deformities
- To decrease period of immobilization by permitting early weight bearing

Care and Handling of Casts

1   Prevent paralysis, schemia or necrosis caused by pressure of the cast on a nerve by observing for edema and circulatory impairment
2   Provide physical comfort for the client
3   Make sure that dents do not form on a wet cast and thus create pressure areas

c Prevent cracking from undue pressure.

d Prevent flat spots in the cast caused by pressure on the bed. For example, when the client has a long leg cast, place pillows under knees to maintain the angle of the cast and under lower leg to prevent pressure and flattening of heel area.

5 Keep the cast uncovered so heat and moisture can dissipate and air can circulate.

6 If the cast is near the client's groin, protect this area with plastic to avoid soiling the edges of the cast.

INTERVENTION: Assessing a Casted Extremity

1 Explain the rationale for the procedure to the client.

2 Encourage the client to notify you if he or she feels any unusual sensations or changes in sensations in the casted extremity.

3 Check the client's fingers or toes to make sure they are relatively pink in color.

4 Feel the client's fingers or toes to make sure they are relatively warm.

5 Ask what the client feels when you touch his or her toes. The client should have normal sensation and be able to identify which digit you are touching. He should *not* have a "pins-and-needles" sensation.

6 Assess for capillary refill by applying pressure to one of the client's toenails or fingernails. After you stop the pressure, observe the nail to see how rapidly the color returns. Compare one of your nails to the client's nail as a check on how quickly color should return.

7 Ask the client to move the fingers or toes that are affected by the cast. The client should be able to move them without difficulty.

8 Ask the client to identify the exact location of any pain. Assess for ischemia or nerve paralysis.

9 Check for any drainage from a wound under the cast. Note the color and amount of drainage. Mark the circumference of the stain on the cast as a gauge for any increases in the amount of drainage.

EVALUATION

EXPECTED OUTCOMES

1 No complications from casting procedure (e.g., pressure from cast impingement on tissues or swelling, which causes circulatory or nervous impairment). *If either of above occur*, follow these alternative nursing actions.

ANA: Assess for signs of complications and notify physician.

ANA: Do not wait for signs to get worse. As the nerve damage progresses, the client may be less aware of any unusual sensations.

ANA: Document all changes in status.

ANA: If pain is main complaint, assess location and degree *before* giving medication.

Nurse-Client Teaching

1 Explain the safety and comfort measures the client should follow while wearing a cast.

2 Explain what the client will experience as the cast dries and what you will be doing during that time.

3 Tell the client to report any pain, changes in sensation, itching, etc.

4 Tell the client how to care for the cast after discharge from the hospital.

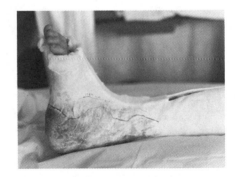

Mark the circumference of stain on cast to gauge increase in amount of drainage.

ANA: If pain is over a bony area, cast may be cut by physician to relieve pressure and prevent necrosis.

2 Dry cast without cracks or indented areas. *If not, or if the cast becomes dented while wet,* follow these alternative nursing actions:
ANA: Notify the physician immediately. The physician may choose to change the cast, to reshape the cast if the dent is at an edge, or to cut a window out at the dented area.

3 Minimal discomfort from pain or edema. *If not,* follow these alternative nursing actions:
ANA: Notify the physician.
ANA: Prepare to have the cast bivalved to relieve pressure.

UNEXPECTED OUTCOMES

1 Client complains of numbness, discomfort, and/or pain.
ANA: Notify physician immediately.
ANA: Reevaluate condition of casted extremity.
ANA: Reassess circulation, movement and sensation (CMS's).

2 Cast cracks from improper drying procedure or stress.
ANA: Notify physician and prepare for new cast application.
ANA: Reassure client.

Charting

- Positioning of cast
- Client's complaints and nursing responses
- Color, warmth, movement, and sensation in casted extremity
- Presence, location, and amount of drainage from wound
- Client's acceptance of the cast

ACTION: SPLINTING A FRACTURE

ASSESSMENT

1 Note location of fracture.
2 Determine whether the fracture is open or closed.
3 Note presence and amount of hemorrhage.
4 Note position of the client who has the fracture.

PLANNING

GOALS

- Immobilization and alignment
- Minimal pain and injury to soft tissue
- Prevention of complications (hemorrhage, edema, shock, emboli, etc.)
- Maintenance of circulation and neurological status

EQUIPMENT

- Splint materials: pieces of wood and/or pillows, magazines, blankets
- Padding materials: pieces of cloth and/or towels, blankets
- Strapping materials: strips of cloth, rope, tape

Rationale for Action

- To immobilize extremity and protect bone fragments
- To decrease pain, thereby reducing potential for shock
- To prevent fat emboli from large bone fractures
- To minimize edema and injury to soft tissues (muscles, blood vessels, and nerves)
- To prevent muscle spasms and increased pain

Clinical Alert

Do not try to reduce dislocations because vascular and neurological damage may occur.

INTERVENTION: Applying a Splint

1 If the client's life is in danger, move the client to a safe place.
2 Control hemorrhage by applying direct pressure and by using pressure dressings.
3 Explain the rationale for the intervention to the client.
4 Move the affected extremity as little as possible.
   a Splint legs in an extended position.
   b Splint arms in a flexed or extended position.
5 Pad joints, bony prominences, and skin areas as much as possible to prevent skin damage. Make sure that the padding does not affect the client's circulation, e.g., don't put padding in the axilla.
6 If splint material is not available, use the client's body for support.
   a Splint the legs together.
   b Splint an arm to the torso.
   c Splint toes or fingers together.
7 Reinforce soft splint materials (pillows, blankets) with something to make them more firm, such as magazines.
8 Strap the splint and extremity together tightly so that the extremity is immobile. Try to include the proximal and distal joints in the splint.
9 Check the client's circulation by assessing pulse, capillary refill, color, and temperature.
10 Get the client to medical facility as soon as possible.

INTERVENTION: Applying and Removing a Jewett-Taylor Brace

1 Notify appropriate person or department to measure for the brace following physician's order.
2 Explain procedure to client.
3 Obtain assistance in applying the brace.
4 Logroll client to side-lying position. Do not allow spine to torque.
5 Place posterior uprights on back so contour of brace matches contour of client's back. Spinal column is centered between the two uprights.
6 Logroll client back to supine position, maintaining back of brace in correct position by holding on to brace while turning. Do not allow spine to torque.
7 Check under client's back to ensure that spinal column is still centered between back uprights.
8 Place anterior portion of brace on client so lateral borders of pubic pad are resting on top of pelvic crests.
9 Fasten the two bottom straps simultaneously; then fasten the two top straps simultaneously. Ensure that you use equal force in pulling on each side of the back brace.
10 Check the position of the brace with the client in a sitting position. Ensure that the back uprights are properly positioned and the bottom of the pubic pad is resting on the top of the pubic bone. Brace should not ride up on client when he or she is moving.

Types of fractures.

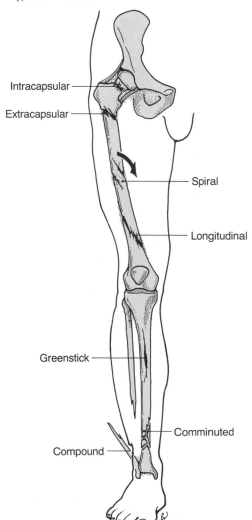

Intracapsular

Extracapsular

Spiral

Longitudinal

Greenstick

Comminuted

Compound

11 To remove the brace, undo all four straps but do not remove the anterior half of the brace.
12 Logroll client to side-lying position. Do not allow the spinal column to torque.
13 Remove posterior half of brace.
14 Logroll client to supine position and remove anterior half of brace.

EVALUATION

EXPECTED OUTCOMES

1 Minimal pain and injury to soft tissues. *If not*, follow these alternative nursing actions:
   ANA: Reassure client and move as little as possible.
   ANA: Support soft tissues until medical facility is reached.
2 Minimal complications, such as hemorrhage and edema, shock, emboli. *If not*, follow these alternative nursing actions:
   ANA: Loosen splint if necessary to relieve edema.
   ANA: Apply direct pressure or a pressure dressing if hemorrhaging occurs.
   ANA: Elevate the extremity if possible.
3 Circulation and neurological status maintained. *If not*, follow these alternative nursing actions:
   ANA: Loosen straps slightly.
   ANA: Check for padding, straps, or splint material that is impinging on a major nerve or blood vessel. Correct the problem.

UNEXPECTED OUTCOME

Extremity still moves in the splint.
   ANA: Apply more padding if possible.
   ANA: Tighten straps slightly. Observe client's circulation and feelings or sensation closely.

Charting
- Location of the fracture
- Time splint applied
- Materials used in splinting
- Circulatory and neurological status of the extremity
- Any changes in client's condition
- Client's comfort and reactions to the fracture
- Presence and treatment of open wound or bleeding

Rationale for Action
- To immobilize a joint or extremity
- To provide support to an injured extremity or surgical site
- To prevent a client from injuring her or himself in a fall
- To restrain a child's elbow to prevent the child from reaching an incision
- To promote client safety when ambulating or sitting in a chair
- To secure a dressing in place

ACTION: APPLYING BINDERS, BANDAGES, AND RESTRAINTS

ASSESSMENT

1 Assess need for binders, bandages, or restraints.
2 Identify appropriate type of binder, bandage, or restraint needed.
3 Assess area under and surrounding a binder or restraint to ensure it is not restrictive.
4 Evaluate binders and bandages for tightness and evenness of pressure.
5 Evaluate the affected extremity for circulation, sensation, and movement.

PLANNING

- Affected joint or extremity is immobilized.
- Incisional area is supported.
- Edema is decreased.
- Client is prevented from falling.
- Child is prevented from reaching incisional site.

EQUIPMENT

- Triangular bandage
- Kerlix gauze
- Safety belt
- Elbow restraints
- Immobilizer
- Posey jacket
- Safety belt
- Ace bandages of appropriate size for area to be immobilized
- Scultetus binder

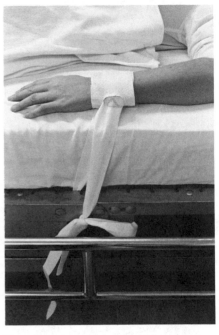

Tie soft wrist restraints on bed frame, not siderail.

INTERVENTION: Using Wrist Restraints

1 Obtain physician's order for soft restraints if required.
2 Obtain Kerlix gauze or cloth restraint with flannel padding.
3 When using Kerlix gauze, make a clove hitch to place over wrist or ankle and secure under bed.
4 When using cloth restraint, place padded section over the wrist or ankle, wrap restraint around the wrist, and slide the strap through

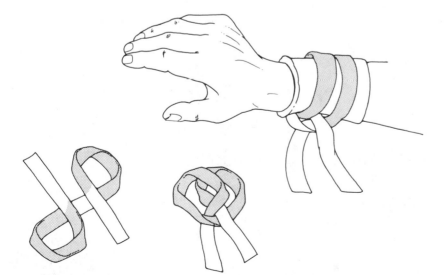

The Clove Hitch restraint prevents circulatory impairment while maintaining client safety.

345

the slit in the wrist area. Tighten the strap securely but maintain adequate circulation. Fasten strap under the bed frame using a square knot.

5 Check limbs every two hours for adequate circulation.
6 Change client's position every two hours.
7 Release restraints every two hours.
8 Put extremities through range of motion every two hours.

INTERVENTION: Using Elbow Restraints

1 Obtain elbow restraints (many types are available).
2 Explain necessity of restraints to parents.
3 Place restraints over elbow of both arms. You may need to insert a tongue blade into pockets of restraint.
4 Wrap restraints snugly around the arm. Secure by tying the restraints at the top. Many restraints have ties long enough to cross under the child's back and tie under the opposite arm.
5 For small infants and children, tie restraints to their shirts.
6 Release the restraints every two hours to allow joint mobility.
7 Assess position of restraints, circulation, and sensation every hour.
8 Provide diversionary activity for small child.
9 Encourage parents or hospital personnel to hold child to promote a feeling of security.
10 Document use of restraints in nurses' notes.

INTERVENTION: Applying a Safety Belt

1 Obtain safety belt. (Belts usually have a buckle to prevent slipping and to provide a snug fit.)
2 Explain necessity for safety belt to client.
3 Apply safety belt as follows:
  a If client is ambulating, place belt around client's waist.
  b If client is on a guerney, CircOlectric bed, or Stryker frame, fasten belt around client's abdomen.
  c If client is in a wheelchair, place belt around client's abdomen and under arm rests, and secure in back.
4 If strap does not have a buckle, tie the belt in a square knot to allow for quick removal in an emergency.

INTERVENTION: Applying a Posey Restraint

1 Obtain physician's order for restraint if required.
2 Explain necessity for restraint to client and family.
3 Place front part of jacket over client's chest, and instruct client to lean forward slightly.
4 Cross the lower and upper straps and tie straps to frame of bed or behind wheelchair.

▶ A physician's order is necessary if leather restraints are used. Also, a key is needed to lock and unlock the buckle.

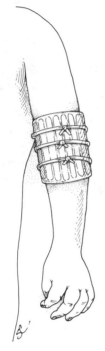

Elbow restraints are frequently used for children.

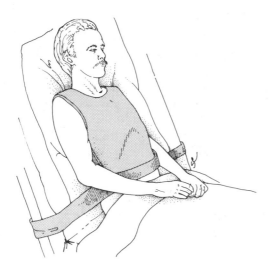

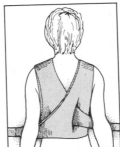

Posey restraints are most often used for safety of the client.

5 If jacket has slits in the side, pass the straps through the slits and then secure them to the bedframe or wheelchair.
6 Observe client frequently to ensure proper fit of the jacket.
7 Document use of restraints in nurses' notes.

INTERVENTION: Applying a Sling

1 If commercial slings are not available, obtain a triangular cloth or bandage.
2 Explain use of sling to client.
3 Place one end of triangular cloth over the shoulder on the uninjured arm.

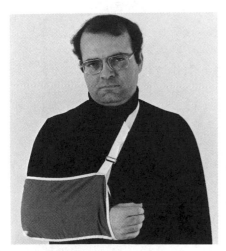

(a) The purpose of this type sling is to support the entire arm and hand.

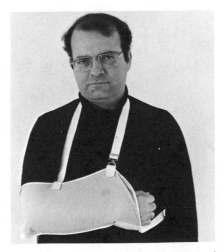

(b) This type of sling supports the arm and hand as well as immobilizes the shoulder.

4 Place sling against the body and under the injured arm.
5 Place the apex, or point, of the triangle toward the elbow.
6 Bring the opposite end of the triangle around the injured arm and over the injured shoulder.
7 Tie the sling at the side of the neck.
8 Fold the apex of the triangle over the elbow in the front and secure with a safety pin.
9 Assess for client comfort and for support of the affected arm.
10 Monitor for adequate circulation every two hours.

INTERVENTION: Applying a Circular Bandage

1 Gather necessary roller bandages. The number and size of the bandages is dependent on the extent and area of the extremity to be bandaged.
2 Explain the use of the bandage to the client.
3 Elevate the extremity to prevent the bandage from becoming too tight after wrapping.
4 Begin to wrap the extremity at the distal end. Anchor the bandage with at least two circular turns. A moderate amount of tension should be maintained on the bandage during the application.
5 Continue to unroll the bandage and overlap the previous circle until the designated area is covered.
6 Secure the bandage with tape, safety pin, or metal clip.

A circular turn is used for anchoring and securing a bandage.

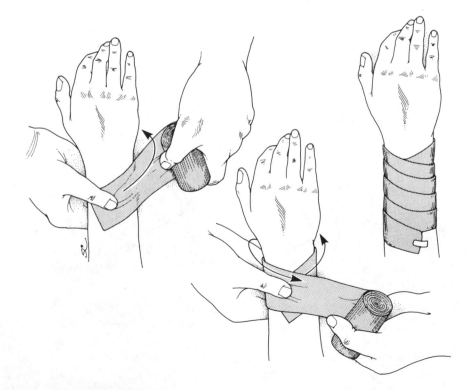

7 Observe for even, tight fit of the bandage and ensure the bandage is not occluding circulation.

8 Assess extremity every two hours for circulation, and ensure that the bandage is wrinkle-free.

9 Rewrap bandage at least every eight hours.

INTERVENTION: Applying a Spiral Bandage

1 Gather necessary roller bandages.

2 Explain necessity for bandage to client.

3 Elevate the extremity to be bandaged.

4 Anchor the bandage with two circular turns at the distal end of the extremity.

5 After anchoring the bandage, begin the spiral turns by moving up the extremity on the first turn, then straight around the extremity toward the back and then down the extremity. Complete the turn by going around the extremity.

6 With each turn of the bandage, overlap the preceding turn by at least one-half of the bandage width.

7 After wrapping the extremity, assess for adequate circulation, evenness of pressure, and comfort of client.

8 Secure bandage with tape, safety pin, or metal clip.

9 Assess client for circulation, fit of bandage, and comfort every two to four hours.

10 Ensure bandage is rewrapped every eight hours.

INTERVENTION: Applying a Figure Eight Bandage

1 Gather necessary bandages.

2 Explain necessity for bandage to client.

3 Anchor bandage around the distal end of the extremity using circular turns.

4 Make a circular turn around the foot and ankle.

5 Make a spiral turn down over the ankle and around the foot.

6 Continue to make alternate turns around the ankle and foot. Overlap the preceding bandage by at least one-half or two-thirds of the bandage.

7 Wrap the entire area below and above the involved joint.

8 Assess extremity for circulation and evenness of pressure as well as comfort of client.

9 Assess extremity at least every four hours and rewrap every eight hours.

INTERVENTION: Applying a Scultetus Binder

1 Obtain binder from appropriate department. Most facilities now use commercial velcro binders or supports in place of the scultetus binder.

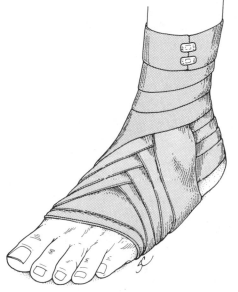

A figure eight turn is used to bandage around joints and is often used to support and limit joint movement.

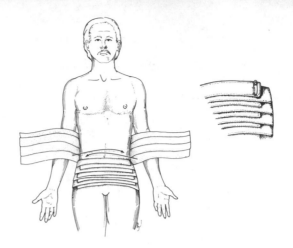

A scultetus binder used on the abdomen provides support after major surgery.

2 Explain use of the binder to the client.

3 Place the client on his or her back.

4 Examine the binder to ensure that the tails are pointing toward the top of the abdomen.

5 Ask client to raise hips, and then slide the binder under the client's hips at about the top of pubic area.

6 Start the binder application by bringing the bottom tails up toward the waist to anchor the binder.

7 For each successive tail, overlap the preceding tail by at least 1.2 cm, using a spiral effect.

8 Pull each tail tightly to the side and maintain pressure with your hand while you bring the other tail across. Alternate sides of the binder as you move each tail up toward the client's waist.

9 Secure the top of the binder with a safety pin.

10 Assess client's ability to move freely, take in a deep breath, and feel secure pressure over abdominal incision or fundal area.

11 Assess effectiveness of binder every four hours and rewrap every eight hours. Many clients use this binder only when ambulating.

EVALUATION

EXPECTED OUTCOMES

1 Affected joint or extremity is immobilized. *If not*, follow these alternative nursing actions:
ANA: Assess if type of bandage is effective or if an alternate type of bandage would provide more support.
ANA: Assess the need for a possible cast or immobilizer in place of the bandage. Notify physician of findings.
ANA: Evaluate if the bandage is applied tightly enough to immobilize the extremity.

2 Incisional area is supported. *If not*, follow these alternative nursing actions:
ANA: Evaluate the effectiveness of the scultetus binder.
ANA: Assess if the binder is properly positioned at the hip level and waist level to provide support.

ANA: Ensure that tails are brought toward the waist in a spiral-like manner.

ANA: Assess if the binder is too loose for the client. The binder will loosen if the end of each tail is not tucked in.

3 Edema is decreased. *If not*, follow these alternative nursing actions:

ANA: Reevaluate use of the bandage for decreasing the edema.

ANA: Remove bandage and apply ice with physician's order.

ANA: Elevate the bandaged extremity to increase venous return and decrease fluid accumulation.

ANA: Rewrap the bandage to ensure a tight fit.

4 Client is prevented from falling. *If not*, follow these alternative nursing actions:

ANA: Evaluate the procedure for securing the client in bed or wheelchair. Were the ties securely fastened under the bedframe or behind the wheelchair? Did the belt or restraint fit the client or was it too large?

ANA: If necessary, use two types of restraints to prevent the client from falling, i.e., posey jacket and wrist and ankle restraints.

5 Child is prevented from reaching the incisional site. *If not*, follow these alternative nursing actions:

ANA: Make sure the elbow restraints are tight enough and extend over the elbow.

ANA: Tie the one elbow restraint to the opposite elbow restraint by placing the tie under the child's back and securing the tie with the upper tie on the opposite restraint.

ANA: Check that the restraint is large enough to completely immobilize the elbow. If not, obtain a larger size or use two restraints and tie them together securely.

UNEXPECTED OUTCOMES

1 Client successfully gets out of the posey restraint.
   ANA: Put one posey restraint on frontwards and one posey restraint on backwards. Secure both of the restraints under the bedframe.

2 Client unties restraints while in wheelchair.
   ANA: If you used a half-bow to secure the restraint, retie in a square knot.

3 Client is too large for the scultetus binder.
   ANA: Fold a drawsheet in half lengthwise and place under client. Position the edges at the waist and pubic area. Pull tightly on the drawsheet and secure the edges with safety pins.

4 Client is disoriented and keeps attempting to get out of bed.
   ANA: If, after trying all types of restraints, you are unable to prevent the client from injuring him or herself, obtain an order for leather restraints.

   ANA: When applying leather restraints, pad the wrists and ankles carefully to prevent abrasions and lesions from occurring.

   ANA: Keep the key accessible to the staff in case of an emergency and the restraints need to be unlocked.

Clinical Alert

When you are tying the knots, be sure the knots can be untied quickly in emergencies.

Charting

- Type of bandage or restraint applied
- Condition of extremity following application
- Effectiveness of bandage or restraint

351

ACTION: CARING FOR CLIENTS WITH AMPUTATIONS

Rationale for Action

Amputation

1 To prevent life-threatening conditions caused from peripheral vascular disease, diabetic neuropathy, and gangrene or infections
2 Following traumatic injury when partial or complete disarticulation unable to be reversed with microsurgery
3 Tumor removal

Care of Amputee

1 Prevent infection
2 Prevent edema
3 Prevent contractures
4 Provide a viable site for prothesis application

Nurse-Client Preoperative Teaching

1 Exercises to develop quadricep muscles
2 Explanation of phantom pain phenomena

Nurse-Client Teaching

1 Tell the client to keep the stump clean and dry at all times.
2 Remind the client not to allow pressure areas to develop from wrinkled dressings.
3 Tell the client to maintain total range of motion of the joint above the amputation.
4 Remind the client not to traumatize the stump with heat lamps, hard objects, pressure, or moisture.
5 Explain the conditions that may necessitate changing the shrinker bandage.
6 Remind the client to change positions frequently.

ASSESSMENT

1 Note time of surgery.
2 Note intactness of incision.
3 Assess client's level of range of motion and muscle strength.
4 Assess client's perceived need for the interventions.
5 Note condition of client's skin: pressure areas, edema, etc.
6 Assess for signs of hemorrhage or infection.
7 Assess for phantom limb pain.

PLANNING

GOALS

- Stump with full range of motion
- Adequate muscle strength in both extremities for optimal use of the prosthesis
- A smooth conical stump that fits into a prosthesis comfortably
- Emotional acceptance of disability.

EQUIPMENT

- Bedboard
- Elastic bandage: two or three 4- to 6-inch bandages, sewn together if possible
- Elastic bandages: one or two 3- to 4-inch bandages for upper extremity

INTERVENTION: Positioning and Exercising

1 Explain the rationale for the intervention to the client.
2 Place a bedboard under mattress, preferably at the time of surgery, so that the client does not sag into the mattress and develop contractures.
3 For first 24 hours, elevate foot of bed. (Do not place pillow under stump as this leads to hip contracture.)
4 Place client in prone position every shift for at least one hour.
5 Explain the importance of the exercises to the client. Tell client that because the flexor muscles are stronger than the extensors, the stump will be permanently flexed and abducted unless the client practices the range of motion exercises.
6 Teach the client quadriceps setting exercises if he or she has a below-the-knee amputation.
   a Extend the client's leg and try to push the popliteal area of the knee into the bed. You may also try to move the patella proximally.
   b Tell the client to contract his or her quadriceps and to hold the contraction for ten seconds.
   c Tell the client to repeat this procedure four or five times.
   d The client should repeat the exercise at least four times a day.

7   Teach stump extension exercises.
    a Tell the client to lie in a prone position with his or her foot hanging over the end of the bed.
    b Ask the client to keep stump next to the client's unaffected leg, to extend stump and to contract gluteal muscles.
    c Tell the client to hold the contraction for ten seconds.
    d Tell the client to repeat this exercise at least four times a day.
8   Teach adduction exercise.
    a Place a pillow between the client's thighs.
    b Ask the client to squeeze the pillow for ten seconds and then to relax for ten seconds.
    c Ask the client to repeat this exercise at least four times a day.
9   Have the client keep track of time spent with the stump flexed and then spend an equal amount of time with the stump extended.

INTERVENTION: Applying a Shrink Bandage

1   Explain the rationale for the intervention to the client.
2   For amputations above the knee, apply three- to four-inch shrink bandages as illustrated.
    a Ask the client to hold the loops of bandage at the top of the thigh.
    b Apply pressure evenly so that the tissues are shaped properly.
    c Apply the bandage smoothly, making sure there are no wrinkles to cause pressure areas.
    d Extend the bandage as high as possible into the groin to prevent formation of an abrasion or loose roll of tissue which can hamper the fit and use of a prosthesis.

▶ Apply shrink bandage only when ordered by the physician.

A shrink bandage applied to an amputation molds the stump so that it can fit comfortably into a prosthesis.

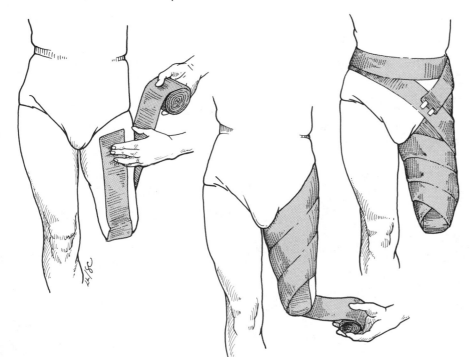

353

e If you use spica turns, make sure that the stump is not pulled into a flexed position by the bandages.

3 For amputations below the knee, apply a shrink bandage using same principles, anchoring bandage on thigh.

4 Carefully observe the bandages you have applied to ensure proper tension and molding of the stump.

5 Rewrap bandages three to four times a day.

EVALUATION

EXPECTED OUTCOMES

1 Stump exhibits full range of motion and adequate muscle strength. *If not*, follow these alternative nursing actions:

ANA: Observe the client to see which positions he uses most often. Assess stump for continued flexion and/or abduction.

ANA: Explain why the client should practice full range of motion exercises and demonstrate exercises again if necessary.

ANA: Show the client how to position the stump to attain optimal stump movement. Help the client assume these positions several times a day.

ANA: Notify the physician and physical therapist about the problem and ask them to reinforce your teaching.

2 A smooth conical stump that fits into a prosthesis comfortably. *If not*, follow these alternative nursing actions:

ANA: Examine the bandage and adjust if necessary.

ANA: Remind the client to notify someone if the bandage becomes loose or slips.

ANA: Tell the other people who are caring for the client about the problem and explain proposed solution.

ANA: Examine the stump every one to two days to see if its shape has improved.

UNEXPECTED OUTCOMES

1 Stump edema occurs even with application of shrink bandage.

ANA: When on bedrest elevate foot of bed to increase venous blood flow and decrease edema.

ANA: Assess for possible complications of infection or obstruction in blood flow.

2 Shrinkage of stump is delayed or doesn't occur as expected.

ANA: Notify physician, who may wish to apply a stump cast.

ACTION: ASSESSING TRACTION

ASSESSMENT

1 Determine type of traction to be used.

2 Note the amount of weight ordered.

3 Note any conditions requiring special treatment.

4 Assess for circulation, movement and sensation of affected extremity.

Charting

- When bandage was changed and range of motion exercises completed
- Condition of client's skin and incision
- Extent of range of motion
- Any changes in how the bandage has been applied
- Client's response to seeing the stump and assisting with its care

Rationale for Action

- To maintain correct alignment of bone ends
- To prevent unnecessary injury to soft tissue
- To prevent ischemia and necrosis which can be caused by continued pressure on the soft tissues

PLANNING

GOALS

- Extremity is in correct alignment
- Bone ends are approximated but do not override
- Skin of affected extremity is intact
- Client maintains correct position in bed
- Client has no complaint about the traction mechanism

INTERVENTION: Assessing the Intactness of Skin Traction

1. Examine the material (tape, foam rubber, or plastic) that attaches the weights to the extremity.
   a. Material should be held in place, not slipping.
   b. Material should fit comfortably, neither too loose nor too tight.
2. Examine all bony prominences of the involved extremity for abrasions or pressure areas.
3. Examine the extremity farthest from the traction.
   a. Note any presence of edema.
   b. Make sure all pulses are present.
   c. Check temperature and color to see if both are normal.
4. Observe for possible circulatory impediment from traction slings encroaching on popliteal space or axilla.
5. Ask the client to move the extremity that is farthest from the traction.
   a. Note if full range of motion is present.
   b. Ask the client if he or she has any decreased or unusual sensations.
6. Examine the rope and weights to see that the pull goes directly through the long axis of the fractured bone.
7. Check the traction mechanism.
   a. Weights should hang free from the floor and bed.
   b. Knots should be secure in all ropes.
   c. Ropes should move freely through pulleys.
   d. Pulleys should not be constrained by knots.

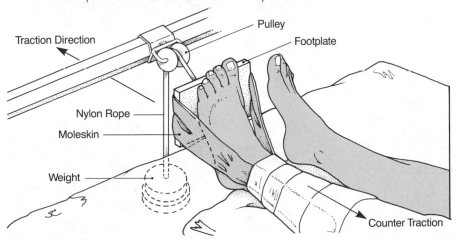

Traction Direction

Pulley

Footplate

Nylon Rope

Moleskin

Weight

Counter Traction

Buck's extension, a type of skin traction, is used to maintain bones in correct alignment.

8 Make sure the client is positioned correctly in bed. The client should not be pulled down to the end of the bed since this would negate the traction.

9 Place sheepskin or an alternative material under the affected extremity to prevent pressure areas.

10 Foot plates should be provided to the affected side to prevent footdrop.

INTERVENTION: Assessing the Intactness of Skeletal Traction

1 Check the pin and the wound area surrounding the pin.
   a Pin should be immobile.
   b Wound should be clean and dry.

2 Assess for infection at the pin site. Note any fever, local pain, redness, heat, or drainage.

3 Examine all bony prominences for pressure areas or abrasions.

4 Assess distal extremity for pulses, temperature, color, and edema.

5 Check for normal range of motion and sensation in the affected extremity.

6 Check the ropes and weights to make sure the force goes directly through the long axis of the fractured bone.

7 Check the traction mechanism.
   a Weights should hang free from the floor and bed.
   b Knots should be secure in all ropes.
   c Rope should move freely through pulleys.
   d Pulleys should not be constrained by knots.

▶ Complex traction mechanisms may not have one rope that provides a direct force through the extremity. Traction that is pulled from several directions can still create the proper amount and direction of force.

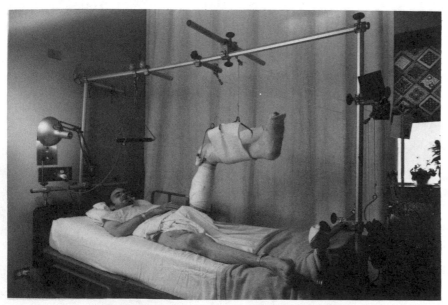

(a) Skeletal traction is immobilization of the bone through insertion of a pin.

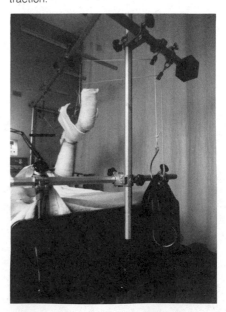

(b) Weights are counteracted by the client's weight and must be freehanging to exert traction.

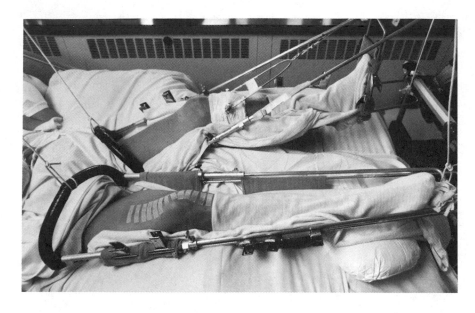

(c) Thomas splint reduces and immobilizes bone and maintains alignment.

8 Make sure the client is positioned correctly in bed. The client should not be pulled down to the foot of the bed since this would negate the traction.

9 Check the placement of the foot rest. The client's foot should be correctly positioned to prevent footdrop.

EVALUATION

EXPECTED OUTCOMES

1 Extremity is in correct alignment. *If not*, follow these alternative nursing actions:

ANA: Notify the physician at once.

ANA: Prepare to have the physician or orthopedic technician adjust the traction mechanism.

ANA: Prepare to x-ray the extremity to assess alignment after traction has been adjusted.

2 Bone ends are approximated and do not override. *If not*, follow these alternative nursing actions:

ANA: Continue traction therapy and reassess healing in one week.

ANA: Healing may be sufficient enough to allow application of a cast.

3 Skin of affected extremity is intact. *If not*, follow these alternative nursing actions:

ANA: Reposition more frequently.

ANA: Request modular water bed, flotation mattress, sheepskin, or eggcrate mattress.

ANA: Rub pressure points with vitamin E four times a day.

ANA: For severe decubiti, use Karaya or special decubiti kit.

357

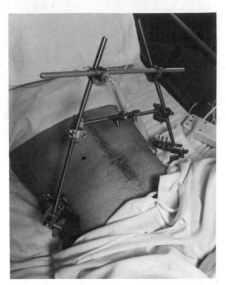

The Hoffman Colles Frame provides bone alignment for fractures and eliminates the need for traction.

Charting
- Alignment of traction is maintained
- Integrity of the skin
- Temperature, color, pulse, and range of motion in extremity
- Specific complaints by client and nursing actions taken to solve problems
- Client's comfort and overall feelings about traction

Rationale for Action
- To provide optimal mobility for a client who is confined to bed
- To gradually introduce gravity forces to clients who have been in a horizontal position for extended periods of time
- To retain or increase the stress of weight-bearing for clients who are on bedrest
- To provide mobility and ambulation for very obese clients

4 Client maintains correct position in bed. *If not,* follow these alternative nursing actions:

ANA: Obtain assistance and pull the client up in bed. You will probably need two people to move the client and one person to move the weights. You want to maintain the traction without placing extra force on the extremity during the moving process.

ANA: Shorten the rope on the weights slightly so that the weights are higher, but not so high that they get stuck in the pulley. You will need two people to help you: one person to maintain the traction and one person to move the knot up and shorten the rope.

5 Client has no complaint about the mechanism of traction. *If so, or if client complains of changed sensation in the affected extremity,* follow these alternative nursing actions:

ANA: Notify the physician at once.

ANA: Check to see if the traction is applying pressure to the extremity.

UNEXPECTED OUTCOMES

1 There is a change in the temperature, color, or pulses of the extremity.

ANA: Notify the physician at once.

ANA: If the client has a fractured femur, measure the size of the thigh with a tape measure every 15 to 30 minutes. Look for areas of ecchymosis. (It is possible to sequester several units of blood in the thigh if a vessel has been torn.)

ANA: Assess the client for circulatory shock.

2 Client has incipient footdrop and decreased range of motion in affected foot.

ANA: Tell client to practice range of motion exercises for the ankle every hour that client is awake.

ANA: Tell client to practice active range of motion exercises on the ankle if necessary.

ANA: Use a footboard to keep the client's foot in the correct position.

ACTION: PROVIDING CARE FOR CLIENTS ON A NELSON BED

ASSESSMENT

1 Assess client's vital signs, including peripheral pulses and circulation.
2 Determine symptoms of orthostatic hypotension.
3 Determine client's ability to maintain balance.
4 Assess client's knowledge of the bed and its function.
5 Ascertain client's previous experience with the bed.

PLANNING

GOALS

- Optimal functioning of body systems is maintained by putting body in positions of normal activity.
- Clients with total hip replacement ambulate without flexion of the affected hip.
- Clients with spinal surgery ambulate without torsion of the spine.
- Serum calcium levels of clients on bedrest remain within normal levels.
- Clients on bedrest are able to change from a horizontal to a vertical position without symptoms of orthostatic hypotension.
- Clients on bedrest maintain or attain normal movement of ankles, knees, and hips.

EQUIPMENT

- Nelson bed
- Safety restraining straps
- Braces, walkers, cane, or additional equipment needed by client for ambulation

INTERVENTION: Preparing and Placing Client on a Nelson Bed

1 Explain the function of bed to client.
2 Adjust seat section of the bed to the height of the individual client. This is most easily done before client is put into the bed, but it may be done afterward.
   a Unscrew knobs at each side of the bed at the area marked "To adjust for patient height."
   b Slide head section until knob position corresponds to the height of the client as printed on the side of the bed.
   c Tighten knobs securely.
3 Place client on the bed.
4 Familiarize client with bed controls for section changes.
   a Tilt: whole bed goes up at head end
   b Head
   c Knee
   d Foot: whole bed goes up at foot end
5 Instruct client how to change height position of bed.
6 Instruct client how to control UP and DOWN for each section.

INTERVENTION: Placing the Bed in Chair Position

1 Explain the procedure to client.
2 Put the siderails in UP position.
3 Adjust the footboard to client's need.
   a To move toward client, push the footboard forward by holding the middle of the supporting legs.

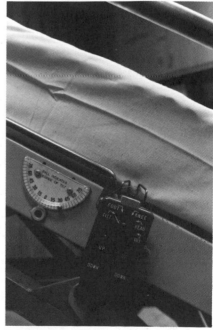

The Nelson bed provides position variation. The control knobs allow clients to change position.

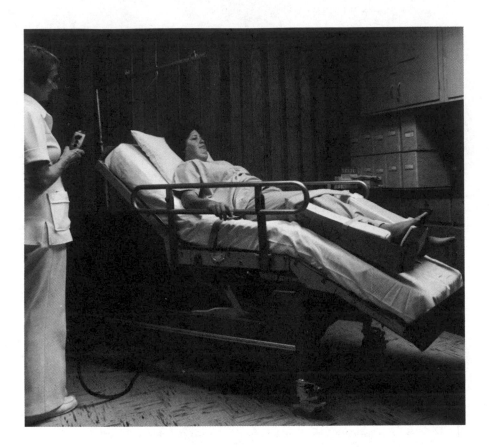

The Nelson bed in sitting position.

b To move away from client, tilt the footboard slightly forward and then pull downward to the desired position.

c The client's weight will lock the footboard in position.

4 Adjust the castors at the foot of the bed so they are parallel to the bed and locked in place.

5 Put safety straps around client if necessary.

6 Put head section up to vertical position.

7 Put knee section down until the foot of the bed is vertical.

8 Lower the bed by choosing HEIGHT and DOWN until the footboard is on the floor.

9 To return the bed to a horizontal position, reverse the procedure.

INTERVENTION: Placing the Bed in a Contour Position

1 Explain the procedure to client.

2 Put the siderails up.

3 Put the head of bed up to a comfortable position.

4 Put knee section down as desired.

5 Use FOOT control to tilt the whole bed back (head end down).

6 Adjust all parts as necessary for comfort.

7 To return to a flat position, reverse the procedure.

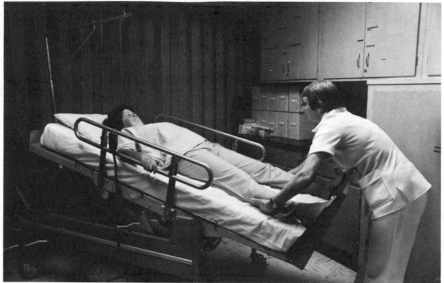

(a) The first step in assisting a client out of bed is to pull client to footboard.

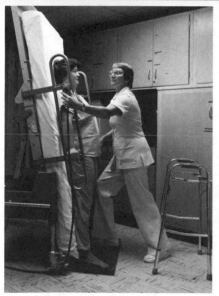

(b) Put bed in vertical position and support client with your knee against client's knee.

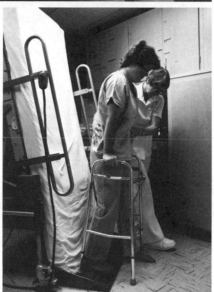

(c) Assist client to step from bed with support of walker.

INTERVENTION: Tilting Bed into Vertical Position

1 Explain the procedure to client.
2 Align and lock the foot casters parallel to the bed frame.
3 Place the bed in flat position.
4 Put height up to highest position.
5 Put the footboard down to farthest position.
6 Slide client down until client's feet are on the footboard.
7 Apply safety restraining straps.

8 Put the siderails up.
9 Select TILT and put the bed up to full tilt (82 degrees) or to a level the client can tolerate.
10 Stay at the bedside until client is comfortable in a tilted position and is able to handle the controls.
11 To place client back to a horizontal position, reverse the procedure.

INTERVENTION: Placing the Bed in Trendelenburg Position

1 Explain the procedure to client.
2 Place the mattress flat.
3 Set the controls to FOOT, and press UP button.
4 To place client back to flat position, set controls to FOOT and press DOWN button.

EVALUATION

EXPECTED OUTCOMES

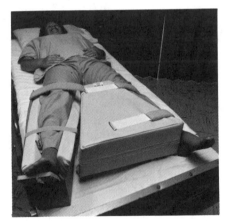

The Charnley pillow is used to keep hips in abduction and in external rotation.

1 Client with total hip replacement ambulates without flexion of the affected hip. *If not*, follow these alternative nursing actions:
ANA: Assess need for changing Charnley pillow or brace used to keep hips in abduction and externally rotated.
ANA: Review client teaching regarding ambulation and hip movement.
ANA: Answer client's questions regarding the procedure and try to allay any fears that are expressed.
ANA: Assess client's understanding about function of the bed.
2 Client with spinal surgery ambulates without torsion of the spine. *If not*, follow these alternative nursing actions:
ANA: Assess client's understanding about function of the bed.
ANA: Review client teaching regarding ambulation and spine torsion.
ANA: Answer client's questions regarding the procedure and try to allay any fears that are expressed.
ANA: Before attempting to move client out of bed, apply brace if ordered to prevent torsion of spine.
3 Client has normal serum calcium levels. *If not*, follow these alternative nursing actions:
ANA: If serum calcium is increased, decrease intake of milk and milk products.
ANA: If serum calcium is increased, have client increase intake of cranberry juice (or other acidic fluid) to acidify the urine and decrease formation of renal calculi.
4 Client is able to change from horizontal to vertical position without symptoms of orthostatic hypotension. *If not*, follow these alternative nursing actions:
ANA: Assess client for another cause of hypotension, such as anemia.

ANA: Obtain an order for antiemboli stockings to decrease venous pooling.

5 Client has normal movement of ankles, knees, and hips. *If not*, follow these alternative nursing actions:

ANA: Perform active and passive range of motion every four hours while awake within limitations of client's illness.

ANA: Assess need for physical therapy consultation.

ANA: Encourage client to do active ROM every 1 to 2 hours p.r.n.

UNEXPECTED OUTCOMES

1 Client experiences syncope when position is made more vertical.

ANA: Lower the head of the bed at once.

ANA: Check blood pressure and pulse every 5 to 10 minutes until normal.

ANA: When raising bed next time, raise client to lower degree of tilt and keep client in that position for a longer time period.

ANA: Increase degree of tilt in small increments, checking blood pressure and pulse with each increment.

2 Client falls from the bed.

ANA: Assess client's ability to maintain balance.

ANA: Use safety straps until sure of client's abilities to maintain balance.

ANA: Strap client's legs if they are weak before changing bed's position.

ANA: Have client checked by physician.

ANA: Obtain x-rays if ordered.

ANA: Complete incident report.

3 Client is fearful of the movement of the bed.

ANA: Fully explain the reasons for using the bed.

ANA: Answer all client's questions.

ANA: Let client control movement of the bed. Stay while client moves bed. Strap client in place while moving bed. Change bed positions slowly.

ACTION: PROVIDING CARE FOR CLIENTS ON A STRYKER FRAME

ASSESSMENT

1 Determine client's level of movement and sensation.
2 Evaluate client's ability to understand explanations.
3 Assess condition of traction apparatus.
4 Evaluate ability of client to assist with turning.

PLANNING

GOALS

- Clients turn horizontally from supine to prone to supine without torsion or abnormal flexion/extension of the spinal column

Charting

- Bed position used
- Degree of tilt
- Time client was in a specific position
- Vital signs
- Emotional reaction of client
- Signs and symptoms of untoward reactions
- Reaction of client according to the specific problem present
- Use of straps

Rationale for Action

- To provide for optimal movement of clients with spinal cord injuries
- To provide for optimal care of clients who should not move voluntarily

▶ Stryker parallel frame is older model frame. Stryker wedge frame is newer model frame.

▶ Stryker wedge frame can be adjusted for the height of the client.

▶ The same linen fits both the old and the new Stryker frame.

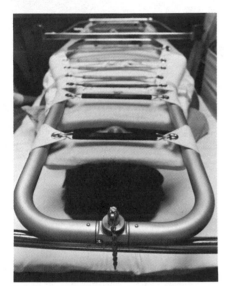

The Stryker frame is used to turn clients horizontally from supine to prone position. Often used for clients with spinal cord injuries.

- Optimal skin care provided to clients who cannot turn normally
- Pressure areas and decubitus ulcers are prevented
- Optimal nursing care is provided to clients with skin grafts or other conditions.

EQUIPMENT

- Stryker frame, either wedge turning or parallel frame
- Arm rests and footboard
- Soft goods: mattress, canvases, linen, straps
- Stryker bedpan
- Safety straps
- Pillows and sheepskins
- Traction equipment

INTERVENTION: Placing Client on Stryker Wedge Turning Frame

1 Explain procedure to client.
2 Show client Stryker frame before placing on frame.
3 Position the posterior frame at the bottom of the turning circle.
4 Place client supine on the posterior frame using the three-man carry transfer method.
5 If client is on a back board, place client and board on the posterior frame.
6 Attach the anterior frame.
7 Turn client and remove the back board.
8 Reverse procedure and turn client to back.

INTERVENTION: Turning Client on Stryker Wedge Frame from Supine to Prone

1 Explain procedure to client. This procedure requires only one person.
2 Position sheepskin, pillows, or comfort aids on top of client.
3 With client on the posterior frame, open the turning circle and put the head end of the anterior frame on the securing bolt and fasten it with the nut.
4 Fasten the foot end of the anterior frame with the nut, making sure that client's legs and feet are correctly positioned.
5 Have client clasp hands around the anterior frame. If client is unable to do this, put a safety strap around the whole frame at elbow level to keep arms contained.
6 Close the turning circle until it locks automatically.
7 Move the arm rests down out of the way of the turn.
8 Pull out the bed turning lock.
9 Turn the frame toward client's right until it locks automatically. The narrow side of the wedge (at the client's right) will always turn down. The frame will automatically lock when the bottom frame is horizontal.
10 Open the turning circle, unscrew the nuts, and remove the upper posterior frame. Relock the turning circle for safety.

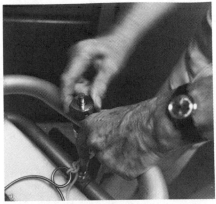

(a) Before turning, fasten nut securely at the head and the foot of the frame.

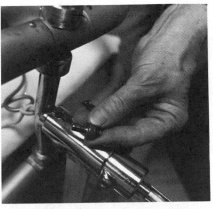

(b) Pull out turning lock before beginning the turning process.

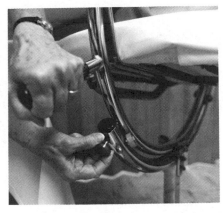

(c) Hold handle while pulling knob before beginning to rotate frame.

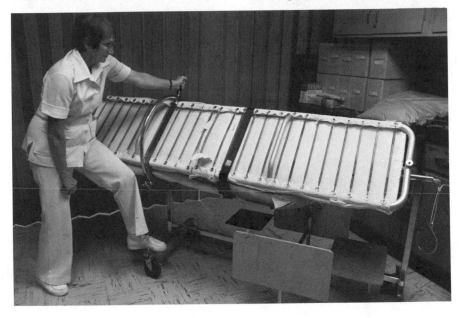

(d) Clients can be securely turned from supine to prone position on the Stryker frame.

11 To turn client on Stryker wedge from prone to supine, reverse procedure for turning from supine to prone. Remember that the narrow side of the wedge (on client's right) always turns down so client cannot slip out.

INTERVENTION: Turning Client on Parallel Stryker Frame

1 Place pillow lengthwise over client's legs to prevent their moving during turning.
2 Attach the anterior frame to the main frame using the two nuts on the turning circle. Make sure client is held firmly between the frames.
3 Put three safety straps around the frame at level of knees, waist, and elbows. Tighten securely.

4 With a person at each end of the frame, pull out the locking pins at the center of each end, turn the frame slightly to hold the lock open, and then quickly finish turning the client. The bed will automatically lock when the bottom frame is horizontal.

5 Remove the top frame and reposition client for comfort.

INTERVENTION: Assisting Client with Bedpan

1 Explain procedure to client.
2 Place client in a supine position.
3 Drop the center section of the posterior frame by releasing the hooks/rubber bands from the sides of the frame.
4 Protect linen by putting plastic or towels around the edges.
5 Insert the bedpan into the opening and hold securely with hands or with the arm supports.
6 Remove the bedpan, clean client, and reattach the center section of the frame.

INTERVENTION: Attaching Fixed Traction to Stryker Wedge Frame

1 Explain procedure to client. Client's body forms counterweight.
2 Attach the rope to the frame of the Stryker through the hole in the center pin of the disc.
3 Apply a traction halter or belt to client.
4 Attach the rope from the frame to the halter or belt.
5 Determine the number of centimeters the end of the frame must be elevated to provide for sufficient traction. Determine client's weight, and use the table provided in operating instructions to obtain the number of centimeters.
6 Lift up the head or foot of the Stryker, depending on type of traction. Put the stop pins into the holes corresponding to the elevation needed.
7 Check that client's body is positioned so feet or head is free to maintain traction.

INTERVENTION: Attaching Skeletal Traction to Stryker Wedge.

1 Explain procedure to client.
2 Attach the rope to weights by placing it through the hole in center of the disc and laying it over the pulley.
3 Attach the rope to the skeletal traction and tape all knots. Traction is applied to head or lower extremities.
4 Assess that weights are clear of frame and remain above the floor.

EVALUATION

EXPECTED OUTCOMES

1 Client is turned horizontally without torsion or abnormal flexion/extension of the spinal column. *If not*, follow these alternative nursing actions:

ANA: Assess that client's body is held firmly between the frames.

ANA: Adjust the turning circle to hold client firmly with adequate pressure.

ANA: Use pillows or blankets to hold legs firmly during the turn.

2   Client receives optimal skin care and does not develop decubiti. *If not*, follow these alternative nursing actions:

ANA: Assess for wrinkles in pads, canvas, or linen.

ANA: Assess the turning schedule to see if client has remained in one position too long.

ANA: Arrange the turning schedule to provide frequent turning but still accommodate meals and visiting hours.

ANA: Use additional padding as needed.

3   Client receives optimal nursing care for skin grafts or similar conditions. *If not*, follow these alternative nursing actions:

ANA: Use trochanter rolls, etc., to limit movement of legs.

ANA: Adjust the turning' circle to prevent lateral movement of client during turning.

ANA: Provide ROM exercises every four hours to those extremities that can receive it.

ANA: Obtain physician's order for physical therapy consultation.

UNEXPECTED OUTCOMES

1   Client expresses fear of being turned.

ANA: Encourage client to lie on the frame and be turned before being placed on it for treatment. This is helpful especially for preoperative clients.

ANA: Carefully explain each step of the turning process and the use of each piece of equipment.

ANA: Let client express fears and concerns.

ANA: Carefully answer all questions in a way that the client can understand.

2   Client experiences unusual pain or discomfort when turned.

ANA: Have client describe details of pain.

ANA: Assess client's neurological status and compare it to the client's status before turning.

ANA: Ensure that the traction apparatus is intact.

ANA: Assess for psychological component of pain.

ANA: Notify physician if pain persists or if there is a change in neurological status.

Charting

- Length of time client spends on each side
- How client tolerates the turning procedure
- Complaints of physical discomfort without lying in one position for an extended time
- Status of the traction apparatus
- Neurological status of client without turning

ACTION: PROVIDING CARE FOR CLIENTS ON A CIRCOLECTRIC BED

ASSESSMENT

1   Determine client's level of movement and sensation.
2   Evaluate client's ability to understand procedure.
3   Assess ability of client to control own turning.
4   Obtain vital signs, especially blood pressure and pulse, to assess for postural hypotension when placed in upright position.

Rationale for Action

- To provide for optimal movement of clients requiring extended immobility due to injury or disease
- To provide optimal care of clients who should not move voluntarily

367

Clinical Alert

The CircOlectric bed *must not* be used for client who cannot bear weight because of spinal cord injuries.

The CircOlectric bed provides optimal position change for clients with restricted mobility.

PLANNING

GOALS

- Client turns from supine to prone to supine without excess movement
- Optimal skin care provided for clients unable to turn normally

EQUIPMENT

- CircOlectric bed
- Bed linen
- Stryker bedpan

PREPARATION

1 Learn the mechanical aspects of operating the CircOlectric bed.
2 Hand control unit has two parts: a toggle switch designated FACE or BACK and a push-button switch for actual movement.
3 Bed is operated by selecting FACE or BACK position and pressing button until bed is in desired position.
4 A crank is stored in a tray at the head of the bed to adjust the bed if the electricity is off.

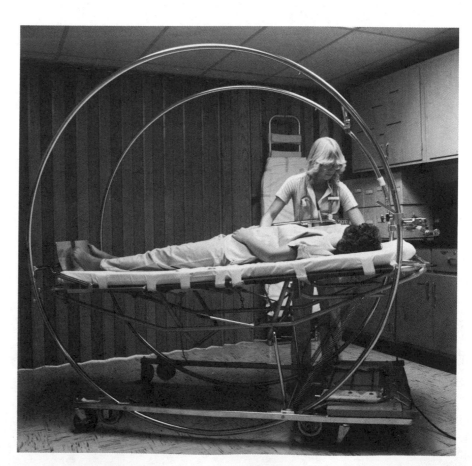

5 Two wheel locks are located on opposite corners of the bed.
6 Two automatic stops are on the bottom rail of the bed. They should be set whenever the anterior frame is not in use.
   a The setting stop, on the client's right side, prevents rotation beyond an upright sitting position.
   b The standing stop, on the client's left side, prevents rotation beyond a semi-erect position.
7 The gatch lever, at the client's right hip, changes the posterior frame from a flat to a semi-sitting position.

INTERVENTION: Placing Ambulatory Client on Bed

1 Explain procedure to client.
2 Demonstrate movement of bed using controls.
3 Place bed in vertical position.
4 Have client step backward onto the footboard with back toward the posterior frame.
5 Rotate bed backward to desired position.
6 Adjust client's position so that hips are at level of gatch.

INTERVENTION: Placing Nonambulatory Client on Bed

1 Explain transfer to client.
2 Demonstrate bed movement to client if client is able to understand explanation.
3 Position bed/gurney parallel to CircOlectric bed.
4 Alert client when you are ready to move him or her to CircOlectric bed.
5 Transfer client using standard sheet or three-man carry method.

INTERVENTION: Turning Client from Supine to Prone

1 Explain procedure to client.
2 Move the footboard from client's feet to foot of bed.
3 Place the anterior frame through the large rings one end at a time.
4 Attach the anterior frame on bolt at head of client and secure with nut.
5 Adjust the footboard of the anterior frame to client.
6 Attach the anterior frame to foot of bed with bolt and nut as at head of bed.
7 Adjust the support bar (at the head of the anterior frame) so chest of client is held firmly but comfortably.
8 Adjust the security collar knobs against the support bar.
9 Adjust the headbands to client's forehead and chin.
10 Put client's arms into the slings attached to the anterior frame.
11 Double-check all attachments and release all stops.
12 Turn client to slightly head down position.

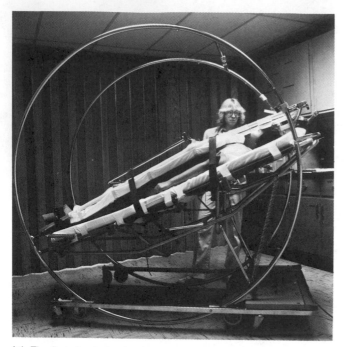

(a) The first step in turning is to secure the anterior frame.

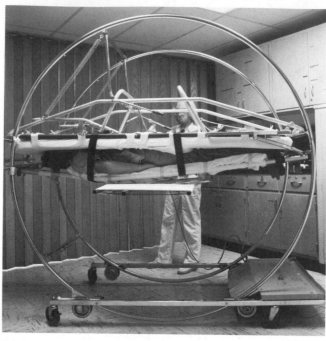

(b) The second step is to stop the bed while it is in prone position with head slightly down.

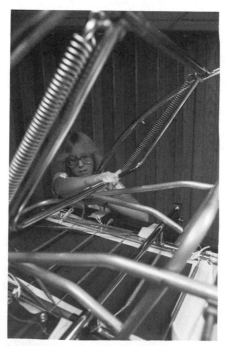

(c) The third step is to raise the posterior frame by pulling the support bar outward.

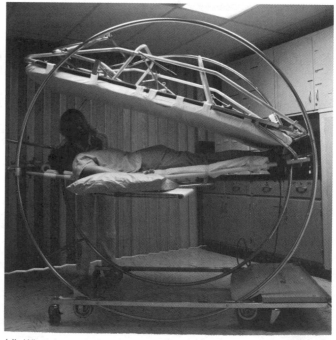

(d) When frame locks with support bar the position change is completed.

13 Raise the posterior frame by removing the nut, pulling the support bar in the frame outward, and lifting the frame until it locks with the support bar.

14 Gatch the posterior frame to remove pressure from client's feet.

15 Rotate bed backward to a prone or a slightly upright position.

16 To turn client from a prone to a supine position, reverse the procedure.

INTERVENTION: Assisting Client with Bedpan

1 Explain procedure to client.

2 Place client on the posterior frame in a flat or semi-sitting position.

3 Pull apart the elastic cords under the posterior frame and remove the round mattress insert.

4 Insert the bedpan into the opening and hold it there with the elastic cord.

5 Place absorbent pads at edges of opening to prevent soiling linen (optional).

6 Remove the bedpan when client is finished and replace the mattress insert.

EVALUATION

EXPECTED OUTCOMES

1 Client is able to turn from supine to prone to supine without excess movement. *If not*, follow these alternative nursing actions:
ANA: Ensure that client is held firmly between frames and does not slip.
ANA: Use extra support measures for client as needed, i.e., arm slings, straps, padding.

2 Client receives optimal skin care. *If not*, follow these alternative nursing actions:
ANA: Assess for wrinkles in pad, canvas, or linen.
ANA: Ensure that client does not remain in one position for more than one to two hours.
ANA: Use additional padding as needed.
ANA: Provide back care with each turn.
ANA: Change damp or soiled gown and linens as needed.

UNEXPECTED OUTCOMES

1 Client expresses fear of turning.
ANA: If possible, give complete preoperative teaching. Encourage client to lie on bed and be turned.
ANA: Carefully explain each step of the turning process and the use of each piece of equipment.
ANA: Allow client to express fears and concerns.
ANA: Carefully answer all client's questions in a way that the client can understand.

Charting

- Length of time client spends on each side
- How client tolerates the turning procedure
- If applicable, how client tolerates being in a relatively vertical position.
- Complaints of physical discomfort without turning or without being in one position for a period of time
- Status of condition for which client is on CircOlectric bed

ANA: Change positions slowly to allow client to adjust to turning position.

2 Client experiences unusual pain or discomfort when turned.

ANA: Have client describe details of pain.

ANA: Assess client's neurological status and compare to client's status before turning.

ANA: Assess for psychological component of pain.

ANA: Call physician if pain persists or if there is a change in neurological status.

TERMINOLOGY

abduction Movement of a bone away from the midline of the body or body part, as in raising the arm or spreading the fingers.

adduction Movement of a bone toward the midline of the body or part.

circumduction Movement of a bone in a circular direction so that the distal end scribes a circle while the proximal end remains stationary, as "winding up" to throw a ball.

dorsiflexion Flexion of the foot at the ankle joint; the foot and toes are turned upward, as in standing on the heel.

eversion Turning outward; movement of the foot at the ankle joint so that the sole faces outward.

extension A movement that increases the angle between two bones, straightening a joint.

flexion A movement that decreases the angle between two bones, bending a joint.

fracture Any break or crack in a bone.

hyperextension Continuation of extension beyond the anatomical position, as in bending the head backward.

inversion Turning inward; movement of the foot at the ankle joint so that the sole faces inward.

plantar flexion Extension of the foot at the ankle joint; the foot and toes are turned downward toward the sole of the foot, as in standing on tiptoe.

pronation Rotation of the forearm so that the palm faces backward or downward; movement of the whole body so that the face and abdomen are downward.

protraction Movement of the clavicle (collar bone) or mandible (lower jaw) forward on a plane parallel to the ground.

retraction Movement of the clavicle or mandible backward on a plane parallel to the ground.

rotation Movement of a bone around its own axis, as in moving the head to indicate "no" or turning the palm of the hand up and then down.

sprain Injury caused by wrenching or twisting of a joint that results in tearing or stretching of the associated ligaments.

strain Injury caused by excessive force or stretching of muscles or tendons around the joint.

supination Rotation of forearm so that the palm faces forward or upward; movement of the whole body so that the face and abdomen are upward.

CHAPTER 11
Alterations in Body Temperature

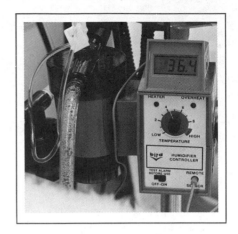

This chapter presents a conceptual basis for understanding alterations in body temperature. The temperature of the human body is regulated and maintained by a group of interrelated feedback systems. When these homeostatic mechanisms are altered by disease or environmental conditions, the body may need assistance to regain its normal temperature.

ANATOMY AND PHYSIOLOGY OF TEMPERATURE CONTROL

Temperature control of the body is a homeostatic function that balances heat production and loss to maintain body temperature within a fairly constant range. The body uses neuronal pathways to collect, organize, and transmit temperature information. These pathways also transmit physiological responses to produce temperature adjustments. The main integrative function is carried out by the hypothalamus.

The hypothalamus is the body's thermostat, and it functions to maintain the body as close as possible to a constant or "set point" temperature. Information reaches the hypothalamus by indirect and direct means; that is, indirectly through receptors and directly by circulating blood. The hypothalamus triggers body response in the tissues and vasomotor tone in the organs to produce shivering, sweating, and changes in convection, conduction, and evaporation. The body uses these physiological processes to alter temperature.

LEARNING OBJECTIVES

Describe the mechanisms responsible for the body's heat loss and heat production.

List at least three adaptive processes which maintain the body temperature within a normal range.

Outline the steps necessary to prepare for the administration of hot, moist applications.

Compare and contrast the application of three types of warm soaks.

State at least three precautions the nurse must be aware of when providing dry heat to clients.

Discuss safety factors which need to be assessed while administering a tepid sponge bath or ice application.

Describe major nursing interventions performed for clients requiring a cooling blanket.

List three safety factors utilized to prevent skin irritation for infants in a radiant warmer.

375

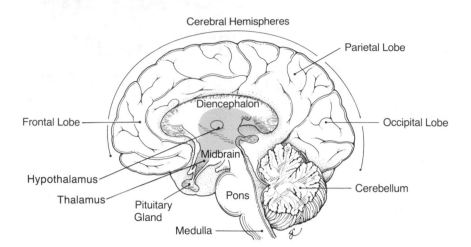

Cerebral Hemispheres

Parietal Lobe

Diencephalon

Frontal Lobe

Occipital Lobe

Midbrain

Hypothalamus

Cerebellum

Thalamus

Pons

Pituitary
Gland

Medulla

The hypothalamus, in the diencephalon portion of the brain, controls the body's thermostat.

The body continuously strives to maintain a constant optimal temperature. As heat is gained through metabolism, exercise, or environmental factors, the body throws off excess warmth through convection, conduction, and/or evaporation. In contrast, upon sensing a loss of heat (cold), the body triggers one or more processes to produce heat (thermogensis), conserve it, or dissipate it. Although these dynamic processes cannot be observed, their resulting effects, such as violent shivering, are readily evident. The hypothalamus continuously makes adjustments varying in intensity to maintain the core body temperature.

Our body works to maintain a neutral thermal environment. We consciously and unconsciously alter levels of activity in response to the physiological stimulus from the body's thermostat, the hypothalamus. When we sense cold, we huddle or curl up to decrease heat lost from the body surface. When warm, we extend our bodies and separate our limbs. There are sensors in the hypothalamus and in the dermis that are distributed widely over the body surface. These sensors react to changes in temperature. In fact, the hypothalamus is sensitive to very minute changes, as slight as 0.01° C in the circulating blood.

Adjustment Processes An important adjustment process is heat conservation. When the body perceives a cooling sensation, heat conserving and heat producing mechanisms are activitated. Vasomotor constriction, a heat conserving mechanism, removes warmed blood from the surface area of the skin. This reduces heat loss to the cooler exterior through conduction. Sweating removes heat from the body through the process of evaporation. The piloerector muscles contract, raising all the body hairs, to create an insulating (nonconductive) layer of air around the body. The latter reaction produces ''goose flesh'' and may lead to the behavioral response of huddling, curling up, or adding clothing to modify the microenvironment.

An emotional reaction can also produce a vasomotor response. Psychological perception of danger triggers the body's alarm system causing epinephrine to be released. This results in vasoconstriction on the periphery of the body, piloerection, and increased respiratory rate.

Heat production, or thermogenesis, is a progressive adaptive process. A mild cold stimulus causes an increase in respiratory rate. This is the result of the increased oxidation process going on in muscles as they are tensing. More oxygen is consumed, shivering begins as muscle tension increases, and heat is produced. This process continues until the temperature, as sensed by the thermostat hypothalamus, is high enough or has reached the set point.

A second kind of thermogenesis, nonshivering thermogenesis, also activates metabolic processes. Production of noradrenalin, mediated through neuroendocrine control, stimulates the metabolism of brown fat. Oxygen consumption is raised during this process, heat is produced, and body temperature increases. Brown adipose tissue has a special, different kind of cell structure normally present in newborns. Newborns, incapable of shivering, still are able to produce body heat through metabolic processes. Brown adipose tissue reserves are felt to decrease with age, which perhaps explains why we feel extremes of cold more severely as we grow older.

In contrast, when the body perceives excess heat, opposite measures are activitated. Sources of excess body heat may be internal, (excessive muscle activity) or external (a very warm environment). The adaptability of the multiple systems to maintain temperature within the critical range is again demonstrated when mechanisms are activated to dissipate heat. The thermostat of the hypothalamus and the peripherally situated warmth receptors provide neurologic information to set the cooling mechanisms in motion. Peripheral vasodilatation occurs and warmed blood is brought to the surface of the body. Surface vessels dilate, promoting radiation of heat away from the body. Behavioral responses are to remove insulative layers and to extend our bodies to increase the surface area for greater heat conduction. Heat conservation mechanisms are reduced, muscle activity is decreased, and heat production is minimized.

When mild thermoregulatory activities are ineffective, sweating will begin. Sweating is stimulated by thermal signals from circulatory and integumentary receptors. Sweat glands are innervated by the cholinergic sympathetic nervous system. Thus, emotions such as anxiety and fear can trigger sweating.

One of the most effective mechanisms for heat loss is evaporation. As internal temperature increases, the sweating and vasodilator responses work together. Behavioral responses to heat include a decrease in activity manifested by apathy and inertia, and decreased hunger sensations. Heat dissipation processes become more efficient as the heat load persists. Then, as the body approaches normal temperature, the activities decrease and the dynamic process for thermoregulation continues.

Some processes associated with heat production may also promote heat loss, and vice versa. For example, physical exercise produces heat, but it also allows a larger body area to be exposed for heat dissipation. Exercise also disturbs the insulative thin-air layer around the body.

All thermoregulatory activities require functional pathways for receptors and effectors. Physiological systems must be healthy and intact to respond to the constant adjustments. The behavioral/intellectual systems must also function effectively to be able to manipulate the immediate environment to maintain body temperature. Our ability to adapt to alterations in temperature is affected by many external factors such as pathogens, medications, physical disorders, and general health conditions related to age, circulation, physical fitness, nutrition, etc.

Conditions That Affect Adaptive Processes Pathogens in the form of viruses and bacteria can produce fever, generally a temperature of over 38.3° C. Fever caused by a pathogenic process is a thermoregulation disorder in which the set point is displaced upward. In response, the body perceives it is cold and seeks to conserve heat (i.e., bundling up) and to raise its temperature (i.e., shivering). The basal metabolic rate increases approximately 7% to 8% for every degree Fahrenheit of temperature elevation. Age, the duration and amount of temperature increase, and the overall disease condition are variables influencing the body's reaction.

Medications can alter the set point of the hypothalamus as well as affect one's ability to shiver or to exert vasomotor control. Drugs such as Thorazine, Demerol, or Phenergan may suppress the brain's temperature regulatory center.

Disorders of or damage to a major adaptive system can make it more difficult for the body to cope with even small changes. For example, the skin is a major organ in the cooling and heating of the body. A severe inflammation or skin infection may render this system unresponsive to temperature fluctuations.

Other health conditions that affect the adaptive processes are poor circulation to the skin, which makes heat dissipation difficult; dermatitis, which decreases the ability of temperature sensors and circulation to respond; and an insufficient amount of muscle mass, which decreases thermogenesis. A very thin person or one with a muscle wasting disease may not have sufficient muscle mass to be able to shiver. Neurological systems of elderly persons may not be able to transmit or process sensory information. Clients with a pathologic condition of the thyroid may be over or under normal levels yet not be euthermic. A person whose immune responses are deficient may not be able to adequately exhibit a febrile response. Interruptions of the hypothalamus through increased intracranial pressure grossly alter body temperature itself as well as the ability to thermoregulate. Finally, clients with decreased or absent body functions, or underdeveloped or very aged systems would also have difficulty responding to alterations.

In addition to these internal sources, the environment itself influences the body's ability to adapt to alterations in temperature. For example, a person undergoing a surgical procedure may suffer extreme exposure in a cold operating room. The client may be without covering for an extended period of time and have the abdomen opened to this environment, causing loss of core body heat. Other external conditions may cause cooling problems even if the cooling is mostly peripheral or surface. Peripheral cooling produces vasomotor changes or vasoconstriction. Continued cool blood from the periphery can eventually reduce the core to subnormal temperature. This cooling process will cause alterations of activity in most organ systems. With extended cooling stress, the thyroid is stimulated and produces an increase in metabolic rate.

In conclusion, alterations in body temperature are influenced by the body systems' integrity, age, particular disease process, and temperature stresses that a healthy person in a moderately neutral environment may experience. Many of these alterations can have temporary as well as chronic qualities. Persons may need assistance for a relatively short time or for the rest of their lives. It is apparent that assistance is often needed to maintain body temperature. Nursing attention and action can make a difference in many situations vital to the client's comfort, healing, and coping. These are supportive and preventive measures. They are also therapeutic as the nurse continues to obtain information about the client's situation, responses, and adaptability.

GUIDELINES FOR MANAGING CLIENTS

Body temperature control is a dynamic process in which there is no absolute constant.

- The body continuously makes adjustments to maintain a core temperature.
- The body's core temperature remains relatively constant only when total heat loss equals total heat influx.
- Internal body temperature is regulated by three independent regulating systems: shivering, vasomotor control and sweating.
- Individuals can maintain constant internal temperature largely independent of the ambient air temperature.
- Body temperature in all parts is not uniform or constant. Warmth and coolness are continuously shifting to maintain a constant core temperature in response to external and internal stimuli.

Body temperature regulation involves multiple body systems and hormonal regulation.

- Neurological, endocrine, musculoskeletal, cardiovascular, respiratory, and integumentary systems are directly involved in temperature control.
- Temperature receptors are distributed widely over the body surface and at various internal points.
- The hypothalamus is the primary temperature regulating center.
- Homeostatic systems for temperature control vary with age as many systems decrease in efficiency.

379

Heat transmission occurs in various ways.

- Skeletal muscle contraction is the major source of heat production in the adult.
- Heat moves passively from a warmer to a cooler area.
- Evaporation across high temperature gradients with low humidity produces the most effective transmission of heat.
- Moist heat is conducted more efficiently than dry heat.

Heat applications produce widespread effects.

- Warm applications of short duration produce vasodilitation of peripheral vessels, a decrease in general heat production, and an increase in mobility of leukocytes.
- Application of heat to one body area will produce heat over other body parts.
- Intermittent warmth to an area allows warmth receptors to fully respond with each treatment.

ACTION: APPLYING MOIST HEAT

Rationale for Action
- To conduct heat through moist application
- To produce local vasodilatation
- To improve tissue metabolism in an infected area
- To increase circulation away from congested area
- To promote comfort for an injured area
- To increase mobility of leukocytes
- To decrease heat loss due to evaporation by using waterproof materials (moisture barriers)
- To apply medication
- To hasten suppuration and soften exudate from a wound
- To assist in redistribution of heat to other body parts

ASSESSMENT

1 Assess skin condition for possible complications such as erythema, burns, and blisters related to previous applications of moist heat.
2 Determine if sterile technique is required.
3 Establish the most therapeutic method for application of moist heat.
4 Before applying heat, obtain and assess vital signs, especially respirations on debilitated clients.

PLANNING

GOALS

- Increased circulation to affected area.
- Increased warmth (if sensation is present) occurs.
- Suppuration occurs in inflamed areas.
- Decrease or relief of pain is experienced.

EQUIPMENT

- Terry towel or wool pieces for hot packs
- Plastic drape or absorbent pad for moisture barrier
- Container for warming solution
- Petroleum jelly for skin protection
- Safety pins
- Bath blanket or terry towel for securing pack
- Heating pad
- Bath thermometer
- Kerlix

ADDITIONAL EQUIPMENT

For Sterile Compresses
- Sterile solution
- Sterile 4 × 4 absorbent pads or cloth
- Sterile forceps or gloves
- Sterile towel or ABD pad for covering compress

For Sterile Soaks
- Sterile basin
- Sterile solution
- Sterile towel
- Sterile dressing (if needed)

INTERVENTION: Preparing for Hot Moist Applications

1   Check orders for type of hot moist treatment ordered, length of treatment, and time interval between treatments.
2   Gather specific equipment for type of hot moist pack ordered.
3   Place material in a warming solution (usually water).
4   Determine amount of time elapsed since last application.
5   Considering age of client, body part involved, and type of treatment, determine safe temperature of application to prevent burning.
6   Explain treatment to client and need for alteration in ambulation.
7   Determine if client is able to identify alterations in sensation if they were to occur.
8   Inspect skin surface for possible complications associated with heat treatments.
9   Take baseline vital signs.
10 Bring equipment to bedside and provide privacy.
11 Wash your hands.
12 Lubricate skin with petroleum jelly.

▶ In most hospitals, the water temperature is controlled at a temperature not to exceed 48.9° C to prevent client injury.

INTERVENTION: Applying Hot Moist Pack

1   Follow interventions for Preparing for Hot Moist Applications.
2   Place moisture-proof pad under affected area to keep bed linens dry.
3   Wring out towel or wool pieces as dry as possible.
4   Place towel or wool pieces over affected area for several seconds.
5   Remove material and check skin for erythema.
6   Ask client if temperature of pack is comfortable.
7   Replace moist pack over affected area.
8   Wrap entire surface involved with plastic drape.
9   Place towel or bath blanket over plastic wrap.
10 Place heating pad or Aqua K-pad over plastic drape (optional).
11 Secure blanket or towel with safety pins or kerlix.

381

12 Take vital signs.

13 Assess client for possible complications of heat treatment, i.e. diaphoresis, flushed face, palpitations.

14 Time the treatment (usually 20 minutes).

15 When treatment is completed, remove pack, inspect area for erythema or tissue damage, remove petroleum jelly, dry client, and apply dressing if ordered.

16 Reposition client in comfortable position and determine any side effects from treatment.

INTERVENTION: Applying Warm Sterile Soaks

1 Follow steps 1 to 11 for Preparing for Hot Moist Applications, omitting step 4.

2 Open sterile basin, maintaining sterility and keeping basin positioned on sterile wrapper.

3 Pour warmed sterile solution into basin. Temperature of solution should be from 105° to 110° F (40.5° to 43.3° C) unless otherwise specified. Test temperature by pouring small amount in a container and checking with thermometer.

4 Remove old dressing.

5 Slowly immerse body part into basin, checking client's reaction to temperature of solution before fully immersing.

6 During treatment, keep solution temperature constant by adding warm solution every five minutes. You may need to discard some solution by dipping it out with a sterile graduate.

7 Continue soak for 20 minutes.

8 Remove body part from solution, assess alterations in condition, and dry area with sterile towel.

9 Apply dressing if ordered, using sterile technique.

10 Position client for comfort and elicit any reactions associated with heat application.

INTERVENTION: Applying Clean Moist Compress

1 Follow steps 1 to 10 in Preparing for Hot Moist Applications.

2 Wring out compress with forceps because solution is hot, usually 110° F.

3 Place compress on skin surface for a few seconds and then lift up to inspect skin.

4 Change compress frequently to ensure warmth.

5 Apply heating pad or Aqua K-pad over compresses to maintain temperature and prevent need for constant compress changes.

6 Maintain treatment for specified time.

7 Remove compress, dry skin, and observe for changes in condition.

8 Reposition client for comfort.

▶ When heating pad is used with warm, moist applications, temperature should not exceed 105° F (40.5° C) in order to prevent burning.

INTERVENTION: Applying Hot Sterile Moist Compress

1. Follow steps 1 to 10 in Preparing for Hot Moist Applications. Omit step 4.
2. Warm sterile solution.
3. Place sterile gauze dressing in sterile basin, and pour warm solution over the gauze.
4. Remove old dressings and cleanse wound of exudate.
5. Wring out gauze dressing, using sterile forceps.
6. Place gauze dressing over wound.
7. Wrap sterile towel around dressing.
8. Place plastic drapes over towel.
9. Apply heating pad or Aqua K-pad (105 to 110° F) (40.5 to 43.3° C).
10. Wrap towel over heating pad and secure with tape or pins.
11. Change compress every one to two hours.
12. Apply sterile dressing to wound between treatments of moist compress if indicated.
13. Remove moist compress and observe for changes in condition.
14. Apply sterile dressing.
15. Reposition client for comfort.

INTERVENTION: Providing a Sitz Bath

1. Check physician's order for sitz bath.
2. Take linen and thermometer to bathroom.
3. Fill clean tub about one-third full with warm water.
4. Check to see that temperature of water is between 105° to 110° F or 40.5° to 43.3° C.

▶ Use of Sterile Forceps

1. Grasp forceps by handles, keeping tips down.
2. Using forceps, pick up gauze dressing by edges.
3. Keeping one forcep stable, wind the gauze dressing around the tip of the forcep.
4. When dressing is dry, unwind and place over wound.

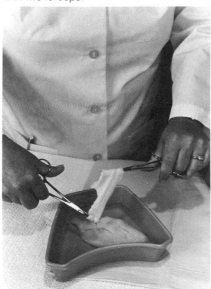

Wring sterile solution out of gauze dressing with two forceps.

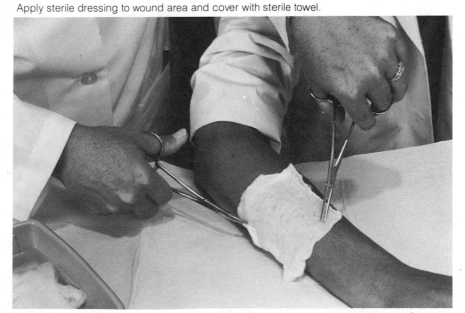

Apply sterile dressing to wound area and cover with sterile towel.

5 Place towel or inflatable ring, if appropriate, on tub bottom and bathmat on floor beside tub.
6 Explain purpose and procedure to client.
7 Instruct client to undress and put towel or bath blanket around shoulders for warmth.
8 Assist client into tub, supporting back with rolled towels.
9 Check water temperature to see that it is comfortable.
10 Remain with client during sitz bath, about 20 minutes.
11 Assess client for any untoward reactions. If client feels dizzy, faint or weak remove him or her immediately. Ring for assistance if necessary.
12 When sitz bath is completed, assist client from tub.
13 Assist with drying and dressing and accompany client to room.
14 Discard soiled linen, clean tub and record procedure on client's chart.

EVALUATION

EXPECTED OUTCOMES

1 Increased circulation occurs to the affected area. *If not*, follow these alternative nursing actions:
   ANA: Observe for circulatory compromise caused by edema resulting from vasodilatation.
   ANA: Remove hot, moist application and elevate extremity.
   ANA: Check for presence of peripheral pulses.
   ANA: Medicate for pain as needed.
2 Increased warmth occurs to area of application. *If not*, follow these alternative nursing actions:
   ANA: Assess client's sensation (ability to feel warmth).
   ANA: Ensure that temperature of hot application is not below 105° F (40.5° C).
3 Suppuration progresses when inflamed area is receiving warm moist applications. *If not*, follow these alternative nursing actions:
   ANA: Observe for cellulitis, which can occur if suppuration does not progress.
   ANA: Assess lymph glands for lymphangitis, which occurs when microorganisms spread to other cells.
4 Pain is decreased with application of heat. *If not*, follow these alternative nursing actions:
   ANA: Observe wound for infection.
   ANA: Observe surrounding skin for erythema or burning.
   ANA: Obtain order for change in type of heat application if indicated.

UNEXPECTED OUTCOMES

1 Affected extremity throbs with increased circulation.
   ANA: Elevate the extremity above the level of the heart to increase venous return.

ANA: Determine if application material is too heavy and is putting too much pressure on wound.

2 Pain in affected area is increased.

ANA: Assess if application is too hot.

ANA: Ensure that temperature is not over 110° F (43.3° C) if a heating pad is used.

3 Client refuses to keep application intact.

ANA: Elicit reason for uncooperative behavior. Determine if client is uncomfortable.

ANA: Explain rationale for treatment.

4 Pack is difficult to secure due to affected area and/or activity of client.

ANA: Use a roll of kerlix (wide gauze) to wrap and mold the pack to the body.

ANA: Use a small sheet to wrap around the trunk.

ANA: Have a person (parent for child) hold the pack in place only if absolutely necessary.

Charting
- Type of solution used
- Length of time of application
- Type of heat application
- Condition and appearance of wound
- Comfort of client

ACTION: APPLYING WARM DRY HEAT

ASSESSMENT

1 Observe client's skin for possible reaction to previous heat treatments.
2 Assess vital signs, especially temperature, to determine if overheating occurs.
3 Observe for and remove ointments and creams, which are non-heat-conductive materials.
4 Assess pain relief obtained from heat treatment.
5 Check cast for dampness.

Rationale for Action
- To increase circulation to compromised area of the body
- To provide comfort and relaxation
- To promote drying of wound, cast, etc.
- To warm a body part
- To promote healing

PLANNING

GOALS

- Body part is warmed.
- Drying of cast is accomplished.
- Relaxation of muscle spasm occurs.
- Healing is accomplished.

EQUIPMENT

- Electric heating pad
- Hot water bottle
- Aquathermic pad
- Heat lamp or heat cradle
- Overall radiant warmer
- Bedding to ensure client comfort and alignment during treatment
- Coverings for pads or hot water bottle

Clinical Alert
Application of warm pads is contraindicated for comatose or paralyzed clients because their circulation is impaired. Heat applications can cause burns.

INTERVENTION: Preparing for Dry Heat Application

1. Review physician's order to determine treatment area, type of application, and temperature of treatment.
2. Gather equipment and check it for safety factors, i.e., frayed cords, water leaks, etc.
3. Bring equipment to client's room.
4. Explain procedure to client.
5. Cover heating pad, hot water bottle, or Aquathermic pad with protective covering.
6. Follow specific intervention protocols, depending on type of application ordered.

INTERVENTION: Using Heat Lamp or Infrared Lamp

1. Follow steps 1 to 4 in Preparing for Dry Heat Application.
2. Ensure that a 60-watt bulb is used for heat lamp or the infrared element is in place for infrared treatment.
3. Wash your hands. Identify client by checking name band.
4. Position cast or cleanse the affected area well and dry thoroughly to prevent burning.
5. Place small lamp 20 to 60 cm or large lamp 60 to 76 cm away from client.
6. Check for any discomfort, burning reaction, or other untoward reaction every five minutes.
7. Instruct client not to change position or touch lamp.
8. Remove lamp after 20 minutes, and check area for erythema, burning, or untoward reaction.
9. Reposition client for comfort.
10. Return equipment to proper storage area.

INTERVENTION: Using a Heat Cradle

1. Follow steps 1 to 4 in Preparing for Dry Heat Application.
2. Ensure that 25-watt bulbs are used.
3. Place cradle over affected area, 20 to 60 cm from client.
4. Cover client and cradle with bath blanket to prevent exposure and chilling.
5. Remove heat cradle after 10 to 15 minutes.
6. Observe skin for erythema, burning, or untoward effects.
7. Reposition client for comfort.
8. Return equipment to proper storage area.

INTERVENTION: Providing Warmth Using Infant Radiant Warmer

1. Check caster locks to make certain that each caster is in locked position.
2. Adjust procedure table to desired position.
3. Plug line cord into a three-wire receptacle.

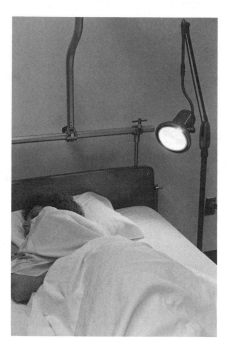

Use a 60-watt bulb in a heat lamp that is used for healing. Place heat lamp at arm's length from the client to prevent burning.

4 Turn power switch on; the red pilot light and the alarm indicator should glow. Turn alarm switch on to test alarm system.
5 Turn manual knob to automatic.
6 Install skin or rectal probe in controller and set switch to either rectal or skin, depending on which probe is being used.
7 Warm unit for seven minutes.
8 Adjust temperature to degree ordered by physician; temperature is dialed on digital temperature set switch.
9 Place infant in warmer.
10 Attach skin probe.
   a Place 1-cm skin probe with polished surface touching skin to left of the umbilicus.
   b If desirable, use a rectal probe in place of the skin probe.
11 Monitor placement of skin probe.
   a Inspect infant's skin under probe at regular intervals.
   b Change probe location if irritation begins to appear.
   c Do not use adhesive tape or pads as they may cause skin irritation or allergic reactions.
12 Allow three to five minutes for probe to reach infant's temperature.
13 Activate audible alarm by setting switch to *ON*. If the infant's temperature exceeds 38.8° C, the audible alarm sounds and the visible alarm light flashes.
14 When the infant is removed from the warmer, provide preventive maintenance of warmer, such as cleaning thoroughly and inspecting all parts.

INTERVENTION: Applying Hot Water Bottle

1 Follow steps 1 to 4 in Preparing for Dry Heat Application.
2 Fill water bottle two-thirds full, using water temperature of no more than 110° F (43.3° C).
3 Expel air from bottle and secure top.
4 Test bottle for water leak by turning upside down.
5 Cover water bottle with protective covering.
6 Place on skin surface, and remove after a few seconds to check skin for erythema or burning. Replace bottle on skin surface.
7 Remove water bottle after one hour. Observe skin for untoward effects.
8 Reposition client for comfort and return bottle to appropriate storage area.

INTERVENTION: Using an Aquathermic Pad

1 Follow steps 1 to 5 in Preparing for Dry Heat Application.
2 Check that reservoir container is two-thirds full of distilled water and is free of air bubbles.
3 Place the reservoir container on bedside stand, and plug into electrical outlet. Be sure that reservoir is not placed below bed level as the water will not circulate through the system.

1 There are several different radiant warmers, or infant care centers, available. Follow the manufacturer's operating instructions for safety and to determine if a manual or proportional controller is used.
2 General operating instructions and protocols are presented here.

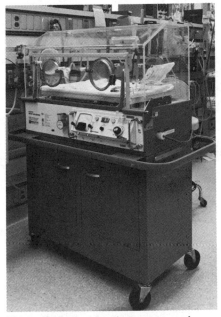

The Isolette Infant Incubator, a type of infant warmer used to maintain optimal body temperature.

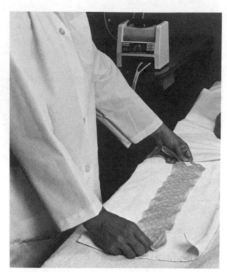

The Aquathermic Pad provides hot, dry heat at a consistent temperature. It is regulated by a special electrical unit.

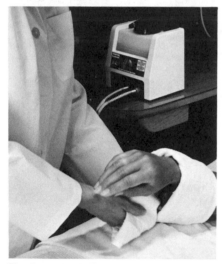

The Aqua K-Pad is wrapped and applied to the appropriate area.

4 Turn on switch. Allow water to circulate through pad to warm pad. Ensure that temperature does not exceed 105° F (40.5° C).

5 Place pad on affected area. If arm or leg is used, pad may be tied around extremity using kerlix or towel and tape. Do not use pins to secure pad as pins may puncture pad, and cause a leak.

6 Remove pad after 15 to 20 minutes. Observe area for erythema, pain, or any untoward reaction.

7 When pad is used to keep dressings or soaks warm, continue treatment longer than 20 minutes if ordered. Treatment may be continuous when used for clients with back pain.

8 Place pad on bedside stand until next treatment or return pad to proper storage area.

9 Reposition client for comfort.

EVALUATION

EXPECTED OUTCOMES

1 Body part is warmed. *If not*, follow these alternative nursing actions:
ANA: Ensure that client is covered adequately with bath blanket.
ANA: Assess that distance from heat source is correct, i.e., heat lamp is no further than 60 to 76 cm from affected area.

2 Drying of cast is accomplished. *If not*, follow these alternative nursing actions:
ANA: Continue with heat treatment until cast is shiny, indicating that it is dry.
ANA: If room is cold and/or humid, increase room temperature to at least 72° F (22.2° C) and use dehumidifiers if possible. Cast drying is delayed under these conditions.
ANA: Do not move casted area with your fingers as indentations in the cast can lead to decubiti formation.
ANA: Elevate casted extremity above level of heart to prevent edema formation.

3 Relaxation c. muscle spasms occurs. *If not*, follow these alternative nursing actions:
ANA: Assess client for alterations in type or intensity of spasms. Notify physician of any changes.
ANA: Obtain order for moist heat application if necessary.
ANA: Check that temperature of heat application is on correct setting. If set too low, heat application may not be therapeutic.

4 Healing is accomplished. *If not*, follow these alternative nursing actions:
ANA: Ensure that all previously applied solutions or ointments are removed through adequate cleansing before heat is applied.
ANA: Observe affected skin surface area for erythema, burns, or untoward reactions, and stop treatment immediately.
ANA: Make sure heat treatments are applied for specified time periods and length of treatment.

DRY HEAT APPLICATION TABLE

APPLICATION	USE	PRECAUTIONS
Heat Lamp	Provide heat to skin surface or mucous membrane	Use only 60-watt bulb
	May be used in drying casts	When used to dry casts, be aware that cast may be dry on outside only
Infrared Lamp	Provide heat to skin surface or mucous membrane	Be aware that heat penetrates only 3 mm of body tissue
Heat Cradle	Supply heat to abdomen, perineum, or chest	Use only 25-watt bulbs
		Ensure that temperature inside cradle does not exceed 125° F
Aquathermic Pad	Supply heat to small body part or to portions of back	Ensure that temperature does not exceed 105° F
		Do not secure with safety pins
Heating Pad*	Supply heat to any body surface	Do not secure with safety pins as could cause shock if wire were hit
		Set temperature control on medium
Hot Water Bottle*	Supply heat to small surfaces Molds easily to area	Do not use water over 110° F

*Generally not used in hospitals due to safety problems, i.e., burns and electrical malfunctions.

UNEXPECTED OUTCOMES

1 Client experiences discomfort with heat.

ANA: Remove heat application.

ANA: Reduce the control settings.

ANA: Examine client for burns (tissue damage) or malfunctioning equipment.

2 Client's internal (core) temperature rises above normal or desired value.

ANA: Remove the heat source.

ANA: Avoid chilling the client.

ANA: Take client's vital signs frequently, including temperature, until returned to normal.

3 Client turns up equipment control settings on own volition.

ANA: Explain reasons why settings must not be changed, i.e., burns.

ANA: Reset and observe settings frequently.

ANA: Assess for tissue damage.

ANA: Discuss reasons why client may have not been sensing the true temperature of the equipment (peripheral receptors become depressed after a time and pad may not feel hot).

4 Client is losing too much body fluid from a full body warmer (exposure to heat produces sweating and evaporative heat loss).

ANA: Give fluids unless contraindicated.

ANA: Use fluid retaining material between client and ambient air (e.g., saran wrap) to allow heat to come through but retard fluid and heat loss through evaporation.

389

Charting

- Appearance of area before and after application
- Length of time of application
- Type of application used
- Client's response to application

Rationale for Action

- To promote vasoconstriction
- To decrease edema
- To reduce pain
- To decrease temperature
- To decrease or stop bleeding

▶ Oral and axillary temperatures tend to be *less* accurate indicators of the true internal body temperature.

▶ Alcohol is infrequently used due to its drying effect; however, due to efficiency of action, it should be used when the temperature needs to be decreased quickly.

5 Client is burned by presence of creams and/or ointments on the skin.

ANA: Remove creams or ointments.

ANA: Assess skin carefully for damage.

ANA: Obtain order for and apply cooling measures such as ice bag to area.

ACTION: USING COLD APPLICATIONS

ASSESSMENT

1 Determine the purpose for the cool application, e.g., injury, fever.
2 Determine client's ability to tolerate cold application.
3 Obtain baseline vital signs and assess any hazards to client's vital functions with the application of cold.
4 Determine if antipyretic medications have been administered (type, amount, time, and response) in addition to the cold application.
5 Determine fluid and electrolyte status, especially in client with elevated temperature.
6 Assess condition of skin before and after application to determine if alterations occur.
7 Take rectal temperatures every 15 minutes throughout procedure.

PLANNING

GOALS

- Edema is slowed or reduced locally.
- Client's internal (core) temperature is reduced.
- Pain is reduced or alleviated.
- Bleeding is reduced or alleviated.

EQUIPMENT

- Water source or source of coolant (e.g., water, ice, or alcohol) for equipment
- Basin or tub for sponge baths
- Washcloth and towels
- Thermometer
- Ice cap, ice bag, ice collar, ice glove, freeze bag
- Plastic drape or absorbent pad

INTERVENTION: Providing Tepid Sponge Bath

1 Review order for type of bath to be given; water, ice, or alcohol.
2 Note temperature of solution ordered and length of application.
3 Gather equipment and bring to client's room.
4 Provide privacy and explain procedure to client.
5 Wash your hands.

6 Remove clothing from body to allow for cooling and observation. Utilize bath blanket for privacy.

7 Observe skin surface before cold wrap is applied, and take vital signs, especially temperature.

8 Monitor body color and vital signs every 5 to 15 minutes during cooling.

9 Emerse washcloths or material for sponging in ordered solution, generally 70° to 80° F (21° to 27° C).

10 Place cloths on forehead, back of neck, axilla, groin, and wrists (blood circulation is near the surface).

11 Depending on type of bath, change wraps or soaks every five minutes. This prevents wraps from holding body heat.

12 Sponge client for 20 to 30 minutes, then stop, and reassess client's condition.

13 Do not allow shivering to occur. Stop the treatment or modify it to prevent shivering.

14 Cool the ambient air to 68° to 72° F (20.0° to 22.2° C) if possible.

15 Promote movement of ambient air (fanning) if possible.

16 If using alcohol, promote ventilation of the room and observe carefully for client's response.

17 When temperature has decreased to desirable level, replace light covering over client and reposition client for comfort.

18 Elicit client's response to cool treatment.

19 Take vital signs every one to two hours until temperature is stabilized.

20 Provide high calorie intake as increased temperatures cause an increased metabolic rate. Carbohydrates, proteins, and 2500- to 3000-cc fluid intake is essential for maintaining homeostasis.

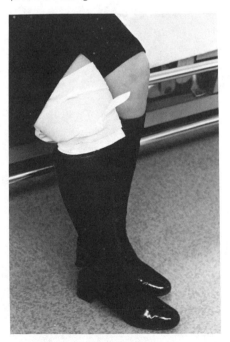

Apply cold pack to decrease edema and promote healing.

INTERVENTION: Using an Ice Application

1 Review order for type and length of treatment.

2 Gather equipment for specific application: ice bag, ice collar, freeze bag, or ice glove.

3 Wash hands.

4 Fill container, if needed, two-thirds full with crushed ice, express air, and secure top shut.

5 Place absorbent covering over ice applicator.

6 Take equipment to client's room and identify client by checking identaband.

7 Explain procedure to client.

8 Provide privacy as needed.

9 Take baseline vital signs, if needed, and observe the skin surface where ice is to be applied.

10 Remove ice pack after one hour or when absorbent cover becomes wet. Observe skin for any untoward effects such as bluish, purple appearance or a feeling of numbness.

11 Reposition client for comfort, and provide warmth if needed.

12 Reapply ice pack in one hour if necessary.

EVALUATION

1 Edema is slowed or reduced locally. *If not*, follow these alternative nursing actions:

ANA: Elevate extremity above level of heart.

ANA: Ensure that body surface is sufficiently covered with cold application to cause vasoconstriction.

ANA: Apply cold treatment every other hour until edema has dissipated.

2 Client's internal (core) temperature is reduced. *If not*, follow these alternative nursing actions:

ANA: Discuss use of antipyretic medications in addition to cold application with physician if not already being administered.

ANA: If temperature cannot be controlled with less extreme methods, obtain physician's order for hypothermia cooling blanket.

ANA: Remove all heat producing measures, such as bed linen and gowns.

3 Pain is reduced or alleviated. *If not*, follow these alternative nursing actions:

ANA: Elevate extremity above level of heart, if possible, to reduce blood flow to the affected area.

ANA: Continue ice application every other hour.

ANA: Obtain order for and administer analgesics. Analgesics may have potentiating effects if antipyretic medication is also being administered; therefore, observe client carefully for hypothermic effects.

4 Bleeding is reduced or alleviated. *If not*, follow these alternative nursing actions:

ANA: Reassess area for possible "bleeders," which may need cautery or ligation.

ANA: If bleeding continues for extended time or large blood loss is observed, notify physician immediately.

ANA: If bleeding occurs in an extremity, elevate the extremity above the level of the heart to decrease blood flow to the area.

ANA: Continue with cold application as cold constricts the arterioles and increases the viscosity of the blood, assisting in the control of bleeding.

UNEXPECTED OUTCOMES

1 Client begins to shiver.

ANA: Stop the procedure and/or warm the solution a few degrees.

ANA: Monitor temperature because shivering causes an increase in the metabolic rate leading to an increase in heat production.

2 Client feels cold.

ANA: Apply warmth to soles of feet.

ANA: Place bath blanket over affected area.

3 Internal (core) temperature drops too low.

ANA: Monitor the temperature frequently, every 30 to 60 minutes.

ANA: Warm the client slowly.

ANA: Take vital signs every 15 to 30 minutes.

ANA: Support vital functions if needed.

4 Skin becomes irritated or mascerated from sponging or cooling measures.

ANA: Remove cold application from the area and use alternate surface site.

ANA: Apply petroleum jelly or oil to area when using cold applications.

ANA: Do not massage or rub the area as this action can cause tissue damage.

5 Total numbness occurs at the site of the cold applications.

ANA: Warm the area immediately by placing body surface in 110° F (43.3° C) water. Remove extremity from water when red flush appears.

ANA: Apply loose dry dressing if area appears broken down.

ANA: Observe circulation closely for any alterations.

ANA: Observe for signs of frostbite.

6 Pain occurs at the site of cold applications.

ANA: Remove cold application.

ANA: Warm the site a few degrees.

ANA: Inspect for tissue damage.

7 Client becomes nauseated or disoriented from alcohol fumes.

ANA: Discontinue using alcohol; remove it from area.

ANA: Provide ventilation in room.

ANA: Assess vital signs.

8 Client's skin becomes very cyanotic and/or mottled.

ANA: Discontinue cooling.

ANA: Assess vital signs.

ANA: Warm the site a few degrees.

ANA: Observe site for signs of frostbite.

Charting
- Cold application used to reduce temperature
- Effectiveness of treatment
- Response of client to procedure
- Vital signs taken during application

ACTION: USING A HYPOTHERMIA BLANKET

ASSESSMENT

1 Evaluate if client's temperature can be reduced by less intensive measures.

2 Assess skin condition, especially of the face, ears, hands, and feet, before, during, and following treatment.

3 Determine client's ability to tolerate treatment.

4 Obtain and record baseline data, i.e., vital signs, neurological signs, mental status, peripheral circulation.

5 Assess that the cooling blanket and machine are functioning properly.

Rationale for Action
- To reduce body's internal (core) temperature
- To provide hypothermia for operative procedures
- To decrease metabolic processes, thereby preventing irreversible states

▶ Uses for Hypothermia Blanket
- Cardiovascular surgery
- Neurosurgery
- Persistent hyperthermia
- Thyroid crisis

▶ Classifications of Hypothermia
- Mild   32° to 37° C
- Moderate 28° to 32° C
- Deep   20° to 28° C
- Profound   0° to 20° C

▶ Hypothermia blanket can be used for increasing client's temperature. Set machine temperature control knob at desired temperature.

▶ Alcohol Solutions
20 percent alcohol
  Mix one quart 50% alcohol with 1½ quarts distilled water.
  Mix one quart 70% alcohol with 2½ quarts distilled water.

▶ There are two separate temperature control knobs, one for automatic and one for manual operation.

6   Evaluate EKG findings throughout treatment.
7   Assess fluid and electrolyte balance (especially potassium level).
8   Evalute fluid intake and output throughout treatment.
9   Assess for shivering.

PLANNING

GOALS

- Client's internal (core) temperature is reduced.
- Skin remains free of injury during use of the cooling blanket.
- Shivering is avoided.
- Cooling blanket functions properly.

EQUIPMENT

- Cooling blanket, top and/or bottom, machine
- Glass thermometer, sphygmomanometer, stethoscope
- Thermometer probe

INTERVENTION: Preparing a Cooling Blanket

1   Gather equipment.
2   Check that electrical plugs are grounded.
3   Ensure that amount of coolant is sufficient. If not, add 20 percent isopropyl alcohol solution through the reservoir cap.
4   Connect the cooling pad to the machine.
    a   Push back the collar. Insert the male tubing connector of the cooling pad into the inlet opening. Release the collar.
    b   Repeat connection using the outlet opening.
    c   If two pads are being used, connect the second pad in the same manner.
5   Turn the unit on by moving the master temperature control knob to the desired temperature. The pads from the machine reservoir fill automatically.
6   Add the alcohol mixture to the reservoir as the pads fill. Observe the reservoir sight gauge to determine fluid level.
7   Set the master temperature control knob to either automatic or manual operation.
8   When using automatic control, insert the thermister probe plug in the electronic control thermister probe jack.
    a   Insert the probe into client's rectum.
    b   Check that client's temperature control knob is at the desired temperature.
    c   Observe that the automatic mode light is on.
    d   Check that the pad temperature limits are set at desired safety limits.
9   When using manual control, set the master temperature control knob to the desired temperature.
    a   Insert the probe into client's rectum.
    b   Observe that the cool mode light is on.

c Watch that the cool limit warning light does not illuminate. This light indicates that unit temperature is below 37° C.

d Monitor the fluid thermometer, which indicates temperature of pad, to ensure pad temperature is maintained at desired level.

INTERVENTION: Using a Cooling Blanket

1 Place the cooling blanket on bed and connect it to the machine. Precool blanket to 5° to 10° C.
2 Follow the steps in Preparing a Cooling Blanket.
3 Place a sheet or a thin bath blanket over the cooling blanket.
4 Obtain baseline client data before starting treatment. (See assessment for particular data.)
5 Place client on the cooling blanket. Wrap client's hands and feet in towels to prevent frostbite or skin damage.
6 Set the temperature control to 37° C and begin lowering temperature 1° C every fifteen minutes until 33° or 34° C.
7 Monitor temperature every fifteen minutes.
8 Observe client for signs predicting onset of shivering: EKG muscle tremor artifact, visible facial muscle twitchings, hyperventilation, and verbalized feelings.
9 If manifestations of shivering occur, administer IV medication, usually chlorpromazine.
10 While client undergoes hypothermia, monitor vital signs every 30 minutes during reduction of temperature control and then every two hours.
11 Monitor EKG it client has cardiac disease or hypokalemia.

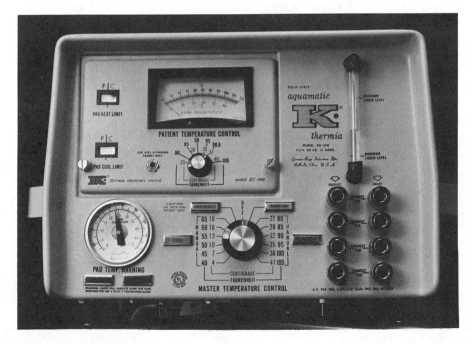

Maintain and monitoring temperature control while using a cooling or heating blanket is important to prevent complications.

12 Observe obese clients for fluid balance and hemodynamic changes.

13 Remove and clean rectal probe every four hours.

14 Check the automatic temperature control every four hours for accuracy by taking temperature with glass thermometer.

15 Apply thigh-high support stockings to client to prevent venous stasis.

16 Turn, cough, and deep breathe client every 30 minutes.

17 Monitor client's skin condition and massage bony prominences every two hours.

18 To discontinue hypothermia, gradually increase temperature from 30° to 37° C over six hours.

19 Monitor vital signs every 15 minutes.

20 Observe for edema due to increased cell permeability, acidotic shock due to shivering, fluid imbalance, and hyperthermia.

EVALUATION

EXPECTED OUTCOMES

1 Client's core temperature is reduced. *If not*, follow these alternative nursing actions:

ANA: Check the master temperature control to see what limits are set. May need to decrease lower limit. Do not set below 30° C without checking with physician.

ANA: Place a top pad on client to provide greater body surface area in contact with pads.

ANA: Place a blanket over the top pad to insulate and provide a more effective and rapid control of temperature.

ANA: Attach small pads to the extra connections on the machine to provide cold areas to body where the arteries are close to the surface, such as groin, axilla, and neck.

2 Skin remains free of injury during use of the cooling blanket. *If not*, follow these alternative nursing actions:

ANA: Make sure client is turned every 30 minutes.

ANA: Lubricate skin with petroleum jelly to provide protection.

ANA: Wrap client's hands and feet securely to prevent frostbite.

ANA: Massage bony prominences at least every hour.

ANA: Ensure that the master control temperature is not set too low.

3 Shivering is avoided. *If not*, follow these alternative nursing actions:

ANA: Obtain physician's order and medicate with IV chlorpromazine.

ANA: Increase machine temperature slightly.

ANA: Notify physician as a light anesthetic agent may be required.

ANA: Monitor for signs of hypokalemia, hypoglycemia, or altered neurological status.

4 Cooling blanket functions properly. *If not*, follow these alternative nursing actions:

ANA: Check that the plug is not disconnected from the outlet.

ANA: Check that the alcohol level is sufficient and that unit freezing has not occurred.

ANA: Check that the thermister probe is properly connected.

ANA: Check that the cool limit on the pad is not set too high.

ANA: Check that there is no constriction through pads or tubing.

UNEXPECTED OUTCOMES

1   Client's core temperature decreases rapidly and falls below 37° C.

ANA: Turn off cooling blanket.

ANA: Take top blanket off if you are using one.

ANA: Monitor temperature every 15 minutes to detect additional temperature decrease.

ANA: If temperature continues to drop the blanket can be turned on to the warming control and the client can be warmed.

2   The rectal temperature probe does not seem to be accurate.

ANA: Assess client's skin condition for cold, presence of peripheral pulses, and ability to feel pressure.

ANA: Take client's temperature every two hours with glass or electronic thermometer to evaluate the accuracy of the thermister. The type of thermometer, oral or rectal, will depend on the condition of the client.

ANA: Calibrate the thermister to ensure that the temperature reading of the thermister is accurate.

Charting

- Client's temperature and method of taking temperature
- Any untoward effects of the treatment, i.e., shivering
- Setting of the cooling blanket
- Whether the top blanket is used
- Skin condition
- Skin treatments done prior to use of cooling blanket
- EKG interpretation if client is monitored

CHAPTER 12
Alterations in Urinary Elimination

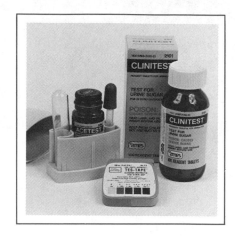

The urinary system removes nitrogenous end products of protein metabolism, waste substances, drugs, and toxins and controls the fluid, electrolyte, and acid-base balances of the body. Effective elimination is essential to maintain well-being and to preserve life itself.

This chapter presents the conceptual basis for alterations in urinary elimination. It includes planned nursing interventions and skills necessary to facilitate and maintain the urinary function.

ANATOMY AND PHYSIOLOGY OF THE URINARY SYSTEM

The primary structures of the urinary system are the kidneys, ureters, bladder, and urethra. Each kidney produces urine, which is carried to the bladder by a ureter that is about 25 cm long and 0.6 cm in diameter. Peristaltic waves, pressure, and gravity propel urine through the ureters so that it can be discharged into the bladder.

The bladder serves as a reservoir for urine until the urge to void takes place. When the act of micturition, or urination, occurs, urine passes through two sphincters and is transported from the bladder to the external environment by the urethra.

The anatomical position of the bladder and the structure of the urethra differ in males and females. The bladder in both sexes is posterior

Female genitourinary system.

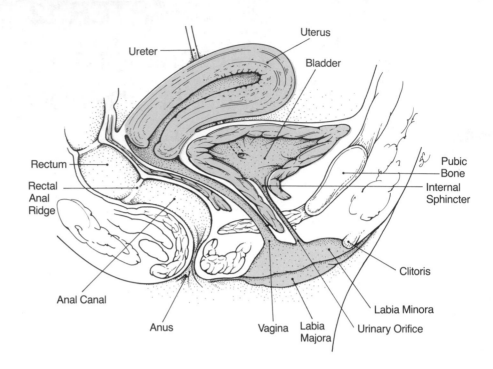

Ureter

Uterus

Bladder

Rectum

Pubic Bone

Rectal Anal Ridge

Internal Sphincter

Anal Canal

Clitoris

Anus

Vagina

Labia Majora

Labia Minora

Urinary Orifice

Male genitourinary system.

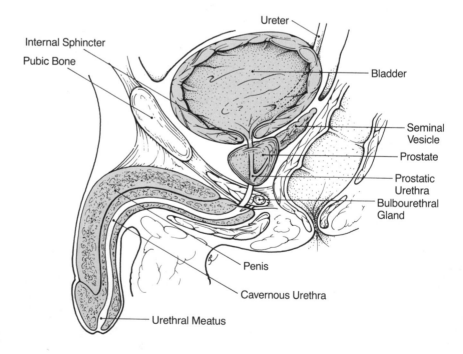

Internal Sphincter

Pubic Bone

Ureter

Bladder

Seminal Vesicle

Prostate

Prostatic Urethra

Bulbourethral Gland

Penis

Cavernous Urethra

Urethral Meatus

to the symphysis pubis. In a female, however, the bladder is anterior to the vagina and the neck of the uterus. In a male the bladder is anterior to the rectum.

The urethra, bladder, ureters, and kidney pelves are lined with a continuous layer of mucous membrane. Because there is no break in the continuity of the lining, bacteria introduced into the normally sterile system can spread rapidly throughout the tract. When the bladder is empty, the lining falls into folds which provide pockets where bacteria can multiply. Since the membrane is highly vascular, septicemia can result as these bacteria multiply.

The Production of Urine   Nephrons, the functional units of the kidneys, produce urine. Each nephron consists of a malpighian, or renal corpuscle, and a renal tubule, which is surrounded by a capillary bed. Each kidney has approximately a million nephrons.

Urine formed in the renal tubule enters a collecting duct. The collecting ducts from a number of nephrons attach to a single, larger collecting duct, which empties urine into the kidney calyx through a papilla. The urine collects in the renal pelvis until enough accumulates to flow into the bladder. If movement of urine from the pelvis is interrupted, infection or formation of calculi may occur.

Filtration of blood plasma occurs within the renal corpuscle. Two arterioles circulate blood to and from a capillary network called the glomerulus. Because the inlet to the glomerulus is larger than the outlet, hydrostatic pressure in the capillary network is higher than the pressure in other capillaries of the body. This high pressure causes filtration to occur.

Alterations in pressure change the rate of filtration. The afferent and efferent arterioles control the flow of blood and maintain the appropriate pressure in the glomerulus by constricting and dilating. Other factors that influence the rate of filtration from the glomerulus are the plasma colloidal osmotic pressure and the pressure in the Bowman's capsule into which the filtrate passes.

Due to the pressure in the glomerulus, certain substances are filtered from the blood through the capillary walls into the Bowman's capsule, which surrounds the glomerulus. These substances, which include water, amino acids, electrolytes, glucose, and waste products, form a filtrate that closely resembles blood plasma. This filtrate leaves the Bowman's capsule through the renal tubule.

The renal tubule is comprised of three parts: the proximal convoluted tubule, the loop of Henle, and the distal convoluted tubule. As the filtrate traverses the tubule, some substances are removed through mechanisms such as active transport and osmosis. Other substances are added to the filtrate through excretion. (A summary of the functions of the segments of a tubule appears in Table 1.)

The process of urine formation in all the nephrons of both kidneys reduces 120 ml of filtrate produced each minute to 1 ml of urine. The average daily urine output is, therefore, about 1500 ml. Alterations in the rate of filtration, the filtrate, or functions of the tubule may result in changes in the volume of urine or its constituents.

TABLE 1 TUBULAR ALTERATIONS OF FILTRATE

Proximal tubule and descending limb	Obligatory water reabsorption, which accounts for about 80% of the absorption of water, occurs in the proximal tube and descending limb. Glucose, amino acids, vitamins, and sodium are actively reabsorbed. Chloride, sulfate, phosphate ions, and urea are passively reabsorbed. Bicarbonate is actively reabsorbed in relation to systemic pH. Water is reabsorbed with these substances, leaving the filtrate osmotic pressure unchanged.
Loop of Henle	Sodium is actively transported from the filtrate in the ascending limb into the medullary interstitial fluid, thus raising its osmotic pressure. This rising pressure causes more water to be reabsorbed from the descending limb and the collecting duct and results in the concentration of the urine.
Distal tubule and collecting ducts	Facultative or optional reabsorption of water, which accounts for about 10% to 15% of the absorption of water, occurs in the distal tubule and collecting ducts. Sodium is actively reabsorbed in exchange for secreted potassium or hydrogen. As water continues to be reabsorbed, the filtrate becomes more concentrated and its volume is greatly reduced.

MICTURITION

Micturition is a reflex act which occurs in response to pressure changes within the bladder. When urine begins to collect, the muscular walls of the bladder are relaxed, with little change in pressure. After about 300 ml of urine accumulate, the bladder walls tighten, and pressure increases. This rising pressure stimulates receptors in the bladder wall, which send impulses to the spinal cord. After 400 to 500 ml of urine are collected, the bladder walls contract and the internal sphincter relaxes, causing a sense of urgency to void. When urine enters the urethra, the external sphincter relaxes and voiding occurs.

Micturition can occur sooner if the tone of the bladder is increased, because of such factors as emotional stress or infection. Micturition can be delayed by voluntary contraction of the external sphincter or voluntary relaxation of the perineum and contraction of the abdominal muscle. Once the volume of urine reaches about 700 ml, however, most individuals lose their ability to prolong micturition.

If an individual is unable to void, as much as 1000 ml of urine can accumulate in the bladder. When a large volume of urine is retained, the bladder's lining and blood vessels can be damaged from the increased stretching and pressure. When this happens, an individual experiences pain, restlessness, chilling, flushing, headache, diaphoresis, and a rise in blood pressure.

ALTERATIONS IN URINARY ELIMINATION

Alterations in urinary elimination can result from changes in the intake and output of fluids, obstructions to the flow of urine, changes in the secretion of the antidiuretic hormone (ADH), and changes in blood volume.

Alterations in the Intake and Output of Fluids   The average person takes in approximately 2600 ml of fluid each day: 1200 ml from drinking, 1100 ml from the water content of food, and 300 ml from changes in metabolism. An increase or decrease in fluid intake will result in a parallel increase or decrease in urine output.

Healthy individuals rarely experience decreases in urine output because they take in more fluids whenever they're thirsty. Individuals who are ill, however, often experience decreases in urine output because they are unable to respond to the thirst response, their intake is limited due to testing that requires n.p.o. preparations, or their IV fluid intake is not properly maintained.

Fluid is lost from the body not only from urine, but also through respiration, perspiration, and feces. On a daily basis, most individuals lose approximately 2400 ml of fluid: 1500 ml through urine output, 200 ml through respiration, 600 ml through perspiration, and 100 ml through the elimination of feces. Individuals who are ill may also lose fluids through vomiting, bleeding, wound drainage, and secretions.

Alterations Caused by Obstructions   A decrease in the output of urine may also be caused by an obstruction to the flow of urine from the bladder. If the obstruction is large enough, the bladder will not empty completely. Instead, it will retain fluid and, over a period of time, become distended. Individuals who have obstructions in the urinary tract experience the need to void more frequently. When they do void, however, they eliminate only very small amounts of urine.

Alterations Caused by Changes in the Secretion of the Antidiuretic Hormone
Changes in the rate of secretion of ADH also alter urine output since this hormone controls the amount of water that is reabsorbed in the distal renal tubules and collecting ducts. Common factors that increase the secretion of ADH and reduce urine output include emotional stress, accidental or surgical trauma, pain, hemorrhage, anesthesia, and drugs such as morphine and barbiturates. Factors that reduce the secretion of ADH and thus increase urine output include alcohol, caffeine, cold, and increased carbon dioxide in the blood.

Alterations Caused by Changes in Blood Volume   Because the production of urine is influenced by the volume of blood filtrate, decreases in this filtrate lead to reductions in the output of urine. Hemorrhage, severe dehydration, and shock reduce the flow of blood through the glomeruli and cause decreases in the filtrate. If the volume of the filtrate is reduced substantially, severe oliguria, or even anuria, may occur.

Other factors that may increase or decrease the output of urine include pathophysiologic states of the kidneys or other body systems, drugs, treatment modalities, diet, and metabolic rate.

▶ Urine output that is less than 30 ml per hour is a sign of potential renal failure.

403

GUIDELINES FOR MANAGING CLIENTS

The primary purpose for performing nursing interventions associated with urinary elimination is to maintain the integrity of the urinary system, which allows the body to eliminate toxic waste products, and thereby promote homeostasis.

Scrupulous aseptic techniques during catheter insertion prevents bladder infection.

- Hand washing before and after caring for clients reduces cross contamination.
- Maintaining a sterile closed urinary collection system decreases the risk of ascending contamination to bladder.
- Utilizing aseptic technique prevents contamination when opening a closed system for clot removal.
- Securing catheters to the skin minimizes to-and-fro motion.
- Maintaining urine collection bag below the level of the bladder prevents retrograde flow of urine to the bladder.
- Reviewing the chapter on Alterations in Fluid and Electrolytes provides the conceptual and practical basis for interventions associated with alterations in urinary elimination.

Rationale for Action
- To help clients void when they are unable to ambulate
- To obtain a nonsterile urine specimen for laboratory studies

ACTION: PROVIDING A BEDPAN AND URINAL

ASSESSMENT

1 Determine client's usual voiding pattern.
2 Assess client's ability to assist with the procedure.

PLANNING

GOALS

- Client voids 200 to 500 ml of urine without discomfort or difficulty

EQUIPMENT

- Bedpan or urinal
- Toilet tissues

INTERVENTION: Placing a Bedpan and Urinal

1 Provide privacy.
2 Elevate the head of the bed, or position client on the edge of the bed or in a chair.
3 Warm a metal bedpan or urinal by running warm water around the insides of the receptacle.
4 Instruct the client to sit on the bedpan or urinal. If the client needs assistance, follow these steps:

Using a bedpan

a Raise the client's hips and slip your arm under the client or turn the client on his or her side. Roll the client onto the pan.

b Place a rolled towel or blanket under the client's sacrum.

Using a urinal

a Place the base of the urinal flat on the bed between the client's thighs.

b Position the client's penis into the urinal.

5 Place the signal light and toilet tissue within easy reach.

6 When the client has voided, remove the receptacle and assist with wiping as necessary.

7 Provide an opportunity for the client to wash his or her hands.

8 Reposition the client for comfort.

EVALUATION

EXPECTED OUTCOME

1 Client voids 200 to 500 ml of urine without discomfort or difficulty. *If not*, follow these alternative nursing actions:

ANA: Inquire as to what techniques the client uses to stimulate voiding.

ANA: Use any of the following techniques to stimulate voiding:

- Run water.
- Stroke client's abdomen, and thighs.
- Push downward on the abdomen.
- Massage the lower abdomen.
- Place a hot water bottle on the abdomen.
- Pour warm water over the perineum.
- Give client a Sitz bath.
- Apply cold to the lower abdomen.
- Place a cotton ball, saturated with ammonia, in the bedpan or urinal.
- Place client's hands in water.

ANA: Assess for bladder distention.

ANA: Assess for signs of urinary tract infection.

ANA: Notify physician and obtain order for catheterization.

UNEXPECTED OUTCOME

Client is unable to turn and has difficulty raising hips.

ANA: Use a fracture pan rather than a bedpan. Powder the fracture pan. Insert the fracture pan with the flat side under the client's buttocks.

ACTION: COLLECTING AND EVALUATING URINE SPECIMENS

ASSESSMENT

1 Assess client's ability to understand instructions and to obtain specimens properly.

▶ **Clinical Manifestations of·Urinary Tract Infection**

- Frequency and urgency when voiding
- Dysuria
- Cloudy urine with or without sediment
- Hematuria
- Elevated temperature
- Flank pain

Charting

- Amount, color, appearance, and odor of urine
- Techniques effective in stimulating voiding

Rationale for Action

- To obtain a clean (nonsterile) urine specimen for diagnostic laboratory studies that include culture and sensitivity tests
- To obtain a urine specimen that is free of contamination when the client is unable to control the act of micturition because of age or physical disability
- To prevent urinary infection by obtaining a urine specimen without interrupting a closed urinary drainage system
- To determine the specific microorganism causing a urinary tract infection
- To obtain a urine specimen for use in a diagnostic urinary workup i.e., glucose, acetone, blood and specific gravity
- To obtain urine specimen for routine hospital admission or as a preoperative urine sample
- To provide a method for ensuring collection of all urine when a 24-hour urine collection is ordered

▶ Contaminated specimen is the single most common reason for inaccurate reporting on urinary cultures and sensitivities

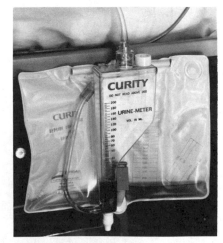

Calibrated drainage bag for a closed urinary drainage system.

2 Determine the purpose for which the specimen is being obtained.
3 Identify the best method for obtaining the specimen.
4 Assess parents' understanding of the purpose for the procedure.
5 Before obtaining a receptacle, determine the type of specimen needed: sterile specimens for culture and sensitivity tests; clean specimens for urinalysis.
6 Check to see if the closed urinary system has a port for obtaining a specimen.

PLANNING

GOALS

- Midstream urine specimen provides noncontaminated specimen.
- Noncontaminated urine specimen obtained from the closed urinary drainage system.
- Urine specimen accurately reflects microbial population in bladder urine without contamination of the specimen.

EQUIPMENT

- Cleaning swab and alcohol or bactericidal soap
- Sterile specimen container
- Label for container

ADDITIONAL EQUIPMENT

For Closed Drainage System
- Syringe with 25-gauge needle
- Sterile specimen container
- Antimicrobial swab

For Infant or Child Specimen
- Cleansing solution
- Towel
- Restraints
- Pediatric urine collector
- Diaper
- Appropriate specimen containers

INTERVENTION: Collecting Midstream Urine Specimens

1 Instruct client to clean his or her urinary meatus.
For a male:
  a Wash hands.
  b Cleanse end of penis with cleaning swab.
  c Initiate urine stream.
  d After single stream achieved, pass specimen bottle into stream and obtain urine sample.

For a female:

a Wash hands.

b Spread labia minora with nondominant hand.

c Cleanse vulvar area with disinfectant swab, beginning above the urethral oriface and moving posteriorly.

d Initiate urine stream. Keep stationary, holding labia open *throughout* the voiding process.

e After single stream achieved, pass specimen bottle into the stream and obtain sample.

2 To prevent contamination of specimen with skin flora, instruct the client to remove the bottle *before* the flow of urine stops and *before* releasing the labia or penis.

3 Label the specimen and take it to the laboratory within 15 minutes. If this is not possible, refrigerate the specimen.

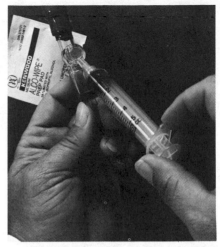

Needle is inserted at aspiration port to withdraw urine specimen from closed drainage system.

INTERVENTION: Collecting a Urine Specimen from a Closed Urinary Drainage System

1 Identify correct client by checking name on identaband.

2 Explain the procedure and the rationale for the procedure to the client.

3 Assemble all equipment.

4 Wash your hands.

5 Wipe the aspiration port of the drainage tubing with the antimicrobial swab.

6 Insert the needle into the aspiration port. Allow urine to accumulate in the tubing. (2 ml of urine is sufficient for a specimen.)

7 Aspirate the urine sample by gently pulling back on the syringe plunger, and then remove the needle.

8 Wipe the aspiration port with the antimicrobial swab.

9 Empty the syringe into the sterile urine container. (Sometimes the urine is sent to the laboratory in the syringe.)

10 Label the container and take it to the laboratory within 15 minutes. If this is not possible, refrigerate the specimen.

Place a pediatric urine collector over child's perineum for urine collection.

INTERVENTION: Collecting a Specimen from Infant or Child

1 Cleanse and dry child's perineum.

2 Remove paper backing from adhesive on urine collector.

3 Apply urine collector to child's perineum, avoiding extension over anus to prevent contamination.

a *Male*: Place opening of the collector over the child's penis and scrotum.

b *Female*: Place the opening of the collector over the child's urinary meatus.

4 Place a diaper on the child to help hold the collector in place.

5 Restrain an active child, if necessary.

6 Check the collector every 15 minutes until a specimen is obtained.

7 Remove the collector and place a clean diaper on the child.

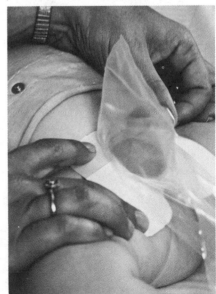

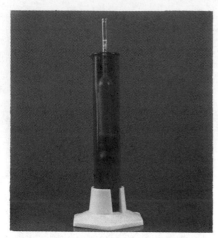

Equipment for measuring specific gravity includes a cylinder and urinometer.

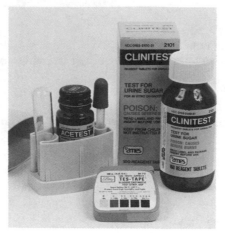

The Clinitest and Tes-Tape are used to evaluate glucose concentration in the urine; Acetest is used to evaluate acetone level in the urine.

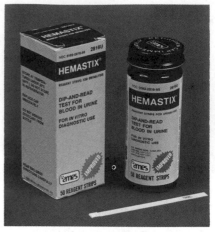

Hemastix is an in vitro diagnostic test for determining blood in the urine.

INTERVENTION: Monitoring Specific Gravity

1 Obtain fresh urine specimen.
2 Fill cylinder with 20 to 30 cc of urine (about three-fourths full).
3 Place cylinder on a flat surface.
4 Place urinometer into cylinder and spin with your fingers so the urinometer floats free and does not touch the side of the cylinder.
5 Take the reading just before the spinning stops by checking the upper curved portion of the urine level to the scale on the urinometer. The scale measures from 0.000 to 0.040.
6 Empty and wash cylinder, and rinse urinometer with water.
7 Document findings in nurses' notes or on urine flow sheet.

EVALUATION

EXPECTED OUTCOMES

1 Noncontaminated urine specimen obtained. *If not*, follow these alternative nursing actions:
   ANA: Teach the client the proper techniques for obtaining a specimen. If the client is unable to cooperate, you must perform the procedure for him or her.
   ANA: Assess the need for an alternate intervention to obtain urine specimen, e.g., catheterization.
   ANA: Repeat procedure.
   ANA: Teach a family member how to help you obtain a specimen.
2 Noncontaminated urine specimen is obtained from the closed urinary drainage system. *If not*, follow these alternative nursing actions:
   ANA: Instruct nursing personnel in how to obtain a urine specimen maintaining sterility.

ANA: Obtain a new urine specimen and send it to the laboratory.

ANA: Do not keep the urine specimen longer than 15 minutes without refrigeration.

UNEXPECTED OUTCOMES

1 Infection in urinary tract occurs.

ANA: Verify that the urinary drainage system is being maintained properly and has not been opened.

ANA: Notify physician of clinical manifestations of urinary tract infection.

ANA: Maintain schedule of antibiotic medications to ensure therapeutic blood levels.

2 Bacteremia develops secondary to urinary tract infection.

ANA: Administer antibiotics as ordered.

ANA: Encourage client to force fluids to flush out bladder.

ANA: Obtain frequent vital signs and physical assessment data.

ANA: Based on client's need, follow treatment modalities for specific nursing interventions.

3 Infant specimen is lost because collector does not adhere or is the wrong size.

ANA: Obtain a new collection bag and repeat the procedure.

ANA: Obtain appropriate size bag and repeat the procedure.

4 Specimen cannot be obtained with a collection bag.

ANA: Obtain an order for catheterization. (Catheterized specimen may be obtained only if absolutely necessary for diagnostic studies.)

Charting

- Method used to obtain specimen
- Color, consistency, and odor of urine
- Amount of urine obtained (Record this amount on the intake and output record also.)
- Type of specimen obtained
- Mode of obtaining specimen from port
- Time of urine collection
- Time specimen sent to laboratory

ACTION: COMPLETING URINARY CATHETERIZATION

ASSESSMENT

1 Determine how catheterization will be accomplished.
2 Assess the client's bladder for distention.
3 Assess the client's physical ability to cooperate with positioning.

PLANNING

GOALS

- Client catheterized without difficulty.
- Sterile urine specimen obtained.

EQUIPMENT

- Disposable catheter kit with appropriate size catheter (size 8 to 10 French for child, size 14 to 16 French for adult female, and size 18 to 20 French for adult male)
- Closed drainage set, if placing an indwelling catheter
- Betadine solution
- Additional lighting

Rationale for Action

- To prevent or relieve bladder distention
- To promote urinary elimination
- To obtain a sterile urine specimen
- To obtain accurate measurements of the bladder function
- To provide continual urinary bladder drainage
- To instill medication
- To measure the amount of residual urine
- To monitor the output of a critically ill client
- To facilitate studies of the urinary system
- To prevent skin breakdown in incontinent, bedridden clients

409

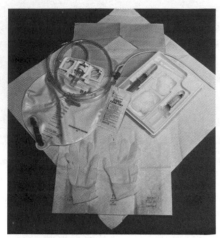

Disposable catheter kit includes necessary equipment for performing a catheterization.

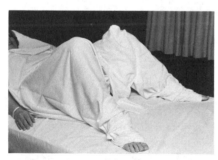

After washing perineum, place client in lithotomy position and drape as illustrated.

INTERVENTION: Inserting a Foley Catheter

1 Assemble equipment.
2 Identify client by checking identaband.
3 Explain procedure and rationale to the client.
4 Wash your hands.
5 Place the client in a dorsal-recumbent position.
6 Place an absorbent pad under buttocks.
7 Fold back top bedding to midthigh. Cover legs to decrease sense of exposure and to avoid chilling. Cover client's chest and abdomen with a blanket.
8 Give perineal care with soap and water. (This is a good time to visualize the urinary meatus if you are catheterizing a female. You may need additional lighting.)
9 Wash your hands. Open outer plastic wrap. Drape client.
10 Using aseptic techniques, assemble the equipment in the catheter kit. Use the outside wrap as the sterile field.
11 Put on sterile gloves, maintaining sterility, and place outside wrap and drape underneath the client.
12 Connect catheter to drainage bag if the catheter has not been previously connected.
13 Pour antiseptic solution over absorbent cotton balls.
14 Squeeze water soluble lubricant onto sterile surface.
15 Position fenestrated drape over the client and expose the genitalia.
16 Cleanse the client's meatus:
    For a female:
    a Separate the client's labia minora with your nondominant hand.
    b With your dominant hand, *use forceps* to pick up an absorbent ball that has been saturated with antiseptic solution.
    c Cleanse the client's meatus with one downward stroke of the forceps. Discard the absorbent ball.
    d Repeat step C at least three to four times.
    e Continue to hold the client's labia apart until you insert the catheter.

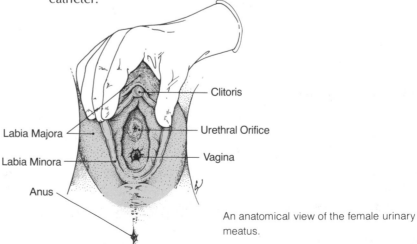

An anatomical view of the female urinary meatus.

For a male:

   a Hold the client's penis upright with your nondominant hand. Hold the sides of the penis to prevent closing the urethra.

   b With your dominant hand, *use forceps* to pick up an absorbent cotton ball that has been saturated with antiseptic solution.

   c Cleanse the client's meatus with one downward stroke of the forceps. Discard the absorbent ball.

   d Repeat step C at least three to four times.

   e Continue to hold the penis until you insert the catheter.

17 Discard the forceps.

18 With your sterile gloved hand, lubricate the catheter tip.

19 Guide the catheter gently through the urethra until the urine begins to drain. (Insert the indwelling catheter 5 cm beyond the point at which urine begins to flow.)

20 Inflate the retention balloon by releasing the clamp on the prefilled balloon at the drainage end of the catheter. (If the catheter does not have this automatic feature, inject the entire contents of the pre-filled syringe into the side arm of the catheter used for balloon inflation.)

21 Retract the catheter until you feel resistance. Release pressure.

22 Tape the catheter with one-inch tape.
For a female: Tape the catheter to the side of the leg.
For a male: Tape the catheter to the abdomen to prevent pressure on the penoscrotal angle.

23 If placing an indwelling catheter, attach drainage bag to bed frame.

24 If obtaining a specimen by straight catheterization, collect the specimen in a sterile container before removing the catheter.

25 Cleanse the client's perineum of the Betadine solution.

26 Reposition the client for comfort.

27 Remove all equipment and discard disposable trash.

28 Wash your hands.

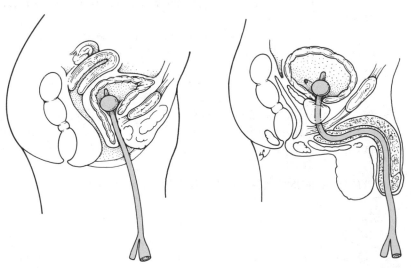

Foley catheter placement is maintained for both males and females with inflated retention balloon.

EVALUATION

EXPECTED OUTCOMES

Client catheterized without difficulty and sterile urine specimen obtained. *If not*, follow these alternative nursing actions:

ANA: For a male:
- Hold penis vertical to client's body.
- Insert catheter while applying slight traction by gently pulling upward on the shaft of the penis.
- If you encounter resistance, rotate the catheter, increase the traction, and change the angle of the penis slightly.
- When urine begins to flow, lower the client's penis.

ANA: For a female:
- Place the client in a lithotomy position.
- Ask the client to hold her legs apart so that you will have better access to the urethral meatus.
- Before cleansing the client, identify the area of the urethral meatus.
- Repeat the catheterization procedure using a new catheter kit or new gloves and a new catheter if the kit has not been contaminated.

UNEXPECTED OUTCOMES

1 Catheter is inserted in the vagina of a female client.
ANA: Follow these steps:
- Leave the catheter in place until a new, sterile catheter is inserted in the urinary meatus.
- Reposition the client if needed and locate her urethral meatus.
- Obtain a new catheter and new gloves if the catheter kit has been contaminated.
- Locate the client's urinary meatus before inserting the catheter.
- Repeat the catheterization procedure.

2 Catheter is contaminated when inserted.
ANA: Obtain a new catheter and repeat the catheterization procedure.
ANA: If the sterile field has been contaminated, obtain a new catheter kit. Repeat the catheterization procedure.

3 Catheter comes out with bag still inflated.
ANA: Notify physician and obtain an order for a Foley catheter with a 30-cc bag.
ANA: Assess client for signs of urethral trauma, e.g., bleeding, pain.
ANA: Obtain a new catheter and repeat the catheterization procedure.

ACTION: ADMINISTERING SUPRAPUBIC CATHETER CARE

ASSESSMENT

1 Observe for urine flow through catheter.
2 Observe for excessive bleeding through catheter or at insertion site.

Charting
- Type of catheterization
- Amount, color, and odor of urine obtained
- Size of catheter used
- Client's tolerance of procedure

3 Check suture site to make sure it is clean, dry, and intact.

4 Check to make sure straight drainage is maintained.

5 Determine if client is maintaining an intake of at least 2000 ml of fluid daily.

6 Assess client for pain or bladder distention.

PLANNING

GOALS

- Catheter remains patent; bladder drains completely.
- Client voids spontaneously after routine clamping procedure.
- Client remains free of infection.

EQUIPMENT

- Closed drainage system, including Foley catheter, tubing and bag
- Catheter clamp
- Dry sterile dressing and tape if ordered

INTERVENTION: Providing Suprapubic Catheter Care

1 Observe client for urinary drainage.
  a First 24 hours: Check the client every hour to detect early signs of an obstruction.
  b Second day: Check the client every eight hours.
  c Third day: Check the client when the catheter is unclamped.

2 Maintain a closed drainage system.

3 Keep the dressing dry around the site of insertion. Apply a new dressing every morning.

4 Monitor clamping protocol after the third postoperative day according to physician's orders.
  a Explain the clamping procedure and ask the client to help you monitor the clamping.

Rationale for Action

- To decrease urinary tract infections after genitourinary surgery
- To provide urinary elimination when urinary tract obstruction prevents elimination from bladder and/or urethra
- To promote early spontaneous voiding after surgery

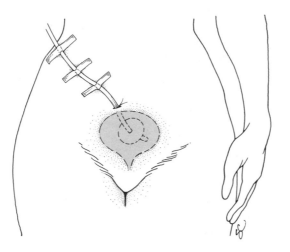

Placement of a suprapubic catheter, which is connected to a closed urinary drainage system.

413

b Instruct client to notify you if he or she feels fullness in the bladder during clamping.
c Clamp the catheter for three to four hours, depending on client's level of discomfort.
d Ask the client to attempt to void while catheter is clamped.
e After client voids, open the collection tube clamp and collect the the residual urine for five minutes.
f Empty the drainage bag and record the amount of urine obtained, both the residual urine and the voided urine.
g Send a urine specimen to laboratory after the first clamping.
5 Continue clamping protocol every three to four hours. (For the first few days the catheter may be open to drainage from bedtime until six in the morning.)
6 When the client is voiding normally, clamp throughout the night in preparation for removal of the catheter.
7 When the client's residual output is less than 100 ml in two successive checks, notify the physician for removal of the catheter.
8 Dispose of the catheter after obtaining physician's order for removal.
9 Apply a bandaid or a small two- by two-inch dressing over the insertion site if ordered by physician.

EVALUATION

EXPECTED OUTCOMES

1 Catheter remains patent; bladder drains completely. *If not*, follow these alternative nursing actions:
   ANA: Obtain order for irrigating suprapubic catheter.
2 Client voids spontaneously after routine clamping procedure. *If not*, follow these alternative nursing actions:
   ANA: Continue to follow protocol for clamping until client is able to void spontaneously.
   ANA: Keep physician informed of client's inability to void spontaneously.
3 Client remains free of infection. *If not*, follow these alternative nursing actions:
   ANA: Monitor client for clinical manifestations of urinary tract infection including elevated temperature, cloudy, foul-smelling urine with sediment present and bladder spasms.
   ANA: Inform physician of possible urinary tract infection and obtain order for urinary antibiotic.
   ANA: Force fluids to at least 2000 ml per day unless contraindicated by diagnosis. Give cranberry juice or fluids high in ascorbic acid.
   ANA: Clarify physician's order for protocol regarding clamping catheter or keeping the catheter open to straight drainage.

UNEXPECTED OUTCOME

Suprapubic catheter was not sutured in place and becomes dislodged.
ANA: Place sterile dressing over puncture site. Do not attempt to replace the catheter.

ANA: Notify physician immediately.

ANA: Have new suprapubic catheter ready for insertion.

ACTION: IRRIGATING AND INSTILLATING MEDICATIONS IN THE BLADDER

ASSESSMENT

1 Determine presence of active bleeding, i.e., dense, dark red drainage.
2 Note rate of urine flow from bladder.
3 Assess client for distended bladder.
4 Determine if client is feeling any discomfort.

PLANNING

GOALS

- Blood clots removed from client's bladder.
- Medications instilled easily into client's bladder.

EQUIPMENT

- Irrigation set (A new set needed for each irrigation.)
- Sterile gloves
- Sterile normal saline irrigant (or solution as ordered)
- Absorbent pad
- Sterile tube plug

ADDITIONAL EQUIPMENT

For Instilling Medications Through a Closed Urinary System
- Syringe with Luer-Lok and 25-gauge needle
- Alcohol or Betadine solution and swabs
- Appropriate medication for irrigation or instillation
- Clamp for catheter tubing if clamp is not a normal component of urinary drainage system

For Continuous Bladder Irrigation
- Irrigating solution
- Tubing

INTERVENTION: Irrigating by Interrupting a Closed Urinary System

1 Assemble equipment tray.
2 Check client's ID band.
3 Explain procedure and rationale to client.
4 Wash your hands.
5 Place client in a comfortable position. The dorsal-recumbent position is the most convenient if the client can tolerate this position.
6 Palpate client's bladder to check for distention.

Rationale for Action
- To remove blood clots
- To relieve bladder spasms
- To instill medication
- To ensure patency of drainage system

7   Open tray on the overbed table. Maintain the sterility of the inside cover of the tray.
8   Place an absorbent pad below the end of the catheter to form a working field.
9   Pour irrigant into solution container.
10 Place syringe in container. Do not contaminate the syringe tip.
11 Place catch basin on pad to form the working field. (Always keep syringe tip and irrigant uncontaminated.)
12 Swab the catheter drainage tube junction with an alcohol sponge.
13 Put on gloves (as soon as tubing is touched, gloves are contaminated).
14 Disconnect catheter from drainage tube and place sterile protective cap over the end of the drainage tube.
15 Place catheter over the edge of the catch basin. Do not allow end of catheter to contact covers, underpad, exposed skin surfaces, or drainage tube.
16 Instill 30 to 50 ml of irrigant into the client's bladder with gentle but firm pressure. Aspirate irrigant from bladder.
17 Remove the protective top from the drainage tube and wipe it with an alcohol sponge.
18 Wipe the catheter with an alcohol sponge.
19 Connect the catheter to the drainage tube.
20 Ensure straight drainage from tubing to drainage bag. Curl excess tubing loosely on the bed and secure the tubing to the linen.
21 Tape catheter to the inner thigh for a female and to the abdomen for a male.
22 Remove and discard equipment.
23 Make sure the client is clean and comfortable. Place the call light within easy reach.
24 Subtract any irrigating solution still remaining in the urinary drainage system from the client's intake and output record.

INTERVENTION: Irrigating by Maintaining a Closed Urinary System

1   Follow steps 1 through 8 above.
2   Fill large Luer-Lok syringe with the amount of irrigating solution ordered.
3   Place the needle into the syringe.
4   Swab the injection port with alcohol or Betadine solution.
5   Insert the needle into the injection port.
6   Pinch off tubing leading to the bag.
7   Inject solution slowly to prevent back pressure into bladder.
8   Remove the syringe and needle from the injection port.
9   Cleanse the port with alcohol or Betadine swab.
10 Remove equipment from room.
11 Subtract any irrigating solution still remaining in urinary drainage system from client's intake and output record.

INTERVENTION: Instilling Medications through a Closed Urinary System

1 Wash your hands.
2 Assemble equipment and draw up ordered medication in syringe.
3 Scrub port site on Foley catheter tubing with alcohol or Betadine solution.
4 Clamp drainage tubing so that medication will be retained in the client's bladder.
5 Insert the needle at an angle into the injection port.
6 Instill medication slowly.
7 Withdraw the needle and cleanse the port site with an alcohol or Betadine swab.
8 Keep tubing clamped for 15 to 20 minutes.

INTERVENTION: Maintaining Continuous Bladder Irrigation

1 Obtain irrigating solution from pharmacy.
2 Connect tubing to irrigating solution container, using aseptic technique.
3 Place irrigating solution container on IV pole and prime tubing as you would prime an IV.
4 Cleanse the third lumen of the three-way indwelling catheter with an alcohol swab.
5 Connect tubing to third lumen using aseptic technique.
6 Adjust drip rate to deliver prescribed hourly rate of irrigant.
   a With clear drainage, drip rate should be approximately 40 to 60 drops per minute.

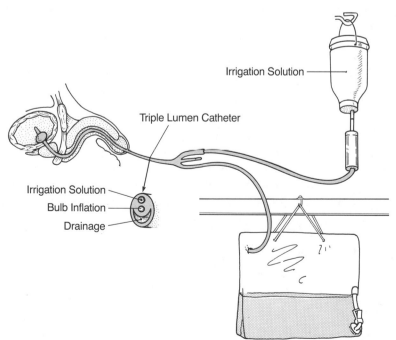

Maintaining continuous bladder irrigation requires a triple lumen catheter.

Irrigation Solution

Triple Lumen Catheter

Irrigation Solution
Bulb Inflation
Drainage

b With drainage that is bright red or contains blood clots, the drip rate should be increased to clear the drainage and flush out clots.

7 Monitor urine output to maintain patency of system.

EVALUATION

EXPECTED OUTCOMES

1 Blood clots removed from client's bladder. *If not*, follow these alternative nursing actions:

ANA: Repeat procedure as often as necessary to evacuate clots and to control bleeding.

ANA: Notify physician of excessive number of clots in the system and the need for repeated irrigations.

2 Medications instilled easily into client's bladder. *If not*, follow these alternative nursing actions:

ANA: If you feel resistance in the urinary system when you insert the syringe through the injection port, assess patency of system by observing urine flow through the system.

ANA: Assess for bladder spasms.

ANA: Irrigate client's bladder with sterile saline to determine patency of system. (A physician's order may need to be obtained before performing this procedure.)

3 Continuous flow of antibacterial solution instilled into client's bladder to prevent or to treat urinary tract infection. *If not*, follow these alternative nursing actions:

ANA: Check flow adjuster clamp to ensure it is open.

ANA: Check for kinks in tubing or client lying on tubing.

ANA: If flow of solution is obstructed, follow procedure for bladder irrigation if physician allows.

4 Continuous flow of solution maintained to evacuate clots and prevent catheter obstruction. *If not*, follow these alternative nursing actions:

ANA: Stop flow of irrigant. Irrigate catheter to reinstitute flow.

ANA: If you are unable to reinstitute flow, notify physician for further orders.

5 Maintenance of solution infusion rate, depending on reason for irrigation. *If not*, follow these alternative nursing actions:

ANA: May need to raise or lower IV standard with attached irrigation bag to assist in regulating flow using gravity.

ANA: Move the flow adjuster clamp to a new site on the tubing if flow is slower than ordered. Tubing may be collapsed due to constant pressure from clamp.

ANA: If infusion rate slows, may indicate clots are blocking flow. Irrigate catheter following physician's orders.

UNEXPECTED OUTCOMES

1 Irrigation solution is not returned because of an obstruction in the system.

ANA: Follow these steps:

- Aspirate the solution from the catheter, using moderate "pull back" pressure.
- If the irrigant does not return, palpate the client's bladder and instill 30 to 50 cc of irrigating solution to agitate and clear any clots.
- If irrigant does not return, reconnect urinary system and observe for 30 minutes. Bladder spasms can block the flow of urine through the system.
- If irrigant does not return, cleanse client's urinary meatus and the catheter tubing with Betadine solution. Gently insert the Foley catheter further into the client's bladder. If the lumen opening of the catheter is against the wall of the bladder, it will obstruct the flow of urine.
- If irrigant still does not return after performing the above procedures, notify physician for further orders.

2 Irrigation solution is not returned because of the client's pain and anxiety which causes "clamping down" and creates an obstruction in the outflow opening to the catheter.

ANA: Help client practice relaxation techniques.

ANA: Place a heating pad or warm towel over client's abdomen to ease bladder spasms.

ANA: Reposition client to reduce pressure on the catheter.

ANA: If you are still unable to obtain the irrigant, notify physician for medication to relieve client's pain and/or bladder spasms.

3 Client experiences excessive bladder spasms.

ANA: Obtain order from physician to place a heating pad on the client's abdomen.

ANA: Obtain physician's order for urinary antispasmodic.

4 Bright red drainage continues even when solution flow rate is increased.

ANA: Notify physician for orders.

ANA: Continue to infuse solution at a rapid rate to cleanse client's bladder until you obtain physician's orders.

ANA: Assess client for signs of anemia and/or significant blood loss. Take vital signs, observe capillary filling pressure, and observe mucous membranes for signs of anemia, hemorrhage or shock.

ACTION: APPLYING EXTERNAL CATHETER AND DRAINAGE SYSTEM

ASSESSMENT

1 Determine clients who are at risk for urinary tract infection but require means of preventing incontinency.
2 Assess need for providing a way to prevent incontinency in bedridden clients.
3 Assess genital area for signs of irritation and edema during use of condom catheter.
4 Assess activity level of clients to determine when leg bag or a continuous drainage system is necessary.

Charting
- Solution administered
- Rate of administration
- Description of urinary output, including color and presence of clots
- Any signs of discomfort or cramping
- Amount of actual urine output (total urine output minus amount of irrigant instilled)

Rationale for Action
- To provide a means for preventing incontinence
- To provide a means of collecting urine in a system which allows for client ambulation
- To prevent urinary tract infections in clients who are at risk but require a method of catheterization to maintain continency

419

PLANNING

GOALS

- Client remains continent
- Urinary tract infection is prevented
- Client ambulation is allowed while catheterized

EQUIPMENT

- Soap, water, towel
- Commercial condom catheter
- Leg bag or continuous drainage system
- Alcohol wipes

INTERVENTION: Applying a Condom

1 Gather equipment, condom catheter, soap, towel, and basin with warm water.
2 Explain procedure to client.
3 Wash genital area with soap and water and dry area thoroughly.
4 When commercial condom catheters are used, apply protective coating to skin on penile shaft and allow to dry completely (30 seconds).
5 Peel off paper from both sides of the adhesive liner that accompanies the commercial product.
6 Spirally wrap the adhesive liner around the penile shaft behind the glans.
7 Take the latex condom catheter and place the prerolled latex sheath so the funnel is against the glans.
8 Unroll the latex sheath up the penis until it is completely over the adhesive liner.
9 Gently squeeze the condom against the liner to seal it after the sheath is completely rolled over the penis. Do not wrinkle the latex as wrinkles cause urine to leak through the catheter.
10 Attach the condom to a drainage system. The drainage system can be a leg bag or a continuous drainage system depending on the activity level and condition of the client.

INTERVENTION: Attaching Catheter to Leg Bag

1 Obtain order for leg bag from physician.
2 Gather leg bag and alcohol swab.
3 Disconnect drainage tubing from indwelling or condom catheter.
4 Wipe the leg bag and catheter connectors with alcohol.
5 Connect the tip of the leg bag into the catheter.
6 Place the cap from the leg bag tip on the collection tubing.
7 Secure the leg bag to the lower leg by placing the rubber strap through the bag and around the leg. Secure the strap by placing the button through the opening in the strap.

8 When removing leg bag, disconnect the catheter from the leg bag and wipe each connection end with alcohol wipes.

9 Take the leg bag cap off the drainage tubing and replace it on the leg bag.

10 Connect the catheter to the drainage tubing.

EVALUATION

EXPECTED OUTCOMES

1 Urinary tract infection prevented. *If not*, follow these alternative nursing actions:

ANA: Obtain physician's order for and collect clean catch specimen if signs of urinary tract infection.

2 Client remains continent. *If not*, follow these alternative nursing actions:

ANA: Reassess method used for applying condom to ensure tight fit.

ANA: Assess need for smaller catheter size.

3 Genital area remains free of inflammation. *If not*, follow these alternative nursing actions.

ANA: Remove condom catheter as much as possible and allow air to reach penile shaft.

ANA: Apply external padding and keep penis free from use of catheters until irritation has cleared.

UNEXPECTED OUTCOMES

1 Incontinency continues even with use of condom catheter.

ANA: Assess method used for applying condom.

ANA: Improvise ways in which catheter can be placed to provide wrinkle-free application

2 Condom catheter falls off.

ANA: Use additional method of adhesion, such as tincture of benzoin evenly spread around penile shaft.

ANA: Assess need for a smaller size condom catheter (pediatric size may be indicated for adult client).

Charting
- Condom catheter applied
- Size of catheter used
- Condition of genital area
- Type of protective coating applied to skin
- Whether catheter connected to leg bag or continuous drainage
- Amount, color, and odor of urine obtained
- Client's tolerance of procedure

ACTION: CARING FOR CLIENT WITH A URINARY DIVERSION

Rationale for Action
- To provide a pouching system that prevents an erythematous and excoriated skin surface
  To assist the client in learning self-care of the urinary diversion
  To assist the client in working through an altered body image
  To promote urinary drainage through sterile catheterization techniques

ASSESSMENT

1 Assess the location of the stoma on the client's abdomen. Check abdomen for creasing, firmness, softness, contour, scars, folds, and incisions.

2 Identify whether client has had ileal or sigmoid conduit urinary diversion.

3 Observe stoma color. The color should be the same as the mucous membrane lining the mouth. A pale stoma may indicate anemia. A dark-to-dusky color may indicate interference with blood supply to stoma.

4 Assess the client's mental alertness and ability to learn.
5 Assess skin for erythema, and excoriation before deciding the necessity of using a skin barrier.
6 Listen for bowel sounds.
7 Before deciding which type of pouching system to use, consider the client's age, manual dexterity, size of stoma, and availability of pouches at health facility.
8 Recognize need to collect sterile urine specimens to monitor urinary tract for infection.

PLANNING

GOALS

- Client accepts need for urinary diversion and strives toward acceptance.
- Client demonstrates proficiency in management of urinary diversion.
- Peristomal skin is clean and intact.
- Urine is collected in pouch system keeping client dry.

EQUIPMENT

- Sterile drape
- Sterile gloves
- Sterile lubricant
- #14 Robinson or Foley catheter
- Prep solution
- Sterile saline or water
- Underpad
- Sterile specimen container with label
- New urinary pouch
- Supplies to apply new pouch
- Plastic bag for used supplies

ADDITIONAL EQUIPMENT

For Application of Urinary Pouch
- Clean postoperative pouch with spigot at bottom to empty urine
- Night drainage bag
- Items to clean stoma, e.g., soft cloth or gauze sponges
- Plastic bag for disposal of used equipment
- Tissue for drying skin
- Tissue or tampon for wicking stoma
- Underpad to protect bedding from leakage
- Scissors with sharp point
- Protective barriers such as skin prep, skin gel, or protective barrier film (If excoriation or sensitivity is present, a skin barrier such as Stomahesive, Reliaseal, or Holliseal is needed.)
- Skin bond cement
- Stoma measuring guide
- Micropore or dermicel tape

INTERVENTION: Using a Catheter to Obtain a Specimen from an Ileal Conduit

1 Place sterile drapes.
2 Put on gloves.
3 Apply lubricant to catheter.
4 Prep stoma with solution and then rinse.
5 Remove top from specimen container and place end of catheter into container.
6 Insert tip of catheter into stoma 5 to 7 cm.
7 When flow of urine completed (usually not more than 20 to 40 cc), clamp catheter with fingers and remove.
8 Return lid to specimen container, apply label, and send to lab.
9 Remove completely any residual prep solution and lubricant.
10 Continue with pouching procedure.

INTERVENTION: Applying a Urinary Diversion Pouch

1 Place underpad under client.
2 Prepare new urinary pouch for application at conclusion.
3 Remove old pouch and discard in plastic bag.
4 Wash skin with warm water. If large residual of cement on skin, remove with solvent.
5 Measure stoma site with measuring guide.
6 Trace size of stoma on adhesive backing on pouch.
7 Cut panel 0.3 to 0.6 cm larger than stoma.
8 Remove paper from adhesive on pouch. Apply thin coat of skin bond cement to adhesive area. Set aside.
9 Wicking stoma with tissue or tampon, apply protective barrier to healthy skin. (If skin is excoriated, apply skin barrier. Do not use protective barriers on excoriated skin because they contain alcohol and will cause burning and pain.)
10 Let dry thoroughly.
11 Wick stoma to keep urine off skin; then apply thin coat of skin bond cement to skin.
12 Let dry thoroughly.
13 Center and apply pouch to dry skin.
14 Smooth tape to skin.
15 "Pix-frame" sides of tape with 2.5 cm tape.
16 Attach to gravity drainage bag.
17 Give client written set of instructions.

EVALUATION

EXPECTED OUTCOMES

1 Client accepts need for urinary diversion and strives toward acceptance. *If not*, follow these alternative nursing actions:
ANA: Allow client time to grieve over change in body image.
ANA: Arrange for visit with another ostomy client to demonstrate total rehabilitation.

Specific steps of stoma care for client with a urinary diversion. Steps include preparing a new urinary pouch, removing the old urinary pouch, wicking the stoma, preparing the skin and applying new pouch.

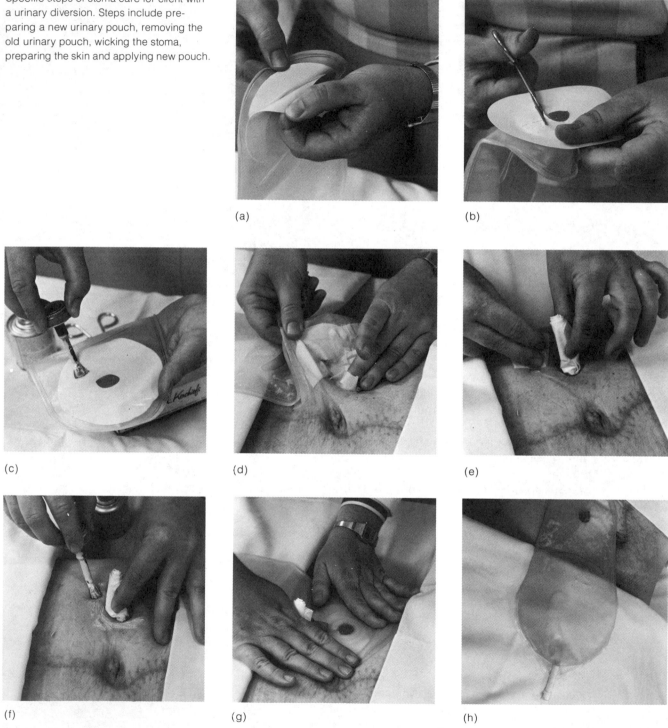

(a)

(b)

(c)

(d)

(e)

(f)

(g)

(h)

ANA: Review management with client and again stress ability to live normal life with stoma.

ANA: Refer to health care professional specializing in ostomy management.

2 Urinary tract is kept free of infection. *If not*, follow these alternative nursing actions:

ANA: Instruct client that the only way to monitor urinary tract is to obtain catheterized specimen. Any specimen taken from pouch or night drainage bag is contaminated.

ANA: Make sure any specimen that is obtained from client for urinalysis and/or culture and sensitivity is a catheterized specimen. If not, notify physician for urine culture and sensitivity order.

ANA: Check pH of urine. Acid urine is least likely to become infected. Vitamin C and cranberry juice are easy ways to keep urine acid.

ANA: Instruct client not to be concerned if urine is clouded with shreds of mucus. The intestine produces mucus which is excreted with the urine through the conduit (sigmoid conduits produce more mucus).

ANA: Encourage client to drink eight glasses of fluid per day to maintain peristaltic action of ureters, thereby preventing reflux of urine.

ANA: If more than 50 cc of urine present in the ileal conduit when catheterized, notify physician. Stasis of urine may occur due to urine being stored in conduit. (This does not act like a reservoir or bladder, but should just conduct urine to outside of body.)

3 Urine is collected in pouch system, keeping client dry. *If not*, follow these alternative nursing actions:

ANA: If leakage occurs at one site, reexamine that area for a crease or dip in skin that allows urine to pool in that area. May need to fill in area with Karaya paste to prevent pooling.

ANA: If leakage occurs along side of appliance, apply belt to minimize leakage.

ANA: If leakage is due to a flush or recessed stoma, client may need to be fitted with convex faceplate to push stoma up into pouch.

ANA: If leakage is due to dissolving of skin barrier, several changes may be necessary. Simply changing the appliance more frequently may solve problem. It also may be necessary to change skin barriers. Reliaseal is a good skin barrier because it absorbs the urine instead of being dissolved by it. Another possibility is to eliminate the skin barrier and place adhesive pouch on skin.

4 Client demonstrates proficiency in management of urinary diversion. *If not*, follow these alternative nursing actions:

ANA: Reassess pouch procedure and simplify where possible.

ANA: Include a family member when teaching pouch management so relative can assist client at home.

ANA: Refer to home health care facility for follow-up care.

ANA: Inform the client where supplies may be purchased when discharged.

5 Peristomal skin is clean and intact. *If not*, follow these alternative nursing actions:

ANA: Assess if problem is due to leakage. Reevaluate method of application or type of appliance.

ANA: Assess if problem is due to yeast sensitivity. Make sure skin is totally dry before applying pouch. To treat yeast sensitivity, apply light dusting of Mycostatin powder to dry skin before applying pouch.

ANA: Assess if problem is due to allergic dermatitis. Use a skin barrier such as Stomahesive, Holliseal or Reliaseal, and/or use a skin care salve like Sween Cream to heal and protect the skin.

ANA: Assess if problem is due to urine getting on skin or stoma. If this is the cause, pouch may need to be cut smaller so it remains only 0.3 to 0.6 cm larger than stoma. (Stoma may shrink first six months.)

UNEXPECTED OUTCOMES

1 Inability to insert catheter into conduit.

ANA: Insert catheter into stoma but do not force. At times the abdominal musculature will tighten. This will usually relax client a few seconds, allowing the catheter to slide in.

2 No urine obtained from conduit.

ANA: If the conduit is functioning correctly, there should be very little urine in it. Sometimes, rotating catheter or turning client to right side will start flow of urine. Remember only 3 to 5 cc is needed for culture and sensitivity.

3 Crystals appear on stoma.

ANA: If client is wearing reusable equipment, change to disposable appliance since crystals are usually due to poor hygiene in pouch. Apply half-strength vinegar compresses 20 minutes daily.

4 Overgrowth of rough skin around stoma.

ANA: Reassess appliance for correct size. (Usually, existing opening is too large.) Also, be sure client is connected to a bag large enough to prevent urine from backing up on stoma.

ANA: Apply a skin barrier like Stomahesive to press skin down.

ANA: Apply half-strength vinegar compresses 20 minutes daily and full-strength vinegar in pouch for 15 minutes q HS before attaching to drainage.

5 Odor in pouch.

ANA: Odor usually due to alkaline urine in pouch turning to ammonia. Client keeps urine acidic by taking vitamin C, 500 mg b.i.d. to t.i.d., and drinking cranberry juice. Other citrus juices should be avoided, as they form an alkaline ash.

ANA: Wash urinary equipment clean with mild soap and water and rinse in vinegar weekly.

ANA: Inform client that certain foods and drugs, such as asparagus and vitamin B complex, give an odor to the urine. The pouch should be emptied frequently if these substances are ingested.

ANA: Cloudy and strong odor to urine may be due to urinary tract infection. Advise physician and collect sterile urine specimen.

Charting

- Color and amount of urine obtained from catheterization
- Amount of residual urine
- Catheter size used for catheterization
- Peristomal skin condition
- Client's acceptance of stoma
- Type and method of drainage pouch applied

CHAPTER 13
Alterations in Bowel Elimination

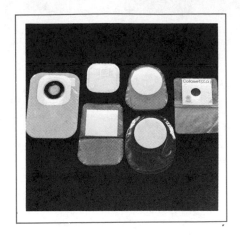

This chapter presents the conceptual basis for alterations in bowel elimination. It includes planned nursing interventions and skills necessary to promote elimination and to preserve the integrity of the integumentary system if diversionary procedures become necessary.

ANATOMY AND PHYSIOLOGY OF THE GASTROINTESTINAL SYSTEM

The gastrointestinal system converts food into products that can be used as nutrients on the cellular level and disposes of wastes incurred in the process. The primary structures in this system include the mouth, esophagus, stomach, small intestine, and large intestine.

The mouth, esophagus, and stomach are the structures of the upper gastrointestinal tract, where the process of digestion begins. The small intestine, where digestion is completed and most absorption takes place, is a 12-foot tube composed of the duodenum, jejunum, and ileum. The large intestine is made up of the cecum, colon, and rectum. The cecum contains the ileocecal valve and the appendix. The colon is divided into the ascending, transverse, descending, and sigmoid colon. The rectum extends from the sigmoid colon to the anus. The terminal inch of the rectum is called the anal canal and is guarded by the internal and external sphincter muscles. The chief functions of the colon are to reabsorb water and sodium and to store wastes.

LEARNING OBJECTIVES

List four precautions which must be carried out when obtaining stool specimens for parasite identification.

Outline the essential steps in administering a tap water or saline enema to an adult client.

Compare and contrast stoma care for an ileostomy and colostomy client.

Outline the essential steps for performing a colostomy irrigation.

State the conditions under which ostomy irrigations are contraindicated.

Explain at least 3 precautions necessary when applying a fecal ostomy pouch.

Discuss the corking and intubating procedure for clients with a continent ileostomy.

Describe the precautions necessary when performing digital stimulation to remove a fecal impaction.

Digestion is accomplished mechanically and chemically. Food is mechanically churned through the intestinal tract by sharp contractions, or peristaltic waves, of the circular and longitudinal muscles of the intestinal wall. Muscular sphincters and valves are located at strategic points throughout the intestinal tract. These structures help propel the food bolus or feces at appropriately timed intervals in a process called rhythmic segmentation. The sphincters and valves, when functioning properly, prevent reflux of contents. Peristaltic waves, coupled with rhythmic segmentation, allow maximal contact between food and the bowel wall so that chemical reactions can accomplish digestion and absorption can take place.

The chemical aspects of digestion in the small intestine begin in the duodenum with the introduction of pancreatic juices and bile. Pancreatic juices are rich in enzymes, which work to break down proteins and fats and to complete the transformation of starch to sugar. Bile, secreted by the liver, aids in the emulsification and absorption of fats. These substances work in an alkaline medium which combines with the acidity of chyme to provide a neutral pH in the duodenum, thereby protecting the duodenal mucosa.

In the 20 feet of jejunum and ileum, approximately 3000 ml of digestive enzymes are secreted. These enzymes, which are secreted by the mucus glands of the intestines, complete the digestive processing of

Anatomy of gastrointestinal tract.

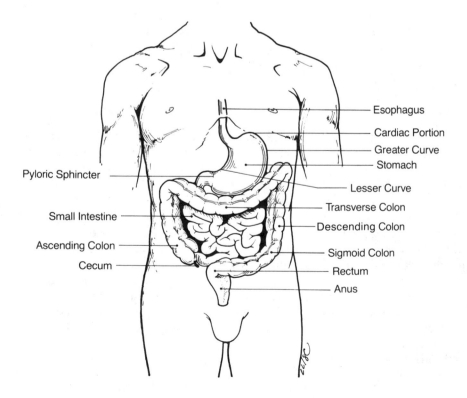

Esophagus

Cardiac Portion

Greater Curve

Stomach

Lesser Curve

Pyloric Sphincter

Transverse Colon

Small Intestine

Descending Colon

Ascending Colon

Sigmoid Colon

Cecum

Rectum

Anus

food prior to absorption. Again, the alkaline nature of these secretions works to protect the mucous membrane of the intestinal tract.

The peristaltic activity of the gastrointestinal tract, as well as its secretory functions, is governed, to a large degree, by parasympathetic and sympathetic nerve fibers. Stimulation of the parasympathetic system increases the activity of the intestinal tract, while stimulation of the sympathetic nervous system inhibits activity in the tract. The internal anal sphincter, however, is activated by sympathetic stimulation, while the external anal sphincter is under voluntary control.

Absorption, another primary function of the small bowel, is the passage of prepared materials from the gastrointestinal lumen to the blood and cells. Most absorption in the small intestine results from the churning action of the bowel. Chyme is continually exposed to the circular folds of the mucosal surface, which is lined with threadlike projections called villi. Villi serve as the sites of absorption of fluid and nutrients. The duration of contact between chyme and the mucosal surface of the bowel is very important in absorption. Hypermotility in the small intestine can result in decreased contact with the mucosal wall and deficient absorption; hypomotility can result in increased absorption of fluids as well as problems with elimination.

The circulatory system delivers nutrients to tissue cells and transports the waste products of metabolism. The small bowel and colon are supplied by the superior and inferior mesenteric arteries. Blood that contains absorbed nutrients is carried from the gastrointestinal tract by the superior and inferior mesenteric veins, which become a part of the portal system delivering blood to the liver. Each villus on the intestinal wall contains a network of small capillaries which absorb sugar and amino acids and a central lymph channel which absorbs fatty acids and glycerol. When circulation is compromised, absorption is decreased and cells are lost.

By the time chyme reaches the ileocecal valve—the junction between the small and large intestines—most nutrients have been absorbed. While three liters of fluid pass through the small bowel, only 500 ml actually pass through the ileocecal valve. The semiliquid material received by the large intestine consists of living and dead bacteria, undigested food and residue, and cell debris. As material is slowly passed along the colon by peristaltic-like mass movements, fluid is absorbed. These movements occur relatively infrequently (perhaps two or three times per day) and are stimulated by the entrance of food into the stomach by the gastrocolic reflex.

Absorption of fluid in the colon takes place primarily in the ascending and transverse colon. Fecal masses are stored in the sigmoid colon and move into the rectum with mass peristaltic movement. When the rectum fills and becomes sufficiently distended, centers in the sacral part of the spinal cord facilitate a defecation reflex which contracts the rectum and relaxes the internal and external anal sphincters. The resulting urge, facilitated by higher centers, leads to contraction of the abdominal, perineal, and diaphragmatic muscles. Willful defecation is a coordinated, learned habit. Voluntary inhibition of the act returns the stool to the sigmoid colon.

ALTERATIONS IN BOWEL ELIMINATION

By-products of digestion must be continually eliminated to maintain normal body function. Alterations in normal elimination can result from changes in motility, obstruction of the lumen of the bowel, circulatory deficiencies, and surgically-induced alterations to the structures of the intestinal tract.

Changes in Motility Motility in the gastrointestinal system is the ability to move spontaneously. Normal motility of the bowel provides peristaltic activity, which pushes and churns food and chyme through the upper tract and feces through the lower tract at timed intervals.

Hypermotility may be caused by direct stimulation or irritation of the autonomic nervous system, as well as by inflammatory processes in the gastrointestinal tract. Stimulation of parasympathetic nerves promotes peristalsis and increases bowel muscle tone. Increased peristalsis speeds the propulsion of chyme through the upper tract, resulting in deficient absorption of nutrients. When increased peristalsis speeds the propulsion of feces through the lower tract, diarrhea occurs.

Stimulation of the autonomic nervous system may be psychic in origin. Anxiety, for example, may be mediated through either parasympathetic nerves with resultant diarrhea or through sympathetic nerves with resultant constipation. The action on the parasympathetic nervous system of certain drugs may also cause hypermotility of the intestine. Antihypertensive drugs, such as reserpine, and cholinergic drugs can cause diarrhea by their stimulation of parasympathetic nerves.

Hypermotility caused by the stimulating effect of an irritant on intestinal peristalsis may arise from infectious agents, chemical agents, or inflammatory disease processes. The most common intestinal irritants are the products of certain bacteria which release toxins in the digestive tract. Chemical agents which irritate the intestinal mucosa include cytotoxic drugs, castor oil, and quinidine. Ulcerative and inflammatory disease processes include diverticulitis, tuberculous lesions, ulcerative colitis, and Crohn's disease.

Hypomotility may be caused by direct stimulation or blockage of the autonomic nervous system, intestinal muscle weakness, and chemical agents which inhibit peristalsis and induce flaccidity in the intestinal tract. Decreased peristalsis causes chyme to move sluggishly through the upper tract so that fluids are overabsorbed. Decreased peristalsis also slows the propulsion of feces through the lower tract and causes constipation, fecal impaction, and obstruction.

Stimulation or blockage of the autonomic nervous system may be congenital in origin, as is the case in Hirschsprung's disease, where the absence of parasympathetic nerve ganglia results in failure of peristalsis in the affected portion of the bowel. The effects of trauma or toxins on the autonomic innervation of the intestine, which occur with paralytic (adynamic) ileus, inhibit motility to the point of obstruction.

Intestinal muscle weakness which results from disease processes, old age, or a lack of essential vitamins (notably the B group) or electrolytes (particularly postassium) may all contribute to hypomotility. Certain drugs, such as codeine and morphine, can also cause hypomotility by relaxing the smooth muscles of the digestive tract and by increasing spasms of the intestinal sphincters.

Obstruction of the Lumen of the Bowel Obstruction of the lumen of the bowel may be partial or complete. The severity of the obstruction depends on the region of the bowel that is affected, the degree to which the lumen is occluded, and the degree to which the circulation in the bowel wall is disturbed.

A small bowel obstruction which occurs as a consequence of persistent vomiting (reverse peristalsis) can cause severe disturbances in the electrolyte balance of the body. Large bowel obstructions, even if complete, are not as dramatic, provided that the blood supply to the colon is not disturbed.

The causes of intestinal obstruction are varied. In rare instances, obstruction may result when a foreign body, such as a large fruit stone or a mass of parasitic worms, becomes lodged in the bowel. More frequently, intestinal obstructions are caused by strictures, adhesions, hernias, volvulus, intussusception, polyps, neoplasms, and fecal impactions.

The physiology of an obstruction in the lumen of the bowel is generally the same, regardless of the cause. As the lumen of the bowel is blocked, the body attempts to overcome the obstruction by increasing peristalsis. During this process, liquid feces move past the site of obstruction and cause diarrhea and increased obstruction which leads to obstipation. Within several hours peristalsis is reduced and the bowel becomes flaccid. As intraluminal pressure builds up, fluid is retained and absorption decreases. The increased intraluminal pressure then leads to the compression of the bowel wall and its capillaries, which causes necrosis of the bowel wall.

An ileostomy is a surgical opening from the ileum through the abdominal wall.

Circulatory Deficiences An adequate circulatory flow is essential for maintaining the structure of the bowel and for carrying on cellular nutrition. Any interruption of the arterial blood supply inhibits the bowel function. An occlusion of the circulatory flow, also called an intestinal infarction, results in gangrene of the bowel unless surgical intervention is carried out. A partial occlusion of the mesenteric arteries due to atherosclerosis can cause abdominal angina, a condition that occurs when the blood supply is increasingly interrupted.

Surgically-Induced Alterations in the Structure of the Bowel When alterations in bowel elimination become life-threatening and medical management fails, surgical intervention becomes necessary. Diversionary surgical procedures of the bowel include ileostomy, cecostomy, and colostomy.

An ileostomy is a surgically created opening from the ileum through the abdominal wall. The entire large intestine is bypassed and/or re-

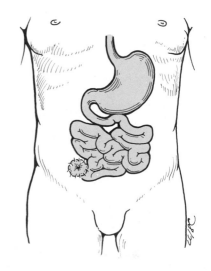

moved and the distal ileum is brought through the abdominal wall to form a stoma. The discharge from an ileostomy contains water and many digestive enzymes which have not yet been absorbed by intestinal villi. Strict attention should be paid to skin protection around the ileostomy stoma to prevent breakdown caused by the digestive enzymes.

A cecostomy is a surgically created opening from the cecum through the abdominal wall. This procedure is generally a temporary method of decompressing the bowel to relieve obstruction. Frequently, a catheter is left in the opening. This catheter requires frequent irrigation to ensure a patent lumen. If a catheter is not left in the opening, the cecostomy opening should be pouched in the same manner as an ileostomy.

A colostomy is a surgically created opening from the colon through the abdominal wall. In a colostomy the diseased portion of the colon is bypassed and/or removed and a healthy portion of colon is brought to the outside of the abdomen to form a stoma. Colostomies are named after the section of the colon surgically altered. The location of the colostomy dictates the type of drainage as well as the proper method of management.

An ascending colostomy will probably have liquid to semisoft effluent, which may flow throughout the day and night. The discharge from an ascending colostomy will contain some digestive enzymes caused by this portion of the colon's proximity to the small intestine. It will also contain a great deal of water, since much of the water-absorbing portions of the colon are bypassed. The stoma is usually located on the right lower quadrant of the abdomen. A drainable pouch with good skin protection is required for management of an ascending colostomy.

The discharge from a transverse colostomy is soft or semisolid. The stool contains water that has not yet been absorbed from the large intestine. Since the discharge from a transverse colostomy may flow periodically throughout the day and night, a drainable pouch is required. Close attention should be paid to skin protection to prevent peristomal skin from becoming waterlogged and irritated.

The discharge from a descending or sigmoid colostomy is formed and firm, since most of the water has been absorbed by the time the feces reaches these portions of the colon. The flow of output from a descending or sigmoid colostomy may be controlled by diet, the careful use of stool softeners, or colostomy irrigations. Once control has been gained, a small, closed-ended pouch may be used to cover the stoma. Not everyone with a descending or sigmoid colostomy is a candidate for regulation. A drainable pouch with appropriate skin barriers is necessary for a nonregulated descending or sigmoid colostomy.

A loop colostomy is often performed in the transverse or ascending colon to allow the remaining portion of the colon to rest before anastomosis. This type of colostomy is frequently temporary. The surgical procedure for a loop colostomy requires the surgeon to lift a loop of healthy bowel through the abdominal wall and to place a rod of some type behind the loop to stabilize the bowel on the abdomen. During the surgery or shortly afterwards, the surgeon opens the loop to allow fecal

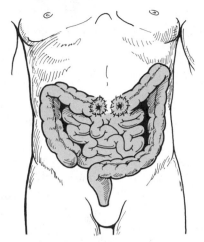

Double Barrel Colostomy

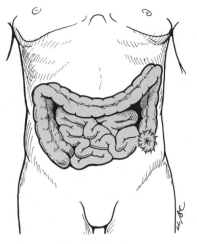

Sigmoid Colostomy

A double-barrel colostomy is a temporary procedure. A sigmoid colostomy is always permanent.

elimination. When the bowel adheres to the abdominal wall, usually five to seven days after the operation, the surgeon removes the rod.

A double-barrel colostomy, which is always temporary, is one in which there are two stomas. The proximal stoma, which connects to the rest of the digestive tract, is the functioning part of the colostomy. The distal stoma, which connects to the rectum, is the nonfunctioning part of the colostomy. The proximal stoma discharges fecal material, while the distal stoma discharges mucus.

An "end" colostomy means the rectum has been removed. This type of colostomy is always permanent and may occur anywhere along the colon, although it is usually located in the sigmoid or descending colon.

GUIDELINES FOR MANAGING CLIENTS

When diversionary surgery becomes necessary, nursing interventions are utilized to properly diagnose dysfunctions, to enhance the forward flow of flatus and feces, to relieve obstructions, and to protect the integumentary system. As you perform interventions, refer to these guidelines:

Stool specimens are tested for many substances to diagnose illness.
- Parasites, ova, bacteria, viruses, chemicals, as well as occult blood, are frequently identified.
- Bleeding from a gastric ulcer or perforation may be a slow process which can be easily detected by examining a client's stools.

The presence of flatulence indicates malfunction of the gastrointestinal system.
- Flatulence may occur after abdominal surgery, when excess air is swallowed during intubation or when liquids are sucked through a straw.
- Dietary indiscretions can lead to increased intraluminal gas production and to the development of flatulence.

433

Enema fluids are designed to be returned by normal bowel action or to be returned by the colon.

- An effective enema depends on proper administration and the type of fluid used.

Daily colostomy irrigations may be initiated for the purpose of controlling elimination.

- In a descending or sigmoid colostomy daily irrigations establish regularity with no bowel movements occurring between irrigations.
- Daily irrigations are generally not taught to clients with temporary colostomies.
- Irrigations of the colon are contraindicated if peristalsis is absent, if perforation is suspected, or if the client has an ileostomy. In these cases an irrigation may bring about severe diarrhea, which can lead to dehydration and circulatory shock.
- Keeping the stool soft with irrigations may help to manage colostomy care for the client with a stenosed stoma.

Chemical composition and consistence of effluent play a large role in the selection of skin barriers and pouches to be used in ostomy care.

- Breakdown of peristomal skin may be caused by improperly fitting pouches, leakage of stool on the skin, hair follicle irritation, misuse of skin barriers, bacterial or fungal infections, perspiration, or allergic reactions.

Rationale for Action
- To obtain stool specimens for diagnosing dysfunction in bowel elimination
- To assess for perforation or bleeding from a gastric ulcer

ACTION: COLLECTING A STOOL SPECIMEN

ASSESSMENT

1 Determine the purpose for the test and whether the specimen must be sent to the laboratory immediately.
2 Determine the eliminatory status of the client, i.e., liquid vs. formed stools, etc.

PLANNING

GOALS

- Specimen meets laboratory requirements for diagnostic testing
- Client does not experience undue discomfort or embarrassment during procedure

EQUIPMENT

- Waxed sterile cardboard container with cover
- Tongue blade
- Label for container
- Clean bedpan or bedside commode

INTERVENTION: Collecting Adult Stool Specimens

1 Explain the procedure to the client.
2 Before collecting stool specimen, ask the client to void. Tell client not to void on the specimen.
3 Clean out all urine from the bedpan or bedside commode.
4 Raise the head of the bed so that the client can assume a squatting position on the bedpan, or help client sit on the bedside commode.
5 Provide privacy until the client has passed a stool.
6 Remove the bedpan or bedside commode. If necessary, help the client clean perineum.
7 Use tongue blade to obtain and place a small portion of the formed stool in a container. (For some tests you may need to collect the entire specimen.)
8 Clean bedpan or bedside commode.
9 Label container with client's name.
10 Fill out laboratory request for appropriate test.
11 Take specimen to laboratory immediately.

INTERVENTION: Collecting Stool for Parasites

1 Collect exudate, mucus, and blood with all specimens.
2 Keep specimens at body temperature to be examined within 30 minutes so that organisms can be seen in their active stages. (Loose, fluid stools are likely to contain trophozoites or intestinal amoebas and flagellates.)
3 There is usually no need to maintain well-formed or semiformed stool specimens at body temperature or to examine them quickly even though they may contain ova or cystic forms of parasites.
4 Collect complete stools after purgative medication.
5 When the presence of tapeworms is suspected, all stools in their entirety must be examined in order to find the head of the parasite.
6 Do not give barium, oil, and laxatives containing heavy metals that interfere with the extraction process (so that ova or cysts are not revealed) for seven days prior to stool examination.
7 Use only normal saline solution or tap water if an enema must be administered to collect specimens. Do not use soap suds or other substances.
8 Do not contaminate the specimen with urine as it kills amoeba.
9 Collect three random, normally-passed stool specimens to ensure accurate test results.

INTERVENTION: Collecting Stool for Bacteria

1 Collect exudate, mucus, and blood with all specimens.
2 Place a small amount of feces in a sterile test tube and send to the laboratory immediately after collection. If there is any delay, the specimen must be iced.
3 Send entire specimen to the laboratory immediately after collection if required for specific test. If there is any delay, the specimen should be kept cold.

Testing for Occult Blood

1 Smear small amount of stool on a filter paper or individual packet.
2 Place two drops of each of the following solutions on the stool:
 • Guaiac solution.
 • Glacial acetic acid.
 • Hydrogen peroxide.
3 Observe for blue or green color change within 30 seconds.
4 Color change indicates positive reaction.
5 Document results of test.

435

4 Report and calculate on the basis of daily output any stool specimens that are to undergo chemical analysis.

INTERVENTION: Collecting Infant or Child Stool Specimen

1 Place a clean, disposable diaper on the child.
2 Check diaper frequently so that you obtain a specimen that is not contaminated with urine.
3 If child is passing liquid stools, place a plastic liner inside the diaper. Use cotton swabs to procure the specimen.

EVALUATION

EXPECTED OUTCOMES

1 Specimen meets laboratory requirements for diagnostic testing. *If not*, follow these alternative nursing actions:
   ANA: Check lab reference for correct collection procedure and secure new specimen according to specific instructions.
2 Client does not experience undue discomfort or embarrassment during procedure. *If otherwise*, follow these alternative nursing actions:
   ANA: Place a bedpan or other collection device under the toilet seat to obtain specimen. If client is confined to bed, pull sheets over client's legs and draw curtains around the bed until procedure is completed.
   ANA: Medicate for pain, especially following anal-rectal surgery, before attempting to collect stool specimen.

UNEXPECTED OUTCOMES

1 Client is unable to pass adequate stool for specimen collection.
   ANA: Request physician's order to give a normal saline or tap water enema.
2 Client passes liquid stools.
   ANA: Obtain a plastic container with a cover and several large cotton swabs. Dip cotton swabs into the liquid stool. Place swabs in plastic container. After procedure, pay close attention to skin care. A protective ointment may be necessary to protect skin from liquid stools.

ACTION: INSERTING A RECTAL TUBE

ASSESSMENT

1 Palpate the client's abdomen to determine the degree of abdominal distention.
2 Assess discomfort caused by flatulence.
3 Note quality and rate of respirations.
4 Note the presence or absence of hemorrhoids.

Charting
- Time specimens collected
- Time specimens sent to laboratory
- Number of specimens sent to laboratory
- Description of stool: color, amount, odor, and any purulent patches or blood noted
- Condition of perianal skin, if client is having diarrhea
- If serial stool specimens are needed, record each specimen on the Kardex card as well as the chart

Rationale for Action
- To promote removal of flatulence in the digestive tract following abdominal surgery
- To promote removal of flatulence which occurs with excessive swallowing of air
- To stimulate expulsion of flatus in the lower digestive tract
- To prevent abdominal distention caused by flatulence, which can interfere with diaphragmatic muscle contraction and cause dyspnea

PLANNING

GOALS

- Relief of abdominal distention and increased comfort
- Relief from dyspnea if flatulence has caused respiratory distress

EQUIPMENT

- Rectal tube: size 22 to 24 French for adults and size 12 to 18 French for children
- Small plastic bag or stool specimen container
- Hypoallergenic paper tape
- Water-soluble lubricant
- Bed protector

▶ Chewing gum, sucking on candy, drinking liquids through a straw, and smoking tend to promote the swallowing of air and increase abdominal distention.

INTERVENTION: Inserting a Rectal Tube

1 Explain the procedure to the client.
2 Place the client on left side, in a recumbent position.
3 Tape the plastic bag around the distal end of the rectal tube or insert the tube into the stool specimen container.
4 Vent the upper side of the plastic bag to prevent inflation.
5 Lubricate the proximal end of the rectal tube with water-soluble lubricant.
6 Gently insert the tube into the client's rectum, past the external and internal anal sphincters (two to four inches in adults, one to three inches in children.)
7 With adults, gently tape the tube in place, using hypoallergenic paper tape. With children, hold the tube in place manually.

Clinical Alert

Prolonged stimulation of the anal sphincter may result in a loss of the neuromuscular response. The prolonged presence of a catheter may cause pressure necrosis of the mucosal surface.

Insert rectal tube past the external and internal anal sphincters.

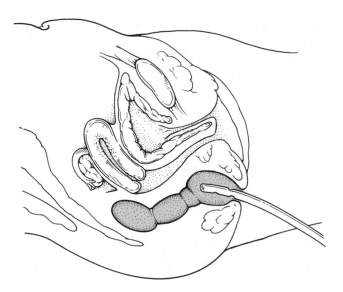

437

8   Leave the tube in place no longer than 20 minutes.
9   Remove the tube and provide perianal care as needed.
10 Help the client assume a comfortable position.
11 Clean the tubing. Remove and discard the plastic bag.

EVALUATION

EXPECTED OUTCOMES

1   Relief of abdominal distention and increased comfort. *If not,* follow these alternative nursing actions:
    ANA: Reposition client at an angle that raises the lower part of his or her body, e.g., in a prone position with the foot of the bed raised. Instruct client to circle, raise, and lower his or her legs.
    ANA: Reinsert the tube after two to three hours.
    ANA: Remove the tube and check for feces that may be clogging the outlet. Clean tube and reinsert.
2   Relief from dyspnea if flatulence has caused respiratory distress. *If not,* follow these alternative nursing actions:
    ANA: Ambulate if client's condition permits.
    ANA: Place client on left side in Fowler's position.

UNEXPECTED OUTCOME

Fecal impaction low in rectum prevents rectal tube insertion.
    ANA: Perform digital examination with gloved finger and water-soluble lubricant. Break up impaction if present.

ACTION: ADMINISTERING AN ENEMA

ASSESSMENT

1   Review client's present and past eliminatory status.
2   Determine the purpose for the enema so that you know what type of solution to use and how much to administer.
3   Perform digital examination if fecal impaction is suspected.
4   Decide if you will need another person to help hold the client while you administer the enema.
5   Palpate the client's abdomen to assess the degree of abdominal distention.
6   Determine the degree of sphincter control by asking client about his or her ability to control bowel movements.

PLANNING

GOALS

- Increased comfort and relief from abdominal distention
- Clear returns if preparing client for diagnostic examination, surgery, etc.
- Relief from fecal impaction
- Complete return of solution plus feces.

Charting
- Time rectal tube inserted
- Time rectal tube removed
- Presence, absence, or change in abdominal distention
- Client's reaction to procedure
- Any unexpected outcomes and measures taken to treat these outcomes

Rationale for Action
- To relieve constipation
- To relieve fecal impactions
- To cleanse the bowel prior to surgery, childbirth, or diagnostic examination
- To evacuate the bowel in clients with neurologic dysfunction
- To provide nutrients
- To introduce an exchange resin

Clinical Alert
Vagal nerve stimulation from enemas, digital examination, or rectal tube placement may cause cardiac arrhythmias.

EQUIPMENT

- Water container with attached rectal tube (size 22 to 32 French for adults, size 14 to 18 French for children, and size 12 or infant enema syringe with bulb for infants)
- Normal saline, tap water, soap solution
- Water-soluble lubricant
- Clean bedpan with cover or potty chair for children
- Bed protector
- Skin care items, e.g., soap, water, towels

ADDITIONAL EQUIPMENT

For a Retention Enema
- Oil: adult 150–200 cc, child 75–100 cc, 91° F
- Small French catheter size 14 to 20
- Barrel from 50 to 100 cc adapter syringe
- Commercially prepared enema may be used

INTERVENTION: Administering an Enema to an Adult

1 Explain the procedure to the client. Explain the benefits of relaxing and taking periodic deep breaths.
2 Place bed protector under client.
3 Place client on left side in a lateral, recumbent position.
4 Fill water container with 750 to 1000 cc of lukewarm solution, 105° to 110° F.
5 Allow solution to run through the tubing so that air is removed. (If air is instilled during the procedure, the client will experience discomfort.)
6 Lubricate the tip of the tubing with water-soluble lubricant.

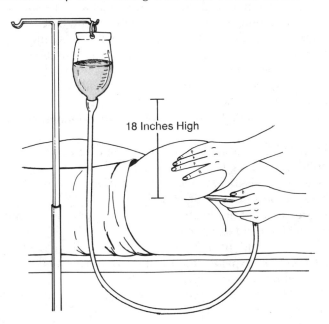

18 Inches High

Types of Enemas

- **cleansing** Stimulates peristalsis through irritation of colon and rectum and by distention from volume. *Agents*: Saline and soap suds.
- **oil** Lubricates the rectum and colon and softens feces. *Agents*: mineral oil, salad oil, liquid petrolatum.
- **carminative** Promotes expulsion of flatus. *Agents*: 1–2–3 enema (30 g of magnesium sulfate, 60 g of glycerin, and 90 ml of warm water); milk and molasses (180 ml to 240 ml of equal amounts).

Place enema solution container no more than 18 inches above the rectum.

▶ **Soap-suds enema**: dilute 5 ml of castile soap in 1000 ml of water. Mild soap solutions stimulate and irritate intestinal mucosa. Strong soap solutions can cause severe irritation of the mucous membrane of the colon.

● **Tap water enemas**: give with caution to infants or to adults with altered cardiac and renal reserve. Tap water is a hypotonic solution which can increase the blood volume if it is absorbed from the colon.

● **Hypertonic enemas**: for normal saline enemas, use a smaller volume of solution. Hypertonic solutions draw fluid into the colon from the body tissues. These solutions are mildly irritating to the mucous membrane of the colon.

Clinical Alert

Solutions that are too hot or too cold or solutions that are instilled too quickly can cause cramping, damage to rectal tissues, and extreme shock.

7 Gently insert tubing three to four inches into the client's rectum, past the external and internal sphincters. (Avoid traumatizing hemorrhoids during insertion.)
8 Raise the water container to a maximum height of 18 inches.
9 Allow solution to flow slowly. If the flow is slow, the client will experience fewer cramps. The client will also be able to tolerate and retain a greater volume of solution.
10 Hold the tubing in place in the client's rectum at all times. Keep a bedpan nearby.
11 After you have instilled the solution, gently remove the tubing.
12 Elevate the head of the bed so that the client can assume a squatting position on the bedpan.
13 Provide privacy until the client has expelled the total volume of the instilled solution.
14 Remove and cover bedpan.
15 Assist client with perineal care and help client to assume a comfortable position.
16 Measure returns to make sure the client expelled the total volume of the solution.
17 Clean all equipment.

INTERVENTION: Administering an Enema to a Child or Infant

1 Explain procedure to child and/or family. Take time to calm a frightened child and to answer the child's questions.
2 Place bed protector under child.
3 Place child on left side or in knee-chest position.
4 Fill water container with 100° F solution (500 ml or less for child, 250 ml for an infant).
5 Allow solution to run through the tubing so that air is removed.
6 Lubricate tip of tubing or infant enema syringe with bulb.
7 Gently insert a size 12 to 18 French catheter or syringe into child's rectum (one to one and one-half inches for infants, two to three inches for children).
8 Elevate water container no more than 12 to 18 inches.
9 Allow solution to flow slowly for 10 to 15 minutes.
10 After you have instilled the solution, gently remove the tubing or syringe.
11 Retain solution 10 to 15 minutes for cleansing enemas.
12 Hold child's buttocks together or tape them with hypoallergenic paper tape. If child is toilet trained, place a potty chair nearby.
13 Place the child on a potty chair or bedpan.
14 If there are no contraindications, you may gently massage child's abdomen to help child expel returns.
15 If the child wants to be left alone while expelling returns, provide privacy. Child must expel the total volume of the instilled solution.
16 Remove and cover the potty chair or bedpan.
17 Clean the child's perineal area and help child assume a comfortable position.

18 Measure returns to make sure the child expelled the total volume of the solution.
19 Clean all equipment.

INTERVENTION: Administering a Retention Enema

1 Prepare client the same as for any enema.
2 After introducing catheter, attach adapter syringe barrel to catheter.
3 Introduce oil slowly through syringe barrel to avoid stimulating peristalsis.
4 Remove catheter gently.
5 Explain to client that oil should be retained for 1–3 hours before it is expelled.
6 A cleansing enema may need to be given to remove oil and stimulate defecation.

INTERVENTION: Administering Disposable Commercially Prepared Enema

1 Read directions on enema container.
2 Lubricate with water-soluble lubricant if necessary. (Usually rectal tube is self-lubricated.)
3 Prepare client as for any enema.
4 After inserting rectal tube, squeeze the container and empty entire 120 cc of hypertonic solution.
5 Instruct client to hold solution five to seven minutes.
6 Continue to follow procedure for care of client undergoing an enema.

EVALUATION

EXPECTED OUTCOMES

1 Increased comfort and relief from abdominal distention. *If not,* follow these alternative nursing actions:
  ANA: Remove rectal tube and reinsert.
  ANA: Repeat enema.
  ANA: Ambulate client if ambulation not contraindicated.
2 Clear returns if preparing client for diagnostic examination, surgery, etc. *If not,* follow these alternative nursing actions:
  ANA: Repeat enema. If, after three enemas, returns are still not clear, notify physician.
3 Relief from fecal impaction. *If not,* follow these alternative nursing actions:
  ANA: Obtain orders for oil retention enema.
  ANA: Obtain orders for catheter.
  ANA: Utilize digital stimulation and manual extraction of feces if not contraindicated by diagnosis of cardiac or neurological involvement.
4 Complete return of solution plus feces. *If not,* follow these alternative nursing actions:

ANA: May need to repeat with same type of enema.

ANA: May need to give an enema with a stronger solution.

ANA: Client may be dehydrated and absorb solution. Do not be concerned that fluid is not expelled.

UNEXPECTED OUTCOMES

1 Client expels solution prematurely.

ANA: Calm client and ease client's distress by reassuring him or her as you clean the equipment. Place bedpan under the client. Place client in semi-Fowler's position with knees flexed. Hold the rectal tube in client's rectum between thighs. Slow the water flow and continue with the enema.

2 Client complains of extreme weakness or feeling faint. You observe a change in client's mental alertness.

ANA: Remove tubing. Assess vital signs. If you suspect cardiac dysrhythmias, remove bedpan and notify physician.

3 Client complains of severe and sudden abdominal pain, nausea, and distention.

ANA: Remove tubing and notify physician of possible perforation.

4 The flow of water is impeded or an obstruction is felt.

ANA: Withdraw tube slightly and reinsert.

ANA: Gently perform a digital examination for the possibility of fecal impaction. Break up impaction if present. Secure physician's order to give a retention enema, followed by a cleansing enema two to three hours later.

5 Client cannot return enema solution.

ANA: Gently massage client's abdomen if not contraindicated. Insert enema tube. Lower the enema bag below the level of the bed. Notify physician for further orders.

Charting

- Time enema given
- Volume and type of solution used
- Results obtained: amount, consistency, and color of returns
- Any unexpected outcomes and measures taken to remedy problems
- Client's reactions to procedure

Rationale for Action

- To provide a means for escape of flatus
- To evacuate the colon of stool
- To regulate discharge from the colon when colostomy is in sigmoid or descending portion

ACTION: IRRIGATING A COLOSTOMY

ASSESSMENT

1 Assess the permanence of the colostomy and the client's prognosis.
2 Identify the location of the colostomy along the large intestine.
3 Listen for bowel sounds.
4 Palpate the client's abdomen for distention.
5 Assess for stomal complications, i.e., peristomal hernia, stenosed stoma, or prolapsed stoma.
6 Note any presence of disease in the client's bowel.
7 Assess the client's ability to sit for a prolonged period of time.
8 Note the client's age and bowel habits prior to surgery.
9 Ask the client how he feels about colostomy management.
10 Assess the client's mental alertness and ability to learn.

PLANNING

GOALS

- Client develops a positive attitude toward living with a colostomy.
- Client becomes proficient in colostomy care.
- Bowel elimination is regulated.
- Complete return of solution plus soft or formed feces.

EQUIPMENT

- Water container with cone or size 18 French catheter (The danger of perforation of the colon is much greater when irrigating a colostomy with a catheter. The use of an irrigation cone usually results in safer administration and better water flow.)
- Water at 105°–110° F (500 ml for the first irrigation; 1000 ml thereafter)
- Irrigating sleeve and a belt cut long enough to reach the water level of the toilet
- Items to clean skin and stoma, e.g., wash cloths or gauze sponges
- Plastic bag for disposal of old pouch device
- Clean pouch and closure
- Skin barriers
- Water-soluble lubricant

Observing the colostomy is one of the first indications of acceptance.

INTERVENTION: Performing a Colostomy Irrigation

1 Explain procedure to client. Explain the benefits of relaxing and taking periodic deep breaths.
2 Remove and dispose of old pouch.
3 Clean stoma and skin with warm water and soft cloth.
4 Apply irrigation sleeve.
5 Fill container with 1000 ml lukewarm water.
6 Remove air from tubing.
7 Suspend container on bathroom hook.
8 Lubricate cone tip or tip of catheter.
9 Help client sit on toilet. Place sleeve into toilet or chair.
10 Insert cone into stoma, parallel to floor. (Insert catheter two to four inches into stoma. Never force catheter insertion.)
11 Start water slowly and allow to run into stoma. (Peristomal hernias may increase the difficulty of an irrigation.)
12 The height of the water container and the rate of water flow can affect the results obtained by an irrigation. When the client is in a sitting position, the bottom of the container should be even with client's shoulder. It should take 10 to 15 minutes for 1000 ml of fluid to be instilled in a colostomy.
13 Close off or fold over the top of the sleeve.
14 Allow client to remain seated while client returns the majority of the stool.
15 Rinse sleeve with water. Dry bottom and close end of sleeve.

Nurse-Client Teaching

1 Help client to develop a positive attitude toward living with a colostomy.
2 Establish a time for irrigation that will meet the client's needs after discharge from the hospital. Ask client to adhere to this time on a daily basis.
3 If possible, show the client the irrigation equipment the day before you perform the intervention.
4 Follow the same steps closely during every irrigation.
5 Gradually teach the client to assume responsibility for his or her colostomy care.

443

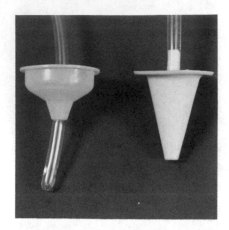

(a) Irrigation cone and catheter.

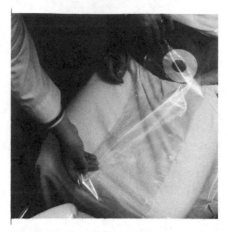

(b) Position irrigation sleeve opening around stoma and place the end in toilet.

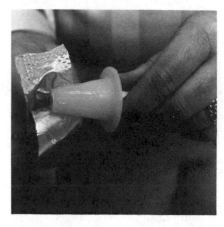

(c) Lubricate cone tip with generous amount of water soluble lubricant.

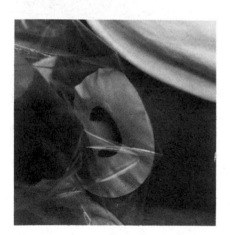

(d) Insert cone gently into stoma.

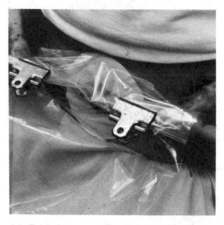

(e) Fold sleeve over and close with clamp.

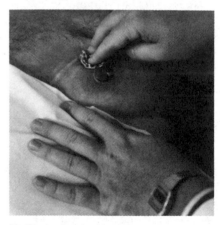

(f) Clean client's skin thoroughly following irrigation.

16 Ask client to wear sleeve in this manner for 30 to 45 minutes. Client may return to bed, walk around, or proceed with other activities during this time.

17 Remove sleeve and set aside for rinsing.

18 Clean client's skin and stoma with warm water.

19 Assemble and apply skin barriers and clean pouch.

20 Rinse irrigation sleeve and hang to dry.

21 Put away all supplies and reorder as needed.

INTERVENTION: Performing Bed Irrigation of a Colostomy

1 Position client comfortably in bed.

2 Close off the bottom of the irrigation sleeve and allow it to rest in a bedpan at the client's side.

3 Follow steps 1 through 12 on page 443.

4   Wait about 30 to 35 minutes to allow most of the irrigation fluid to return.
5   Open the bottom of sleeve into the bedpan.
6   Remove sleeve and set aside for cleansing.
7   Clean client's skin and stoma with warm water.
8   Apply appropriate pouch and skin barriers.
9   Place client in a comfortable position.
10 Rinse sleeve and hang to dry.
11 Put away all supplies and reorder as necessary.

EVALUATION

EXPECTED OUTCOMES

1   Client develops positive attitude toward living with a colostomy. *If not*, follow these alternative nursing actions:
    ANA: Discuss with client the care and management of a stoma. Through this discussion, decide what problems the client is encountering, and reassess your plan of action.
    ANA: Arrange visit between ostomy visitor and client to demonstrate the rehabilitation possible following surgery.
    ANA: Refer client to health specialist skilled in teaching ostomy management.
    ANA: Refer client to ostomy club.
    ANA: Refer client for psychological support.
    ANA: Allow client to grieve over change in body image.
2   Client becomes proficient in colostomy care. *If not*, follow these alternative nursing actions:
    ANA: Repeat intervention and nurse-client teaching until client is able to perform the procedure.
    ANA: Bring family member into teaching plan to help client with management.
    ANA: Refer to home health care practitioner to help client after discharge.
    ANA: Reassess stoma construction and location to be sure there is no physical problem with management. (If client cannot see stoma, client cannot learn self-management.)
3   Bowel elimination is regulated. *If not*, follow these alternative nursing actions:
    ANA: Inform client of foods to avoid and/or to eat to help regulate elimination.
    ANA: Establish a time for irrigations that will prevent unexpected eruptions.
    ANA: Reassess irrigation procedure. Make sure the client receives a sufficient amount of solution and that all solution is returned.
    ANA: Be sure to irrigate daily at approximately the same time.
    ANA: Place client on a low residue diet while learning irrigation. Once bowel content is established, have client add foods at 2 to 3 day intervals. Eliminate foods that cause spillage. (If a client wants to eat something that causes spillage, have client wear a pouch.)

4   Complete return of solution plus soft or formed feces. *If not*, follow these alternative nursing actions:

ANA: Gently massage client's abdomen.

ANA: Repeat irrigation using one-half the amount of solution.

ANA: After the second irrigation, insert a catheter into the client's stoma. Attach catheter to an irrigation bag and lower the bag below the level of the stoma.

ANA: If client is uncomfortable and unable to expel solution, notify physician.

ANA: Make sure client retains 1000 cc tap water for at least 10 to 15 minutes.

ANA: Be sure cone or dam fits tightly enough to prevent water from running out.

ANA: Instruct client to drink at least 8 glasses of fluid daily.

UNEXPECTED OUTCOMES

1   Stool leaks out under irrigation sleeve.

ANA: Apply dampened Karaya washer around the faceplate at the opening of the irrigation sleeve.

ANA: Tighten belt slightly.

2   Water does not flow easily into colostomy stoma.

ANA: Change angle or position of cone slightly.

ANA: Check for kinks in tubing from container.

ANA: Check height of water container.

ANA: Ask client to relax and to take deep breaths.

ANA: Instill small amounts of water to loosen stool.

3   Client experiences cramping, nausea, or dizziness during irrigation.

ANA: Stop flow of water leaving cone or catheter in place. Do not resume until cramping has passed.

ANA: Check water temperature. Water that is too hot can cause dizziness.

ANA: Check height of water bag. Water that flows too rapidly can also lead to same problem.

4   Inability to run water into colostomy.

ANA: Perform digital exam to assess construction of stoma, since cone or catheter is probably against wall of bowel.

ANA: Rotate cone or catheter to different position to start flow.

5   No return of stool or water from irrigation.

ANA: Apply drainable pouch.

ANA: Have client increase fluid intake.

ANA: Repeat irrigation next day.

6   Continual spillage of stool between irrigations.

ANA: Reassess type of colostomy — only those in descending or sigmoid colon are to be irrigated.

ANA: Be sure client uses and retains 1000 cc of tap water. (Too little water does not provide complete elimination. Too much water causes the bowel to become flaccid and work poorly.)

ANA: Assess client's past bowel habits prior to surgery. Clients who have had very irregular bowel habits or frequent stools may not be candidates for irrigation.

7 Poor returns due to constipation and/or fecal impaction.

ANA: Assess client's diet. More bulk foods may need to be added.

ANA: Assess medications client is taking. (Drugs such as codeine, iron, and vincristine can be very constipating. Stool softeners and/or mild laxative may be needed.)

ANA: Assess client's fluid intake. Increasing the amount of fluids may be necessary.

ANA: Perform a digital exam to check for impaction. If impaction or severe constipation persists, colostomy may be irrigated with 30 cc soap, 60 cc oil and 500 cc water. (Warn client that this can cause severe cramping.)

ANA: Secure physician's order to add liquid Colace or mineral oil to irrigating solution. A red rubber catheter may be used to put the liquid medication nearer to the obstruction.

8 Diarrhea occurs.

ANA: Do not irrigate colostomy. Apply drainable pouch.

ANA: If client is receiving radiation therapy, which usually causes diarrhea, stop irrigation until therapy is completed.

ANA: Assess client's medications. (Drugs such as antibiotics or chemotherapy drugs can cause diarrhea.)

ANA: If diarrhea is excessive and/or prolonged the client needs to be monitored for potassium loss and have diet adjusted accordingly.

Charting
- Time irrigation administered
- Amount and type of solution used
- Results obtained: amount, color, and consistency of returns
- Condition and color of stoma (It should be healthy red.)
- Condition of peristomal skin
- Amount of client participation
- Client's reaction to procedure
- Nurse-client teaching

ACTION: APPLYING A FECAL OSTOMY POUCH

ASSESSMENT

1 Observe stoma color. Usually color is dark pink to red. Blanching, darkening or lightening of the color may indicate circulation problems.
2 Before deciding which type of pouch to apply, inspect client's abdomen for creasing, firmness, softness, contour, scars, folds, and incisions.
3 Before deciding which type of skin barrier to apply, inspect the client's peristomal skin for signs of erythema, excoriation, ulceration, and fistula formation.
4 Before deciding which type of pouching system to use, consider the client's learning abilities, age, and manual dexterity.

PLANNING

GOALS

- Colostomy pouch remains intact without leakage for one to three days; ileostomy pouch for four to seven days.
- Pouching system provides maximal skin protection.
- Pouching system remains odorproof for three to five days.
- Client gradually assumes an active role in applying pouch.

Rationale for Action
- To collect effluent for the accurate assessment of output in the hospital
- To collect effluent for the comfort of the client
- To contain drainage and odors so that the client feels he or she is socially acceptable
- To protect peristomal skin from erythema, excoriation, infection, and fistula formation
- To protect the client's clothing

447

► The surgical construction of the stoma, the contour of the abdomen, and the firmness of the abdomen dictate the types of skin barriers and pouches used.

- If the stoma is flush with the peristomal skin, a thin, occlusive skin barrier and a thin faceplace is needed to prevent leakage. Peristomal skin is skin that surrounds the stoma for an area between two to five inches.
- If the stoma protrudes nicely above the skin, a broader range of skin barriers and pouches may be applied.
- If the abdomen is very soft and large, a convex faceplate may be needed to prevent leakage.
- If the abdomen is firm and small, a flat faceplate may be used.

► Patch testing should be done before applying new products on clients with a history of allergic responses.

► Pouch application for a fecal ostomy is not a sterile procedure. Wash your hands thoroughly before and after this procedure to prevent cross contamination to other clients. Gloves are not needed unless infection is present. Using gloves may contribute to the client's feelings of social unacceptability.

EQUIPMENT

- Clean pouch (A drainable pouch should be used for all fecal ostomies except regulated descending or sigmoid ostomies.)
- Skin barriers, e.g., Skin Gel, or Skin Prep (An occlusive skin barrier with the correctly sized opening should be used for all clients with fecal ostomies.)
- Warm water, 105° to 110° F
- Warm water
- Soft cloths
- Plastic bag for disposal of old pouch
- Tail closure for drainable pouch
- Deodorant (optional if pouch is odorproof)
- Hypoallergenic paper tape (optional)

INTERVENTION: Applying a Fecal Ostomy Pouch

1 Prepare the clean pouch.
   a Measure the stoma with a measuring guide.
   b Trace a circle one-sixth to one-eighth inch larger than stoma on the paper covering the adhesive backing.
   c Cut the stoma pattern, and apply cement or double-faced adhesive disc according to the type of pouch being applied. Pouches applied with adhesive can be left in place for seven days unless leakage or skin irritation occurs.
2 Prepare occlusive skin barrier. Make sure the opening of the barrier is the same size as the stoma to prevent contact between the stoma and the skin. If using Karaya ring, rub moisture into ring until the ring turns sticky. If using Stomahesive or Reliaseal, cut opening to fit stoma as was done for the pouch.
3 Empty the old pouch. (Pouches should be emptied when one-third to one-half full of feces or flatus to prevent destruction of the pouch seal.)

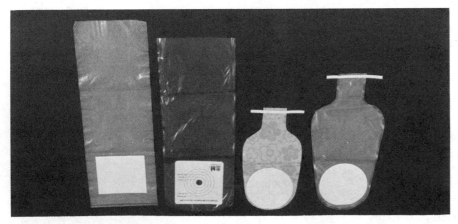

(a) Ileostomy pouches are available in different styles; note the flowered one usually worn by females.

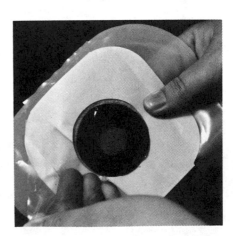

(b) Prepare Karaya ring for placement by taking off protective cover.

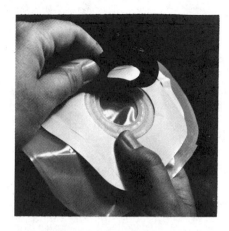

(c) Remove Karaya ring from pouch before applying to skin.

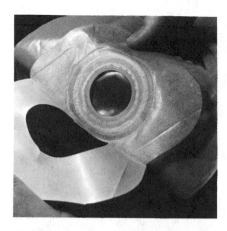

(d) Remove paper from adhesive backing and the new pouch is ready for application.

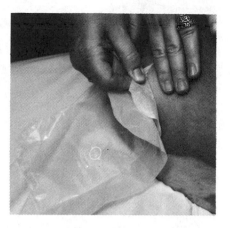

(e) Remove old pouch gently to protect skin.

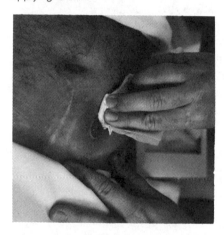

(f) Clean peristomal area with warm water and a soft cloth. Dry thoroughly before applying the pouch.

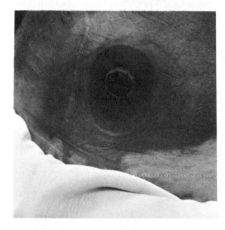

(g) Observe stoma and peristomal area for color and ulceration.

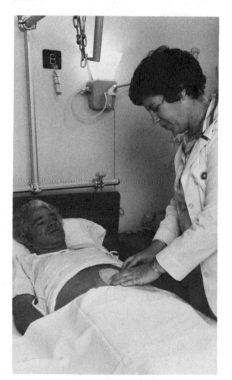

(j) Client teaching is important to help the client adjust to an ostomy.

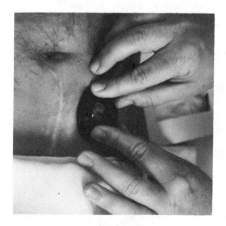

(h) Apply Karaya ring, a skin barrier, flush to stoma.

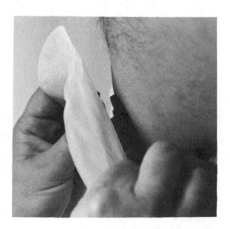

(i) Place pouch on Karaya ring. Ring is cut ⅛ to ¼″ larger than stoma.

Nurse-Client Teaching

The new ostomate will probably experience all of the stages of grief in an effort to become accustomed to his or her new body image. Good nurse-client communication techniques are essential for the psychological and psychosocial rehabilitation of the ostomate.

1 Help the client to develop a positive attitude toward living with an ostomy by practicing a nonjudgmental, accepting attitude toward the client.
2 As you demonstrate the procedure, explain the use of skin care items, the criteria used in pouch selection, the importance of appropriate skin care, and the importance of wearing a well-fitting pouch.
3 Follow the same steps closely during every pouch change.
4 Gradually allow the client to assume responsibility for ostomy care.

4 Gently remove the old pouch. If it is disposable, discard it. If it is reusable, set it aside for cleaning.
5 Clean the client's skin and stoma gently with warm water and a soft cloth. (Oily substances should be kept away from areas of pouch application as they interfere with the adhesive.)
6 Dry client's skin well with a soft cloth.
7 Observe skin and stoma for changes in size, ulcerations, or color. (Skin should be a healthy red.)
8 If *not* using occlusive skin barrier, spray the skin with skin prep, allow it to dry, and spray again.
9 Apply a skin barrier such as Stomahesive, Hollihesive, Crixiline, Reliaseal, or Karaya washer or rings.
10 Center and apply clean pouch. Pouch should be applied away from fresh incision lines to decrease infection. The opening of the faceplate of the pouch should be ⅛ inch larger than the stoma to prevent rubbing, cutting, or trauma to the stoma. The pouch is applied either directly on the skin or on the Karaya ring if used.
11 Press the adhesive around the stoma to form a seal. Do not allow adhesive to wrinkle in order to prevent leakage.
12 Insert deodorant, either liquid or tablet, if bag not odorproof.
13 Close and secure the end of the pouch with tail closure.
14 "Picture-frame" the faceplate of the pouch with hypoallergenic paper tape (optional).
15 Attach belt to faceplate of pouch (optional).
16 Check supplies and reorder as necessary.
17 Clean and store all reusable items.

EVALUATION

EXPECTED OUTCOMES

1 Pouch remains intact without leakage. *If not*, follow these alternative nursing actions:
  ANA: Reassess abdomen and pouching system for weak points.
  ANA: Remind other health personnel to empty the client's pouch whenever it is one-third to one-half full of flatus or feces.
2 Pouching system provides maximal skin protection. *If not*, follow these alternative nursing actions:
  ANA: Reassess abdomen and pouching system for weak points.
  ANA: Apply an occlusive skin barrier to allow the peristomal skin to heal.
  ANA: Change the pouch a little more frequently (once per day or every other day) until the peristomal skin is healed.
3 Pouching system remains odorproof for three to five days. *If not*, follow these alternative nursing actions:
  ANA: Reassess client's ability to cleanse and care for colostomy or ileostomy.
  ANA: Reassess method of cleansing reusable bags.
  ANA: Tell client how to deodorize bag if not using odorproof appliance. Liquid deodorant is applied to a cotton ball or piece of tissue and placed in bottom of pouch through the emptying spout.

ANA: Discuss the use of different appliances which are odorproof.

4 Client gradually assumes an active role in applying pouch. *If not*, follow these alternative nursing actions:

ANA: Give the client more time to work through the grief process.

ANA: Use good nurse-client communication techniques to assist the client through the grief process.

ANA: Involve a family member or a significant person in the client's life in the care of the ostomy.

ANA: Make referrals as necessary to visiting nurses' associations or extended care facilities.

ANA: Provide written instructions and nurse-to-nurse demonstrations if client is to have colostomy care administered by a health care professional after discharge from the hospital.

UNEXPECTED OUTCOMES

1 The stoma appears dark, dusky, or black.

ANA: Notify the surgeon at once of a diminished blood supply to the stoma.

2 The stoma becomes ulcerated or cut.

ANA: Examine the pouching system to determine the cause: the faceplate of the pouch may be rubbing or cutting into the stoma.

ANA: Slightly enlarge the opening of the faceplate to the pouch to avoid traumatizing the stoma.

ANA: Notify the surgeon, since this outcome may indicate a recurrence of disease.

ACTION: INTUBATING A CONTINENT ILEOSTOMY

ASSESSMENT

1 Gently palpate client's lower abdomen to determine the fullness of the internal pouch.
2 Observe client for full pouch. Internal pouch is visible under the skin as the pouch enlarges.
3 Observe client closely for signs of obstruction, e.g., nausea, abdominal distention, etc.

PLANNING

GOALS

- Continent ileostomy pouch is completely drained
- Client experiences no pain during the procedure
- Continence is maintained

EQUIPMENT

- Silastic catheter No. 28
- 500-ml collection container (glass or metal)
- 50-ml syringe
- Water-soluble lubricant

Charting

- Type of pouch and skin barrier used
- Time pouch applied
- Time pouch emptied
- Amount, color, and consistency of stool emptied from pouch
- Presence or absence of flatus through the stoma
- Client participation in pouch application
- Condition of peristomal skin and stoma
- Condition of incision line, i.e., any redness or swelling
- Condition of abdomen, e.g., distention, etc.

Rationale for Action

- To promote a positive body image by eliminating the need for an external stoma and pouch for clients with continuous liquid stool drainage.
- To provide a means by which liquid stool is evacuated at designated times during the day
- Clients with Crohn's disease are not candidates for pouch ileostomies as the disease is a multiple-focus disease and often affects the terminal ileum, the area from which the pouch is created

▶ The Koch pouch is made by sewing together a loop of the terminal ileum. About four inches of the distal ileum is doubled back into the pouch to create a nipple valve. Pressure from feces forces the valve closed and prevents constant drainage.

451

Nurse-Client Teaching

1 Help the client develop a positive attitude toward living with an ostomy by practicing good nurse-client communication techniques and by acting in a non-judgmental, accepting way toward the client.

2 Demonstrate and discuss the proper methods and rationale for intubation.

   a For the first six months after surgery, intubation is carried out every two to four hours to keep the drainage below 250 cc and prevent strain on the suture line.

   b Between six months to one year after surgery, intubation is performed three to four times a day because the internal pouch capacity can reach between 500 to 1000 cc.

3 Demonstrate and discuss alternative methods of care when complications arise.

4 Demonstrate the procedures for intubation until the client can care for his or her intubation.

5 Instruct the client to chew food well. This is especially important for fibrous foods. Undigested food may cause bacterial buildup in pouch which could cause distention and rupture.

6 Instruct the client to avoid eating gas-forming foods.

7 Have the client maintain an intake of eight glasses of fluid per day.

8 Tell the client how to apply an external drainable pouch with appropriate skin barriers.

- Dressing gauze or a 5-cm square bandaid
- Tissues
- Coverlet dressing
- Catheter cork

INTERVENTION: Irrigating and Corking Pouch

1 During surgery, a catheter is inserted into the client's stoma to maintain a continuous outflow of ileal content.

2 This catheter remains in place for 10 to 14 days after surgery.

3 During the immediate postoperative period, the catheter is irrigated manually every two hours to prevent clogging.

4 The irrigant is never aspirated for fear of traumatizing the internal pouch.

5 If there is no return flow, there may be a pouch obstruction.

6 After 10 to 14 days, the drainage system is removed from the pouch catheter and the catheter is corked.

7 The pouch catheter is uncorked every hour to allow the ileal contents to drain spontaneously.

8 Catheter is recorked for the next hour.

9 Process is carried out from 8:00 A.M. to 10:00 P.M.

10 From 10:00 P.M. to 8:00 A.M. the catheter is attached to gravity drainage and irrigated every two hours.

11 Corking is gradually increased by 15-minute intervals until corking reaches two hours.

12 When corking reaches two hours, pouch is corked at night as well as day. Pouch must be emptied every two hours around the clock.

13 Pouch catheter is removed five days after corking is accomplished around the clock. Intubation and drainage are instituted.

INTERVENTION: Intubating a Continent Ileostomy

1 The client should learn how to drain the pouch as soon as the catheter is discontinued.

2 Have client drain on toilet or position the collection container lower than the stoma to promote drainage by gravity.

3 Lubricate the tip of the catheter with a water-soluble lubricant.

4 Gently insert and advance the catheter about two inches into the stoma, angling the catheter into the internal pouch.

5 Use gentle pressure to pass the catheter through the nipple valve. (Some resistance may be met as the valve is compressed shut by fecal material collecting inside the pouch.)

6 Allow the internal pouch to empty (usually takes five to ten minutes).

7 Remove the catheter and wash it with hot, soapy water.

8 Clean the client's skin and stoma with warm water.

9 Dry the client's skin well.

10 Cover the stoma with gauze dressing or bandaid.

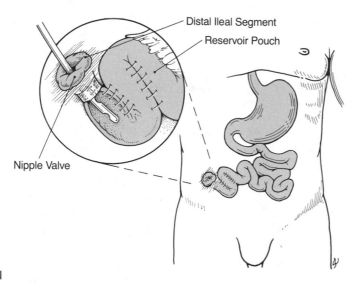

Distal Ileal Segment

Reservoir Pouch

Nipple Valve

Insert catheter through nipple valve approximately two inches into Koch pouch.

EVALUATION

EXPECTED OUTCOMES

1 Continent ileostomy pouch is completely drained. *If not*, follow these alternative nursing actions:

ANA: Reposition client to allow for increased drainage.

ANA: Gently massage over nipple valve area if not contraindicated to increase fecal flow.

ANA: Manipulate catheter by rotating and withdrawing and then inserting further.

ANA: Have client bear down if not contraindicated.

ANA: Irrigate pouch, as thick effluent may be causing some blockage.

2 Client experiences no pain during the procedure. *If otherwise*, follow these alternative nursing actions:

ANA: Instruct in relaxation technique.

ANA: Assess nipple valve functioning. If pain occurs with catheter insertion, change to smaller catheter size. If pain persists, notify physician.

ANA: Assess the volume of feces in pouch to determine if pain is related to increased volume in pouch.

ANA: Assess for associated nausea and abdominal distention as gastrointestinal obstruction can occur. If obstruction occurs, keep client n.p.o. Nasogastric tube is inserted for a few days.

3 Continence is maintained. *If not*, follow these alternative nursing actions:

ANA: Insert catheter, drain pouch, and measure volume to determine if incontinence is caused by overdistention of pouch.

ANA: Notify physician if incontinence continues or is unrelated to volume increases.

ANA: Pouch the area over the nipple valve to prevent embarrassment to the client.

453

1 The catheter will not advance past the nipple valve.
ANA: Tell the client to take a deep breath and turn the catheter at the same time.
ANA: Have the client lie down and relax for a while.
ANA: Have the client take a warm bath and relax.
ANA: Try squeezing a little water or air through the valve with a syringe attached to the catheter.
ANA: Notify the physician.
2 The catheter drains very slowly or becomes blocked with undigested food.
ANA: Irrigate the catheter with 30 to 40 ml of normal saline or tap water.
ANA: Milk the catheter by squeezing it several times.
ANA: Tell the client to cough a few times before inserting the catheter.
ANA: Gently press the client's abdomen.
ANA: Remove the catheter and wash it thoroughly. Then reinsert it into the internal pouch.
ANA: Instruct the client to chew foods well, especially fibrous foods.
3 Effluent thickens, making intubation and draining difficult.
ANA: Tell the client to drink eight to ten glasses of liquid per day.
ANA: Give the client water, prune juice or grape juice to drink.
ANA: Irrigate the internal pouch with 30 ml of normal saline or tap water.
4 Client develops peristomal skin problems from mucus accumulation under dressing.
ANA: Wash and dry the client's skin and expose it to air for 20 minutes several times a day.
ANA: Use a waterproof ointment under the dressing.
5 Client experiences fullness in pouch due to the buildup of flatus (not feces).
ANA: Tell the client to avoid gas-forming foods such as dried beans, cauliflower, and cabbage.
6 Client develops incontinency from diarrhea.
ANA: Identify cause of diarrhea and treat accordingly.
ANA: Pouch stoma with an external drainable pouch that allows intubation through the end of the pouch.

Charting
- Time of intubation
- Amount, color, and consistency of stool emptied from pouch
- Ease of entry into internal pouch
- Amount and type of solution used, if pouch irrigated
- Condition of peristomal skin
- Condition and color of stoma
- Whether continency is attained
- Amount of client participation
- Client's reaction to procedure
- Nurse-client teaching

Rationale for Action
- To assure proper placement and advancement of the tube
- To maintain a patent lumen to decompress the bowel
- To prevent mucosal damage upon removal of the tube

ACTION: PLACING, IRRIGATING, AND REMOVING A MILLER-ABBOTT TUBE

ASSESSMENT

1 Determine the client's level of consciousness.
2 Determine the client's knowledge of the procedure.
3 Auscultate the client's abdomen for the presence of bowel sounds.
4 Palpate abdomen for distention.

5 Note the amount, color, and odor of drainage.

6 Locate the tube in the client's gastrointestinal tract through fluoroscopic examination.

PLANNING

GOALS

- Proper placement and advancement of the tube
- Relief of abdominal distention through suction
- Maintenance of a clear tube lumen throughout the intubation period
- Removal of the tube without trauma to intestinal mucosa

EQUIPMENT

- Water-soluble lubricant
- Ice in basin
- Miller-Abbott tube
- Stethoscope
- Piston syringes: 5 ml, 10 ml, 50 ml
- Emesis basin
- Tissues or wash cloth
- Towel
- 1-ml mercury
- Normal saline solution
- Items for oral hygiene

INTERVENTION: Placing a Miller-Abbott Tube

1 Tell the client what he or she can expect during and after insertion.

2 Explain how the client can help with the insertion.

3 Agree on a signal that the client can use to stop the procedure for a moment or two.

4 Test the patency of the balloon and measure the capacity by filling it with air. Then completely deflate the balloon (20 to 50 ml of air used).

5 Label the adapters at the proximal end of the tube. One adapter should be labeled for suction; the other should be labeled Balloon.

6 Place the client in a high-Fowler's position with neck flexed.

7 Spread the towel "bib-fashion" over the client's chest.

8 Measure the tubing, using the distance from the client's earlobe to the bridge of the nose plus the distance from the bridge of the nose to the bottom of the sternum.

9 Wrap a piece of tape around the tube and mark the distance you measured.

10 Chill the tube; then lubricate the distal end sparingly.

11 Instruct the client to breathe through his or her mouth. Remove dentures.

12 Gently insert the tube into the client's nostril. Advance the tube gently but firmly, instructing the client to swallow as you advance the tubing past the pharynx.

Clinical Alert

If the client is suffering from a small bowel obstruction, the drainage from the tube will be yellow and fecal-smelling. If the client is suffering from a complete bowel obstruction, the drainage will be clear and may approach 3000 ml per day.

▶ A Miller-Abbott tube is a double-lumen tube that is six to ten feet in length. This tube is used to decompress the bowel proximal to an obstruction or, on rare occasions, to assess gastrointestinal bleeding. One lumen drains secretions. A balloon containing air and/or mercury is attached to the end of the other lumen to stimulate peristalsis. The tube progresses through the duodenum, jejunum, and ileum by gravity and peristalsis.

Clinical Alert

Do not secure the tube to the client's nose until tube has been advanced to the desired position. This will halt the progress of the tube and may lead to bowel injury or intussusception.

13 Advance the tube to the premarked area on the tube. Observe for aspiration of secretions. (Advancement of the tube more than two to four inches at a time can create knots and kinks in the tubing which may prevent relief from the obstruction or cause intussusception of the bowel.)

14 Determine the placement of the tube in the client's stomach using either one of the following measures:
   a Instill 5 ml of air in the suction portion of the tube while you listen with a stethoscope over the stomach area. If you hear a "whoosh" sound, the tube is in the stomach.
   b Using a syringe, aspirate for stomach contents through the suction portion of the tube.

15 Instill mercury into the balloon portion of the tube to help the balloon through the pyloric valve.

16 Reposition the client on right side.

17 Order a fluoroscopy to determine if the balloon has passed the pyloric valve.

18 When the balloon has passed the pyloric valve, inject air into the balloon portion of the tube.

19 Reposition the client every two hours, turning from right to left side and back to high-Fowler's position. Encourage ambulation. Repositioning and ambulation will help the balloon through the gastrointestinal tract.

20 Attach the tube to suction any time after the balloon has passed the pyloric valve.

21 Advance the tube one to two inches every hour, or two to four inches every two hours. When the client is in bed, coil and pin extra tubing to the bed. When the client is standing, coil and pin tubing to the gown.

22 When the tube reaches the desired position, secure it with tape to the client's nose or forehead. Make sure that the tubing is not putting pressure on the lumen of the nostril.

23 Administer oral hygiene at least once every four hours since colonic bacteria travel to the client's mouth by "wick action."

24 To irrigate, slowly instill 30 to 60 cc normal saline in the suction portion of the tube and then aspirate contents of the tube.

INTERVENTION: Removing a Miller-Abbott Tube

1 Removing a tube that has not reached the ileocecal valve.
   a Explain what the client should expect as you remove the tube.
   b Aspirate and ensure that the mercury and air are removed from balloon portion of the tube.
   c Gradually remove the tube a few inches every five to ten minutes.
   d Give client oral hygiene immediately.

2 Removing a tube that has passed the ileocecal valve.
   a Explain what the client should expect as you remove the tube.
   b Allow the tube to advance through the rectum.
   c Secure the tube at the rectum.

d Cut the tubing at the nose.

e Remove the remaining portion of the tube from the rectum with the aid of peristalsis.

f Provide perineal care.

EVALUATION

EXPECTED OUTCOMES

1 Proper placement and advancement of the tube. *If not*, follow these alternative nursing actions:

ANA: Assess that tube is not kinked or coiled by pulling back on the tube and then allowing it to advance again.

ANA: Ensure that the tube is not pinned to gown or bed in such a way as to prevent advancement.

ANA: If indicated, add more mercury if more weight is required.

ANA: Reposition client to aid in advancement of the tube. If not contraindicated, ambulate client to assist in advancement of tube.

2 Relief of abdominal distention through suction. *If not*, follow these alternative nursing actions:

ANA: Irrigate the tube through the suction portion of the tube.

ANA: Insert rectal tube for 20 minutes.

3 Maintenance of clear tube lumen throughout the intubation period. *If not*, follow these alternative nursing actions:

ANA: Irrigate tube.

ANA: Notify the physician for additional orders.

4 Removal of tube without trauma to intestinal mucosa. *If not*, follow these alternative nursing actions:

ANA. Observe stool for occult blood and notify physician.

Charting

- Time and date tube inserted
- Ease of insertion
- Amount, consistency, color, and odor of drainage obtained from suction
- Oral care given
- Records of intake and output
- Dates and times irrigated
- Amount of irrigant used
- Time intervals tubing is pulled during removal
- Number of inches tubing is pulled during removal
- Unexpected outcomes and measures taken to correct outcome
- Client's reactions to all phases of nursing intervention

A Miller-Abbott tube is used for intestinal decompression.

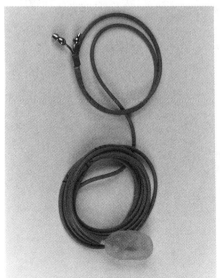

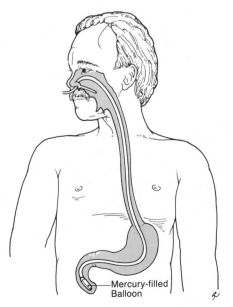

Mercury-filled Balloon

Suction is applied after balloon passes pyloric valve; tube is advanced in increments of one to two inches every hour.

1 Client has reflux esophagitis from decreased competence of the gastroesophageal sphincter caused by the presence of the tube.
   ANA: Elevate the head of the bed 30 degrees.
2 Client develops irritation and inflammation of the oral cavity.
   ANA: Allow the client to gargle frequently with warm saline solution.
3 Client becomes extremely distressed during removal of the tube.
   ANA: Have the client use relaxation techniques during tube removal.
   ANA: Distract the client's attention away from the procedure.
4 The client becomes very nauseated during removal of the tube.
   ANA: Administer antiemetic medication.
   ANA: Remove the tubing from the client's sight as quickly as possible after removal.

ACTION: ESTABLISHING A REGULAR BOWEL EVACUATION

ASSESSMENT

1 Evaluate client's diet.
   a Amount of high-bulk foods.
   b Amount of fluid intake daily.
2 Evaluate client's physical status.
   a Ability to ambulate, i.e., spinal cord injury, CVA.
   b Ability to perform bed exercises, abdominal exercises.
   c Extent of disease process.
3 Assess effectiveness of drugs such as stool softeners, bulk formers, suppositories.
4 Assess time of day client usually evacuates bowel.
5 Identify client's ability to adapt and psychological readiness for the program.
6 Identify position most effective for bowel evacuation.
7 Assess consistency of stool for abnormal findings (diarrhea or fecal impaction).
8 Assess when client had last bowel movement.
9 Assess for abdominal distention.

PLANNING

GOALS

- Client establishes regular bowel evacuation program.
- Client does not become impacted.
- Client is able to evacuate bowel at a time convenient for his or her life-style.
- Client is able to perform own bowel program.

EQUIPMENT

- Nonsterile gloves
- Lubricant

Rationale for Action

- To promote regular bowel evacuation
- To prevent constipation
- To remove a fecal impaction
- To establish a bowel program to which the client can easily adapt

- Commode
- Absorbent pad
- Specific enema if ordered
- Washcloth and towel
- Medications if ordered
- Bedpan

INTERVENTION: Removing a Fecal Impaction

1. Obtain physician's order if client is at risk for possible complications from vagal stimulation (i.e., cardiac or spinal cord injured client).
2. Gather equipment.
3. Explain procedure to client.
4. Provide privacy.
5. Wash your hands.
6. Obtain baseline pulse and blood pressure.
7. Place client on left side.
8. Place absorbent pad on bed.
9. Place bed pan next to client's buttocks.
10. Place glove on hand and lubricate fingers well.
11. Ask client to take a deep breath and exhale slowly as your index finger is gently inserted into rectum.
12. Gently remove the hardened stool.
13. Allow client to rest between digital removal if any untoward effects such as palpitations, faint feeling, etc., are exhibited.
14. Obtain vital signs if client complains of any discomfort.
15. Wash and dry buttocks thoroughly.
16. Dispose of equipment.
17. Send stool specimen to lab if ordered; otherwise, dispose of stool in toilet.
18. Wash your hands.
19. Position client for comfort.
20. Wash your hands.

▶ **Clinical Alert**

Vagal stimulation can result from manual removal of feces; therefore, it should be used only as a last resort and with a specific physician's order.

INTERVENTION: Providing Digital Stimulation

1. Digital stimulation, given one half hour after dinner or breakfast, is usually required for spinal cord injured clients.
2. Gather equipment.
3. Explain procedure to client.
4. Provide privacy.
5. Place client in position for bowel evacuation (bedpan, commode, toilet).
6. Place glove on hand or finger cot on index finger and lubricate well.
7. Insert finger into rectum 4 to 14 cm.
8. Move your finger from side to side in a circular motion to slightly stretch the rectal wall. Move toward the spine and not the bladder to prevent injury to the bladder.

459

9 Continue stretching the rectal wall for one to three minutes until the internal sphincter muscle relaxes.
10 Work with client to discover an associated stimulus to help establish a good bowel routine.
11 Use abdominal massage, coughing, deep inhalations, and tightening of abdominal muscles, in conjunction with digital stimulation, to assist in bowel evacuation.
12 Repeat digital stimulation for one to three minutes at five minute intervals up to 20 minutes if a bowel movement does not occur.

INTERVENTION: Developing a Regular Bowel Routine

1 Explain procedure to client.
2 Identify time of day client usually evacuates bowel.
3 Evaluate diet, exercise, former use of medications for bowel evacuation.
4 Administer the following drugs:
   a Stool softener (Colace or Parlax) daily.
   b Bulk former (Metamucil) q.d. to t.i.d.
   c Mild laxative (Senokot, Doxidan) eight hours before program.
   d Suppository (glycerin or Dulcolax) just before digital stimulation.
5 Perform digital stimulation one half hour after dinner or breakfast.
6 Place client on toilet or commode. (Use bedpan if client is on bedrest.)
7 Provide privacy and sufficient time for evacuation.
8 Wash and dry perineal area if client unable to do so.
9 Place client in wheelchair or bed and position for comfort.
10 Wash your hands.
11 Wean client away from suppositories and laxatives when spontaneous bowel movements occur with digital stimulation.

INTERVENTION: Administering a Suppository for Bowel Program

1 Wash your hands.
2 Gather equipment.
3 Explain procedure to client.
4 Provide privacy.
5 Place glove on hand or finger cot and lubricate well.
6 Insert suppository (usually glycerin) with pointed end first, and place high in rectum beyond external and internal sphincter.
7 Push the suppository against the side of the rectal wall. Ensure it is not placed into fecal mass as it will be ineffective. Place client on toilet or commode.
8 If bowel movement does not occur, perform digital stimulation.
9 Repeat with stronger suppository (Dulcolax) after 20 minutes if there are no results.
10 Allow client to retain Dulcolax suppository for 20 minutes. If no results, do digital stimulation again.

▶ Good bowel training program must include:
1 Initiation of defecation on demand with digital stimulation and abdominal massage.
2 Evacuation at same time each day.
3 Proper diet.
4 Daily physical exercise regimen.
5 Client and family education.

11 Repeat bowel training program next day. If after third day there are no results, notify physician for orders.
12 Following bowel evacuation, cleanse and dry perineal area.
13 Wash your hands.
14 Position client in wheelchair or bed.

EVALUATION

EXPECTED OUTCOMES

1   Client establishes regular bowel evacuation program. *If not*, follow these alternative nursing actions:
    ANA: Alter diet to include more fruits and vegetables.
    ANA: Increase fluid intake to 3000 cc daily unless contraindicated.
    ANA: Obtain order from physician to administer stool softeners and bulk formers in greater quantity.
    ANA: Increase physical activity, especially exercise of the abdominal muscles.
    ANA: Ensure that client begins bowel training program one-half hour after a meal to make use of normal peristalsis and the gastro-colic and duodenal reflexes.
2   Client's bowel movement is regular. *If not*, follow these alternative nursing actions:
    ANA: Complete digital stimulation and use of multiple suppositories for three days. If no bowel movement by then, a laxative or enema may need to be prescribed.
    ANA: If client has a spinal cord injury, observe for signs of autonomic hyperreflexia (goose pimples, pounding headache, hypertension, perspiration above level of spinal cord injury).
    ANA: If clinical manifestations of autonomic hyperreflexia occur, discontinue digital stimulation, apply Nupercainal or Xylocaine ointment around anus and rectum. This will anesthetize the area and decrease the stimulation that caused the response. Wait ten minutes for symptoms to decrease and then gently remove the feces.
3   Client is able to evacuate bowels at a convenient time. *If not*, follow these alternative nursing actions:
    ANA: Evaluate length of time for entire program and help client plan an appropriate time period for evacuation.
    ANA: Alter daily routine to allow necessary time for effective bowel elimination.
    ANA: Reinforce the need for an unhurried time for proper bowel evacuation.
4   Client is able to perform own bowel training program. *If not*, follow these alternative nursing actions:
    ANA: Instruct client on ways he or she can assist with the bowel training program, such as inhaling deeply, coughing, and tightening abdominal muscles.
    ANA: Encourage client to become responsible for own care (unless physically unable to do so). The program will be more effective if the client is an active participant.

ANA: Instruct family members in bowel training routine.

ANA: Refer client to home health care agency for visiting nurse services.

UNEXPECTED OUTCOMES

1 When digital stimulation is performed, client exhibits reflex spasm and prevents stool expulsion.

ANA: Apply local anesthetic around rectum and anus.

ANA: Wait for spasm to relax and then proceed with stimulation.

2 Client develops diarrhea.

ANA: Identify and treat cause of diarrhea.

ANA: Observe dietary intake for possible cause. Provide for bulk.

ANA: Hold the laxatives and stool softeners temporarily.

ANA: Provide yogurt and milk.

ANA: Obtain physician's order for Kaopectate. Administer 2 tsp after each loose stool for 24 hours.

ANA: Readjust medications for bowel training program as needed.

3 Client exhibits signs and symptoms of vagal response during removal of fecal impaction.

ANA: Immediately discontinue procedure.

ANA: Place client in shock position.

ANA: Monitor vital signs every five to fifteen minutes until condition is stable.

ANA: Notify physician for medication order such as atropine.

Charting

- Type and number of suppositories used
- Digital stimulation used
- Approximate time used for digital stimulation
- Amount, consistency, characteristics of stool
- Protocol for bowel evacuation for client
- Untoward complications of bowel training program
- Nursing interventions needed to correct complications

CHAPTER 14
Alterations in Fluid and Electrolytes

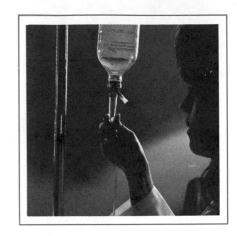

This chapter discusses the role that fluid and electrolytes play in maintaining the fluid balance within the body. It also outlines common nursing actions that can be utilized to restore homeostatic balance to the client.

ANATOMY AND PHYSIOLOGY RELATED TO FLUID AND ELECTROLYTES

Fluids and electrolytes do not exist independently. They exist in a state of dynamic equilibrium which demands a stable composition of the various elements that are essential to life. The primary elements that control this state of equilibrium are fluids, or body water, and electrolytes, most of which are minerals.

Fluids Body fluids are primarily water. Depending on the amount of body fat, a person's total body weight is usually made up of between 50 and 70 percent water. Since fat is essentially water-free, an obese adult's body weight will be 50 percent water. In a leaner individual the percentage of body weight due to body water is closer to 70 percent.

Body water is divided into three compartments: intracellular fluids, extracellular fluids, and intravascular fluids. The majority of the body water is located inside the cell. Most extracellular fluid is found in the

LEARNING OBJECTIVES

Describe the role the kidney plays in maintaining fluid and electrolyte balance.

Compare and contrast the clinical manifestations associated with overhydration and dehydration.

List the steps in preparing the IV bottle.

Describe the steps in the procedure for performing a venipuncture using a wing-tipped needle and an over-the-needle catheter.

Calculate an IV flow rate using a standard formula.

Describe the reason for hanging the partial fill bottle higher than the primary IV bottle.

Describe the procedure for obtaining a CVP reading.

Explain safety checks utilized to ensure proper blood is administered to client.

Differentiate between the clinical manifestations associated with bacterial, allergic, and hemolytic blood transfusion reactions.

interstitial spaces surrounding body cells. Only a small percentage of the body's total water is located in the intravascular fluid compartment, or the body's plasma.

Communication between these fluid compartments varies. Intracellular body water does not move out of the cell readily. In contrast, body water in the intravascular and interstitial spaces can diffuse easily and is similar in electrolyte composition. The diffusion of fluid from the vascular compartment to the interstitial spaces back to the blood is controlled by a variety of factors such as hydrostatic pressure, osmotic pressures, and the diameter of the vessels.

The overall maintenance of body water is the result of adjustments made between the gains and losses of water that occur on a daily basis. The major sources of water coming into the body are fluids or solid foods. A small amount of water is also produced as a by-product of cellular metabolism. Most fluid leaves the body through urinary excretion. Water is also lost by fecal elimination, sweating, and diffusion and evaporation through the skin and the lung.

The major organ of excretion is the kidney. Because the kidney handles the end-products of cellular metabolism, as well as the intake of fluids, it must excrete a minimum of 500 to 600 cc of urine every 24 hours. Depending on the amount of fluid intake, this amount usually varies from 600 to 1600 cc.

The regulation of the volume and concentration of body fluids is handled by two mechanisms: thirst and urinary excretion. Thirst is stimulated by receptors in the central nervous system. Under normal circumstances, an individual will ingest fluids when these receptors are activated. During an illness or an altered level of consciousness, the thirst response may change, causing such conditions as hypovolemia and increased tonicity or concentration of the extracellular fluids.

Urinary excretion through the kidney is directed or influenced by two regulatory systems. The first regulatory system involves the antidiuretic hormone (ADH). By increasing and decreasing ADH, this system helps to regulate the balance of fluids in the body.

When extracellular body fluids become concentrated, osmoreceptors located in the hypothalamus stimulate the release of ADH from its storage place. ADH then acts on the kidney, causing it to retain more water.

As this retained water circulates through the extracellular fluid department, the concentration of body fluids is reduced. The osmoreceptors, sensing this change, slow the secretion of ADH, which then acts on the kidney, causing it to excrete more water.

Other conditions that can stimulate the secretion of ADH and lead to increased water retention by the kidney include hemorrhage, decreased cardiac output, trauma, pain, fear, surgery, and dehydration. Drugs such as morphine, barbiturates, and nicotine and some anesthetics and tranquilizers will also increase the secretion of ADH. The secretion of ADH can be inhibited by alcohol, decreased concentration of body fluids, and hypervolemic states.

The second system that regulates urinary excretion involves the hormone aldosterone. Like ADH, aldosterone is secreted by the adrenal cortex and regulates the levels of sodium in the body. Because sodium is exchanged for either potassium or hydrogen, aldosterone indirectly affects the levels of potassium and hydrogen as well. Secretion of aldosterone is increased in response to several stimuli which include decreased sodium and increased extracellular potassium, hypovolemia, and physical or emotional stress.

When the level of sodium is lowered, or when hypovolemia occurs, the receptor-like area in the glomerulus of the nephron releases an enzyme substance called renin. As renin circulates in the body, it converts a plasma protein in the liver into a vasoconstrictor substance called angiotensin I. When this substance enters the lungs it is converted into angiotensin II. Angiotensin II acts directly on the adrenal cortex and increases the level of aldosterone secretion. Aldosterone then stimulates the kidney's tubule cells to retain sodium and to secrete either hydrogen or potassium. The sodium that is retained in the body increases the overall concentration of extracellular fluids, which stimulates the osmoreceptors in the hypothalamus to increase the secretion of the hormone ADH. The hypersecretion of ADH, in turn, causes the kidney to retain more water.

Electrolytes In partnership with body fluids are substances called electrolytes. These substances, mostly minerals, contribute to body function in many ways and are essential to life.

Electrolytes are distributed throughout the body, both intracellularly and extracellularly. In the extracellular compartment, the main electrolytes are sodium, chloride, and bicarbonate. Intracellular electrolytes are potassium, magnesium, phosphate, and sulfate.

Electrolytes, in body fluids, possess an electrical charge when placed in water. Electrolytes with a positive charge are called cations. Negatively charged electrolytes are called anions. Positive cations and negative anions are attracted to each other because of their opposite electrical charges. When they combine with each other, they form neutral compounds that either remain in body fluids or dissociate and regain their electrical charges. When they do dissociate or ionize, they are referred to as ions. Refer to the Fluid and Electrolyte Summary Chart.

The unit of measure for the body's electrolytes is the milliequivalent. Since electrolytes combine electrochemically because of their electrical charge and chemical activity, the milliequivalent is a more useful measure than a gram or milligram, which indicates weight only. One milligram of hydrogen represents the unit for chemical combining power.

FLUID GAINS AND LOSSES

INTAKE	OUTPUT	
Oral intake 1,500 – 3,000	Urine	600 – 1,600
Cellular catabolism of PRO, CHO AND FAT	Skin	300 – 600 (insensible loss)
	Lung	350 (insensible loss)
	Feces	200
	Sweat	100 – 300

TABLE 1 MAJOR ELECTROLYTES

CATIONS$^+$		ANIONS$^-$	
Na^+	Sodium	Cl^-	Chloride
K^+	Potassium	HCO_3^-	Bicarbonate
Ca^{++}	Calcium	HPO_4^{--}	Phosphate
Mg^{++}	Magnesium		

ALTERATIONS IN FLUID AND ELECTROLYTES

Alterations in fluid and electrolytes may occur as a primary event or as secondary responses to a preexisting disease state or to a sudden, unexpected traumatic episode. When alterations among the fluids and electrolytes exceed the narrow limits consistent with health, the body needs to adjust quickly.

Changes in the composition of body fluids and electrolytes may be relative or absolute. Relative losses or gains can occur when fluids or electrolytes shift from one body space to another. Absolute losses or gains can occur when electrolytes and fluids are lost outside the body or added to the overall body stores by IV fluid and blood replacement because of injury or medical/surgical procedures. Because body elements are in a state of continual change, minor alterations in one element can affect all the other elements within the body's matrix.

In summary, this chapter will examine the methods of identifying fluid losses through the measurements of intake and output, weight, and serum electrolytes. These modalities provide baseline data as well as sequential measurements in the assessment of fluid and electrolyte gains or losses.

In addition to obtaining assessment data, the chapter will discuss methods of providing fluid and electrolytes to clients who have experienced alterations in their homeostasis.

Clients undergoing major surgery or trauma may be subjected to blood loss necessitating replacement therapy. Administration of blood and blood products will be discussed. Clients requiring intravenous therapy frequently have associated nutritional needs that are not always met. The nutritional needs of clients cannot be met by intravenous fluids alone. If the client will need to remain on parenteral therapy, other means of nutritional support must be considered.

GUIDELINES FOR MANAGING CLIENTS

The primary purpose for performing interventions associated with alterations in either fluids or electrolytes is to maintain homeostasis and regulate and maintain essential fluids and nutrients. As you perform nursing interventions, refer to the following guidelines.

Clients subject to severe alterations in fluids and electrolytes will not be able to remain in homeostatic balance.
- Excesses or deficits of fluids and electrolytes may be due to loss of function of the regulatory mechanisms.
- The kidney is an electrolyte computer. If it is functioning correctly, it will supply the body with optimum intravascular volume so that many mild to moderate imbalances will correct themselves.

Excessive losses of either fluids or electrolytes necessitate replacement therapy.
- A daily minimum fluid intake of 1500 cc is essential for fluid balance.
- The kidney has an obligatory urine output and the body has an insensible water loss which must be replaced daily.

▶ Anticipate alterations in fluid, electrolyte, and regulatory mechanisms when any of the following has occurred:

Trauma
Major surgery
Major traumatic injuries, such as crush injuries or thermal burns
Dietary restrictions
Drug therapy involving diuretics, steroids, or nephrotoxic drugs
Abnormal losses of body fluids/electrolytes
High level emotional stress
Disease states directly affecting the regulatory organs, i.e., kidney, lung, skin, GI tract
Disease states indirectly influencing the dynamic equilibrium of the body, i.e., cancer, metabolic disorders, CNS alterations, congestive heart failure.

- Essential electrolytes must be replaced to ensure cellular metabolic processes.

Intake and output are approximately equal when the body's fluid state is in balance.

- A loss of body water greater than intake results in weight loss. A gain of body water greater than output results in weight gain.
- One kg of body weight gain or loss is equal to 1000 cc or one liter of fluid.
- Daily weights reflect fluid gains and losses more accurately than written intake and output records, which are subject to many inaccuracies.
- Fluid imbalances involving the redistribution of fluids, as in burns or gastric surgeries, will not be reflected as changes in body weight.

▶ Some 24-hour intake and output records preprint a 600 to 900 insensible loss in the output column to alert the staff to incorporate this number in their calculations.

Barrier nursing principles related to IV therapy dictate that the skin is the first line of defense against microbial invasion.

- Handwashing decreases the numbers of both endogenous and exogenous microorganisms, reducing the risk of cross contamination of the catheter.
- A vigorous skin prep will decrease endogenous and exogenous organisms at the venipuncture site.

Each time the closed body system is entered the potential for contamination exists.

- Strict attention should be directed to maintaining the infusion system aseptically.
- Once the catheter has been inserted, it should be anchored with tape to prevent rocking motion which may irritate the vein or push bacteria into the bloodstream from the skin.
- The sterile dressing should be applied in such a way that daily dressing changes and venipuncture site inspection can occur without undue problems.
- The IV administration set should be changed every 24 to 48 hours to decrease levels of microbial contaminants in the infusion solution.

ACTION: ASSESSING INTAKE AND OUTPUT

ASSESSMENT

1 Identify client's need for intake and output even if there has been no physician's request.
2 Assess client's ability to keep intake and output fluid records.
3 Evaluate client for any factors that might affect his intake and output, e.g., preexisting disease states, concurrent diagnosed disease, drug therapies, and current physical status.
4 Determine all measurable sources of fluid intake: fluids with and between meals, liquid medications, IV fluids, and IV medications as baseline for urinary output.

Rationale for Action

- To establish a written record of the client's total fluid intake (oral, parenteral, and/or feeding tubes) and fluid output (urine, stool, GI and chest drainage, unexpected loss from a wound, diarrhea, vomiting)
- To plan fluid replacement or appropriate therapy by assessing deficits and/or excesses of fluids and/or electrolytes
- To diagnose specific disease states

467

5 Determine all measurable sources of fluid output: urine, vomitus, diarrhea, and drainage.
6 Determine alterations in nonmeasurable sources of fluid intake and loss: food, increased metabolism, rapid respirations, and excessive perspiration.
7 Check Table 3 for sites to assess hydration status.

PLANNING

GOALS

- Intake and output, though not exactly equal, within 200 cc to 300 cc of each other
- Fluid intake at least 1500 cc unless contraindicated by diagnosis, e.g., CHF, pulmonary edema
- Client's hydration state, vital signs, and mental state normal
- Electrolyte values within normal limits

EQUIPMENT

- Graduated metric container in client's bathroom
- Intake and output fluid balance sheet at client's bedside or in client's chart
- Urinal/bedpan; bedside commode/underseat basin for toilet
- Hourly inline urine measurement device for catheterized clients
- Posted measurement standards for commonly used drinking and eating glasses, mugs, bowls, etc.
- Posted signs, dietary slips, and other communication devices to notify hospital personnel about how client's intake and output is to be measured.

INTERVENTION: Monitoring Intake and Output

1 Determine if client needs intake and output measurements by checking Kardex or client's chart.
2 Measure intake from all sources.
  a Oral fluids
  b IV fluids
  c Fluids with IV meds
  d Tube feedings and water used to clear tubing
3 Measure output from all sources.
  a Foley/French catheters
  b Bedpans/urinals
  c Nasogastric drainage
  d Drainage tubing, i.e., T-tubes
  e Diarrheal stools
  f Draining wounds
  g Vomitus

4 Record intake and output on bedside record each time you take a measurement.
5 Record 24-hour totals of intake and output on bedside record and on graphic sheet in client's chart.
6 Report intake and output measurements to incoming shift.
7 Notify physician of any abnormality which could lead to complications, e.g., hourly urine output less than 25 to 30 cc per hour or 24-hour urine output less than 500 cc.

EVALUATION

EXPECTED OUTCOMES

1 Intake and output, though not exactly equal, are within 200 cc to 300 cc of each other. *If not*, follow these alternative nursing actions:
ANA: Check to see if other hospital personnel are keeping accurate records.
ANA: Talk with client and/or family to find out if they are cooperating with the recording of all intake and output.
ANA: Check for errors made in adding up notations of measurements or for errors in measurement standards.
ANA: Make sure that IV volumes are recorded each shift and that any fluid remaining in the bottle is reported to the next shift.
2 Fluid intake is at least 1500 cc unless contraindicated by diagnosis. *If not*, follow these alternative nursing actions:
ANA: Check to see if client has had access to fluids on diet trays and at bedside and has been given fluid supplements.
ANA: Assess thirst level and client's physical condition. Is client too weak to ask for or to drink fluids by him or herself?
3 Client's hydration state, vital signs, and mental status appear normal. *If not*, follow these alternative nursing actions:
ANA: Assess all factors that might be contributing to fluid imbalance, e.g., hypotension, hypovolemia, stress, or surgery that might have altered hormonal regulation of output, primary kidney disease, cardiovascular disease, or obstructive lung disease (which might affect regulatory mechanisms).
ANA: Check for losses that might not have been noted by other personnel, e.g., excessive diaphoresis, extended high temperature, incontinence of either urine or stool, rapid respiratory rate, or large denuded skin areas with serum loss.
4 Electrolyte values are within normal limits. *If not*, follow these alternative nursing actions:
ANA: Refer to Fluid and Electrolyte Summary chart for specific treatment for electrolyte imbalances.
ANA: Assess signs and symptoms of client (specific symptoms are manifested with specific electrolyte imbalances).
ANA: Establish a baseline so when correction occurs you will be able to reassess.

Charting
- Measurements of intake and output
- Approximate volume of loss
- Dietary intake (food as well as water)
- Time, amount, and description of all measurable intake and output
- Client's state of hydration, including supporting data

469

TABLE 2 INTAKE AND OUTPUT FLOW SHEET

DATE	TIME	IV NO.	IV AMT. STARTED	DESCRIPTION	IV INTAKE	ORAL INTAKE	URINE OUTPUT	OTHER	N/G
1/9/82	9 A			Full liquid breakfast		620			
	9:45 A			Vomitus				400	
	10:30 A	#1	1000						
	12 N						450		
	2:30 P						300		
				7-3 Total	450	620	750	400	100
	6:30 P	#2	1000		550				
	9 P						375		
				3-11 Total	1050	NPO	375		250
1/10/82	2:30 A	#3	1000		450				
	5 A						250		
				11-7 Total	1050	NPO	250		175
				24-hr Total	2550	620	1375	400	525

TABLE 3 BODY SITES FOR ASSESSMENT OF HYDRATION

SITE	EXCESS HYDRATION	DEHYDRATION
HEAD AND NECK		
Face	Eyeballs firm and/or protruding	Eyeballs soft and/or sunken
	Edema, especially around eyes	Poor skin turgor over forehead
Mucous	Excessive salivation	Dry or sticky mucosa
Membranes	Swollen tongue	Shrunken tongue
		Crusted lips
Neck	Jugular vein distention	
TRUNK		
Chest	Moist rales	Poor skin turgor
	Pulmonary congestion	Dry, flaking skin
Abdomen	Ascites (measure girth at umbilicus)	
Sacrum	Edema	Poor skin turgor
EXTREMITIES		
Arms	Edema, particularly of the hands	Poor skin turgor
	Delayed capillary refill	Delayed capillary refill
	Unequal quality of radial pulses	Dry, flaking skin
	Pulse bounding	Pulse weak and thready
Legs	Edema	Poor skin turgor, especially across shins
	Taut shiny skin	Dry, flaky skin, especially on feet
	Weak pedal pulse and/or decreased capillary refill	Weak pedal pulse and/or decreased capillary refill

TABLE 4 OBJECTIVE DATA INDICATIVE OF THE STATE OF HYDRATION

DATA	EXCESS HYDRATION	DEHYDRATION
VITAL SIGNS		
Blood Pressure	Increased*	Decreased
Pulse	Increased rate	Increased rate
Temperature	Unchanged	Elevated
Respirations	Increased rate	Unchanged or increased
LABORATORY FINDINGS		
Urine Specific Gravity	Decreased, approaching 1.010	Increased, approaching 1.025 or greater
Blood Hematocrit	Less than three times the hemoglobin	Greater than three times the hemoglobin
Serum Sodium (Na)	Less than 135 mEq/L	Greater than 145 mEq/L
Hourly Urine Output	More than 60 cc/hr	Less than 30 to 60 cc/hr
Weight	A 5% or greater gain	Mild: 2% loss
		Moderate: 3 – 5% loss
		Severe: 6% or greater loss

*If the heart is no longer able to pump the increased blood volume, and cardiac decompensation occurs, the blood pressure will drop.

ACTION: WEIGHING CLIENTS

ASSESSMENT

1 Assess the need for daily or weekly body weight measurements.
2 Determine appropriate method for obtaining client's weight (bedside scale, bed scale).

PLANNING

GOALS

- Client's weight, depending on status, disease state and therapy, shows expected losses, gains or stabilization.
- Weight is obtained and recorded as ordered by physician.

EQUIPMENT

- Balance beam scale (for clients who are able to stand without assistance)
- Bed scale (for clients who are confined to bed or who are unable to stand)
- Bed scale that is built into the bed
- Floor scale (for clients in wheelchairs)

INTERVENTION: Weighing Clients

1 Ask client to void before weighing.
2 Weigh client in the morning before breakfast.
3 Use the same scale each time you weigh the client.

Rationale for Action

- To establish baseline data to check against total body fluid balance
- To identify excess or deficits of fluid balance
- To establish baseline data for diagnostic tests that involve dye and radioactive material injections
- To determine drug dosage

4 Make sure the client wears the same clothing for each weighing.
5 If the client is bedridden, weigh the linens that are used for covering, such as drawsheet.
6 Change wet gowns or heavily saturated dressings before weighing the client.

EVALUATION

EXPECTED OUTCOMES

1 Client's weight, depending on status, disease state, and therapy, shows expected losses, gains, or stabilization. *If not*, follow these alternative nursing actions:
  ANA: Check to see if the weighing procedure was carried out correctly and with the proper equipment.
  ANA: Assess client for clinical manifestations indicating the onset of fluid/electrolyte disturbance.
  ANA: Check serum electrolyte lab slips for abnormal findings.
2 Weight is obtained and recorded as ordered by physician. *If not*, follow these alternative nursing actions:
  ANA: Assess method of weighing to see if appropriate to client status.
  ANA: Rearrange weighing schedule so that it is completed at the same time every day by a responsible person.

UNEXPECTED OUTCOME

Client is too critically ill to be weighed accurately because of mechanical devices used to sustain life.
  ANA: Estimate weight loss and gain by assessing other factors, e.g., skin turgor, output, presence of edema.

Charting
- Client's weight recorded in weight book or on graphic sheet
- Type of scale used for weighing
- Bed linens, gowns, and/or equipment weighed (record on care plan or on Kardex)

Rationale for Action
- To maintain fluid and electrolyte balance
- To administer medications through the most therapeutic intravenous route
- To provide a ready access for emergency medications, particularly in critically ill clients
- To provide a route for administering blood and blood products
- To provide a route for maintaining the nutritional status of the client
- To obtain information about the status of the right side of the heart, the fluid status, and blood volume of the body

ACTION: ADMINISTERING INTRAVENOUS THERAPY

ASSESSMENT

1 Assess need for IV therapy.
2 Determine client's need for psychological support.
3 Assess need for client teaching about IV therapy.
4 Identify appropriate site for venipuncture. Vein should be superficial, large enough for the needle to be inserted smoothly, readily palpated, and easily followed.
5 Evaluate client for proper placement of cannula.
  a Placement is based on client convenience and functional use (left vs. right hand).
  b If possible, the cannula is not placed in joints that bend, e.g., antecubital space, wrist. When a cannula must be placed in a joint, a splint must be used to immobilize the joint.

c Assess type and size of cannula necessary. (Blood requires a larger size cannula, at least #18.)

6 Determine length of time necessary for therapy so that you can select the appropriate equipment.

7 Assess client's cardiovascular status so that you know which vein to use for IV equipment.

PLANNING

GOALS

- IV therapy initiated and maintained without difficulty
- Catheter inserted into central vein without complications
- Fluids, additives, and medications administered without adverse effects on the client
- Blood and blood products administered through appropriate tubing and equipment
- IV site remains free from redness, edema, and purulent drainage
- IV infusion rate accurately calculated and reassessed throughout the therapy
- IV equipment removed without complications

EQUIPMENT

- Tourniquet or blood pressure cuff
- Antimicrobial wipe (povidone-iodine or iodophors are preferred; alcohol is acceptable if client is allergic to iodine.)
- Sterile cannula or needle: winged-tipped needle; intermittent infusion set or heparin lock; over-the-needle catheter
- IV solution in either bottle or bag, as ordered by physician
- Administration set: drip system, which includes drip chamber and IV tubing
- Extension tubing to lengthen the original tubing or to provide extra ports for the administration of additional medication
- IV pole: free-standing, bed-attached, or ceiling-affixed
- Tape (Check client for adhesive allergy.)
- Sterile two- by two-inch strips or bandaids
- Antimicrobial ointment
- Filter to be used whenever the IV system has been entered to administer drugs or whenever an infusion catheter is to be inserted into a large central vein.

ADDITIONAL EQUIPMENT

For Intermittent Infusion
- Three syringes with needles
- Several extra needles
- Vials of heparin
- Vials of saline solution

Clinical Alert

In conditions of unexplained fever, always suspect IV catheter-related sepsis.

▶ Sterile gloves are recommended for the following conditions:

If client is a severely compromised host.

If the catheter will have to remain in place for an extended period. For example, with a CVP, arterial line, or hyperalimentation line.

If the client has few available veins for venipuncture.

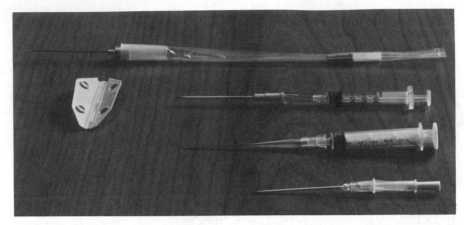

(a) Frequently used types of over-the-needle and through-the-needle IV catheters.

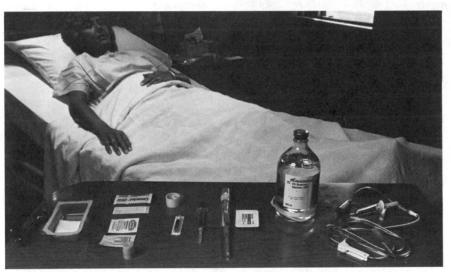

(b) Gather and prepare necessary equipment before beginning venipuncture.

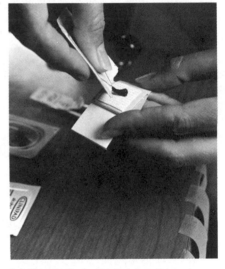

(c) Place antimicrobial ointment on gauze pad before performing venipuncture.

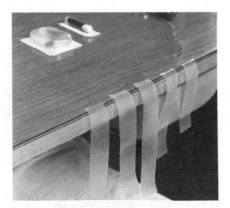

(d) Cut appropriate length strips of tape in preparation for venipuncture.

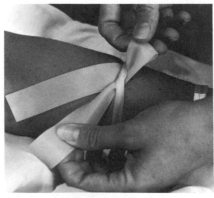

(e) Apply tourniquet proximal to IV puncture site.

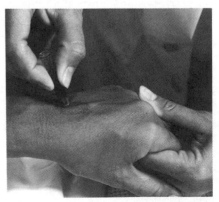

(f) Apply povidone-iodine to puncture site and allow to dry thoroughly.

PREPARATION

For selection of puncture site
- Veins should be superficial, easily palpated and followed, and large enough for a needle to be smoothly inserted.
- Veins should be free of sclerosis, hematomas, and pain
- Veins should be selected according to the IV solution that will be infused. Larger veins are preferable for caustic solutions, blood, and viscous fluid.
- Distal end of veins should be punctured first. Proximal ends should be preserved for further IV therapy.
- Cannula or needle should be placed in the arm that is not used for writing.
- Cannula or needle should not be placed near joints, which require immobilization.

For selection of cannula or needle
- Winged-tipped needles: Used in short-term therapy with adults and in normal therapy with children, infants, and elderly clients who have small or fragile veins.
- For neonates, use a 25- to 27-gauge needle. For older children, use a 21- to 25-gauge needle.
- Intermittent infusion set or heparin lock: Used in short-term therapy to permit the intermittent administration of drugs directly into the client's vein without exposing the client to the expense and annoyance of a continuous intravenous drip. This system allows blood to

▶ Do not shave the venipuncture site. Shaving can facilitate the development of infection through the multiplication of organisms in microabrasions that occur. Hairy sites can be clipped with scissors.

Anatomical sites frequently used for venipunctures.

Dorsal Venous Network
Basilic Vein
Dorsal Metacarpal Veins
Cephalic Vein

Dorsal Plexus
Dorsal Arch
Greater Saphenous Vein

Radial Vein
Accessory Cephalic Vein
Ulnar Vein
Median Cubital Vein
Basilic Vein

be withdrawn and blood transfusions to be performed without the pain of repeated venipunctures.

- Usually a 23–25 butterfly needle with plug adaptor is used.

For selection of IV fluid and tubing for infusion
- Wash your hands before preparing IV equipment.
- Compare the type and amount of solution with physician's orders.
- Check IV solution container for expiration date and for signs of contamination or deterioration.
- Hold in both a dark and bright light to examine for discoloration, cloudiness, or particulate matter, which indicates a problem.
- Examine glass bottles for cracks or leaks; examine bags for tears.
- Inject any required additives through the medication port in the container before inserting IV tubing.
- Select IV tubing according to the viscosity of the solution that will be infused.

For setting up administration set with glass container
- Remove metal cap, metal disc, and rubber diaphragm from IV bottle. If pharmacy has added medications, remove protective additive cap.
- Listen for the escape of air when rubber diaphragm is removed. No air will escape if additives have been previously added.
- Close control clamp on IV tubing administration set.
- With the container placed on a firm surface, squeeze the IV drip chamber and insert the spike through the appropriate area on the bottle cap.
- Invert IV bottle and place it on the IV pole. Release drip chamber until it is one-third to one-half full of fluid.
- Open tubing control clamp and clear the tubing of air over a receptacle such as an emesis basin or a sink. (It may be necessary to remove the adaptor cap at the end of the tubing so that fluid can flow through the tubing.)
- Readjust the adaptor cap or place covered needle over the tubing insertion site to maintain sterility before infusion is established.
- Before taking IV equipment to client's room, tell client what you will be doing and what type of equipment you will be using.

For setting up administration set with plastic container
- Remove outer wrap surrounding IV container.
- Remove plastic protector from the administration set. Since there is no vacuum in the plastic container, you should not hear any escaping air.
- Close control clamp on IV tubing administration set and squeeze the IV drip chamber.
- Insert the spike into the port, holding the neck of the port tightly to prevent slipping and possible contamination of the setup.
- Invert the IV container and release pressure on the drip chamber.
- Hang the IV container on the IV pole.

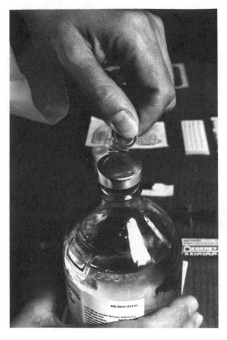

(a) Remove metal cap from IV bottle.

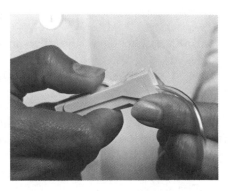

(b) Close control clamp on IV tubing before insertion into IV bottle.

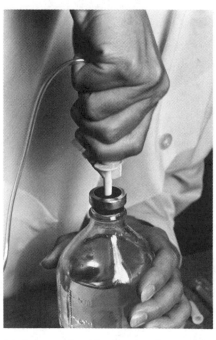

(c) Squeeze the drip chamber. Insert the spike through the rubber stopper of the IV bottle.

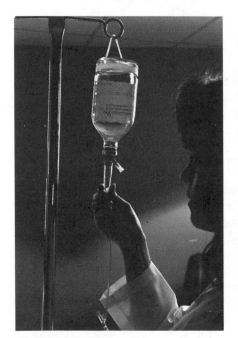

(d) Hang IV bottle on pole.

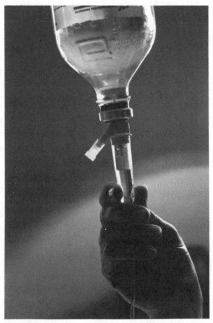

(e) Squeeze drip chamber to fill at least one-third full.

- Open the IV tubing control clamp and clear the tubing of air.
- Readjust the adaptor cap or place covered needle over tubing insertion site to maintain sterility before infusion is established.
- Before taking IV equipment to client's room, tell client what you will be doing and what type of equipment you will be using.

INTERVENTION: Performing a Venipuncture with a Wing-Tipped Needle

1 Assemble equipment in medication room.
2 Take equipment to client's bedside.
3 Hang bottle and place covered end of administration set within easy reach.
4 Position client and adjust lighting as necessary.
5 Cut pieces of tape. Open two-inch by two-inch strips or bandaids and squeeze a dollop of antimicrobial ointment on the sterile surface.
6 Wash your hands again.
7 Select a vein. Inspect both of the client's arms, palpating and visualizing the exact course of the veins. If the client's skin is thick or darkly colored, you may not be able to visualize the veins easily. Instead, palpate them until you find a vein that feels full and superficial.
8 Prepare the site with povidone-iodine or a 70% ethyl alcohol solution if the client is allergic to iodine.
9 Let the iodine or alcohol solution dry on the client's skin before continuing with the intervention.
10 Dilate the client's vein by using one of these methods:
   a Ask the client to open and close his or her fist several times. You may also slap the vein lightly.
   b Place the client in a low or semi-Fowler's position with client's arm over the edge of the mattress for one or two minutes.
   c If the vein is difficult to dilate, apply warm, moist compresses for 10 to 15 minutes.
11 Distend the vein by applying a tourniquet or blood pressure cuff. If using a cuff, pump it to a pressure between the client's systolic and diastolic pressures.
12 Select a winged-tipped needle. (A 20- to 22-gauge needle is adequate for an adult.)
13 Carefully affix the end of the IV administration tubing to the end of the catheter needle. Run fluid through the catheter and needle.
14 Remove sterile cover from needle. Hold winged-tipped needle by its wings.
15 Anchor vein by placing your thumb below the client's vein and gently stretching the skin by pulling down distally.
16 With bevel of the needle up, enter the client's skin at a 45-degree angle. You may use either of these methods:
   a Enter skin at a 45-degree angle next to the vein. Flatten the angle once the needle is under the skin and enter vein from the side.
   b Enter skin and vein in one smooth motion from above. You will

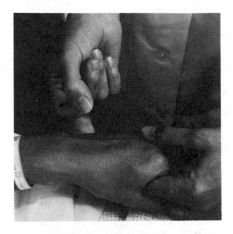

(a) Start venipunctures at distal end of vein to preserve future IV sites.

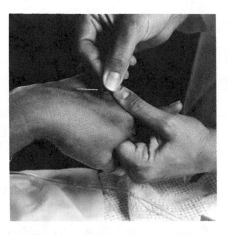

(b) Select a number 20 to 22 gauge winged-needle. For adults keep bevel up and insert needle at 45-degree angle.

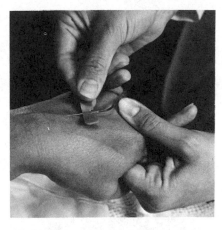

(c) Observe IV tubing for blood backflow indicating the needle is in the vein.

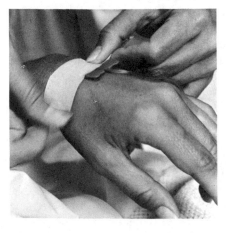

(d) Place tape over needle insertion site to secure it to skin.

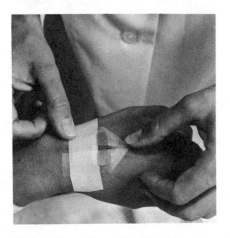

(e) Tape down wings of needle securely to prevent accidental dislodging.

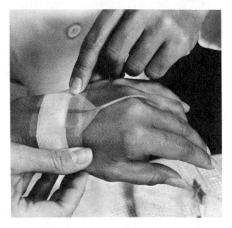

(f) Secure IV site with additional tape, then position tubing.

feel a gentle "pop" or release as the needle enters the vein. Observe for flashback of blood in needle tubing. (This method requires experience and judgment, since it is easy to put the needle through the vein.)

17 Advance needle carefully up the course of the vein.
18 Release tourniquet or blood pressure cuff.
19 Open clamp on IV tubing and observe drip chamber. Fluid should flow easily, and there should be no sudden swelling around the IV site.
20 Reduce flow rate to keep open until you have taped the needle and the tubing in place.
21 Apply antimicrobial ointment to needle site and cover with sterile two- by two-inch strips or bandaids.

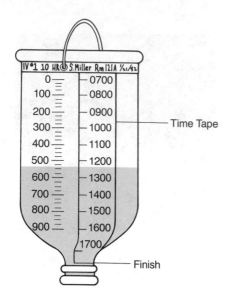

IV #1 10 HR ⊙ S.Miller Rm 121A ⅓₁/₄₂

0	0700
100	0800
200	0900
300	1000
400	1100
500	1200
600	1300
700	1400
800	1500
900	1600
	1700

—— Time Tape

—— Finish

Tape the bottle and indicate the number of ml's to be infused hourly to monitor IV fluid flow rate. For example, a 10-hour bottle will be marked by placing the hour next to each 100 ml increment on the bottle.

▶ Preparation of heparin solution
Solution is usually prepared with 1 ml 1:1000 heparin added to 9 ml of normal saline to produce 100 u/ml solution.

22 Tape winged-tipped needle and tubing to client.
23 Using a watch, set drip rate according to physician's orders.
24 Label IV site with pertinent information, according to hospital policy.

INTERVENTION: Performing a Venipuncture with an Intermittent Infusion Set or Heparin Lock

1 Prepare medication and draw it up into a syringe.
2 Fill a syringe with 2 to 2½ ml of saline.
3 Fill a third syringe with heparin from vial or use a prefilled heparin syringe. (Method will be determined by hospital policy.)
4 If client does not have an intermittent infusion set in place, proceed with venipuncture, selecting veins that are both large enough to receive the bolus of medicine and away from areas of movement, e.g., the elbows and wrists. When taping the set in place, secure the injection port away from the needle insertion site to minimize needle movement when the port is being used.
5 Swab injection port with alcohol or iodophor swab.
6 Insert medication syringe into port.
7 Pull back on syringe plunger and check for flow of blood into syringe. The presence of blood indicates that the needle is placed into the vein, not into surrounding tissues.
8 Inject medication into the vein, timing the flow rate according to physician's orders or drug manufacturer's instructions.
9 Observe client for any adverse reactions.
10 Remove medication syringe.
11 Insert syringe filled with saline.
12 Flush the catheter tubing with saline to clear the line.
13 Remove saline syringe.
14 Insert heparin syringe and inject the heparin to fill the catheter and needle lumen. (The heparin should prevent the catheter from clotting.)
15 Remove syringe and secure the injection port.

INTERVENTION: Performing a Venipuncture with an Over-the-Needle Catheter

1 Prepare IV equipment.
2 Select a moderate to large vein.
3 Just prior to insertion, carefully remove needle cover. Inspect both needle and catheter.
4 With bevel of needle up, insert needle and catheter together as one unit into the client's skin.
5 Insert the cannula into the vein.
6 Advance catheter and needle gently as one unit into the lumen, making sure that both are inside the vein. Observe for backflow of blood in plastic hub of needle.
7 Place small, sterile gauze sponge under hub of the over-the-needle unit.

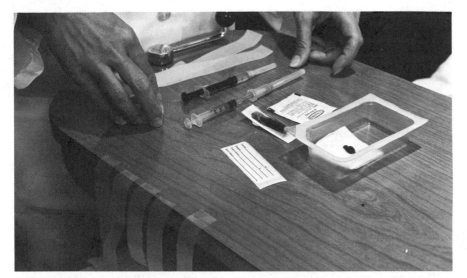

(a) Setting up over-the-needle catheter equipment.

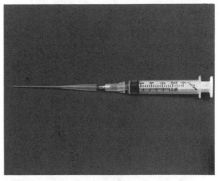

(b) A Medicut is a type of over-the-needle catheter.

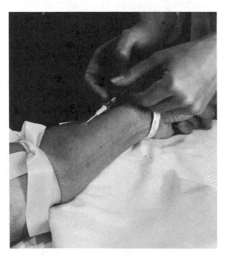

(c) Advance catheter and needle into vein as one unit.

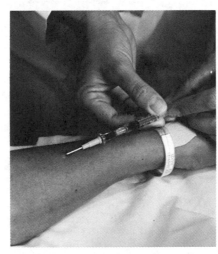

(d) Observe for blood return in plastic hub of needle.

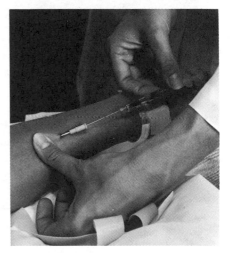

(e) Place fingertip over catheterized vein while gently pulling needle out of catheter.

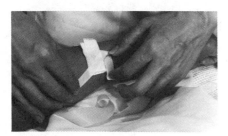

(f) Secure hub of needle to skin by criss-crossing tape over needle hub.

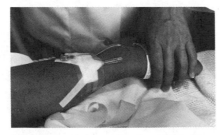

(g) IV tubing is looped and secured with tape to assist in preventing pull on the needle site.

481

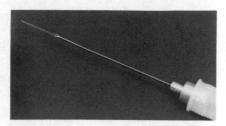

(a) Through-the-needle (inside-the-needle) catheters are used most frequently for long-term therapy and delivery of IV drugs which are irritating to veins.

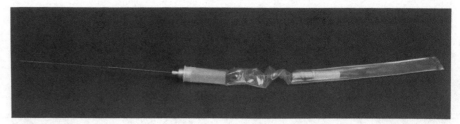

(b) Inside-the-needle catheters are generally inserted by specially trained nurses.

8   As soon as the catheter and needle are fully in place, release the tourniquet.

9   Gently withdraw the needle from inside the catheter with one hand, placing your fingertip firmly above the catheter tip to occlude the vein and prevent sudden bleeding.

10 Connect hub to administration set.

11 Open clamp on set briefly and observe drip chamber. Fluid should flow rapidly without obstruction, and there should not be any sudden swelling at IV site.

12 Reduce flow and proceed with taping, using chevron method.

13 Tape the needle and tubing to the client, using two strips of tape.

INTERVENTION: Regulating the IV Flow Rate

1   Check manufacturer's drip rate calibration on administration set package. Macrodrip sets vary from 10 gtts to 20 gtts to equal 1 ml.

2   Check physician's order for amount of fluid to be delivered per unit of time. Some physicians state one liter to be given over eight hours; others specify hourly flow rate, such as 60 ml per hour.

3   Calculate flow rate. There are several formulas which may be useful. Here is one two-step method.

   a   To find ml to be given per hour:

$$\frac{\text{Total solution}}{\text{No. of hours to run}} = \text{ml per hour}$$

   b   To find drops per minute:

$$\frac{\text{ml/hr} \times \text{drop factor}}{60 \text{ minutes}} = \text{gtts/minute}$$

4   Stand near the drip chamber and count the drops for one minute, using a watch with a sweep hand.

5   Adjust clamp until the chamber drips the desired number of drops.

6   Affix tape to bottle and mark the hourly flow rate.

INTERVENTION: Maintaining an IV System

1   Change IV dressing daily.

2   Examine venipuncture site for redness, edema, or purulent drainage. If any of these conditions are present, discontinue the use of the IV site immediately.

3 Start IV at a different site. (Use of an antimicrobial agent is optional.)

4 Change site of IV insertion every 48 to 72 hours.

5 Change IV tubing every 48 hours.

6 Do not leave any solution hanging longer than 24 hours.

IV CALORIE CALCULATION

In IV solutions, carbohydrates are given in the form of dextrose (glucose) or fructose. With either sugar, one gram provides approximately four calories. Therefore, the amount of calories found in a liter of dextrose or fructose and water can be measured by multiplying the grams of dextrose or fructose by four.

Solution	Amount of gm/liter	× 4	Calories
2.5% dextrose	0.025 g/ml × 1000 =	25 gm × 4	100
5% dextrose	0.05 g/ml × 1000 =	50 gm × 4	200
10% dextrose	0.1 g/ml × 1000 =	100 gm × 4	400
50% dextrose	0.5 g/ml × 1000 =	500 gm × 4	2,000

Normal energy requirements of an active adult are between 1400–1800 calories per 24-hour period. A minimum calorie supply of 600–800 calories per day can help prevent catabolism and metabolic acidosis. If a client is on parenteral therapy while n.p.o., three IVs per day with dextrose and electrolyte additives are usually sufficient, even though the total calorie requirement is not being met.

INTERVENTION: Using a Controller and Pump

1 Identify if type of medication or amount of medication requires use of the controller or pump.

2 Bring equipment to client's room and explain use of the machine.

3 Plug the machine into the electrical outlet.

4 Place IV solution container and tubing on the IV pole.

5 Fill the drip chamber of the IV tubing at least one-third full.

6 Flush the tubing to expel all air bubbles.

7 Raise the IV pole to ensure that the drip chamber is at least 76 cm above the infusion site.

8 Attach the drip sensor device to the IV drip chamber.

9 Lift the door handle and open the door of the controller or pump.

10 Place the IV tubing through the tubing guides on the machine.

11 Close the door and push the handle down.

12 Open the IV control clamp completely.

13 Select the appropriate drops per minute on the dial.

14 Connect the IV tubing to the venipuncture site.

15 Press the power button to the ON position.

16 Press the start button.

17 Count the drops for one full minute to verify that the drop rate is correct as set.

Uses for IV Controllers and Pumps
- Administration of heparin
- Administration of antihypertensive agents
- Administration of IV antibiotics
- Administration of antiarrhythmic agents
- Administration of accurate IV fluid rates

▶ Some types of controllers or pumps have modular units attached that need to be changed every 24 hours. The IV extension tubing and regular IV tubing are attached directly to the modular unit.

▶ If alarm sounds check the following
- Ensure that drip chamber is only one-third full.
- Assess that height of the IV container is at least 76 cm above the venipuncture site.
- Examine the IV tubing in the guides to ensure it is not pinched down.
- Assess that drop sensor is placed properly to sense the drops.
- Evaluate the position of the needle and tubing to prevent kinking.

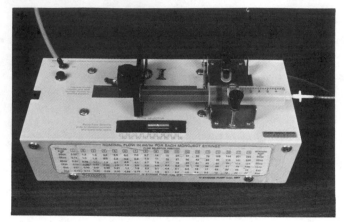

The Harvard pump allows the infusion of small volumes of concentrated drugs over long periods of time.

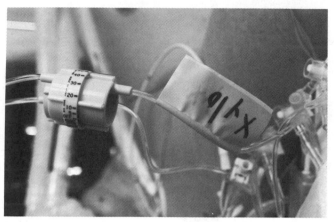

The Dial-A-Flo inline device is a simple method to regulate flow of IV fluids.

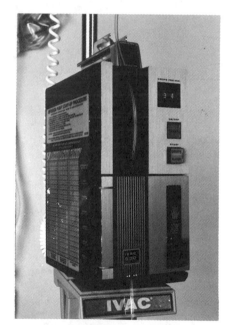

IV fluids can be carefully monitored by an infusion pump such as the IVAC 530. This pump infuses IV fluids up to 99 drops per minute by dialing in the desired number.

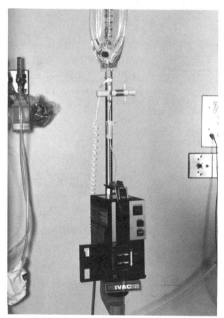

The electronic drop sensors monitor the drops per minute which are set on the IVAC machine.

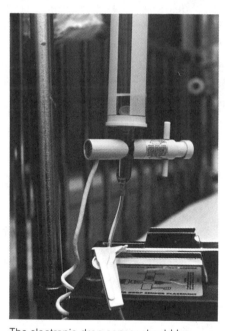

The electronic drop sensor should be placed on the drip chamber below the needle and above the fluid level.

18 Assess the drops being delivered, the condition of the tubing in the guide, and the fluid level in the drip chamber at least every four hours.

19 Change the site of the tubing in the guide at least every eight hours.

20 Listen for the alarm and respond immediately to determine the problem.

INTERVENTION: Using a Harvard Pump

1 Check physician's order for drug, dosage, and amount of fluid to be delivered over specified time.
2 Identify the amount of medication and/or fluid to be delivered per minute.
3 Check the chart on the Harvard pump to identify proper syringe size and machine setting according to amount of drug to be delivered.
4 Set dial on side of pump.
5 Assemble equipment, i.e., syringes, extension tubing, and pump.
6 Draw up medication in syringe. Predilute the medication in another container before withdrawing into syringe.
7 Place extension tubing on the syringe and flush the tubing to expel all air bubbles.
8 Place syringe in holder clamp on pump.
9 Position carriage carefully over plunger of syringe. Ensure that it fits properly or the syringe can break when machine is turned on.
10 Plug machine into electrical outlet at the bedside.
11 Make sure the switch of the pump is set on the infusion site and not on the withdrawal site.
12 Connect the extension tubing to the IV site by either piggy-backing the tubing into the existing IV line or inserting the tubing directly into an IV site.
13 Double check the dials and recalculate the rate of infusion.
14 Turn Harvard pump on.
15 Monitor the amount of fluid infused in the first hour to ensure proper fluid administration.

INTERVENTION: Removing IV Equipment

1 Assemble equipment and sterile pad with two- by two-inch strips of tape or bandage and scissors.
2 Explain procedure to client.
3 Remove tape from tubing and catheter or wings of needle. Hold catheter hub or needle wings while manipulating tape to prevent unnecessary movement that could injure the vein.
4 Remove needle or catheter quickly and smoothly. Don't press down on top of needle point or catheter tip while either is in the vein.
5 Quickly press sterile strips or bandage over venipuncture site and hold firmly until bleeding stops.
6 Apply sterile pad and tape in place.
7 Observe venipuncture site for redness, swelling, or formation of hematoma.
8 Check site again in 15 to 30 minutes.

EVALUATION

EXPECTED OUTCOMES

1 IV therapy is initiated without difficulty. *If not*, follow these alternative nursing actions:

ANA: If needle enters vein but IV will not flow, check position of needle. A slight adjustment may be needed to move the needle away from the vein wall i.e., the needle may need to be angled differently or to be pulled back slightly.

ANA: Consider other factors: The height of the bottle may be too low; the client's position may occlude the vein; the IV tubing may be kinked; or the inline filter may be slowing the flow rate.

2 IV flow is maintained. *If not*, follow these alternative nursing actions:

ANA: Check for flashback of blood into tubing when either IV bottle is lowered or tubing is pinched tight. If you suspect a clot, close clamp on tubing and affix syringe to hub of catheter. Then take a syringe filled with normal saline and try to aspirate the clot. *Never irrigate the tubing as this may force the clot into the bloodstream.* If aspiration is not successful, discontinue IV and start at a new site.

ANA: Check to see if blood flows back into the infusion set tubing when you pull back the plunger of the medication syringe. You may need to leave the needle in the vein for a longer period of time to reduce venous spasm or let go of plunger to decrease pressure. You may also remove the intermittent infusion set and insert a new one in another site.

3 Fluids, additives, and medications are administered without adverse effects on the client. *If not*, follow these alternative nursing actions:

ANA: Stop injecting medication immediately. Give supportive care. Report problem to physician immediately.

4 IV site remains free from redness, edema, and purulent drainage. *If not*, follow these alternative nursing actions:

ANA: Discontinue IV immediately. Restart at new site. Consult with physician (if hospital policy) about the need for additional treatment.

ANA: Remove IV immediately. Send catheter and tubing to lab for culture. Culture drainage. Treat site as infected; clean it and apply topical antimicrobial medication.

5 IV infusion rate is accurately calculated and reassessed throughout the therapy. *If not*, follow these alternative nursing actions:

ANA: If behind in fluids, recalculate fluids for rest of 24-hour span and set drip factor accordingly.

ANA: If ahead in fluids, follow same procedures as above but assess for signs of fluid overload.

6 IV equipment is removed without complications. *If not*, follow these alternative nursing actions:

ANA: If redness, edema, or drainage is present check with physician for orders.

ANA: Apply warm, moist compresses to the site.

ANA: If catheter tip is not intact on withdrawal, notify physician immediately.

UNEXPECTED OUTCOMES

1 Venipuncture attempt does not result in cannulization of vein.

ANA: Remove needle or cannula and needle together as a unit. Apply dressing. Move to other side of body for vein assessment. If necessary, move up proximally on the same vein. Select new site and use fresh needle or catheter and needle. After two attempts, ask more experienced personnel to perform venipuncture.

2 Veins roll and are difficult to enter.
   ANA: Use firmer pressure to anchor skin and vein.

3 Veins are fragile and appear to "balloon" around the needle once the vein has been entered.
   ANA: Loosen tourniquet to reduce pressure in the vein. If possible, use a smaller gauge needle or switch to a winged-tipped needle.

4 Client develops unexplained fever with chills and rising pulse rate.
   ANA: Unexplained fever may be associated with catheter-related sepsis. Contact physician to discuss action.

5 During insertion, the needle enters an artery. This may result in a rapid, backward movement of the syringe plunger and the appearance of bright red blood.
   ANA: Completely remove the syringe and needle. Apply pressure to the puncture site *if possible* for a minimum of ten minutes.

Charting
- Location of insertion site
- Type of intermittent infusion set used
- Time of insertion
- Type and amount of medication given
- Rate medication administered
- Client's response to medication
- Appearance of insertion site
- Time dressing changed
- Any unusual conditions or reactions

ACTION: ADMINISTERING IV MEDICATIONS WITH ADDITIVE SETS

ASSESSMENT

1 Note client's allergies.
2 Note any drug and/or solution incompatibilities.
3 Assess client's general condition to establish a baseline for administering medications.

Rationale for Action
- To maintain a therapeutic level of medication in the client's bloodstream
- To administer medication on larger volumes over a longer period of time
- To prevent complications associated with bolus administration, such as speed shock and vein irritation

PLANNING

GOALS

- With partial-fill bottle client receives intermittent IV drug therapy at the prescribed time and rate of administration.
- With volume control set client receives intermittent IV drug therapy at the prescribed time and rate of administration.
- With secondary bottle set client receives intermittent IV drug therapy or concurrent drug therapy.

EQUIPMENT

- Primary IV set, consisting of IV solution bottle and IV administration set with injection port
- Additive sets
  - Partial-fill additive bottle or bag set: macrodrip administration set, 20 gauge one-inch needle, and extension hook or lowering hanger for primary bottle
  - Volume control set: Soluset®, Metriset®, Volu-Trol®, or Buretrol (depending on need and/or manufacturer)
  - Secondary bottle and administration set: administration set and 20 gauge one-inch needle

487

INTERVENTION: Using a Partial-Fill Additive Bottle or Bag

1   Prepare medication following directions on label. Add to partial-fill bottle aseptically.
2   Spike partial-fill bottle with administration set. Affix the needle to the end of the tubing, and prime both the tubing and the needle. Close the clamp on the tubing.
3   Cleanse the injection port of the primary IV with an alcohol swab.
4   Insert the needle of the partial-fill bottle set and secure in place with tape.
5   Hang the partial-fill bottle on the IV pole. Use the extension hook to lower the primary bottle below the partial-fill bottle.
6   Open the clamp on the partial-fill bottle tubing. The solution in the partial-fill bottle should begin to flow.
7   Using the clamp on the primary IV tubing, adjust the drip rate to the desired rate of administration.
8   Make sure that the partial-fill bottle is higher than the primary IV bottle so the solution will drip until the partial-fill bottle is empty.
9   When the partial-fill bottle and drip chamber are empty, readjust the rate of administration in the primary solution to desired flow.
10   To hang a new partial-fill bottle, prepare the medication and add it to the new bottle aseptically. Remove the old partial-fill bottle and spike the new bottle. Close the clamp on the partial-fill bottle tubing.

(a) Instill medication in the additive bottle before inserting IV tubing. Gently rotate bottle to mix medication.

(b) Hang the additive bottle higher than the primary bottle to allow the primary bottle to begin infusing IV solution when the additive bottle is emptied.

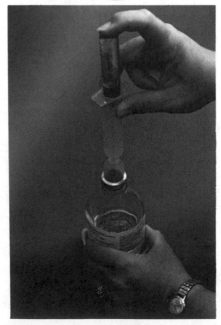

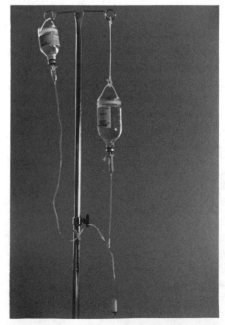

11 Lower the partial-fill bottle below the injection port of the primary IV.

12 Open the clamp on the partial-fill tubing and allow the solution from the primary IV set to enter the tubing, back-filling the tubing to the drip chamber. (This procedure will displace any air left in the tubing.)

13 Replace new partial-fill bottle on IV pole and proceed with administration.

14 Change partial-fill tubing every 48 hours.

INTERVENTION: Using Volume Control Set

1 Obtain volume control set and IV bottle.

2 Close clamps on volume control set, both above and below the volume chamber.

3 Open the air vent by turning the clamp located on top of volume chamber.

4 Spike IV bottle with the volume control set, and then hang the bottle.

5 Open the upper clamp (between the bottle and the volume chamber) and fill the chamber with IV solution so that the chamber is one-third full.

6 Close the upper clamp.

(a) Fill volume-control set to appropriate fluid level by opening tubing clamp between bottle and control set. The air vent must be opened to allow fluid to flow.

(b) To ensure proper fluid flow, check that the rubber diaphragm is not occluding the opening to the drip chamber.

(c) Wipe medication injection site with alcohol; then inject medication while rotating the chamber to thoroughly mix the IV solution and medication.

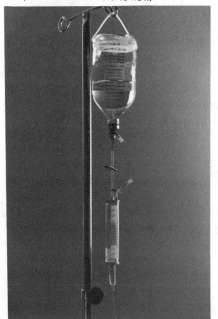

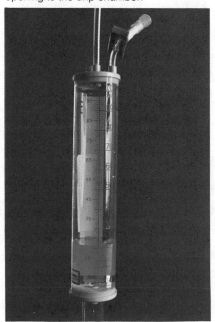

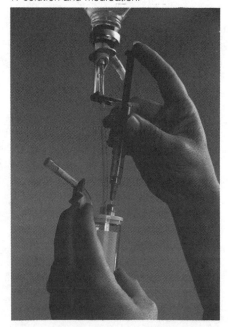

7 Open the lower clamp and squeeze the drip chamber (located underneath the volume chamber) until it is one-half full.

8 Allow the solution to flow down the tubing.

9 Prime the tubing and needle affixed to the end of the tubing. If the volume control set has a membrane filter instead of a floating valve filter, follow the manufacturer's instructions for priming so that you do not damage the filter.

10 Close the clamp.

11 Swab off the injection port (located on top of the volume chamber) with alcohol.

12 Inject prepared medication into chamber and agitate gently to mix medication with solution in chamber.

13 Dilute medication, if necessary, by opening the upper clamp and adding additional fluid from the IV bottle.

14 Swab the injection port on the primary IV tubing and insert needle into the volume control set.

15 Tape securely in place.

16 Clamp off primary IV.

17 Open clamp on volume control set and adjust drip rate to desired rate of administration.

INTERVENTION: Using Secondary Bottle and Administration Set

1 Prepare medication per instructions. Add medication to compatible IV solution in small IV bottle or bag.

2 Label bottle with date, time, medication dosage, and your name.

3 With administration set, spike the bottle.

4 Hang bottle and prime the tubing.

5 Affix and prime a 20-gauge one-inch needle.

6 Close tubing clamp.

7 Swab injection port on primary IV tubing.

8 Carefully insert needle and tape securely in place.

9 Depending on physician's orders, either clamp off primary IV or run in secondary IV solution concurrently with primary IV solution to further dilute the medication.

10 When medication is finished, clamp off tubing, remove needle from injection port, and discard tubing, bottle, and needle.

EVALUATION

EXPECTED OUTCOMES

1 Partial-fill bottle solution drips. *If not*, follow these alternative nursing actions:

Check height of IV bottle. Be sure primary IV bottle is lower than partial-fill bottle. Check position of needle from partial-fill bottle in the injection port to be sure it is in position and has not pierced the IV tubing.

2 Volume control set runs smoothly. *If not*, follow these alternative nursing actions:

ANA: If the drip chamber below the volume chamber fills completely with solution while the drip chamber and tubing are being primed, close both the air vent and upper clamp. Invert drip chamber and volume chamber. Squeeze IV solution back into volume chamber.

3 Secondary bottle set runs smoothly. *If not*, consider these alternative nursing actions.

ANA: Change tubing in primary set if needle from secondary IV punctures primary IV tubing.

UNEXPECTED OUTCOME

Solution in primary IV tubing is incompatible with medication to be administered via secondary additive set.

ANA: Prior to running medication into primary IV tubing, flush tubing with solution that is compatible with medication, e.g., normal saline or 5% dextrose in water. Then proceed with medication administration.

Charting
- Type and amount of medication administered
- Rate medication administered
- Method of administration
- Client's response to medication

ACTION: MONITORING CENTRAL VENOUS PRESSURE

ASSESSMENT

1 Check presence of deformities that would interfere with insertion.
2 Determine client's level of consciousness so full explanation of procedure can be done to allay anxiety.
3 Assess level of anxiety for possible premedication.
4 After insertion, assess proper placement by obtaining x-ray.
5 Assess CVP values in reference to other data such as pulse, blood pressure, respirations, heart sounds, and fluid intake and output.

Rationale for Action
- To provide information about blood volume
- To determine the effectiveness of the heart as a pump
- To provide baseline data about vascular tone

PLANNING

GOALS

- CVP line properly placed in right atrium or vena cava
- Patency of CVP line that accurately reflects pressure in client's right atrium
- Accurate CVP readings so that staff will be able to monitor for fluid shifts and detect early complications of fluid imbalances
- Central venous dressing changed without complications
- Insertion site free of infection and catheter free of thrombosis

▶ Central venous pressure is a measure of the pressure of blood in the right atrium or vena cava. It is measured in centimeters of water pressure, which vary even within the normal range of values cited.

EQUIPMENT

- Routine IV setup with pole
- CVP catheter
- Water manometer
- Three-way stopcock
- Tape

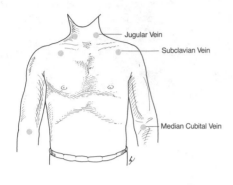

Frequently used sites for CVP catheter insertion.

ADDITIONAL EQUIPMENT

For Central Venous Catheterization

- In-the-needle radiopaque catheter, 14- to 16-gauge needle that is 15 to 20 cm long
- Sterile two- by two-inch and four- by four-inch sponges
- Anesthetic, sterile syringes, and needles
- Sterile gloves, drapes, and sutures

For Changing a Central Vein Dressing

- Mask
- Central catheter dressing kit or sterile gloves, mask(s), drape(s), acetone wipes, 70% alcohol pads, saline or hydrogen peroxide, povidone-iodine ointment, sterile two- by two-inch gauze pads with precut slits
- Tincture of benzoin
- Air-occlusive tape
- Receptacle for soiled dressing, e.g., paper bag, wastepaper basket, plastic bag

INTERVENTION: Assisting a Physician with a Central Venous Catheterization

1 Explain procedure to client.
2 Place client in Trendelenburg's position (approximately 15- to 30-degree angle).
3 Extend client's neck and upper chest by placing a rolled pillow or blanket under the shoulders. Make sure that the side of the client's neck or chest where the CVP line will be inserted is closest to physician.
4 Turn client's head away from the site of the venipuncture.
5 Maintaining sterility, open the glove packet and sterile drape pack. (Physician should wear sterile gloves for this procedure.)
6 Open the povidone-iodine prep pads.

Physician's Actions

a Physician dons sterile gloves for this procedure.
b The physician preps the client's skin, drapes the area, and using a sterile syringe and needle, draws up anesthetic to infiltrate the site.
c Using the large needle and syringe, the physician will insert the needle into the central vein (subclavian or internal jugular).
d Once the vein is entered and the needle is placed correctly, the physician will remove the syringe and advance the catheter through the needle to the desired length. (The needle and catheter must be handled as one unit. The catheter must never be pulled back through the needle as this may shear off a part of the catheter and create an embolus.)
e With the catheter in place, the physician will withdraw the obturator, if one is used, and pull back the needle.
f The physician will then attach the IV tubing to the hub of the needle or to an adapter.
g The physician will finally snap the needle guard around the

needle and suture the catheter into place.

7 As the physician is working, have the client perform Valsalva's maneuver to prevent air-embolism.

8 Both these procedures will help to decrease chances of air embolism.

   a Instruct the client to exhale against a closed glottis.

   b If client is unable to do this, compress the client's abdomen.

9 When the physician has completed this procedure, adjust the infusion drip to the desired rate of administration.

10 Cover the insertion site with povidone-iodine ointment, sterile gauze pads, and tape.

11 After the position of the radiopaque catheter has been checked with an x-ray, dress the catheter insertion site according to hospital policy. (See following intervention for dressing change.)

12 Tape all connections on the tubing.

13 Label the insertion site with the date, nurse's initials, and the time of insertion.

INTERVENTION: Changing a Central Vein Dressing

1 Check the location of the central vein catheter.

2 If located in the client's neck or subclavian area, position the client flat on his or her back to eliminate the risk of air embolism.

3 Turn the client's head away from the insertion site and mask the client's nose and mouth if necessary.

4 Wash your hands thoroughly.

5 Explain the procedure to the client.

6 Mask all personnel.

7 Carefully remove the old dressing and tape without pulling on the catheter or touching the soiled surfaces of the dressing.

8 Discard the old dressing in the receptacle obtained for this purpose.

9 Put on sterile gloves.

10 Using a sterile gauze pad and saline or hydrogen peroxide, clean debris such as dried blood or serum from the insertion site and catheter.

11 After the site is clean, check for signs of infection, inflammation, or infiltration.

12 If skin, insertion site, and catheter look normal, cleanse the skin around the catheter, working from the insertion site outward in a circular motion. (Do not scrub the catheter with acetone solution since it will damage the plastic part of the catheter.)

13 Apply an antimicrobial solution, such as povidone-iodine, working from the insertion site outward in a circular motion.

14 Apply the povidone-iodine ointment directly on the insertion site.

15 Place precut sterile two- by two-inch gauze pads around the insertion site. The catheter should protrude through the center of the pads.

16 Apply tincture of benzoin around the edges of the pads.

17 Change the tubing, if hospital policy requires dressing and tubing to be changed at the same time.

▶ Aseptic techniques must always be used when changing catheter dressings. Catheter dressings should be changed every 48 hours.
If a dressing at the catheter insertion site becomes loose, wet, or soiled, it is considered contaminated and should be changed.

    a Remove gloves and wash your hands. (You may also keep your hands gloved.)

    b Loosen the tubing in the catheter hub. (Policy may dictate that you wipe the hub with an alcohol swab at this time.)

    c Tell the client to hold his or her breath and bear down while you insert the new tubing into the hub of the catheter.

    d Tape the connection.

18 Tape the dressing around the catheter site.

19 Tape the connection of the tubing on the catheter hub to the client's skin. (If a filter is part of the central line tubing, i.e., a hyperalimentation catheter, you may secure the filter to the dressing with tape.)

20 Label the dressing with the date and your initials.

INTERVENTION: Measuring and Monitoring a CVP

1 Discuss the reasons for placing a CVP line in the client with the client's physician. This information will help you interpret the measurements.

2 Determine the desired CVP parameters with the client's physician. Discuss what actions you should take if the client's measurements rise or fall outside these parameters.

3 Establish a baseline by taking the client's vital signs and by checking the client's hydration status.

4 Spike the IV solution bottle with the IV administration set.

5 Prime the tubing with the solution, making certain that no air bubbles are present in the tubing.

6 Close the clamp on the tubing. If you are using a reusable manometer scale, affix a three-way stopcock to one end of the IV tubing.

7 Place tubing into manometer scale and snap stopcock into place below the manometer. If you are using a one-piece disposable manometer and stopcock, affix the unit to an IV pole with a C-shaped clamp.

8 Push the male end of the IV administration set into the female end of the stopcock connecting the IV set to the stopcock.

9 Turning the stopcock so that the manometer and IV solution are open to each other, open the clamp on the IV tubing and fill the manometer with IV solution to between 18 and 20 cm.

10 Close the clamp and rotate the stopcock so that the IV solution is open to the client.

11 With IV solution, prime the rest of the IV tubing that extends from the stopcock and connect tubing to CVP catheter.

12 Place the client flat in bed, without a pillow.

13 Locate the client's right atrium (midaxillary at the fourth intercostal space). Mark this location on the client's skin.

14 Adjust the level of the manometer so that zero on the manometer scale is at the same level as the client's right atrium. (Use a yardstick and carpenter's level if this type of apparatus is not part of the manometer.)

▶ The presence of conditions such as chronic lung disease, hypovolemia, or right-sided heart failure will affect CVP measurements. Assess for these conditions.

▶ When changes occur beyond the values established for the client, check the CVP system and the client's vital signs. If the CVP system is functioning correctly, report changes in values to the physician.

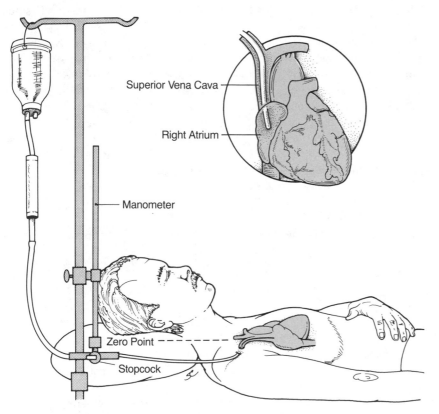

Superior Vena Cava

Right Atrium

Manometer

Zero Point

Stopcock

(a) Take the CVP reading with the "0" point of the manometer at the level of the right atrium.

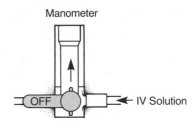

Manometer

OFF ← IV Solution

Solution to Manometer

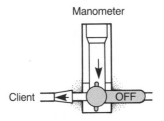

Manometer

Client ← OFF

Manometer to Client

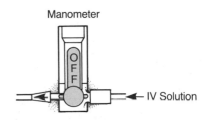

Manometer

OFF

← IV Solution

Solution to Client

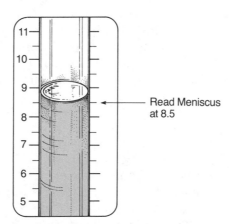

Read Meniscus at 8.5

Take CVP reading at highest level of meniscus and in response to client's breathing.

(b) **Top stopcock**: Fill the manometer by turning stopcock OFF to the client. This allows solution to flow from the bottle to the manometer. **Middle stopcock**: Measure CVP by turning stopcock OFF to IV solution allowing fluid to flow from manometer to client. **Bottom stopcock**: Reinstitute flow from IV bottle to client by turning stopcock OFF to the manometer.

15 Turn the stopcock to the open position for the manometer IV solution, filling the manometer with additional solution if needed.

16 Turn the stopcock to the manometer-client position and watch the level of the solution in the manometer fall to the pressure level existing in the right atrium. (Normally, this pressure should be between 3 and 12 cm. It is important to remember, however, that there are no absolute values and that the trends — the rise and fall — of CVP readings are more important to the individual client than one pressure level reading.)

17 Observe the meniscus at eye level and watch the rise and fall of the fluid column in response to the client's breathing.

18 Take the reading at the highest level of the fluid column.

19 Turn the stopcock off to the manometer and adjust the rate of infusion with the clamp.

20 Return the client to the desired position and record CVP readings.

EVALUATION

EXPECTED OUTCOMES

1 CVP line is properly placed in right atrium. *If you suspect it is not*, follow these alternative nursing actions:

ANA: Repeat x-ray to determine placement.

ANA: Assist while the physician retracts catheter (usually from the ventricle).

2 CVP manometer and line remain open, accurately reflecting pressure in the client's right atrium. *If not*, follow these alternative nursing actions:

ANA: Physician can be notified to irrigate the catheter.

ANA: Obtain order for placing 1000 U heparin in IV bottle in order to prevent clotting at tip of catheter.

3 Accurate CVP readings will be obtained so early complications can be evaluated. *If not*, follow these alternative nursing actions:

ANA: Assess client's level of pain, which could affect reading.

ANA: Assess position of client, which, if changed, could alter CVP reading.

ANA: Check marked area at client's mid axillary level to determine if level is accurate.

ANA: Take client off respirator, instruct him or her to take a deep breath, and repeat reading.

4 Central venous dressing is changed without complications. *If not*, follow these alternative nursing actions:

ANA: If leakage around the catheter has wet the dressing and skin, check all connections. Lower the solution and check for backflow of blood in the tubing. Describe the type of leakage to the physician.

ANA: If an air embolism has occurred because connections are loose or because the client was unable to perform Valsalva's maneuver when the tubing was changed, place the client in Trendelenburg's position with the right part of the chest uppermost and the left part of the chest down. Inform physician of the problem.

Charting
- Location of insertion site
- Type and size of needle or cannula used for insertion
- Time of insertion
- Appearance of needle insertion site
- Name of physician performing catheterization
- Types of solutions used, including all additives listed in sequence used
- Amount of solution infused
- Time x-ray was performed to check position of radiopaque catheter
- Time and date dressing and/or tubing changed
- Initials of person changing the dressing
- Condition of catheter insertion site when dressing changed
- Date and time of CVP reading (record subsequent CVP readings on appropriate forms.)
- Condition of flow rate
- Client's response to treatment
- Any unusual conditions or reactions

UNEXPECTED OUTCOMES

1 Air enters central vein producing air embolism.
   ANA: Inform physician immediately.
   ANA: Place client in a head-down position with the right atrium uppermost. Monitor until physician arrives.
2 CVP system does not drip.
   ANA: Check the entire line for kinks in the tubing. Change client's position. Check to make sure the manometer stopcock is in the IV client position. Lower IV bottle below the client's heart level and check for backflow of blood. Do not irrigate. Report any problem to physician.
3 Client is unable to lie flat because of respiratory problem or other difficulties.
   ANA: Determine how high the client has to be positioned for breathing. Note this position on the Kardex or care plan. Duplicate this exact position every time you take a CVP reading.

ACTION: ADMINISTERING BLOOD TRANSFUSIONS

ASSESSMENT

1 Check order for transfusion in client's chart.
2 Examine client's IV. An 18- or 19-gauge catheter or needle should be placed in a medium or large-sized vein.
3 Take the client's vital signs to establish a baseline.
4 Take and record client's temperature.
5 Assess for signs and symptoms of blood reactions during infusion.

PLANNING

GOALS

• Transfusion of blood is performed smoothly without complications
• Needle remains patent throughout transfusion procedure

EQUIPMENT

• Blood unit and 250-cc bottle of normal saline
• Blood administration set, either straight line or Y-set
• Venipuncture tray, if client does not already have an IV in place. An 18- or 19-gauge needle or 18- to 20-gauge catheter should be used. If blood is to be administered rapidly, a 15-gauge needle should be used.
• An 18-gauge needle if client already has a primary IV line in place
• Alcohol swabs and tape

PREPARATION

• Obtain whole blood unit or packed blood cells unit from blood lab or blood bank.
• Obtain the requisition form for the transfusion.

Rationale for Action

• To provide blood or blood components, such as red blood cells, platelets, blood protein, and plasma, for clients who have a demonstrated deficiency
• To ensure compatibility between the client's blood and the whole blood or packed red blood cells which may be transfused
• To prevent the infusion of fibrin clots and microaggregates (broken-down blood cells)

Clinical Alert
Whole blood and red blood cells, when administered with IV solution, must be given with saline solution.

Blood Transfusions

▶ Routine transfusions should not be warmed. If warming is required, as in massive transfusions, a blood warming coil is inserted into the transfusion line. Immerse coil in a 98.6°-100° F water bath. Once blood is warmed, it must be used or disposed of, as it cannot be returned to the blood bank. Hemolysis of the blood occurs at temperatures above 104° F.

- With lab technologist, check requisition form and lab blood record against the blood unit for essential data: client's name and ID number, blood group and type (ABO and Rh), blood unit number, and expiration date of blood unit.
- With another RN, check the requisition form and the lab blood record with the information on the client's identification band to make sure that all data matches. Essential data includes client's name and ID number, blood group, blood type, blood unit number, and expiration date on the blood unit.
- Sign the form with the other RN according to hospital policy. Remember that blood must be started within 30 minutes from the time it is removed from refrigeration.

INTERVENTION: Administering Blood Through a Straight-Line

1. Rotate the blood unit bag gently to mix the blood cells and plasma.
2. With blood administration set ready, pull back the tabs on the blood unit bag and expose the port.
3. Carefully spike the port and hang the unit.
4. Fill the drip chamber by gently squeezing its flexible sides. Make sure the filter is submerged in the blood.
5. Open the clamp on the tubing, run the blood through the tubing, and cap the tubing.
6. If the client needs a venipuncture, select a vein and insert an IV needle and tubing.

TABLE 5 TRANSFUSION REACTIONS

TYPE	CLINICAL MANIFESTATIONS	NURSING INTERVENTIONS
Bacterial	Sudden increase in temperature	Stop transfusion immediately.
	Hypotension	Maintain IV site; change tubing as soon as possible.
	Dry, flushed skin	Observe for shock. Monitor vital signs every 15 minutes until stable.
	Abdominal pain	Obtain urine specimen. Insert Foley if necessary.
	Headache	Notify physician and obtain order for broad spectrum antibiotic.
	Lumbar pain	Draw blood cultures before antibiotic administration.
	Sudden chill	Send blood tubing and bag to lab for culture and sensitivity.
		Control hyperthermia.
Allergic	Urticaria and hives, pruritus	Stop transfusion immediately if symptoms are severe.
	Respiratory wheezing, laryngeal edema	Monitor vital signs for possible anaphylactic shock.
	Anaphylactic reaction	If symptoms are mild, slow down transfusion and obtain order for antihistamine.
		Monitor for signs of progressive allergic reaction as transfusion continues.
Hemolytic	Severe pain in kidney region and chest	Stop transfusion immediately.
	Pain at needle insertion site	Change IV tubing as soon as possible, maintaining patent IV. If necessary, disconnect IV tubing from needle and run normal saline through IV tubing into emesis basin. Reconnect tubing to needle and obtain new tubing as soon as possible.
	Fever (may reach 105° F), chills	Administer oxygen.
	Dyspnea and cyanosis	Send two blood samples, from different sites, urine sample (cath if necessary), blood, and transfusion record to lab.
	Headache	Obtain orders for IV volume expansion and diuretic (mannitol) to ensure flushing of kidneys to prevent acute renal tubular necrosis.
	Hypotension	Monitor vital signs every 15 minutes for shock.
	Hematuria	Monitor urine output hourly for possible renal failure. Foley catheter may need to be inserted.

7   If the client has a primary IV in place with an appropriate-sized needle, place an 18-gauge needle (or larger needle) in the end of the blood unit tubing.

8   If the primary IV solution is *not* compatible with the blood to be infused, remove the primary IV solution and cap it for sterility.

9   Spike the small bottle of normal saline and run this solution through the tubing.

10 Prime the blood unit tubing.

11 Swab the injection port with alcohol.

12 Insert the needle carefully and tape it into place.

13 Shut off the primary IV and begin the blood transfusion.

14 Give blood slowly for the first 15 minutes, approximately 20 drops per minute which equates to 100 cc/hr.

15 Observe the client closely for adverse reactions such as chilling, backache, headache, nausea or vomiting, tachycardia, tachypnea, skin rash, or hypotension.

16 If there are no adverse effects, administer the blood unit at the prescribed rate.

17 Transfusion of the blood should be completed in less than four hours since blood deteriorates rapidly after a two-hour exposure to room temperature. Most clients can tolerate a flow rate of one unit of packed cells in one-and-a-half to two hours.

18 Continue to monitor the client throughout the transfusion.

19 When you have completed the transfusion, flush the line with normal saline, inject the primary IV solution, and adjust the drip to the desired rate.

Preventing Transfusion Reactions

1   Identify client and blood bottle or bag
    - ID band number matches transfusion record number
    - Name spelled correctly on transfusion record
    - Blood bottle number and pilot tube number are same
    - Blood type matches on transfusion record and blood bottle

2   Check blood with another RN before infusing

3   Ask client about allergy history and report any previous blood reactions

4   Establish baseline vital sign data

5   Start transfusion slowly to observe for severe reactions

6   Maintain aseptic technique during procedure

7   Observe time rules (length of time blood can hang) for administering blood

8   Observe blood bag or bottle for bubbles, cloudiness, dark color, or black sediment, which is indicative of bacterial invasion

9   Do not allow blood to remain at room temperature unnecessarily

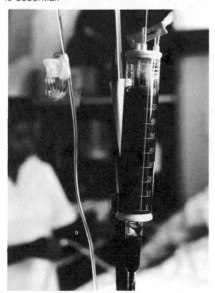

Volume-control set can be used for blood administration but a blood filter in the set is essential.

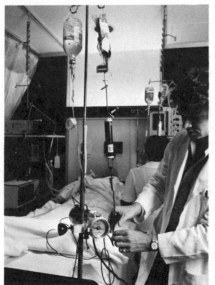

Blood should be warmed when a client is to receive a large volume over a short time period.

20 Remove the blood unit bag and administration set. If you are going to transfuse a second unit of blood, obtain that unit and a new administration set and repeat the procedure described above.

INTERVENTION: Administering Blood Through a Y-Set

1 Obtain blood unit following procedures outlined on page 497.
2 Close all clamps on the Y-set.
3 Spike the small saline bottle, using aseptic technique; then spike the blood bag.
4 Hang both the saline bottle and blood bag.
5 Open the clamp to the saline bottle and squeeze the sides of the drip chamber until the filter is half covered and the drip chamber is full.
6 Open the main clamp and prime the rest of the tubing. To ensure easier flow, remove the cap that protects the end of the IV tubing.
7 When the tubing is primed, replace the cap and close the main clamp.
8 Cleanse the injection port on the primary IV.
9 Affix a large-gauge needle to the end of the tubing and prime.
10 Insert the needle into the injection port and clamp off the primary IV flow.
11 Using saline solution, open the clamp to the saline bottle and turn clamp on the main tubing to begin the flow to clear primary IV tubing.
12 Clamp off the saline bottle and open the clamp to the blood bag.
13 Squeeze the sides of the Y-set drip chamber so that blood covers all the filter.
14 Follow procedure as you did with previous bottle.
15 When the blood bag is empty, clamp off the tubing to the bag, open the clamp to the normal saline bottle and flush the line.
16 Close all clamps and remove the needle from the injection port.
17 Open the clamp on the primary IV and establish the desired rate of administration.

INTERVENTION: Administering Blood Components

1 Obtain blood component from lab or appropriate source.
2 Obtain appropriate administration set.
3 Read directions for proper administration of the solution.
4 Identify rate at which blood component should infuse.
5 Check blood component therapy chart for appropriate rate, risk factors, and possible complications.

EVALUATION

EXPECTED OUTCOMES

1 Transfusion of blood is performed smoothly, without complications. *If not, or if client develops chills, fever, low back pain, headache, nausea, vomiting, tachycardia, tachypnea, or hypotension*, follow these alternative nursing actions:

ANA: Stop the flow of blood immediately. Keep the client's vein open with a slow drip of normal saline. Notify physician and blood bank, according to hospital procedure. (In most cases you will need to obtain blood and urine samples and return the blood unit and the administration set to the lab.)

ANA: Monitor client's vital signs and place client on intake and output.

2 Needle remains patent. *If not*, consider these alternative nursing actions:

ANA: Discontinue needle immediately. Insert new needle into another site and restart blood unit. Treat old site according to hospital procedure.

UNEXPECTED OUTCOMES

1 Transfusion reactions.
   ANA: See chart on transfusion reactions.
2 Blood unit does not flow.
   ANA: Check site where IV needle has been inserted to make sure it is in place. Gently agitate the blood bag to mix the blood cells with the plasma. Raise the blood bag to a higher location on the IV pole. Squeeze the flexible tubing to promote blood flow. Adjust clamp on tubing. As the blood unit passes over the filter, more blood micro-aggregates clog the filter and slow the drip rate.

Charting

Charting content is same as IV administration, with the following additions:

● Vital signs before transfusion begins; 15, 30, and 60 minutes after infusion begins; and then hourly until infusion completed
● Blood bank slip may have space for vital sign information as well
● Your signature on blood slip and trans-fusion record
● Client's response to procedure
● Any unusual clinical manifestations

ACTION: WITHDRAWING BLOOD FOR VENOUS SPECIMENS

ASSESSMENT

1 Check order for blood withdrawal in client's chart.
2 Note specific requirements for the test, e.g., fasting or administration of medications prior to the test.
3 Check to see if the test is routine or urgent.

Rationale for Action

● To obtain specimens of blood that can be used to diagnose the client's illness
● To obtain and transfer specimens with-out destroying red blood cells
● To ensure accurate test results by making sure the client follows all re-quirements for the test, e.g., fasting
● To ensure accurate test results by selecting the right tube for the right test

PLANNING

GOALS

● Preconditions such as fasting are adhered to so blood sample is viable
● Blood sample obtained without complications such as hematoma formation or excessive oozing at the site
● Uncontaminated blood specimen obtained

EQUIPMENT

● 5-cc or 10-cc syringe
● 20-gauge one-inch needle(s)
● 70% alcohol wipe (with blood alcohol specimen, solution of benzal-konium will be needed)
● Appropriate laboratory tubes
● Dry, sterile sponges

TABLE 6 BLOOD COMPONENT THERAPY

TYPE	USE	ALERTS	ADMINISTRATION EQUIPMENT
Fresh Plasma	To replace deficient coagulation factors To increase intravascular compartment	Hepatitis is a risk. Administer as rapidly as possible. Use within 6 hours.	Any straight line administration set
Platelets	To prevent or treat bleeding problems, especially in surgical clients To replace platelets in clients with acquired or inherited deficiencies (thrombocytopenia, aplastic anemia) To replace when platelets drop below 30,000 cu/mm (normal 150,000–350,000 cu/mm)	Administer at rate of 10 minutes a unit (usually come in multiple platelet packs).	Platelet transfusion set with special filter to allow platelets to infuse through filter
Granulocytes	To treat oncology clients with severe bone marrow depression and progressive infections To treat granulocytopenic clients with infections that are unresponsive to antibiotics To treat clients with gram-negative bacteremia or infections where marrow recovery does not develop	Administer slowly, over two to four hours. Give one transfusion daily until granulocytes increase or infection clears. Use within 48 hours after drawn. Give when granulocytes are below 500. Observe for shaking, fever, chills (treat with Tylenol before transfusions). Observe for hives and laryngeal edema (treat with antihistamines).	Use Y-type blood filters and prime with physiological saline. A microaggregate filter is not used as it filters out platelets.

- Plastic adapter (vacutainer)
- Double-ended needle that screws into the adapter

ADDITIONAL EQUIPMENT

For Obtaining Blood Culture
- Two 5-cc syringes
- Povidone-iodine swab-2
- Four 22-gauge sterile needles
- Four alcohol wipes
- Two paired sets of blood culture media
- Tourniquet

For Obtaining Culture of Cannula
- Blood agar plate
- Sterile scissors
- Sterile cotton tip applicator
- Povidone-iodine swab
- Bandaids

TYPE	USE	ALERTS	ADMINISTRATION EQUIPMENT
Serum Albumin	To treat shock	Available as 5% or 25% solution.	Special tubing accompanies albumin solution in individual boxes
	To treat hypoproteinemia	Infuse 25% solution slowly 1 ml/minute to prevent circulatory overload. Administer 100–200 cc (25% solution) for shock clients and 200–300 cc for hypoproteinemia.	
Gamma Globulin	To treat agammaglobulinemia	Pooled plasma contains antibodies to infectious agents.	Given IM
	To act as a prophylaxsis for hepatitis exposure	Administer 0.25 ml–0.50 ml of immune serum globulin per kg of body weight every two to four weeks.	
Coagulation Factors	To treat clients with von Willebrand's disease	Made from fresh-frozen plasma.	Standard syringe or component drip set only
Factor VIII (cryoprecipitate)	To treat clients with factor VIII, hemophilia A	Administer one unit cryoprecipitate for each 6 kg of body weight initially, followed by 1 unit/3 kg of body weight at 6- to 12-hour intervals until treatment discontinued. Administer one unit per five minutes. Observe for febrile reactions: shaking, fever, chills, and headache.	
Factor IX	To treat clients with factor IX, hemophilia B	Administer in 12- to 24-hour cycle. Preparation for administration is 400 to 500 u/vial. Must reconstitute in 10- to 20-cc diluent. One unit/lb. of body weight increases the circulating factor activity by 5%. Serum hepatitis can be transmitted.	Any straight line set

INTERVENTION: Using a Syringe and Needle to Withdraw Blood

1   Identify client by checking client's wristband; introduce yourself and explain the procedure.
2   Place a tourniquet above the client's elbow (if client has an IV in place, place the tourniquet on the other arm). Tighten the tourniquet and tell the client to open and close his or her fist.
3   Cleanse the antecubital fossa (inner aspect of elbow) with an alcohol swab and let the area dry.
4   With needle affixed to the syringe, perform a venipuncture with bevel of the needle pointed up at a 30-degree angle.
5   Pull the syringe plunger back gently and check for placement of the needle in the vein. If placement is correct, release the tourniquet, wait a few seconds to allow fresh blood to flow into the vein and then pull back gently on the plunger.
6   Fill the syringe to the desired amount.
7   Remove the needle from the vein, cover the venipuncture site with a sterile sponge, and press the sponge firmly on the site (client may be able to hold sponge in place).

8 Remove the top from the laboratory tube. Do not touch the inside of the tube or spill its contents.

9 Remove the needle from the blood-filled syringe and gently eject the blood down the side of the tube. Do not allow the blood to foam or splash. Red blood cells can be destroyed if the blood sample is not handled carefully.

10 Replace the tube top and rotate the blood gently to mix the blood with the tube contents.

11 Label the tube promptly. Write the client's name, date, and the time. You may also need to write the initials of the person who drew the specimen if this information is required by hospital policy.

12 Check the client's venipuncture site for oozing. Continue to press the sponge firmly over the site if clots have not begun to form at the site.

13 Take the blood specimens to a designated station or laboratory according to hospital procedure.

INTERVENTION: Using Vacutainer System to Withdraw Blood

1 Obtain plastic adapter, double-ended needle that screws into the adapter, and appropriate vacuum specimen tubes.

2 Screw the double-ended needle into the plastic adapter, with the shorter needle facing the plastic adapter.

3 Prepare the client by explaining procedure. Tighten the tourniquet above the elbow and cleanse the venipuncture site.

4 Place the vacuum tube inside the plastic adapter, with the top of the tube resting against the short needle.

5 Proceed with the venipuncture. Once the needle is positioned inside the vein, hold the plastic adapter steady and press the vacuum tube firmly into the short needle so that it pierces the top of the tube. Blood should begin to spurt quickly into the tube until the tube is filled.

6 Release the tube and set it aside.

7 Remove the needle from the client's vein.

8 Wipe and check site for oozing; press bandaid into place.

INTERVENTION: Collecting a Specimen for Blood Culture

1 Prepare skin with povidone-iodine (alcohol if allergy is present).

2 Withdraw 5 cc from a vein without an IV. Do *not* draw specimen through catheter.

3 Remove needle used for venipuncture and replace with new sterile needle.

4 Swab top of paired blood culture bottles and inject 2½-cc blood into each bottle, changing the needle each time so that a new sterile needle is used for each bottle.

5 In 15 minutes, draw a second sample of blood with a percutaneous stick. (Prepare skin with povidone-iodine solution again)

6 Place in second set of paired blood culture bottles, using single

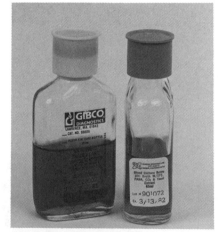

Two bottles, containing different culture media, are used for each blood culture obtained.

sterile needle technique.

7 Label and transport to lab immediately.

INTERVENTION: Obtaining a Culture of Suspected Contaminated Cannula

1 Wash hands and remove catheter, being careful not to touch catheter to any surface as you are removing or once it has been removed.

2 Hold catheter over blood agar plate. With sterile scissors, cut last one to one-and-a-half inches off catheter and let fall onto blood agar plate.

3 With sterile cotton tip applicator, roll the catheter across the surface of the blood agar plate.

4 Replace cover of blood agar plate. Label and transport to lab immediately.

5 Cleanse venipuncture site with povidone-iodine solution and apply bandaid.

EVALUATION

EXPECTED OUTCOMES

1 Blood sample is obtained without complications such as hematoma formation or excessive oozing at the site. *If not*, follow these alternative nursing actions:

ANA: Apply pressure to the site. Raise the client's arm in air and hold it upright. Do not allow the client to bend arm at the elbow as this increases the chance of hematoma formation.

2 Uncontaminated blood specimen is obtained. *If not*, follow these alternative nursing actions:

ANA: Repeat culture specimen maintaining asepsis.

UNEXPECTED OUTCOMES

1 Blood does not flow into the syringe.

ANA: Check the position of the needle in the vein. Pull needle back slightly away from the wall of the vein. Rotate needle gently. Do not pull excessively on the plunger, especially if the vein is small, since this movement may cause the vein to collapse.

2 Blood does not flow into the vacuum tube.

ANA: Check the position of the needle in the vein. If vacuum in the tube is lost or if the vein is not large enough, discard the tube and get another. If there is pressure on the vein for vacuum pull, select a larger vein or use a syringe and needle instead of the vacutainer method.

3 Signs of redness, purulence, or phlebitis at needle insertion site.

ANA: Discontinue IV immediately. Restart in new site. Care for wound as a surgical wound.

ANA: Culture cannula tip.

4 Unexplained fever.

ANA: Unexplained fever may be associated with catheter-related sepsis. Contact physician to discuss appropriate action.

Charting

- Time of blood withdrawal
- Date and name(s) of test(s) for which blood was drawn
- Any unusual conditions in either the client or specimen

	SODIUM	POTASSIUM	CALCIUM	MAGNESIUM	CHLORIDE
Source	Major cation in ECF Supplies 90% of total cations	Major cation intra-cellularly	99% found in bone	Present in bone and cells	⅔ of total anion in blood
Normal Serum Values	135 to 145 mEq/L	3.5 to 5.0 mEq/L	8.8 to 10.5 mg/100 ml	1.5 to 2.5 mEq/L	95 to 109 mEq/L
Function	Responsible for conduction of nerve impulses and muscle contraction. Controls regulation of body water volume through hormonal secretion of ADH.	Controls cellular osmotic pressure. Activates enzymatic reaction. Regulates acid-base balance. Maintains neuro-muscular excitability.	Gives bone its hardness and durability. Mediates neuro-muscular function	Plays essential role in cellular energy metabolism.	Maintains water balance, osmotic pressure, and extracellular cation/anion balance. Maintains acid-base balance. Competes with bi-carbonate for combination with sodium ions.
IMBALANCES	**Hypernatremia**	**Hyperkalemia**	**Hypercalcemia**	**Hypermagesemia**	**Hyperchloremia**
Causes	Water loss exceeding sodium loss in diarrhea, profuse sweating, diabetes mellitus and insipidus, high protein tube feedings Insufficient fluid intake Excessive sodium intake	Renal failure Addison's disease Massive crushing injuries Large surface area burns Myocardial infarctions	Primary hyper-parathyroidism Parathyroid adenoma Multiple myeloma Vitamin D overdose Overuse of antacids Metastatic car-cinomas Paget's disease and other skeletal diseases	Chronic renal failure in which magnesium cannot be excreted Excessive intake of magnesium-based antacids Excessive use of cathartics containing magnesium,	Dehydration Head injuries with neurogenic hyper-ventilation Hyperparathyroidism when kidneys waste phosphates Metabolic acidosis Respiratory alkalosis
CLINICAL MANIFESTATIONS					
Symptoms	Thirst	Weakness Malaise Nausea Muscle irritability	Lethargy Anorexia Nausea	Drowsiness Warm feeling	Fluid retention leading to edema Thirst
Signs	Dry mucous membranes Flushed dry skin Elevated temperature Oliguria	Diarrhea Flaccid paralysis Oliguria EKG changes: Prolonged P-R interval Wide QRS Tented T-wave S-T depression	Vomiting Constipation Dehydration Coma EKG changes: Q-T abnormalities Occasional PVCs	Flushing Perspiration Absent deep tendon reflexes Hypotension Hypothermia Flaccid paralysis Respiratory depression Bradycardia/heart block EKG changes: Widened QRS complex P-R interval Elevated T-waves	Elevated temperature Oliguria

	SODIUM	POTASSIUM	CALCIUM	MAGNESIUM	CHLORIDE
IMBALANCES	Hyponatremia	Hypokalemia	Hypocalcemia	Hypomagnesemia	Hypochloremia
Causes	Water intoxication Dilutional hypo- natremia due to expansion of total body fluid SIADH resulting in water retention Low body sodium levels as a result of extrarenal loss from burns and diarrhea Starvation as a result of terminal and/or chronic illness	Cushing's syndrome Aldosteronism Renal disease Congestive heart failure Use of potent diuretics Nasogastric tube drainage and/or irrigations without proper electrolyte replacement Prolonged vomiting or diarrhea	Hypoparathyroid- ism, vitamin D deficiency, pan- creatitis, magne- sium deficiency Laxative ingestion Surgical intervention involving para- thyroid or thyroid glands	Malabsorption syndrome Starvation diet Bowel resection Chronic alcoholism Diuretic therapy Diabetic acidosis Prolonged naso- gastric tube suction Prolonged IV fluid therapy with magnesium supplements Associated low potassium levels	Associated with low potassium and sodium levels Excessive chloride loss in perspiration Prolonged suction or vomiting Acidosis Edema Excessive urinary losses
CLINICAL MANIFESTATIONS					
Symptoms	Weakness Lassitude Irritability Apprehension Headache	Weakness Muscular irritability Speech changes	Perioral paresthesia	Cramps in leg and foot Insomnia Muscle weakness	(Same as sodium loss)
Signs	Weight loss or edema with weight gain Skin turgor Hypotension Tremors/ convulsions	Decreased reflexes Rapid, weak, ir- regular pulse Abdominal disten- tion leading to paralytic ileus EKG changes: S-T segment depression Flattened T-wave Presence of U-wave	Twitching Carpopedal spasms Tetany Seizures Cardiac arrhythmias	Cardiac arrhythmias Twitching/tremors Seizures Tetany Positive Babinski Nystagmus	Decreased cardiac output Peripheral vaso- constriction Cyanosis Cold, clammy skin Rapid, thready pulse Oliguria

	SODIUM	POTASSIUM	CALCIUM	MAGNESIUM	CHLORIDE
TREATMENT OF IMBALANCES	**Hypernatremia** Increase fluid intake with salt-free solutions	**Hyperkalemia** Limit oral intake of K+ and protein Monitor EKG Facilitate urinary output with diuretics if renal system functioning If renal system not functioning, remove excessive K+ by administering: • Cation exchange resin such as Kayexalate, either rectally or through NG tube. • Give NaHCO₃, calcium salts, or insulin and glucose. • Prepare for peritoneal or hemodialysis.	**Hypercalcemia** Assure adequate hydration q4h with 1000 cc NS to improve dilutional factor of calcium Administer loop diuretics to increase calcium excretion Administer 5 cc oral sodium phosphate q.i.d.	**Hypermagesemia** Alleviate renal insufficiency Administer calcium parenterally as an antagonist	**Hyperchloremia** Treat underlying disease
TREATMENT OF IMBALANCES	**Hyponatremia** Restrict fluids In SIADH, use Lasix IV	**Hypokalemia** Monitor EKG Administer potassium IV or p.o. Do not give more than 20 mEq/L KCl IV in one hour unless monitored and severely hypokalemic	**Hypocalcemia** Administer calcium salts, usually calcium gluconate, IV Give 10–20 ml of a 10% solution, either IV push or in small volume of 5% dextrose Follow initial calcium infusion with 20–30 ml of 10% solution in 1 liter of 5% dextrose Do not use saline solution for infusion Do not use calcium salts with NaHCO₃ Do not give calcium to clients on digitalis. Treat for chronic hypocalcemia with 1.5–3 gms calcium per day	**Hypomagnesemia** Administer magnesium sulfate: 8–16 mEq/L q8h IM for 5 days Give maintenance dose of 8 mEq per day until deficit corrected Keep calcium gluconate on hand for overdose of magnesium	**Hypochloremia** Replace chloride using arginine hydrochloride IV through central venous line Administer L-lysine monohydrochloride p.o.

CHAPTER 15
Alterations in Nutritional Status

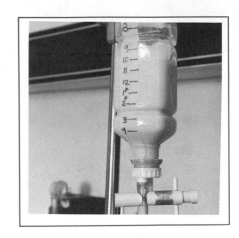

This chapter presents the subject of nutrition and the conceptual basis for administering therapeutic diets. It discusses how the body utilizes foods and the relationship of food to health.

ESSENTIAL NUTRIENTS

Nutrition is comprised of essential nutrients, all of which are necessary for growth and development through the life cycle. The essential nutrients are carbohydrates, fats, proteins, vitamins, minerals, and water. When these are supplied to the body in proper balance, the body utilizes them for energy, growth and development, tissue repair, and regulation and maintenance of body processes.

Carbohydrates Carbohydrates are the chief source of energy and contain carbon, hydrogen, and oxygen. Carbohydrates include sugars, starches, and cellulose. Simple sugars, such as fruit sugar, are easily digested. Starches, which are more complex, require more sophisticated enzyme processes to be reduced to glucose, the end product of carbohydrate metabolism. Glucose, which is converted sugars and starches, appears in the body as blood sugar and is "burned" as fuel by the tissues. Some glucose is processed by the liver, converted to glycogen, and stored by the liver for later use.

LEARNING OBJECTIVES

List the six essential nutrients necessary to sustain life.

Explain the process of digestion; include the primary functions of the gastrointestinal system and accessory organs.

Identify the assessment categories important for a total nutritional assessment.

Describe a sodium restricted diet and list at least three foods high in sodium.

Name and discuss the purpose of at least four therapeutic diets necessary for altered health status.

List at least three diabetic food exchanges that you would teach to a client.

Define what is meant by enteral feeding and outline the steps of inserting a nasogastric tube.

Identify the primary steps (at least ten) of assisting the physician with CVP insertion.

Demonstrate the Valsalva's maneuver.

Ingesting too many carbohydrates crowds out other important foods and prevents the body from receiving the necessary nutrients for healthy maintenance. Too few carbohydrates may lead to loss of energy, depression, ketosis, and a breakdown of body protein. Differences in individual body structure, energy expenditure, basal metabolism, and general health status will determine the amount and kind of carbohydrates that should be consumed for optimal health.

Fats Fats or lipids are the second important group of nutrients. Fats also provide energy. In fact, when oxidized, they are the most concentrated sources of energy and as such, furnish the calories necessary for survival. Fats also act as carriers for the fat-soluble vitamins, A, D, E, and K. Consuming too much fat can lead to weight problems and poor metabolism of food products because the digestive and absorption processes are affected.

Fatty acids are the basic components of fat and comprise two main groups. Saturated fatty acids usually come from animal sources. Unsaturated fatty acids primarily come from vegetables, nuts, or seed sources. In the unsaturated group are three essential fatty acids. These acids are called "essential" because they are necessary to prevent a specific deficiency disease. Also, the body cannot manufacture them, and they are obtained only from the diet. These three acids are linoleic acid, arachidonic acid, and linolenic acid. They are necessary for healthy blood, arteries, nerves, and skin. A deficiency in this group would lead to skin problems and illness.

Proteins Proteins, the third essential group of nutrients, are complex organic compounds that contain amino acids. Protein is critical to all aspects of growth and development of body tissues. This substance is necessary for the building of muscles, blood, skin, internal organs, hormones, and enzymes. Protein is also a source of energy when there is insufficient carbohydrate or fat in the diet. When protein is spared, it is either used for tissue repair and maintenance or converted by the liver and stored as fat.

When proteins are digested and broken down, they form 22 amino acids. These amino acids are then absorbed from the intestine into the bloodstream and carried to the liver for synthesis into the tissues and organs of the body. They are the chemical basis for life, and if just one is missing, protein synthesis will decrease or even stop. All but eight of the amino acids can be produced by the body. These eight must be obtained from the diet. If all eight are present in a particular food, the food is a "complete protein". Foods that lack one or more of these essential amino acids are called "incomplete proteins". Most meat and dairy products are complete proteins, and most vegetables and fruits are incomplete. When several incomplete proteins are ingested, they should be combined carefully so that the result will be a balance yielding complete protein. For example, the combination of beans and rice is perfectly balanced to give a complete protein food.

It is difficult to determine the exact amount of protein needed to supply all of the essential amino acids because there are many variables. Height and weight, level of activity, and nutritional and health status all influence the amount of protein necessary for a healthy body. The National Research Council recommends that 0.42 grams of protein be consumed per day per pound of body weight. It is suggested that a person weighing 56 kg should consume 75 grams of protein; however, recent research shows that this amount can be decreased by about one-third without negative results. It appears that as long as the essential amino acids are included in the diet, the total grams of protein can be reduced.

Protein deficiency can affect the entire body — organs, tissues, skin, and muscles, as well as certain body processes. If a child is deficient in protein, he or she may get kwashiorkor, a disease resulting in physical and mental impairment and, if severe enough, death. If an adult is deficient in protein, his or her stamina, mental state, and ability to withstand stress and infection is affected. Protein deficiency also interferes with recovery from diseases or surgery.

Protein is very plentiful in the body. It is an integral part of all cells and essential for growth and development. Just like fats and carbohydrates, adequate protein must be consumed in balance with other nutrients for human survival.

Water   While not specifically a nutrient, water is essential for survival. Water is involved in every body process from digestion and absorption to excretion. It is a major portion of circulation and is the transporter of nutrients throughout the body.

Body water performs three major functions: it gives form to the body, comprising from 50 – 75 percent of the body mass; it provides the necessary environment for cell metabolism; and it maintains a stable body temperature. For a complete explanation of water and its relationship to electrolytes, refer to Chapter 14.

Almost all foods contain water that is absorbed by the body. The average adult body contains 56 quarts of water and loses about 3 quarts a day. If a person suffers severe water depletion, dehydration and salt depletion can result and can eventually lead to death. A person can survive longer without food than without water.

Vitamins   Vitamins are organic food substances and are essential in small amounts for growth, maintenance, and the functioning of body processes. Vitamins are found only in living things — plants and animals — and usually cannot be synthesized by the human body.

Vitamins can be grouped according to the substance in which they are soluble. The fat-soluble group includes vitamins A, D, E, and K. These vitamins are measured in International Units. Each unit generally refers to the amount of the vitamin needed to produce a change in the nutritional health of a laboratory animal. The water-soluble vitamins include the B-complex vitamins, vitamin C, and the bioflavanoids. These are usually measured in milligrams.

Vitamins have no caloric value, but they are as necessary to the body

▶ **Essential Body Nutrients**

Carbohydrates	Monosaccharides
	Glucose, fructose, galactose
	Disaccharides
	Sucrose, lactose, maltose
	Polysaccharides
	Starch, dextrin, glycogen, cellulose, hemicellulose
Fats	Linoleic acid, linolenic acid, arachidonic acid
Proteins	Amino acids
	Phenylalanine, lysine, isoleucine, leucine, methionine, valine, tryptophan, threonine
Vitamins	Fat-soluble
	Vitamins A, D, E, and K
	Water-soluble
	Vitamins B_1, B_2, B_6, B_{12}, niacin, pantothenic acid, folacin, biotin, choline, mesoinositol, para-aminobenzoic acid, and vitamin C
Minerals	Major elements
	Calcium, chloride, iron, magnesium, phosphorus, potassium, sodium, sulfur
	Trace elements
Water	

as any other basic nutrient. Currently, there are about 20 substances identified as vitamins, but recent research is concerned with identifying even more of these substances since they are so essential to survival.

For many years research groups have attempted to determine basic vitamin requirements for various age groups. The most commonly used are the listings of the Recommended Dietary Allowances (RDA), based on standards established by the National Academy of Sciences.

Minerals Minerals are inorganic substances, widely prevalent in nature, and essential for metabolic processes. Minerals are grouped according to the amount found in the body. Major minerals include calcium, magnesium, sodium, potassium, phosphorus, sulfur, and chlorine, all of which have a known function in the body. Major minerals are measured in milligrams. A second group, trace minerals, are iron, copper, iodine, manganese, cobalt, zinc, and molybdenum. These minerals are measured in micrograms, and their function in the body remains unclear. There remains a third group of trace minerals found in scanty amounts in the body and whose function is also unclear. Minerals form 60–90 percent of all inorganic material in the body, and are found in bones, teeth, soft tissue, muscle, blood, and nerve cells.

Minerals act on organs and in metabolic processes. They act as catalysts for many reactions such as controlling muscle responses, maintaining the nervous system and acid-base balance, transmitting messages, maintaining cardiac stability, and regulating the metabolism and absorption of other nutrients. Even though they are considered separately, all minerals work synergistically with other minerals, and their actions are interrelated. A deficiency in one mineral, therefore, will affect the action of others in the body. It is essential that adequate minerals be ingested because a mineral deficiency can result in severe illness. Likewise, excessive amounts of minerals can throw the body out of balance.

Sufficient minerals can be supplied by an adequate diet. Even though RDAs have not been established on all minerals, a diet that contains all the other nutrients can supply the necessary amount of minerals for the body. Many nutritionists and biochemists, however, recommend a daily basic vitamin-mineral supplement to ensure adequate levels.

ASSIMILATION OF NUTRIENTS

Following the discussion of the essential body nutrients, it is now important to identify how these elements are broken down, absorbed, and utilized in the body. Nutrients, in most cases, are ingested through the mouth, and the body must break down these substances. This process is called digestion. It takes place in the mouth, pharynx, esophagus, stomach, and the small and large intestines.

Gastrointestinal Tract The main functions of the gastrointestinal system are the secretion of enzymes and electrolytes to break down raw materials

▶ The total daily energy requirement for an individual is the number of calories needed to replace the energy loss from the metabolic rate, plus loss from a person's exercise output, emotional and mental state, and diet.

The number of calories ingested should be directly related to maintaining an adequate energy level and supporting the body's metabolic processes.

that are ingested; the movement of the ingested products through the system; the complete digestion of nutrients; and the absorption into the blood, the storage, and the excretion of the end products of digestion.

When nutrients reach the stomach, both mechanical and chemical digestive processes occur. Nutrients are churned, and peristaltic waves move the material through the stomach and, at intervals with relaxation of the pyloric sphincter, into the duodenum. This chemical action creates hydrochloric acid, which provides the proper medium for pepsin to split protein into proteoses and peptones. Other chemical actions produce lipase, a fat-splitting enzyme, rennin, which coagulates the protein of milk, and the intrinsic factor, which acts on certain food components to form the antianemic factor.

As nutrients move into the duodenum and the jejunum, intestinal juices provide a large number of enzymes that break down protein into amino acids, form and convert maltase to glucose, and split nucleic acids into nucleotides. The large intestine provides for the absorption of nutrients and the elimination of waste products. It is here that the formation of vitamins K and B_{12}, riboflavin, and thiamin occurs. Also, there is absorption of water from the fecal mass.

The Accessory Organs   The accessory organs of the gastrointestinal tract also play an important role in the utilization of nutrients. These organs include the tongue, salivary glands, teeth, liver, gallbladder, and pancreas.

The liver is especially important because it has a major role in the metabolism of carbohydrates, fats, and proteins. In the metabolism of carbohydrates, the liver converts glucose to glycogen and stores it. The liver then can reconvert glycogen to glucose when the body requires higher blood sugar. The process of releasing carbohydrates (end products) into the bloodstream is called glycogenolysis.

The liver metabolizes fats through the process of oxidation of fatty acids and the formation of acetoacetic acid. Also, the liver forms lipoproteins, cholesterol, and phospholipids and converts carbohydrates and protein to fats.

Proteins are metabolized in the liver, and deamination of amino acids takes place. Also in this process, the formation of urea and plasma proteins is completed. Finally, the interconversions of amino acids and other compounds occurs in the liver.

The gallbladder's primary function is to act as a reservoir for bile. Bile emulsifies fats through constant secretion (500 – 1000 ml in 24 hours).

The pancreas secretes pancreatic juices that contain enzymes for the digestion of carbohydrates, fats, and proteins. Enzymes are secreted as inactive precursors that do not become active until secreted into the intestine. In the intestine, the enzyme trypsin acts on proteins to produce peptones, peptides, and amino acids; pancreatic amylase acts on carbohydrates to produce disaccharides; and pancreatic lipase acts on fats to produce glycerol and fatty acids.

In summary, the alimentary tract's primary function is to provide the body with a continuous supply of nutrients through utilization of a tract for ingestion and movement of food and fluids, secretion of digestive juices for breaking down the nutrients, and an absorption mechanism for utilizing foods, water, and electrolytes. Nutrients are essential for life, but their simple ingestion into the body is not sufficient for survival. They must be broken down, absorbed, and utilized efficiently if the body is to remain in homeostasis.

NORMAL AND THERAPEUTIC NUTRITION

Normal nutrition is based on recommended daily dietary allowances. These standards are scientifically designed for the maintenance of nearly all healthy people in the United States.

Therapeutic nutrition is a modification of nutritional needs based on the disease condition and/or the excess or deficit of a nutrition state. Combination diets, which include alterations in minerals, vitamins, proteins, carbohydrates, fats, as well as fluid and texture, are prescribed in therapeutic nutrition.

Whether a normal or a therapeutic diet is being considered, a person's cultural, socioeconomic, and psychological influences, as well as the physiological requirements, must be taken into account for effective nutrition; thus, in any given situation, the nutritional requirements must be considered within the context of the total needs of an individual.

Nutritional Problems in the Hospital In a hospital, nutrition is frequently neglected as a viable component of client management. Studies conducted at various medical centers support the claim that clients become more malnourished the longer they remain in a hospital.

For clients who seem to be stable on admission and give no history of nutritionally related food problems, the usual hospital diet is adequate; however, these clients must be reassessed periodically to prevent nutritional problems from developing. A periodical assessment is especially important for clients hospitalized for a long period of time.

For clients identified as having a nutritional problem, a nursing care plan must be developed. To manage these clients correctly, the cause of depletion must first be determined. Research indicates that poor food intake is the leading cause of malnutrition. Reasons for poor food intake include fear, anxiety, or depression prior to or during hospitalization. Some clients may not be capable of feeding themselves or may have poor fitting dentures. Treatment and therapy may limit the capability of a client to eat or interfere with a client's appetite. Also, some clients may have the desire to eat and a good appetite, but shortly after eating a certain food, they have cramps, pain, gas, or diarrhea or feel nauseous and/or vomit. This eventually leads to less food intake. Whatever the source, the cause of depletion must be determined to prevent further malnutrition. As clients become more and more malnourished, they lose the ability to handle foodstuffs metabolically. As their intake decreases below their nutritional requirements, their body cannot generate the epithelium of the gastrointestinal tract from the crypt cells. The villi and microvilli, needed to metabolize and absorb food, flatten and become ineffective. This leads to malabsorption, with resulting malnutrition.

Therapeutic Management After determining the cause and the extent of depletion, the next step is to institute therapeutic procedures that meet the needs of the client. In selecting nutrients, the clinician needs to evaluate the status of the client's gastrointestinal tract to determine if modifications in nutrients are necessary. For example, can the client split intact protein into the peptides and amino acids needed for absorption? Can the client tolerate the osmotic load of monosaccharides or disaccharides? Is the client fat intolerant, or does the client need special fat? Is the client lactose intolerant?

After therapeutic diets have been ordered, it is critical that the nurse be aware of compliance by the client. The nurse is the professional most closely involved with the client and the one who can best determine the client's actual intake. The nurse should ensure that the client is not receiving inappropriate foods from other sources and that the client is actually eating the foods prescribed. If the prescribed diet is not meeting the client's needs, an alternative method of feeding might be considered. For example, if oral feedings prove inadequate, then alternative methods such as feeding by nasogastric, nasoduodenal, or nasojejunal tube should be considered. There are a variety of delivery systems and methods of enteral feeding that are now available for adequate care of the client. The particular choice should be based on the individual client's needs and requirements.

When other methods have failed, parenteral nutrition may be the management of choice. This can be either administered peripherally, using isotonic concentrations of glucose, crystalline amino acids, and fats, or it can be through a central, high-flow vein in which hypertonic glucose, along with crystalline amino acids, fats, electrolytes, vitamins, and trace elements, may be given. This technique requires special handling and management of the client and is the most expensive method of feeding. It should be used only if the intestines do not work adequately, if the client is obstructed or has a fistula, if a bowel rest is required, or if the client is so debilitated that the gastrointestinal tract is nonfunctional.

In this era of sophisticated medical and nursing management, no client should become or remain malnourished or develop any kind of nutritional problem. As health professionals, nurses are responsible for meeting the client's needs. Among these needs are adequate nutritional requirements to maintain status and to be able to successfully deal with or overcome the medical problems for which the client is being treated.

GUIDELINES FOR MANAGING CLIENTS

An adequate diet must include carbohydrates, fats, proteins, vitamins and minerals.

- Carbohydrates are the chief source of energy, and diets not sufficient in carbohydrates lead to a low energy level, use of protein for energy, and ketosis.
- Fats provide the most concentrated source of energy and are carriers for fat-soluble vitamins.
- Proteins are essential for building body tissue and are necessary for tissue repair.
- Vitamins are essential for growth, maintenance, and functioning of body processes.
- Minerals are essential for metabolic processes.

Digestion takes place throughout the gastrointestinal tract.

- The gastrointestinal system breaks down raw materials through the secretion of enzymes and electrolytes.
- Mechanical and chemical digestive processes are necessary for nutritional synthesis.
- Nutrients are absorbed mainly through the small intestine.
- The liver plays a major role in nutritional metabolism.

Nutritional needs are based on a client's disease condition and excess or deficit of a nutritional state.

- Therapeutic diets are used to alter health status.
- Combination diets, which include alteration of all the major nutrients, are prescribed for certain disease conditions.

Alternative methods of providing nutrients must be instituted when clients are unable to ingest or assimilate foods orally.

- Enteral feedings provide life-sustaining nutrients when other oral methods cannot be utilized.
- Parenteral nutrition may be administered peripherally, using isotonic concentrations, or centrally with intravenous catheter placement.

ACTION: PROVIDING APPROPRIATE NUTRITION

Rationale for Action
- To provide a nutritional diet based on individual needs
- To identify the client who exhibits nutritional deficits and to determine an appropriate diet
- To provide nutritional requirements for clients unable to consume oral feedings

ASSESSMENT

1 Appropriate dietary order.
2 Nutritional needs of client.
3 Sociocultural orientation of client.
4 Diet history, eating habits, and food preferences of client.
5 Ability of client to comply with diet regimen.
6 Analysis of appropriate diagnostic tests.
7 Alterations in health status that indicate need for therapeutic vs. regular diet.

ASSESSMENT CATEGORIES	NORMAL	ABNORMAL
1 Appetite	Remains unchanged	Increased or decreased recently Particular cravings
2 Weight	Previous weight maintained Normal for client Appropriate for age and body build	Changed — increased or decreased recently Rapid or slow changes in weight
3 Nutritional intake	Adequate foods and fluids to supply body nutrients Nonallergic response to major food groups No pattern of fad diets Absence of drugs, chemicals, or other substances that influence appetite or metabolism	Elimination of certain food categories that results in limited nutrients Emphasis on some food groups (sugar) to the exclusion of others (vegetables) Allergic response to certain foods Constant use of fad diets to lose weight Use of drugs or chemicals that interferes with appetite nutrient assimilation Presence of emotional disorder (depression, anorexia, manic response) that interferes with food ingestion
4 Meal patterns	3-6 home-prepared meals/day Adequate time and calm atmosphere for meals	Fast-food or packaged foods Missed meals, constant snacking, or over-eating Eating "on the run" or hurried
5 Physical factors	Adequate chewing and swallowing capability Mouth and gums healthy so food can be ingested Physical exercise adequate for calorie intake	Teeth and/or gums in poor condition or ill-fitting dentures Swallowing impairs ingestion Inadequate physical exercise to burn calories
6 Presence of disease	No disease process that interferes with nutrient assimilation No congenital condition or post-surgery condition that interferes with nutrient assimilation	Disease present that interferes with ingestion, digestion, assimilation, or excretion Congenital condition, rehabilitation phase, or post-surgery that interferes with food assimilation
7 Sociocultural-religious factors	Ability to afford adequate foods in all food categories Cultural beliefs that do not eliminate whole food groups Religious beliefs that do not eliminate whole food groups Food does not lose all nutrient value in preparation	Economic position that precludes purchase of adequate foods Religious or cultural beliefs that interfere with receiving balanced diet (macrobiotic diets) Inadequate knowledge, experience, or intelligence to prepare healthy meals
8 Elimination schedule	Regular, adequate elimination of foods Absence of constant flatus, discharge, or mucus	Irregular and/or painful elimination Presence of constant flatus Presence of discharge, blood, or mucus

8   Status of GI tract, including digestion and/or absorption.
    a   Ability of the client to split intact protein into peptides and amino acids needed for absorption.
    b   Ability of the client to tolerate osmotic load of monosaccharides or disaccharides.
    c   Ability of the client to tolerate lactose.
    d   Assessment of client's fluid intake needs.
9   Recommended daily dietary allowances.
10   Essential body nutrients.

PLANNING

GOALS

- Diet is nutritious and appropriate for the client's needs
- The client complies with the diet
- Diet is tolerated physiologically and emotionally by the client

INTERVENTION: Providing Nutrients for the Client

1 Assist physician in determining a diet appropriate for the client's needs.
2 Elicit food preferences of the client.
3 Send request to the diet kitchen for the specific diet and keep diet sheets or diet Rands up to date.
4 Check all diet trays before serving to ensure the diet provided is the one ordered.
5 Ensure that hot food is hot and cold food is cold.
6 Keep food trays attractive. Avoid spilling liquids on tray.
7 Position the client in a chair or up in bed (unless otherwise ordered) to assist in feeding.
8 Assist the client with cutting meat and opening milk cartons as needed.
9 Feed the client if necessary.

EVALUATION

EXPECTED OUTCOMES

1 Client will receive adequate diet, fluids, electrolytes, vitamins, minerals, and trace elements. *If not*, follow these alternative nursing actions.
   ANA: Assess for mechanical problems of eating, i.e., missing or poorly fitting dentures.
   ANA: Assess if the client is very anxious or fearful regarding hospitalization or surgery.
   ANA: Identify if the client is unable to feed self. Is an IV interfering with the client's ability to eat?
   ANA: Assess medications that client is receiving to determine if side effects could possibly be causing poor intake.
   ANA: Assess if there is a history of anorexia.
2 Reasonable compliance to diet is maintained. *If not*, follow these alternative nursing actions:
   ANA: Identify if diet promotes flatus, pain, abdominal cramping, diarrhea, or nausea/vomiting. Alter diet accordingly.
   ANA: Alter diet to adhere to client preferences and/or sociocultural traditions.
   ANA: Assess if anorexia is possibly emotionally based. If so, report to physician for possible psychiatric consultation.

3 Diet is tolerated physiologically and emotionally by client. *If not,* follow these alternative nursing actions:

ANA: Advance to high-calorie density foods.

ANA: Provide between-meal supplements.

ANA: Omit high-water density food selections (low-calorie density).

ANA: Modify meal pattern to six small feedings.

ANA: Provide diet change in oral feeding.

ANA: Provide alternate means of nutritional intake, i.e., tube feeding or hyperalimentation.

UNEXPECTED OUTCOMES

1 Client is unable to assimilate foods metabolically.

ANA: Notify physician of abnormal results of diagnostic tests which identify assimilation problems.

ANA: Assist physician in altering method of feeding (enteral or parenteral).

2 Client vomits or has diarrhea.

ANA: Evaluate allergic responses to food. Review history and physical to determine food allergies which may exist.

ANA: Revert to clear liquid diet, gradually progressing back to regular diet.

ANA: Assess overall health status (e.g., temperature, obstruction, etc.).

Charting
- Appetite
- Food Intake
- Tolerance to diet
- Weight
- I and O fluid status
- Client's subjective response to diet

ACTION: ADMINISTERING THERAPEUTIC DIETS

ASSESSMENT

1 Total condition of client — physical, emotional, and mental status.

2 Appropriateness of prescribed therapeutic diet as related to altered state of health.

3 Ability of client to tolerate diet.

4 Mental state of client in regard to compliance to diet regimen.

5 Refer to general assessment steps in maintaining normal nutritional status.

Rationale for Action
- To maintain balanced nutritional status
- To meet nutritional needs based on alterations in client's health status
- To tolerate foods and nutrients more efficiently

PLANNING

GOALS

- Prescribed diet is appropriate for the client's needs.
- Diet is tolerated by client.
- Client complies with diet regimen.

INTERVENTION: Providing Diets Associated with Carbohydrate Control

1 A hypoglycemic diet is utilized to reduce stimulation of excessive insulin by avoiding highly concentrated carbohydrate foods.

519

DIABETIC EXCHANGE DIETS

FOOD GROUP	UNIT OF EXCHANGE	CALORIES	FOOD ALLOWED
Milk			
Whole	1 cup	170	1 cup whole milk = 1 cup skim milk and 2 fat exchanges
Skim	1 cup	80	
Fruit	Varies according to allotted calories	40	Fresh or canned without sugar or syrup
Vegetables			
A	1 cup	Vary	Green, leafy vegetables; tomatoes
B	½ cup	35	Vegetables other than above
Bread	1 slice	70	Can exchange cereals, starch items, some vegetables
Meat	1 ounce	75	Lean meats, egg, cheese, seafood
Fat	1 teaspoon	45	1 teaspoon butter or mayonnaise = bacon, oil, olives, avocado
Unlimited foods			Coffee, tea, bouillon, spices, flavorings

    a Foods prescribed are high protein, high fat, and low carbohydrate.

    b Foods not allowed are high carbohydrate, for example, sugar, syrup, candy.

2 A diabetic diet modifies the insulin disorder and controls sugar intake.

    a Foods prescribed usually use food exchange method.

    b Foods not allowed are refined sugars.

INTERVENTION: Providing Diets Associated with Protein Control

1 A low-protein diet is utilized for renal impairment (uremia), hepatic coma, and cirrhosis (according to individual requirements).

    a Control end products of protein metabolism by limiting protein intake.

    b Evaluate the number of grams of protein allowed.

    c Eliminate high-protein foods, such as eggs, meat, milk, and milk products.

2 A high-protein diet is necessary for tissue building, correction of protein deficiencies, burns, liver diseases, malabsorption syndromes, undernutrition, and maternity.

    a Correct protein loss and/or maintain and rebuild tissues by increasing intake of high-quality protein food sources.

    b Encourage the eating of high-protein foods, such as fish, fowl, organ and meat sources, and dairy products.

    c Suggest protein supplements (usually ordered by physician), such as Sustagen, Meritene, and Proteinum.

3 An amino acid metabolism abnormality diet is utilized for phenylketonuria (PKU), galactosemia, and lactose intolerance.

    a Reduce and/or eliminate the offending enzyme in the food intake of protein and utilize substitute nutrient foods.

    b Avoid milk and milk products as they constitute the main source of enzymes for the three diseases.

    c Utilize substitutes to meet daily allowances.

INTERVENTION: Providing Diets Associated with Fat Control

1 A restricted cholesterol diet is utilized for cardiovascular diseases, diabetes mellitus, and high-serum cholesterol levels.

    a Control the blood cholesterol level and/or maintain blood cholesterol at a normal level by restricting foods high in cholesterol.

    b Limit high-cholesterol foods, such as egg yolk, shellfish, organ meats, bacon, pork, avocado, and olives.

    c Encourage low-cholesterol foods, such as vegetable oils, raw or cooked vegetables, fruits, lean meats, and fowl.

2 A modified fat diet is utilized according to individual tolerance in malabsorption syndromes, cystic fibrosis, gallbladder disease, obstructive jaundice, and liver disease.

a Attempt to lower fat content in diet to reduce irritation of diseased organs and to reduce fat content where there is inadequate absorption of fat.

b Low-fat diet: Avoid such foods as gravies, fat meat and fish, cream, fried foods, rich pastries, whole milk products, cream soups, salad and cooking oils, nuts, and chocolate. Allow eggs (2 to 3 per week), lean meat, and butter or margarine.

c Fat-free diet: allow vegetables, fruits, lean meats, fowl, fish, bread, and cereal and restrict all fatty meats and fat.

3 A high-polyunsaturated fat diet is utilized for cardiovascular diseases and individuals with high-serum cholesterol.

a Reduce intake of saturated fats and increase intake of foods rich in polyunsaturated fats. (Physician usually prescribes caloric level as well as restrictions.)

b Avoid foods originating from animal sources, selected peanuts, olives, avocado, coconuts, chocolate, and cashew nuts.

c Allow foods originating from vegetable sources (except for those named above), margarine, corn/soybean/safflower oil, fresh ground peanut butter, and nuts (except cashews).

INTERVENTION: Providing Diets Associated with Renal Disease

1 A low-protein diet and essential amino acid diet (modified Giovannetti diet) is comprised of 20 gm of protein and 1500 mg of potassium.

a Prevent electrolytes and byproducts of metabolism from accumulating to a fatal level between artificial kidney treatments.

b Allow foods such as one egg daily, 6 ounces of milk, low-protein bread, fruit, vegetables, butter, oil, jelly, candy, tea, and coffee.

c Restrict foods such as meat, chicken, fish, peanuts, and high-protein bread.

2 A low-calcium diet is utilized to prevent formation of renal calculi.

a Decrease the total daily intake of calcium to prevent further stone formation. Total calcium intake is 400 mg per day instead of 800 mg (normal).

b Allow foods such as milk (one cup daily), juices, tea, coffee, eggs, and fresh fruits and vegetables.

c Restrict foods such as rye and whole grain breads and cereals, dried fruits and vegetables, fish, shellfish, cheese, chocolate, and nuts.

3 An acid ash diet is utilized to prevent precipitation of stone elements.

a Establish a well-balanced diet in which the total acid ash is greater than the total alkaline ash daily.

b Allow foods such as breads and cereals of any type, fats, fruits (one serving), vegetables, meat, eggs, cheese, fish, fowl (two servings), and spices.

c Restrict foods such as carbonated beverages, dried fruits, bananas, figs, raisins, dried beans, carrots, chocolate, nuts, olives, and pickles.

▶ Examples of foods rich in fat-soluble vitamins

- Vitamin A—liver, egg yolk, whole milk, butter, fortified margarine, green and yellow vegetables, fruits
- Vitamin D—fortified milk and margarines, sunshine, fish oils
- Vitamin E—vegetable oils and green vegetables
- Vitamin K—egg yolk, leafy green vegetables, liver, cheese

Examples of foods rich in water-soluble vitamins

- Vitamin C—citrus fruits, tomatoes, broccoli, cabbage
- Thiamine (B_1)—lean meat such as beef, pork, liver; whole grain cereals and legumes
- Riboflavin (B_2)—milk, organ meats, enriched grains
- Niacin—meat, beans, peas, peanuts, enriched grains
- Pyridoxine (B_6)—yeast, wheat, corn, meats, liver, and kidney
- Cobalamin (B_{12})—lean meat, liver, kidney
- Folic acid—leafy green vegetables, eggs, liver

▶ **Definitions of Sodium Restrictions**
Mild: 2 to 3 g sodium
Moderate: 1000 mg sodium
Strict: 500 mg sodium
Severe: 250 mg sodium

▶ **Foods High in Sodium**

- Table salt and all prepared salts, such as celery salt
- Smoked meats and salted meats
- Most frozen vegetables or canned vegetables with added salt
- Butter, margarines, and cheese
- Quick-cooking cereals
- Shellfish, and frozen or salted fish
- Seasonings and sauces
- Canned soups
- Chocolates and cocoa
- Beets, celery, and selected greens (spinach)
- Anything with salt added, such as potato chips, popcorn

4 A low-purine diet is utilized to prevent uric acid stones; also utilized for clients with gout.
  a Restrict purine, which is the precursor of uric acid; 4 percent of urinary stones are composed of uric acid.
  b Allow foods such as milk, tea, fruit juices, carbonated beverages, breads, cereals, cheese, eggs, fat, and most vegetables.
  c Restrict foods such as glandular meats, gravies, fowl, fish, and high meat quantities.

INTERVENTION: Providing Diets Associated with Vitamin Control

1 An increased vitamin diet is necessary for treatment of specific vitamin deficiencies.
  a Provide high-vitamin diet for clients with burns, healing wounds, raised temperatures, and infections. Also used for pregnant clients.
  b Evaluate diseases, such as cystic fibrosis and liver disease, that require water-soluble vitamins.
2 Total low-vitamin diets are not generally prescribed—although specific vitamins might be decreased for periods of illness.

INTERVENTION: Providing Diets Associated with Mineral Control

1 A restricted sodium diet is utilized for hypertension, hepatitis, congestive heart failure, renal deficiencies, cirrhosis of liver, and adrenal corticoid treatment.
  a Correct and/or control the retention of sodium and water in the body by limiting sodium intake. May be done by restriction of salt in the diet or in combination with medications.
  b Restrict salt in cooking or at the table. In clients requiring dietary modification in salt intake any product containing sodium, such as soda bicarbonate, may be prohibited.
2 An increased potassium diet is utilized for diabetic acidosis, extended use of certain diuretic drugs, burns (after first 48 hours), vomiting, and fevers.
  a Replace potassium loss from the body with specific foods high in potassium or a potassium supplement. (Severe loss is managed with intravenous therapy.)
  b Avoid no specific foods unless there is a sodium restriction because some foods high in potassium are also high in sodium.
3 A high-iron diet is utilized for anemias (hemorrhage, nutritional, pernicious), postgastrectomy syndrome, and malabsorption syndrome.
  a Replace a deficit of iron caused by inadequate intake or chronic blood loss.
  b Include foods high in iron content, such as organ meats (especially liver), meat, egg yolks, whole wheat products, seafood, leafy vegetables, nuts, dried fruit, and legumes.

INTERVENTION: Providing Diets Associated with Fiber Control

1 A high-residue (roughage) diet is prescribed for constipation and diverticulosis.
   a Suggest foods high in residue, such as any meat or fish, cheese, fat, milk, whole wheat breads, cereals, and especially unrefined bran.
   b Instruct client that foods low in carbohydrates are usually high in residue.
2 A low-residue diet is utilized for ulcerative colitis, postoperative colon and rectal surgery, diverticulitis (when inflammation decreases, diet may revert to high residue), rheumatic fever, diarrhea, and enteritis.
   a Inform client that low-residue foods are ground meat, fish, broiled chicken without skin, creamed cheeses, limited fat, warm drinks, refined strained cereals, and white bread.
   b Instruct client that foods high in carbohydrates are usually low in residue.

INTERVENTION: Providing Bland Food Diets

1 A bland diet is utilized to promote the healing of the gastric mucosa by eliminating food sources that are chemically and mechanically irritating. Bland diets are used for duodenal ulcers, gastric ulcers, and postoperative stomach surgery.
   a Instruct client that bland diets are presented in stages with the gradual addition of certain foods.
   b Provide frequent, small feedings during active stress periods.
2 Establish regular meals and food patterns when condition permits.

INTERVENTION: Providing Diets Associated with Calorie Control

1 A restricted calorie diet reduces the caloric intake of food below the energy demands of the body so weight loss will occur.
   a Provide psychological support and exercise.
   b Restrict such foods as carbohydrates and fats.
2 An increased calorie diet is utilized to meet the increased metabolic needs of the body. There is usually an increase in protein and vitamins when increased calories are ordered.

INTERVENTION: Providing Diets Associated with Surgery

1 A high-protein preoperative diet is essential for the maintenance of normal serum protein levels during and following surgery.
   a Provide adequate carbohydrates to maintain liver glycogen and adequate amino acids to promote wound healing. This diet also restores nitrogen balance if protein-depleted for burn victims, the elderly, and severely debilitated clients.

▶ **Foods High in Potassium**
- Fruit juices such as orange, grapefruit, banana, raw apple
- Instant, dry coffee powder
- Egg, legumes, whole grains
- Fish, fresh halibut, codfish
- Pork, beef, lamb, veal, chicken
- Milk, skim and whole
- Dried dates, prunes
- Bouillon and meat broths

▶ **Bland Diet Allowances/Requirements**
1 Foods allowed
- Milk, butter, eggs (not fried), custard, vanilla ice cream, cottage cheese
- Cooked refined or strained cereal, enriched white bread
- Jello; homemade creamed, pureed soups
- Baked or boiled potatoes
2 Examples of foods that are eliminated
- Spicy and highly seasoned foods
- Raw foods
- Very hot and very cold foods
- Gas-forming foods (varies with individuals)
- Coffee, alcoholic beverages, carbonated drinks
- High-fat contents (some butter and margarine allowed)

- Total calories: 2800 for tissue repair; 6000 for extensive repair
- Protein:
     50 to 75 g/day early in postoperative period.
     100 to 200 g/day if needed for new tissue synthesis.
- Carbohydrate—sufficient in quantity to meet caloric needs and allow protein to be used for tissue repair
- Fat—not excessive as it leads to poor tissue healing and susceptibility to infection
- Vitamins:
     Vitamin C—up to 1 g/day
     Vitamin B—increased above normal
     Vitamin K—normal amounts

Charting

- Daily weight
- Appetite
- Client's response to diet
- Client's compliance
- Reasons for noncompliance

b Provide a 2500-calorie diet that is high in carbohydrates, moderate in protein with high-protein supplements.

c Instruct client that an elemental diet is low in residue and contains a synthetic mixture of CHO, amino acids, and essential fatty acids with added minerals and vitamins. It is bulk free and easily assimilated and absorbed.

2 A special postoperative surgical diet is necessary to promote wound healing, avoid shock from decreased plasma proteins and circulating red blood cells, prevent edema, and promote bone healing.

a Provide 2800 total calories for tissue repair and 6000 calories for extensive repair.

b Fluid intake is 2000 to 3000/day for uncomplicated surgery and 3000 to 4000/day for sepsis or renal damage. Seriously ill clients with drainage can require up to 7000 cc/day.

3 A postoperative diet protocol progresses from nothing by mouth the day of surgery to a general diet within a few days following surgery. Foods allowed in each phase of the progressive diet include:

a A clear-liquid diet is 1000 to 1500 cc/day and is comprised of water, tea, broth, jello, and juices (avoid juices with pulp).

b A full-liquid diet is clear liquids, milk and milk products, custard, puddings, creamed soups, sherbet, ice cream, and any fruit juice.

c A soft diet is full liquid and, in addition, pureed vegetables, eggs (not fried), milk, cheese, fish, fowl, tender beef, veal, potatoes, and cooked fruit.

d General diet, taking into consideration specific alterations necessary for client's health status.

EVALUATION

EXPECTED OUTCOMES

1 Client complies with prescribed therapeutic diet. *If not*, follow these alternative nursing actions:
ANA: Discuss with client reasons for noncompliance.
ANA: Check method of diet preparation and administration to see if it is attractive and appealing.
ANA: Assess environment to see if it is conducive to eating.
ANA: Modify diet within prescribed limits to enhance toleration.
ANA: Structure nursing care conference to which the physician and dietician are invited to discuss problems and suggest solutions.

2 Client tolerates diet well, and disease symptoms diminish. *If not*, follow these alternative nursing actions:
ANA: Reassess prescribed diet in terms of diagnosis.
ANA: Evaluate impact of medications on therapeutic diet.
ANA: Determine if psychosocial responses interfere with client's compliance with diet.
ANA: Modify diet within prescribed limits to enhance tolerance.
ANA: Structure nursing care conference to which the physician and dietician are invited to discuss problems and suggest solutions.

ACTION: PROVIDING NUTRIENTS VIA ENTERAL FEEDING

ASSESSMENT

1 Assess overall status:
   - Weight change/loss
   - Temperature
   - Presence of sepsis
   - Trauma
   - Mental state
   - Other medically related nutritional problems, e.g., diabetes, hyperlipidemia, alcoholism
2 Evaluate oral intake. Is it adequate, moderate, or altered?
3 Assess nutritional requirements. Are they being met or not being met? Does the client have special needs?
4 Assess status of GI tract. Is it normal, limited, or obstructed? Is there a fistula or ostomy present?
5 Assess capacity to chew and swallow.
6 Check for presence of gag reflex.
7 Evaluate respiratory or thoracic conditions.
8 Check for renal complications.
9 Check for vomiting and/or diarrhea.
10 With high-protein diets, assess for fluid and electrolyte imbalance.

PLANNING

GOALS

- Necessary nutrients are provided to sustain normal weight.
- Client complies and is able to tolerate method of ingesting nutrients.
- Equipment functions efficiently and correct volume is given to client.
- Fluid and electrolyte balance is maintained.

EQUIPMENT

- Syringes, delivery system, method of delivery (flow control), formula or ordered feeding (prepared daily by dietary department)
- Portable suction equipment available
- Number 6, 8, 12 Levin tube
- Water-soluble lubricant
- Feeding equipment, 60-cc asepto syringe or feeding bag
- Hypoallergenic tape
- Tincture of benzoin
- Towel
- Emesis basis
- Stethoscope
- Tongue blade
- Normal saline irrigation solution
- 20-cc syringe or asepto syringe
- Disposable irrigation set (optional)

Rationale for Action

- To provide alternate means of ingesting nutrients for clients with nonfunctional gastrointestinal tract
- To intervene in preexisting or impending nutritional depletion from debilitation
- To provide aggressive management for certain disease conditions (anorexia)
- To provide means of nutrition if there is an inability to swallow or an existing obstruction in upper alimentary canal
- To provide nutrients for client in comatose or semiconscious state
- To provide increased nutrient requirements above oral consumption.
- To provide nutrients for postoperative clients with bowel sounds present

INTERVENTION: Inserting a Nasogastric Tube

1. Check order for tube feeding.
2. Warm feeding to room temperature.
3. Discuss procedure with client.
4. Demonstrate and display items to be used in order to allay client's fear and to gain cooperation.
5. Wash hands.
6. Position client at 45-degree angle or higher.
7. Examine nostrils and select the most patent nostril by having client breathe through each one.
8. Measure from earlobe to tip of nose to xiphoid process of sternum to determine appropriate length for tube insertion. If tube is to go below stomach, add additional 15 to 25 cm. Mark point on tube with tape.
9. Lubricate first 10 cm of tube with water-soluble lubricant and stylet, if used.
10. Insert tube through nostril to back of throat and ask client to swallow. Sips of water may aid in pushing tubing past oropharynx.
11. Continue advancing tube until taped mark is reached.
12. Check position of tube.
    a. Inject 10 cc of air through nasogastric tube and listen with the stethoscope over stomach for a rush of air.

Measure NG tube from tip of earlobe to tip of nose and then to xiphoid process.

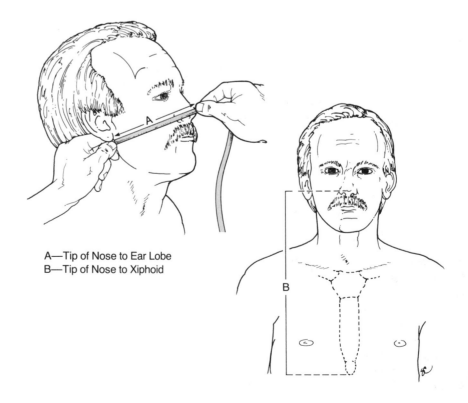

A—Tip of Nose to Ear Lobe
B—Tip of Nose to Xiphoid

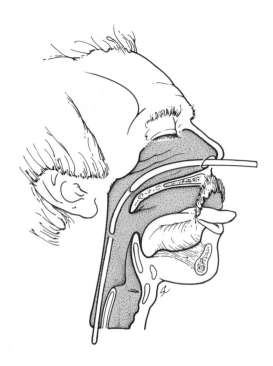

Use flashlight to check nasogastric tube placement by observing if tube is coiled in pharynx.

b Aspirate gastric contents if still unsure (sometimes difficult with small bore tubes).

c X-ray confirmation. If nasoduodenal or nasojejunal feedings are required, client should have an x-ray to confirm correct placement. Passage through the pylorus may require several days.

d Tape tube securely to nose and to cheek.

13 Remain with and talk with client until client's anxiety level is decreased (tube insertion often raises anxiety).

▶ Nurses never insert or withdraw a nasogastric tube for clients with gastric resections. The suture line could easily be interrupted, and hemorrhage could occur.

INTERVENTION: Irrigating a Nasogastric Tube

1 Obtain disposable irrigation set or emesis basin for irrigation solution, 20-cc syringe, and normal saline irrigation solution.

2 Wash hands.

3 Place client in semi-Fowler's position.

4 Check for nasogastric tube placement by instilling air and listening for "whoosh" sound.

5 Draw up 20-cc normal saline into irrigating syringe.

6 Gently instill the normal saline into the nasogastric tube. Do not force the solution.

7 Withdraw the 20-cc irrigation solution and empty into basin.

8 Repeat the procedure twice.

9 Record on I&O sheet the irrigation solution that has not been returned.

INTERVENTION: Administering a Tube Feeding

1 Obtain order from physician for appropriate formula (calories and/or amount).
2 Send requisition for formula to diet kitchen.
3 Check early in shift to ensure adequate formula is available.
4 Warm formula to room temperature using a microwave or set formula in basin of hot water.
5 Assemble feeding equipment. If using bag, fill with ordered amount of formula.
6 Explain procedure to client and assure privacy.
7 Place client on right side in high-Fowler's position.
8 Aspirate stomach contents to determine amount of residual.
9 Return aspirated contents to stomach to prevent electrolyte imbalance.
10 Pinch the tubing to prevent air from entering stomach.
11 Attach syringe to nasogastric tube.
12 Fill syringe with formula. (If using feeding bag, adjust drip rate to infuse over 30 minutes.)
13 Hold tubing no more than 39 cm or 18 inches above client.
14 Allow formula to infuse slowly (between 20 to 35 minutes) through the tubing.
15 Follow tube feeding with water in amount ordered.
16 Clamp end of the tube.
17 Wash tray and return it to client's bedside.
18 Give water between feedings if tube feeding is the sole source of nutrition.

EVALUATION

EXPECTED OUTCOMES

1 Client tolerates feeding well, and weight is maintained or increased. *If not*, follow these alternative nursing actions:
   ANA: Alter concentration of feeding and/or modify formula.
   ANA: Alter rate of feeding and/or change method (from syringe to bag or vice versa).
2 Appropriate residual is obtained from aspiration of stomach contents. *If not*, follow these alternative nursing actions:
   ANA: If no residual, reassess placement of the tube to determine if it is in the stomach.
   ANA: If excessive residual, (over 50 to 100 cc or according to hospital policy), hold current feeding and check for residual in one hour. Pooling in stomach leads to increased risk of aspiration, vomiting, and diarrhea.
3 Client complies with feeding procedure. *If not*, follow these alternative nursing actions:
   ANA: Staffing demands may cause feeding time to be rushed; therefore, allow more time for communication and feeding.
   ANA: Request more counseling time for client or recommend that a dietician confer with client.

▶ If residual is over 50–100 cc (according to hospital policy) hold feeding until residual diminishes.

▶ Usually, drip factor on feeding bags is 20 drops/cc (most bags do not give you calculated drip factor).

▶ All equipment maintained by careful cleaning and handling. Thorough washing, rinsing and drying essential to avoid contamination.

▶ **Variation in Methods**
Gravity drip is difficult with smaller bore tubes or with more viscous formulas. This kind of method may be intermittent or be a continuous slow drip. The latter method is desirable with a peristaltic infusion pump.

4 Intake and output balance is maintained. *If not,* follow these alternative nursing actions:

ANA: Check bedclothes and linen for spillage and leakage.

ANA: Assess for diarrhea (check with client).

5 Nasogastric tube functions efficiently and remains patent. *If not,* follow these alternative nursing actions:

ANA: Irrigate with 20 cc of normal saline solution. Repeat twice.

ANA: Reposition the nasogastric tube and irrigate again.

ANA: If clots are present and obstructing the tube, gently exert pressure with the syringe by pushing in and pulling back on the piston several times until clot is extracted.

ANA: Assess for possible occlusion of the tube; may have to withdraw tube and insert new nasogastric tube.

UNEXPECTED OUTCOMES

1 Client aspirates formula.

ANA: Suction client. Evaluate respiratory status until normal breathing pattern resumes.

ANA: In future feedings, ensure that client is kept at a 30-degree angle or higher for at least 30 minutes following feeding.

2 Vomiting occurs.

ANA: Position client quickly in high-Fowler's position (if not already) to prevent aspiration.

ANA: Suction immediately.

ANA: Assess concentration, amount, and rate with which formula was given.

ANA: Reduce rate of formula infusion in future feedings.

3 Fluid and electrolyte imbalance occurs.

ANA: Reevaluate procedure to make sure stomach contents were replaced after residual was checked.

ANA: Reassess formula concentration and amount of water given.

4 Stress ulcer in the GI tract from permanent tube placement.

ANA: Check to see if the tube can be intermittently placed to avoid constant irritation.

ANA: Give antacids one hour after feeding.

ANA: Obtain gastric aspirant to test for blood before each feeding and monitor results.

ACTION: PROVIDING TOTAL PARENTERAL NUTRITION

ASSESSMENT

1 Assess nutritional needs of clients who are unable to ingest calories normally.

2 Identify the caloric intake necessary to promote positive nitrogen balance and tissue repair and growth.

3 Ensure patency of central venous line.

4 Observe for correct additives in each hyperalimentation bottle.

Charting

- Weight
- Residual obtained
- Nasogastric tube size
- Amount and type of irrigating solution used
- Results of nasogastric tube irrigation
- Rate and volume of feeding
- Urine sugar and acetone
- I & O
- Client's response, behavior, attitude toward feeding
- Client teaching given to encourage self-care

Rationale for Action

- To provide a nitrogen source for clients unable to ingest protein normally
- To provide adequate calories for clients unable to tolerate oral feedings
- To provide nutrients for clients requiring bypass of the gastrointestinal tract
- To provide increased calories where regular IV solutions are insufficient
- To prevent or correct a deficiency of essential fatty acids
- To provide a contamination-free mode of delivering the hyperalimentation solution

5 Observe catheter insertion site for signs of infection, thrombophlebitis, or possible infiltration.
6 Inspect dressing over central line to ensure a dry, noncontaminated dressing.

PLANNING

GOALS

- Solution is infused at prescribed flow rate and tolerated by client.
- Dressing remains dry and intact during interval between changes.
- Catheter is placed correctly with no infiltration.
- Insertion site remains free of infection and inflammation.

EQUIPMENT

▶ **Composition of Hyperalimentation Solutions**

Amino acids—Freamine or Aminosol
Carbohydrates
Vitamins
Minerals
Hypertonic glucose/dextrose (20% to 50%)—calories (1000 to 2000 cal/liter)
Electrolytes
Water
Hyperalimentation solution is prepared in the pharmacy under a laminar flow hood.

- Intracath (20 cm, 16-gauge, radiopaque, polyvinyl chloride) or peripheral line catheter
- Betadine solution
- Betadine ointment
- Alcohol sponges
- Acetone solution (optional)
- Sterile 4- by 4-inch sponges
- Sterile gloves
- Sterile towels for drapes
- 3-cc syringe with 25-gauge needle
- Xylocaine or local anesthetic agent
- Sterile 00 or 000 black silk suture with needle
- IV filter
- Plastic tape/micropore tape, or occlusive dressing material
- IV extension tubing
- 500-cc normal saline IV bag
- Hyperalimentation solution from pharmacy
- IV infusion pump and cassette (for some equipment)
- Bath blanket to provide roll under client's shoulders
- Mask

Clinical Alert
- Do not use hyperalimentation central line for "piggyback" medications or CVP readings.
- Do not add any medications or solutions to hyperalimentation solution.

ADDITIONAL EQUIPMENT FOR CENTRAL VEIN INFUSIONS

- Sugar and acetone testing equipment
- Specific gravity urometer
- Small paper bag
- Betadine swabs
- Sterile gauze pads

INTERVENTION: Assisting with Catheter Insertion

1 Explain procedure to client and teach the Valsalva's maneuver.
2 Assess site for catheter insertion.
3 Review physician's order for correct hyperalimentation solution additives. Check solution content with orders.

4   Assemble IV insertion tray or kit, normal saline solution bottle, IV tubing, extension tubing, and filter.

5   Wash hands, assemble IV equipment and flush IV tubing with IV solution.

6   Place IV tubing through infusion pump. (IV tubing may be placed through an infusion cassette with some equipment.)

7   Place catheter insertion equipment on bedside stand.

8   Position client in head-down position with head turned to opposite direction of catheter insertion site. Place a small roll between client's shoulders to expose insertion site (use Trendelenburg's position of bed).

9   Cleanse insertion area with acetone and then Betadine solution. (If allergic to Betadine, use 70 percent isopropyl alcohol and Neosporin Ointment).

10 Assist physician as needed.

11 Instruct client in Valsalva's maneuver when stylet is removed from catheter and when IV tubing is connected to catheter.

12 Turn on IV infusion pump, using normal saline solution, at slow rate —10 drops/minute—until x-ray ensures accurate catheter placement.

13 Place Betadine (or Neosporin) ointment over catheter insertion site. Apply 4- by 4-inch sterile gauze pad over IV site and occlude dressing with micropore or plastic tape.

14 Order chest x-ray to verify correct catheter placement.

15 Following confirmation of catheter placement, change IV solution to hyperalimentation solution and adjust flow rate as ordered.

16 Observe for signs of air embolism, subcutaneous bleeding, pneumothorax, or allergic responses to protein (chills, increased temperature, nausea, headache, urticaria, dyspnea).

Valsalva's Maneuver

Ask client to take a deep breath and bear down. Apply gentle pressure to the abdomen. This maneuver prevents air from entering the catheter during catheter insertions or tubing changes.

INTERVENTION: Placing a Peripheral Vein Catheter

1   Assess upper extremities for IV catheter site.

2   Review physician's orders, gather equipment, wash hands.

3   Assemble normal saline IV solution tubing and extension tubing, and flush tubing with solution.

4   Wash hands and prepare the skin with Betadine solution and alcohol wipe.

5   Insert peripheral line using technique outlined in Chapter 14.

6   Insert IV tubing into the long line peripheral catheter.

7   Place IV tubing through IV pump and set rate at 10 drops/minute.

8   After assessing patency of peripheral line, hyperalimentation solution may be superimposed in IV line.

9   Set drop factor at prescribed rate.

10 Place Betadine ointment and 4- by 4-inch sterile gauze pad over insertion site.

11 Observe for signs of protein allergy.

Clinical Alert

This is not the site of choice for hyperalimentation catheter insertion, as thrombus formation is a major complication.

The right subclavian vein is the most common site for catheter placement.

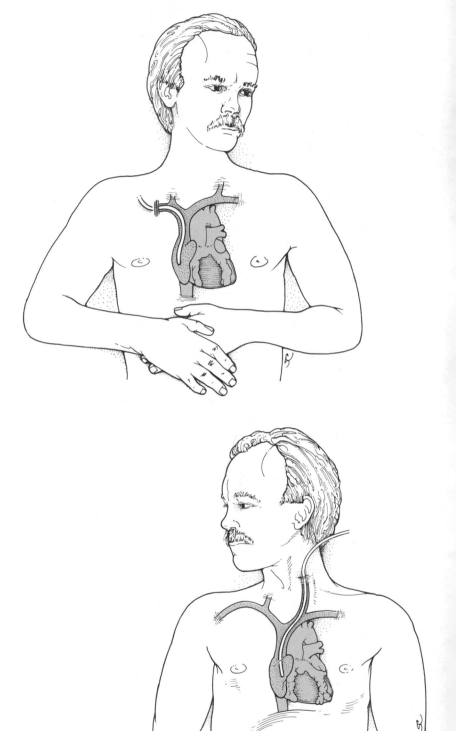

▶ Insertion site: solutions with glucose and protein concentrations of 10% and over must be infused directly into the superior vena cava via the subclavian or internal jugular vein to rapidly dilute the solution and to prevent thrombophlebitis. Usually, the right subclavian vein is used as it flows into the superior vena cava and because it is safe and easy to insert with a catheter.

The jugular vein may be used as an alternate site for catheter.

INTERVENTION: Maintaining Central Vein Infusions

1 Store hyperalimentation solution in refrigerator until 30 minutes before use. (Some pharmacies deliver the solution before each infusion.)

2 Change IV tubing, filter, and infusion pump cassette (if used) every 24 hours. Change should accompany IV fluid bottle change.

3 Change central vein dressing every 24 to 48 hours (generally, dressing change is completed every 48 hours).

4 Monitor IV flow rate every 30 to 60 minutes even though using IV pump. Dextrose solution must be changed every 12 hours to prevent bacterial growth.

5 Check urine specific gravity, sugar, and acetone every four hours.

6 If necessary, administer insulin according to prescribed rainbow coverage.

7 Notify physician of urine sugars of 3+ or 4+ and positive urine acetone.

8 Maintain accurate I and O. Record on special Total Parenteral Nutrition (TPN) sheet at least every four hours.

9 Weigh daily and record on graphic sheet and TPN sheet.

10 Observe for complications such as air embolus, hyperglycemia, osmotic diuresis, infiltration, or sepsis.

INTERVENTION: Changing Parenteral Hyperalimentation Dressing and Tubing

1 Gather equipment and wash hands thoroughly.

2 Add IV tubing and filter to parenteral hyperalimentation solution bottle.

3 Flush tubing to force out air.

4 Place IV tubing through IV pump or insert pump cassette into infusion pump and then prime cassette if used.

5 Prepare dressing material: open 4- by 4-inch sterile gauze pads, Betadine swabs, and ointment, and tear tape into 4-inch strips.

6 Place the client in a head-down position with head turned in the opposite direction of the insertion site. Instruct the client not to talk or cough. (Place mask on client if client cannot cooperate.)

7 Place mask over your nose and mouth and put on sterile gloves.

8 Take off old dressing and dispose of it in paper bag. (Do not touch the insertion site.)

9 Remove gloves and put on new sterile gloves.

10 Cleanse around the insertion site with sterile saline or hydrogen peroxide solution, using a circular movement from inside out, to cleanse the site of dried blood or serum.

11 Observe insertion site for signs of erythema, drainage, or possible thrombophlebitis.

12 Defat the skin around the catheter site with an acetone solution on a 4- by 4-inch sterile gauze pad, using a circular, outward motion.

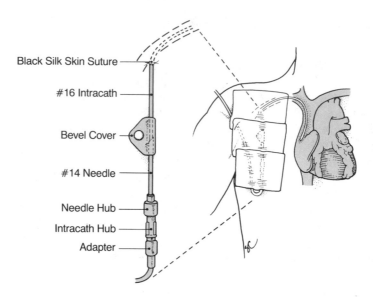

Black Silk Skin Suture

#16 Intracath

Bevel Cover

#14 Needle

Needle Hub

Intracath Hub

Adapter

Tape the dressing around the catheter to maintain an infection-free cannula site.

(Do not allow the solution to touch the plastic tubing as acetone reacts with plastic.)

13 Apply Betadine solution (providone-iodine) in same circular motion, working outward from catheter site. Allow at least two minutes for drying.

14 Cleanse the area with 70 percent isopropyl alcohol to remove Betadine, which can cause burning.

15 Apply providone-iodine ointment directly to the insertion site.

16 Place precut 2- by 2-inch sterile gauze pad around the insertion site, with the catheter protruding through the center of the pad.

17 Apply tincture of benzoin around the edges. Allow 30 seconds for drying.

18 Change the tubing if hospital policy dictates that tubing is changed at the same time as the dressing.

   a Remove gloves and wash hands or keep hands gloved.

   b Loosen the tubing in the catheter hub. Policy may dictate that the hub be wiped with alcohol swab.

   c Tell the client to hold breath and bear down while the new tubing is inserted into the hub of the catheter in order to prevent air from entering the catheter.

   d Tape the connection between the tubing and catheter hub.

19 Tape down the dressing around the catheter site. Tape the connection (tubing-catheter hub) to the skin. If a filter is part of the central line tubing, as with a hyperalimentation catheter, secure the filter onto the dressing with tape.

20 Label the dressing with the date and your initials.

INTERVENTION: Maintaining Hyperalimentation for Children

1 Assess for correct solution. Generally, there is a higher concentration of calcium, phosphorus, magnesium, and vitamins. Usually, a 10

Clinical Alert

When central-line dressings are loose, wet, or soiled, they are considered contaminated and must be changed.

percent solution of dextrose is started. It can be increased to 25 percent if tolerated.

2 Monitor patency of catheter (usually placed through internal or external jugular or scalp veins). Stopcocks are never used. Monitor constant infusion pump and filter.

3 Obtain urine sugar and acetone samples. Usually exogenous insulin is not required as the pancreas adapts to high-glucose loads.

4 Change the dressing every 48 hours and the tubing every 24 hours using aseptic technique. Stockinette can be used to keep scalp dressing secure. Tight-fitting T-shirt can keep chest site secure.

5 Monitor for accurate rate of infusion. Do not "catch up" if infusion is behind. Positive pressure pumps can be used to maintain infusion rates, particularly when small amounts of solution are being infused.

6 Observe the child when ambulating for accidents such as twisting or kinking the tubing, getting the tubing caught in the crib, or stepping on it.

7 Instruct parents on rationale for treatment and methods to prevent accidental dislodging of the tubing.

8 Provide play therapy and sources of stimulation to distract the child from thinking about the catheter.

EVALUATION

EXPECTED OUTCOMES

1 Hyperalimentation solution is infused at the prescribed rate. *If not*, follow these alternative nursing actions:
   ANA: Observe filter to ensure patency. A plugged filter is the most common cause of infusion failure. Replace the plugged filter.
   ANA: Ensure that the next hyperalimentation bottle is ready to be superimposed. If bottle is not ready, add a bottle of $D_{10}W$ until the hyperalimentation solution can be superimposed.
   ANA: Observe for signs of hypoglycemia caused by sudden change in dextrose concentration: weakness, trembling, sweating, hunger.

2 The dressing remains dry and intact during the interval between changes. *If not*, follow these alternative nursing actions:
   ANA: Change the dressing as soon as moisture is observed, following aseptic technique.
   ANA: If the dressing is exposed to moisture or secretions, a plastic, adhesive-like Steridrape or Saran wrap can be applied over sterile dressing.

3 Accurate placement of catheter. *If not*, follow these alternative nursing actions:
   ANA: Obtain and review all chest x-rays following catheter insertion.
   ANA: Infuse only isotonic IV solution into central vein catheters until catheter placement is ensured.
   ANA: If catheter enters heart, notify physician so that catheter can be pulled back until it reaches superior vena cava. Order new chest x-ray.

4   Catheter insertion site remains free of infection, inflammation, or infiltration. *If not*, follow these alternative nursing actions:
ANA: Notify physician immediately so catheter can be discontinued.
ANA: Cut tip of catheter off with sterile scissors and place in sterile container. Send to lab for culture and sensitivity for specific causative organism.
ANA: Cleanse site of catheter insertion with Proviodine and place sterile dressing over site.
ANA: Obtain order for and administer antibiotics as needed.

UNEXPECTED OUTCOMES

1   Infusion rate is set too high or infusion pump not used and IV rate increases inadvertently.
ANA: Observe for signs of hyperglycemia: dry mouth, flushed skin, thirst.
ANA: Monitor urine, sugar and acetone, and specific gravity. Notify physician if a large amount of solution is infused or if S/A is higher than previous reading.
ANA: Readjust flow rate to physician's orders. Continue to monitor for signs of hyperglycemia.
ANA: Institute use of infusion pump with hyperalimentation solution.
2   Infusion rate is less than ordered.
ANA: Adjust flow rate to that which was ordered. Do not attempt to "catch up" the amount not infused as this action could lead to osmotic diuresis from hyperglycemia.
3   Hydrothorax or pneumothorax occurs from inaccurate catheter placement.
ANA: Assess symmetry of chest expansion and breath sounds, and observe for signs of shortness of breath following catheter placement.
ANA: Call physician immediately to alter catheter placement.
ANA: Assess for signs of respiratory distress.
ANA: Set client in Fowler's position if not contraindicated by condition.
ANA: Administer oxygen at 6 l/minute via nasal prongs.
ANA: Obtain chest tube insertion tray and Pleur-evac system.
ANA: Monitor vital signs.
4   Catheter insertion site looks red and/or edematous.
ANA: Inform the physician. Instructions may direct the nurse to discontinue the IV and to culture the IV solution, tubing, and catheter, including the tip.
5   Leakage around the catheter insertion site has dampened the dressing and skin.
ANA: Check all connections. Lower the solution bottle to check for blood backflow in the tubing.
ANA: Inform the physician and describe the type of leakage.

Charting

- Catheter insertion site, size, physician's name, and any difficulty in insertion
- X-ray, following insertion
- Type of hyperalimentation solution and flow rate
- Specific gravity, results of urine sugar and acetone
- Specific gravity results of urine sugar and acetone acid
- If insulin administered, type, amount, and site
- Time of dressing and/or tubing change, date, and condition of catheter insertion site, along with name or initials of person who did the change
- Condition of insertion site
- Client's tolerance of procedure
- Signs of hypoglycemia or hyperglycemia
- Daily weights
- Vital signs every four hours

▶ Special TPN sheets may be used and then charting is done directly on the sheet, not in nurses' notes.

6 Air embolism has occurred because of loose connections or client's inability to perform Valsalva's maneuver at the time of tubing change (coupled with low central venous pressure).

ANA: Observe for cyanosis; hypotension; rapid, weak pulse; elevated CVP; loss of consciousness; or alterations in heart sounds.

ANA: Place client in Trendelenburg's position with the right chest uppermost, left chest down. Inform physician.

ANA: Administer oxygen at 6 l/minute via nasal prongs.

ACTION: ADMINISTERING IV INTRALIPIDS

ASSESSMENT

1 Assess for signs of essential fatty acid deficits; rash; eczema; dry, scaly skin; poor wound healing; sparse hair.

2 Assess pancreatic function.

3 Assess client for predisposing factors that could promote fat emboli such as anemia, coagulation disorders, abnormal liver, or pulmonary function.

4 Assess IV site for patency, erythema, and edema before infusing solution.

PLANNING

GOALS

- Adequate calories and essential fatty acids are provided to clients unable to ingest them by usual means.
- No untoward effects or complications are experienced as a result of procedure.
- Parenteral nutrients are provided without complications.

EQUIPMENT

- IV fat solution: Intralipid 10 percent (soybean oil); Liposyn 10 percent (safflower oil)
- Nonphthalate IV tubing infusion set (to prevent pooling of fat on IV tubing)
- Iodophor sponges

INTERVENTION: Infusing IV Fat

1 Review physician's order and take baseline vital signs as immediate reactions can occur.

2 Obtain Intralipid (refrigerated) from the pharmacy and warm the solution to room temperature or obtain Liposyn (nonrefrigerated) from the pharmacy.

Rationale for Action

- To spare protein in critically ill client
- To provide a source of energy for clients with deficient protein intake
- To provide essential fatty acids

Clinical Alert

Do not administer IV Intralipids to client with acute pancreatitis

▶ Guidelines for IV Fat Infusion

- IV fat solutions are isotonic and provide 1.1 calories/ml of solution.
- 1 ml of Intralipid equals 0.1 g.
- Putting additives into IV bottle is contraindicated as additives might be incompatible.
- Use of an IV filter is contraindicated as the particles are large and the infusion will not pass through the filter and it will become plugged.

▶ IV Lipid Side Effects

- chills
- fever
- flushing
- diaphoresis
- dyspnea
- cyanosis
- allergic reactions
- chest and back pain
- nausea and vomiting
- headache
- pressure over the eyes
- vertigo
- sleepiness
- thrombophlebitis

3 Examine bottle for separation of emulsion into layers or fat globules or for accumulation of froth. Do not use if any of these appear.

4 Wash hands and then swab stopper on IV bottle with iodophor sponge and allow to dry.

5 Attach special IV tubing to bottle, twisting the spike to prevent particles from the stopper falling into the emulsion.

6 Fill drip chamber two-thirds full, slightly open clamp on the tubing, and prime the tubing.

7 Attach the tubing to the IV site and tape connectors to prevent dislodging of the tubing.

8 Infuse fat solutions initially at 1.0 ml/min for adults and 0.1 ml/min for children. Time period for initial infusions varies from 15 to 30 minutes for Intralipid to 30 minutes for Liposyn.

9 Monitor vital signs every ten minutes and observe for side effects during first 30 minutes of the infusion. If side effects occur, stop the infusion and notify the physician.

10 Monitor and maintain the infusion at the following rates:

   a *For adults*
      Intralipid 10 percent — Up to 500 ml every four hours on first day to maximum of 2.5 gms/kg body weight per day. Do not exceed 60 percent of client's total caloric intake per day.
      Liposyn 10 percent — No more than 500 ml/day in four to six hours.

   b *For children*
      Intralipid 10 percent — Up to 1 g/kg in four hours. Do not exceed 60 percent of total caloric intake.
      Liposyn 10 percent — No more than 100 cc/hr.

11 Monitor serum lipids two hours after discontinuing infusion.

12 Monitor liver function tests as impaired liver function can occur following fat infusions.

13 Discard partially used bottles to prevent contamination.

EVALUATION

EXPECTED OUTCOMES

1 Client receives increased calories and essential amino acids without difficulty. *If not*, follow these alternative nursing actions:
   ANA: Reassess client's ability to tolerate fat solution.
   ANA: Notify physician for order to discontinue fat solution and administer hyperalimentation solution.
   ANA: Observe liver function tests.

2 Other peripheral nutrients are provided at the same time without complications. *If not*, follow these alternative nursing actions:
   ANA: Check for compatibility of both solutions.
   ANA: Obtain IVAC controller and place IV tubing through controller mechanisms. Piggyback the additional IV nutrient tubing into the Y

site closest to the catheter hub, maintaining the fat infusion as the primary IV line.

UNEXPECTED OUTCOMES

1 Client develops dyspnea, cyanosis, or allergic reactions such as nausea, vomiting, increased temperature, or headache.
   ANA: Stop IV infusion immediately and notify physician.
2 Client develops hyperlipemia or hypercoagulability.
   ANA: Monitor lab results, particularly liver function tests, and notify physician when any abnormality occurs.
3 Client's serum triglyceride and liver function tests remain elevated.
   ANA: Notify physician for change in lipid order.
   ANA: Generally after 18 hours of infusion the liver function tests and triglyceride level should return to normal.

Charting
- Type of solution infused
- Initial rate and maintenance rate of infusion
- Site of infusion
- Adverse clinical manifestations and appropriate nursing intervention

ACTION: PROVIDING ENTERAL FEEDINGS VIA NEEDLE CATHETER JEJUNOSTOMY TUBE

ASSESSMENT

1 Assess need for obtaining nutritional support by means other than the usual oral route.
2 Assess whether nasogastric, gastrostomy, or jejunostomy tube is inserted via a needle catheter.
3 Observe for signs of abdominal cramping, diarrhea, or electrolyte imbalance following initial enteral therapy.
4 Ensure that correct type and strength of formula has been ordered and delivered to unit.
5 Observe that correct IV tubing is being used to administer feeding and that formula is not being administered into IV site. Vivonex is clear and can be mistaken for IV solution.

Rationale for Action
- To supply nutrients for clients recovering from upper gastrointestinal and abdominal surgery
- To promote wound healing

PLANNING

GOALS

- To provide nutrients for clients unable to ingest or assimilate nutrients by usual methods.
- To restore normal metabolic function and promote wound healing.

EQUIPMENT

- Formula: Ensure (½ strength), Isocal (½ strength), Vivonex (full strength)
- IV tubing (pediatric tubing preferred)
- Micropore or nonallergic tape
- #18 Luer-Lok adapter and plug

The needle catheter jejunostomy tube is a polyethylene catheter that is surgically threaded along the wall of the jejunum. The tube is inserted with a surgical procedure.

**INTERVENTION: Administering Enteral Feedings
Via a Needle Catheter Jejunostomy Tube**

1 Obtain ordered formula for infusion from pharmacy or dietary department.
2 Check the glass irrigating bottle for correct formula and strength. Wash hands.
3 Connect an adapter cap to the glass bottle.
4 Attach pediatric (or adult) IV tubing into the adapter cap on the bottle.
5 Attach a #18 Luer adapter to the jejunostomy tube to adapt it to the IV tubing.
6 Attach the IV tubing to the Luer adapter.
7 Hang the solution bottle on an IV standard as you would an IV bottle.
8 Begin the feeding with a weaker concentration of formula and increase the concentration slowly.
9 Calculate correct drop rate for formula infusion. Start the infusion slowly and gradually increase the flow rate.
10 Change formula bottle every eight hours and entire tubing every 24 hours to prevent bacterial growth.
11 Check that catheter is tightly secured with tape.
12 If feedings are intermittent, disconnect IV tubing, place an adapter into the Luer-Lok adapter, and tape tube securely.

INTERVENTION: Providing Enteral Feedings Through Gastrostomy Tube

1 Obtain formula from pharmacy or dietary department. Same formulas are used as for jejunostomy feeding.

This method of supplying nutrients is also used for babies when they are unable to ingest food orally.

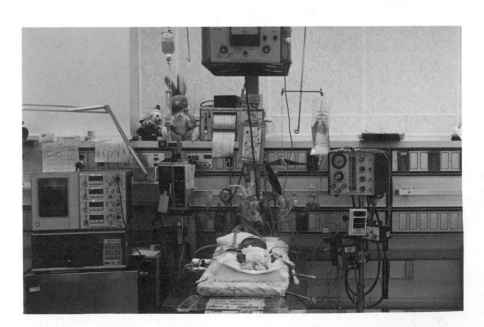

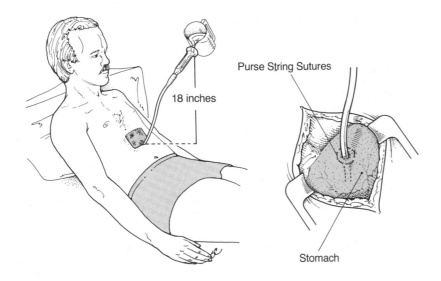

Purse String Sutures

18 inches

Stomach

Administer warmed formula through gastrostomy tube.

2 Assess patency of gastrostomy tube by aspirating gastric contents through a 20-cc syringe attached to the tube.

3 When Ensure and Isocal are used, irrigate gastrostomy tube with 30 cc of normal saline every four hours to prevent formula from coating the lumen of the tube.

4 Warm formula to room temperature.

5 Infuse formula through a 60-cc syringe or by connecting IV tubing to glass irrigating bottle.

6 When using a syringe, attach barrel of syringe to gastrostomy tube, pour formula from graduate into syringe, raise syringe no more than 18 inches above stomach, and allow formula to flow by gravity. Do not force formula through syringe.

7 If glass feeding bottle and IV tubing are used, prepare bottle and tubing according to directions for specific equipment used. Place an adapter on the gastrostomy tube, insert IV tubing into the adapter, and regulate flow rate as ordered.

Infuse formula by gravity flow over a 20-30 minute period. The feeding bottle tubing is inserted into gastrostomy tube with a special adaptor.

EVALUATION

EXPECTED OUTCOMES

1 Client receives increased nutritional support. *If not*, follow these alternative nursing actions:

ANA: Decrease rate and/or concentration of formula if diarrhea, electrolyte imbalances, or abdominal cramping occurs. This prevents utilization of calories.

ANA: Test for urine sugar every four hours, particularly when using Vivonex because of high-carbohydrate content.

2 Wound healing occurs. *If not*, follow these alternative nursing actions:

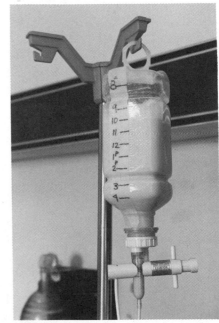

ANA: Reevaluate calories provided by formula to determine if they are sufficient.

ANA: Observe for possible infection or other causes for poor wound healing.

UNEXPECTED OUTCOMES

1 Difficulty distinguishing between Vivonex solution and the regular IV solution is encountered.

ANA: Vegetable dye can be inserted into the Vivonex solution to distinguish it from the regular IV solution. Other formulas are opaque so this is not a problem.

2 Jejunostomy tube becomes kinked and feeding does not infuse.

ANA: Cut the jejunostomy tube above the blockage.

ANA: Attach Luer-Lok adapter to end of tube.

ANA: Reconnect IV tubing and reinstate infusion at ordered rate.

Charting

- Type, strength, and amount of formula
- Tubing and bottle changes
- Time of infusion and amount of solution.
- Any difficulties with gastrostomy tube irrigations

NUTRITIONAL SUPPLEMENT

THE BASIC FOUR FOOD GROUPS

Milk Group

Foods Included
- Milk: whole, evaporated, skim, dry, buttermilk
- Cheese: cottage, cream, cheddar, natural or processed
- Ice cream

Contribution to Diet Milk is a leading source of calcium, which is needed for bones and teeth. It also provides high-quality protein, riboflavin, vitamin A (if milk is whole or fortified), and other nutrients.

Amounts Recommended Some milk every day for everyone. Recommended amounts are given below in terms of whole fluid milk.

	237-ml (8-ounce) cups
Children under 9	2 to 3
Children 9 to 12	3 or more
Teenagers	4 or more
Adults	2 or more
Pregnant women	3 or more
Nursing mothers	4 or more

Part or all of the milk may be fluid skim milk, buttermilk, evaporated milk, or dry milk.

Cheese and ice cream may replace part of the milk. To substitute, figure the amount on the basis of calcium content. Common portions of various kinds of cheese and ice cream and their milk equivalents in calcium are:

16 cc (1-inch cube) cheddar-type cheese = ½ cup milk
½ cup cottage cheese   = ⅓ cup milk
2 tablespoons cream cheese   = 1 tablespoon milk
½ cup ice cream or ice milk   = ⅓ cup milk

Meat Group

Foods Included

- Beef; veal; lamb; pork; variety meats, such as liver, heart, kidney
- Poultry and eggs
- Fish and shellfish
- Alternates: dry beans, dry peas, lentils, nuts, peanuts, peanut butter

Contribution to Diet Foods in this group are valued for their protein, which is needed for growth and repair of body tissues — muscle, organs, blood, skin, and hair. These foods also provide iron, thiamin, riboflavin, and niacin.

Amounts Recommended   Choose 2 or more servings every day.

Count as a serving: 57 to 85 g (not including bone weight) cooked lean meat, poultry, or fish. Count as alternates for ½ serving meat or fish: 1 egg, ½ cup cooked dry beans, dry peas, or lentils; or 2 tablespoons peanut butter.

Vegetable-Fruit Group

Foods Included   All vegetables and fruit. This guide emphasizes those that are valuable as sources of vitamin C and vitamin A.

Sources of Vitamin C

GOOD SOURCES: Grapefruit or grapefruit juice, orange or orange juice, cantaloupe, guava, mango, papaya, raw strawberries, broccoli, brussel sprouts, green pepper, sweet red pepper
FAIR SOURCES: Honeydew melon, lemon, tangerine or tangerine juice, watermelon, asparagus tips, raw cabbage, cauliflower, collards, garden cress, kale, kohlrabi, mustard greens, potatoes and sweet potatoes cooked in the jacket, rutabagas, spinach, tomatoes or tomato juice, turnip greens

Sources of Vitamin A

Dark-green and deep-yellow vegetables and a few fruits, namely, apricots, broccoli, cantaloupe, carrots, chard, collards, cress, kale, mango, persimmon, pumpkin, spinach, sweet potatoes, turnip greens and other dark-green leaves, winter squash

Contribution to Diet   Fruits and vegetables are valuable chiefly because of the vitamins and minerals they contain. In this plan, this group is counted on to supply nearly all the vitamin C needed and over half of the vitamin A.

543

Vitamin C is needed for healthy gums and body tissues. Vitamin A is needed for growth, normal vision, and healthy condition of skin and other body surfaces.

Amounts Recommended   Choose 4 or more servings every day, including:

- 1 serving of a good source of vitamin C or 2 servings of a fair source.
- 1 serving, at least every other day, of a good source of vitamin A. If the food chosen for vitamin C is also a good source of vitamin A, the additional serving of a vitamin A food may be omitted.
- The remaining 1 to 3 or more servings may be of any vegetable or fruit, including those that are valuable for vitamin C and vitamin A.

Count as 1 serving: ½ cup of vegetable or fruit; or 1 medium apple, banana, orange, or potato, half a medium grapefruit, a slice of cantaloupe, or the juice of 1 lemon.

Bread-Cereal Group

Foods Included   All breads and cereals that are whole grain, enriched, or restored; *check labels to be sure.*
Specifically, this group includes bread, cooked cereal, ready-to-eat cereal, cornmeal, crackers, flour, grits, macaroni and spaghetti, noodles, rice, rolled oats, and quick bread and other baked goods if made with whole-grain or enriched flour. Parboiled rice and wheat also may be included in this group.

Contribution to Diet   Foods in this group furnish worthwhile amounts of protein, iron, several of the B vitamins, and food energy.

Amounts Recommended   Choose 4 or more servings daily. Or, if no cereals are chosen, include an extra serving of bread or baked goods, which will make at least 5 servings from this group daily.
Count as 1 serving: 1 slice of bread; 28 g ready-to-eat cereal; ½ to ¾ cup cooked cereal, cornmeal, grits, macaroni, noodles, rice, or spaghetti.

Other Foods

To round out meals and meet energy needs, almost everyone will use some foods not specified in the four food groups. Such foods include unenriched, refined bread, cereal, flour; sugar; butter, margarine, other fats. Often these are ingredients in a recipe, or are added to other foods during preparation or at the table. Include some vegetable oil among the fats used.

CHAPTER 16
Alterations in Aeration

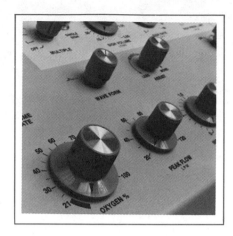

This chapter presents the conceptual basis for alterations in respiration. It includes planned nursing interventions and skills necessary to promote ventilation and respiration.

ANATOMY AND PHYSIOLOGY OF THE RESPIRATORY SYSTEM

The respiratory system provides for the exchange of gases between the blood and the external environment. The respiratory structures in this system include the lungs, trachea, bronchi, nose, pharynx, larynx, intercostal muscles, ribs, and diaphragm.

The nose, pharynx, and larynx are the structures of the upper respiratory tract. These structures filter particles of dust and bacteria. They also humidify and moisten the air as it passes through the respiratory tree. When the upper respiratory tract is bypassed due to intubation and tracheostomy, an artificial humidification process must be carried out.

The trachea is composed of smooth muscle reinforced with C-shaped rings of cartilage lined with a membranous sheath branching into the right and left main stem bronchi. The right main bronchus extends vertically from the trachea. The left main bronchus extends from the trachea at an angle. Because of this division and the ease with which an endotracheal or tracheostomy tube could slip into the right bronchus, a chest x-ray should be taken to ensure proper placement of the tube.

LEARNING OBJECTIVES

Describe the steps for instructing a client in deep breathing and coughing exercises.

Differentiate between the positions used of percussion, vibration, and drainage of upper lobes, lower and middle lobes.

Compare and contrast the differences in suctioning techniques used for naso-oral and tracheostomy-endotracheal suctioning.

Compare and contrast the FIO_2 delivered, and specific nursing interventions required by at least four of the common types of oxygen administration sets.

Describe the nursing actions included in performing tracheostomy care.

List the safety measures which are carried out to promote safe, effective care for clients with chest tubes in place.

Discuss the nursing actions required for managing clients requiring mechanical ventilation.

Compare and contrast the purpose of administering PEEP, CPAP, and IPPB.

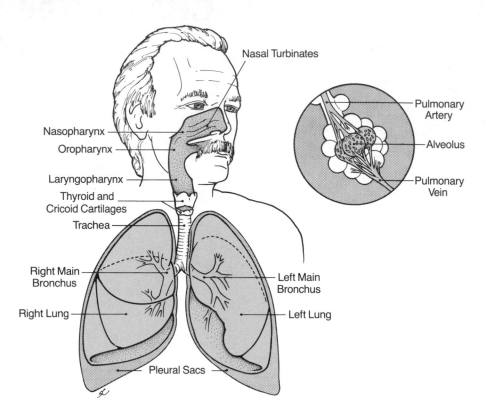

The anatomy of the respiratory system.

The bronchi divide into terminal bronchioles and finally into alveolar ducts, sacs, and alveoli. Each alveolus is surrounded by capillaries which allow the exchange of oxygen and carbon dioxide. Because the alveoli are so important for the exchange of gases, they must be adequately ventilated to prevent respiratory failure.

The Respiratory Cycle Respiration occurs when oxygen is transported from the atmosphere to the cells and carbon dioxide is carried from the cells to the atmosphere. Respiration is divided into four phases. The first phase is ventilation, which is the constant replenishment of air in the lungs. The alveolar pressures increase as the diaphragm descends, the external costal muscles contract, and the chest expands. This process allows air to flow into the lungs. The second phase is movement of oxygen from the alveolar air to the blood and movement of carbon dioxide in the opposite direction. Next, there is transportation of oxygen and carbon dioxide in the blood to and from the cells; oxygen moves out of the blood and into the cells, and carbon dioxide moves from the cells into the blood. The fourth phase of respiration is the regulation of ventilation.

Respiration, then, involves inspiration, or breathing in, and air flows into the lungs; expiration occurs when alveolar pressures decrease so that air can flow out of the lungs. This is normally a passive process, whereas inspiration is an active process. In order for adequate respiration to take place, oxygen must be carried to the cells, and carbon dioxide must be carried away from the cells. Without this exchange of gases, survival is not possible.

ALTERATIONS IN THE RESPIRATORY CYCLE

Alterations in normal respiration can result from biochemical reactions, malfunctions of the circulatory system, obstructions blocking the airways, and inadequate ventilation and gaseous exchange.

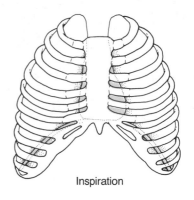

Inspiration

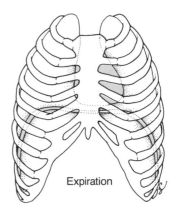

Expiration

Inspiration and expiration are considered the respiratory cycle.

Biochemical Alterations Biochemical alterations are any physiological disturbances in the acid-base balance of the body. Acid-base balance is the ratio of acids and bases in the body necessary in order to maintain a chemical balance conducive to life. Acid-base ratio is 20 base to 1 acid. Acid-base balance is measured by arterial blood samples and recorded as blood pH. Range is 7.35 to 7.45. Acids are hydrogen ion donors. They release hydrogen ions to neutralize or decrease the strength of the base. Bases are hydrogen ion acceptors. They accept hydrogen ions to convert strong acids to weak acids. The body controls the pH balance by use of buffers. Chemical buffers work fastest. Then lungs, cells, and kidneys act as buffers, giving slower but more reliable protection against acid-base imbalance.

When the pH balance is disturbed, the chemical buffers react in an attempt to keep the pH within normal limits. The three primary buffer systems—bicarbonate, plasma proteins, and hemoglobin—all respond to the imbalance. Next to react are the lungs. They take 10 to 30 minutes to inactivate hydrogen molecules by converting them to water molecules. The carbonic acid that was formed by neutralizing bicarbonate is taken to the lungs. There it is reduced to carbon dioxide and water and exhaled. Therefore, when there is excessive acid in the body, the respiratory rate increases in order to blow off the excessive carbon dioxide and water. When there is too much bicarbonate or base in the body, the respirations become deeper and slower. This process builds up the level of carbonic acid. The result is that the strength of the excessive bicarbonate is neutralized. The lungs can only inactivate the hydrogen ions carried by carbonic acid. The other ions must be excreted by the kidneys.

When carbon dioxide is retained through hypoventilation, the condition of respiratory acidosis occurs. This condition, caused by defective functioning of the lungs, refers to the increased carbonic acid concentration, which is accumulated carbon dioxide combined with water. Because the basic problem in respiratory acidosis is a change in the lungs, the kidneys must be the major compensatory mechanism. The kidneys work much slower than do the lungs, so it will take from hours to days for the compensation to take place.

Respiratory alkalosis occurs when an excessive amount of carbon dioxide is exhaled, usually caused by hyperventilation. One of the causes of this condition is hypoxia, which stimulates the person to breathe more vigorously. Hyperventilation results in decreased carbon dioxide. The loss of carbon dioxide results in a decrease in the H^1 concentration along with a decrease in pCO_2 and an increase in the ratio of bicarbonate to carbonic acid. The result is an increase in the pH level. Since the basic problem is related to the respiratory system, the kidneys will compensate by excreting more bicarbonate ions and retaining H^1. This process will return the acid-base balance to a normal ratio.

Circulatory Alterations An adequate cardiac output is essential for the exchange of oxygen and carbon dioxide. Sufficient amounts of blood must be delivered to the pulmonary system for gas exchange to occur. The amount of oxygen that is available to the tissues depends on the oxygen content of the blood as well as the cardiac output.

The pulmonary and cardiac systems work together to maintain normal tissue respiration. These two systems are influenced by the heart and buffer mechanisms which act to maintain normal circulation and blood pressure.

The buffer mechanisms in the body assist in maintaining the exchange of oxygen and carbon dioxide. The capillaries respond to decreased pO_2 or increased pCO_2 levels by vasodilation. When vasodilation occurs, the flow of blood is reduced and the amount of time for gaseous exchange is increased. As the flow of blood decreases, peripheral resistance is lowered and venous return reduced.

Whenever there is a decreased venous return, alterations in cardiac output take place which result in the accumulation of excessive amounts of fluid in the pulmonary system. This excess fluid reduces the space available for O_2-CO_2 exchange and can cause vasoconstriction. When this happens, the blood is shunted to capillaries in better ventilated areas of the lungs to allow for better tissue oxygenation.

Another result of decreased venous return is a drop in blood pressure. Aortic and carotid baroreceptors respond to increases or decreases in blood pressure. A decrease in the arterial blood pressure results in a reflex increase in respiratory rate. The baroreflex mechanism restores the blood pressure to normal. If these mechanisms cannot respond adequately, the blood flow to the tissues will be decreased and normal metabolic activities will be altered.

Alterations in intrapulmonic pressure occur when pressures in the lungs and thorax change and produce altered respiration. Intrapulmonic pressure must be less than atmospheric pressure in order for air to flow into the lungs. If air enters the intrapleural space, the negative pressure is lost, leading to a collapse of the lung and expansion of the thoracic cage.

A pneumothorax is an example of an alteration that can occur when pressure changes in the thorax. As air enters the pleural space, perhaps due to a traumatic injury, the higher atmospheric pressure exerted on the lung forces out air and causes the lung to collapse.

Airway Obstruction Alterations Obstructions which block the airways can cause pathological conditions such as bronchiectasis, atelectasis, or pneumothorax. Whenever an obstruction occurs in the respiratory tract, regardless of cause, a change in the respiratory status of the client occurs.

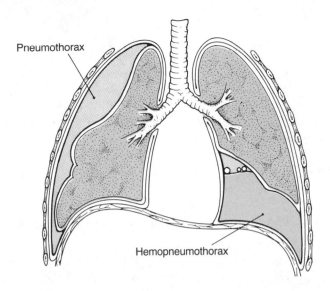

Pneumothorax

Hemopneumothorax

Decreased lung volume occurs when pressure changes in the thorax. When air, blood or fluid enter the pleural space it causes a pneumothorax or hemothorax.

Maintaining a patent airway is essential for respirations to be sustained. Obstruction of the airway can be caused by a mucous plug, particles of food lodged in a small opening, epiglottitis, croup, and laryngeal paralysis.

Pathological changes can affect the mechanics of respiration by interfering with the movement of air into and out of the airways. Tumors can put pressure on the airway and decrease airway space. Edema, accumulated secretions, and spasms of smooth muscle can compromise the bronchioles and increase airway resistance, causing expiratory difficulties. Anatomical alterations such as scoliosis and kyphosis can also restrict the total vital capacity of the lungs.

Ventilation and Gaseous Exchange Alterations   Adequate gas exchange within the lung fields depends on the effective ventilation of air and perfusion of blood in both lungs. The thickness and permeability of the alveolar membrane, the amount of surface area available for diffusion, and the pressure gradient are also factors which affect gas exchange.

Ventilation replenishes the supply of oxygen in the alveoli and removes the carbon dioxide released by the capillaries. If ventilation is not uniform throughout all the lung fields (due to a change in perfusion of one area of the lung), then the rate of oxygen replenishment is reduced, which can lead to hypoxemia.

Ventilation-perfusion problems are usually the result of chronic conditions such as heart failure, asthma, and chronic obstructive pulmonary disease (*COPD*), as well as acute conditions such as pneumonia.

In the normal lung the capacity for diffusion of both oxygen and carbon dioxide is so great and the alveolar capillary membrane so thin that gas exchange occurs long before the blood reaches the end of the pulmonary capillary.

Diseases that cause thickening of the alveolar membrane, such as COPD, will impair this gas exchange and cause hypoxemia and hypercapnia. When the alveolar surface area is decreased in chronic conditions such as COPD, serious problems in gas exchange can occur.

Pressure gradient: the difference in partial pressures of pO_2 and pCO_2 and the alveolar air. The pressure gradients promote the transfer, or inward diffusion, of oxygen from alveolar air to the blood and the outward diffusion of carbon dioxide from the blood to the alveolar air.

549

GUIDELINES FOR MANAGING CLIENTS

Nursing interventions are utilized routinely as preventative measures in most clinical settings. These interventions help prevent respiratory complications for clients on extended periods of bedrest, for clients who are prone to respiratory complications, or for surgical clients who have undergone general anesthesia.

The primary purpose for performing nursing interventions associated with the respiratory function is to improve vital capacity and pulmonary ventilation. As you perform interventions, refer to these guidelines.

Decreasing psychological stress assists in maintaining adequate ventilation.

- Increased anxiety and fear may lead to tachypnea and increased loss of carbon dioxide during respiration. Explain your interventions and the rationale for your actions to alleviate clients' fears.

Adequately ventilated lungs ensure oxygen and carbon dioxide exchange at the alveolar level.

- Position the client in a Fowler's, forward-leaning position to allow the lungs to expand fully and maintain maximum vital capacity with minimal effort.
- Administer oxygen from external sources through nasal cannula or intubation via endotracheal or tracheostomy tube.
- Remove secretions from the airway to enable oxygen to travel to the alveoli. Cleansing the airway may necessitate suctioning, IPPB, aerosol therapy, or chest physiotherapy.
- Administer drugs which stimulate the sympathetic nervous system.
- Provide a cool, moist environment via a croup tent.
- Maintain the diameter of the bronchi and prevent bronchial spasms in order to allow oxygen to reach the alveoli.
- Ensure humidification of the respiratory tree to enable easier removal of secretions and increased oxygen and carbon dioxide exchange.

Maintaining physiological integrity promotes adequate oxygenation of the tissues.

- Splinting caused by pain leads to hypoventilation and alterations in the chemical balance of respiration. Administer pain medications to prevent splinting, promote lung ventilation, and increase tissue oxygenation.
- Support through artificial ventilation methods those clients with dysfunction in the neurological system, such as brain stem injury or myasthenia gravis, or alterations in the chemical regulation of respiration, such as chronic respiratory acidosis. Artificial measures include the use of pressure control or volume control ventilation.
- Utilize chest tubes and waterseal drainage following pneumothorax to promote adequate tissue oxygenation.

Clients Who Have Respiratory Alterations Should Meet Certain Requirements Before Any Action or Intervention is Performed

- Functioning respiratory center in the brain
- Intact nerve cells to regulate respiratory muscles
- Patent airway for exchange of gases
- Alveoli that are able to expand and contract
- Adequate pulmonary capillary bed to allow exchange of gases
- Adequate supply of oxygen
- Functioning cardiovascular system

ACTION: TEACHING DEEP BREATHING AND COUGHING EXERCISES

ASSESSMENT

1 Determine client's physical ability to perform exercise (i.e., to assume Fowler's position, the degree of pain experienced, and the amount of medication needed to control pain).
2 Auscultate breath sounds.
3 Assess quality, rate, and depth of respiration.
4 Note presence of cough reflex. Should be diminished after anesthesia.
5 Note placement of incision in relation to diaphragmatic muscles necessary for breathing. The incision may interfere with lung expansion.

PLANNING

GOALS

- Improved vital capacity and pulmonary ventilation.
- Energy is conserved.
- Loosened secretions and full lung expansion.
- Abdominal breathing more automatic and respirations more efficient and relaxed.

EQUIPMENT

- Hospital bed in upright position or a straight chair
- Pillows for positioning and abdominal support
- Incentive spirometer

INTERVENTION: Instructing Clients in Deep Breathing

1 Explain the rationale for the procedure.
2 Prior to exercise, instruct the client to clear respiratory tract by coughing or suctioning.
3 Position so that client is sitting up in bed as straight as possible, with head and shoulders supported by a firm surface.
4 Demonstrate the deep breathing steps, allowing time for the client to practice each step.
5 Place your hands palm down around the sides of the client's lower ribs.
6 Tell the client to breathe in slowly through nose until chest is expanded and abdominal muscles rise visibly. Watch for contraction of intercostal muscles and diaphragm.

INTERVENTION: Instructing Clients in Coughing

1 Place the client in a sitting position to initiate coughing.
2 Instruct the client to inhale deeply and to cough, using abdominal and other respiratory muscles.

Rationale for Action

- To improve vital capacity and pulmonary ventilation
- To facilitate respiratory functioning through the removal of secretions
- To prevent the build-up of carbon dioxide
- To counteract the effects of hypoventilation and clinical irritation caused by anesthetic agents and anesthesia

Nursing Protocol

Pulmonary Care Sequence:
1 Deep breathing, coughing, and/or suctioning
2 Postural drainage with percussion and vibration (PVD)
3 Coughing and/or suctioning
4 Inhalation therapy and coughing

▶ How often this exercise should be performed will vary according to the client's condition.
1 After abdominal or chest surgery the client should practice this exercise every four hours daily, with five to ten breaths during each exercise.
2 Clients with pulmonary problems such as COPD, cystic fibrosis or high abdominal surgery should practice this exercise every hour, with a minimum of five deep breaths during each practice.

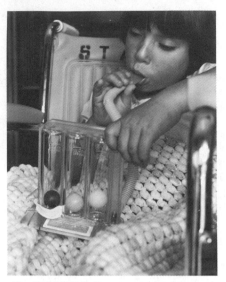

The TRIFLO II facilitates deep inspiration when the client inhales. Inhaling deeply lifts the triflo balls to the top of the chambers. The amount of inspired air ranges from 600 cc/sec (1 ball) to 1200 cc/sec (3 balls).

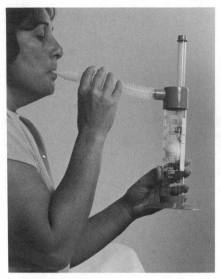

The Respirex spirometer reaches optimal levels of 2700 cc/sec when inspired breath is maintained for 1 second. It reaches up to 5400 cc/sec when maintained for 3 seconds. Ball is suspended at top of chamber during inspired breath.

3   Support any abdominal incision with the palms of your hands on either side of the client's incision. You may also place a rolled pillow firmly against the incision.
4   Encourage the client to cough frequently. Explain why coughing will be beneficial.

INTERVENTION: Teaching Controlled Diaphragmatic Breathing

1   Inform the client that the purpose of this exercise is to learn how to breathe by using abdominal muscles.
2   Place the client in a supine position. (After learning the exercise, the client may assume other positions.)
3   Tell the client to breathe in deeply through nose.
4   Tell the client to purse lips and to forcibly exhale air through the mouth to make a slow "whoosh" sound.
5   Instruct the client to contract (tighten) abdominal muscles while exhaling. The client's chest should move as little as possible.
6   Tell the client to relax and stretch after completing the exercise.
7   Continue accelerating this exercise, gradually increasing the client's diaphragmatic breathing for five to ten minutes, four times a day.

INTERVENTION: Using Flow Incentive Spirometers

1   Obtain specific spirometer ordered.
2   Explain purpose and procedure to client.
3   Have client hold incentive spirometer upright. When spirometer tilts less effort is needed to raise ball.

▶ Pursing the lips creates a resistance against air flowing out of the lungs by increasing pressure within the bronchus. Pursing the lips also prolongs the expiratory phase and slows the respiratory rate so that the lung can be emptied of air.

4 Instruct client to take in a deep breath with lips forming tight seal around mouthpiece of spirometer. Flow rates range from 100 to 2700 cc/second.

5 Encourage client to keep the ball elevated for three seconds to provide for alveolar inflation.

6 Repeat the procedure hourly to maintain alveolar inflation.

7 Cleanse the mouthpiece and filter, if spirometer has filter, with warm water and shake dry.

8 Store in client's bedside unit.

INTERVENTION: Using Volume Incentive Spirometer

1 Obtain specific volume incentive spirometer.

2 Explain purpose and procedure to client.

3 Set the predetermined volume. Volume ranges are 0 to 5000 cc depending on type of spirometer.

4 Check that spirometer is functioning before client begins procedure. Most spirometers function on batteries.

5 Place spirometer on bedside table.

6 Place client's mouthpiece on spirometer.

7 Instruct client to inhale through mouthpiece. As client inhales, air is drawn into system causing piston to rise to preset level. Lights may be illuminated identifying volume obtained or word HOLD may light up when volume is reached.

8 Instruct client to hold breath for 2½ to 3 seconds.

9 Following breathing exercises remove mouthpiece, cleanse with warm water, and store in bedside unit. (Volume incentive spirometers are used for many clients.)

EVALUATION

EXPECTED OUTCOMES

1 Vital capacity and pulmonary ventilation are improved. *If not*, follow these alternative nursing actions:
   ANA: Check chest excursion and reevaluate breathing pattern.
   ANA: Obtain order for incentive spirometer.

2 Client is able to reach predetermined volume level when using incentive spirometer. *If not*, follow these alternative nursing actions:
   ANA: Reassess client's knowledge of procedure and ability to correctly use spirometer.
   ANA: May need to reassess volume to be reached by client and reset volume on spirometer.
   ANA: Have client take few practice breaths before attempting to increase volume with spirometer.

3 Client's energy is conserved. *If not*, follow these alternative nursing actions:
   ANA: Begin procedure over and check client's chest exercises until repetition procedure becomes automatic and on-going.
   ANA: Allow adequate rest periods between exercises.

▶ **Two Types of Incentive Spirometers**

Flow incentive spirometers: require clients to inhale air through the vent at a predetermined rate in order to provide increased lung pressures and alveolar inflation.

TYPES: Incent-O-Net, Inspirator Incentive Spirometer, Triflo II, Uniflo, Air-Eze, L-V-E Lung Volume Exerciser, Respirex

Volume incentive spirometers: preset at a specific volume, the client inhales through the mouth piece and draws air from the spirometer causing a piston to rise to the specific volume.

TYPES: Bartlett-Edwards, Spirocare, U-Mid/Volume Plus

▶ Nebulizer components may be added to certain incentive spirometers to deliver medications to the airway while completing deep breathing exercises.

4 Secretions are loosened and lungs are fully expanded. *If not*, follow these alternative nursing actions:

ANA: Request physician's order for aerosol treatments prior to breathing exercises to relax and open air passages and to loosen mucus.

ANA: Prior to exercises, suction trachea to remove tenacious secretions.

ANA: Use postural drainage to help remove secretions.

5 Abdominal breathing is more automatic and respirations are more efficient and relaxed. *If not*, follow these alternative nursing actions:

ANA: Reinstruct client in abdominal breathing procedure so that it occurs more spontaneously.

ANA: Provide practice sessions several times a day until breathing pattern is established.

UNEXPECTED OUTCOMES

1 Client is unwilling to complete exercise because of fear of pain or dehiscence.

ANA: Elaborate on rationale and necessity for procedure.

ANA: Demonstrate cough exercise after teaching the client inhalation.

ANA: Support the incision area more fully, using the palms of your hands or a firmly rolled pillow to allay fears of dehiscence.

2 Nasal congestion inhibits client's breathing capability.

ANA: Ask client to blow nose prior to the breathing exercise.

ANA: Ask physician to prescribe medications that will open nasal passages.

ACTION: PERFORMING PERCUSSION, VIBRATION, AND DRAINAGE (PVD)

ASSESSMENT

1 Auscultate breath sounds to evaluate lung field. Assess for adventitous sounds, ventilation, and air exchange.

2 Determine rate and depth of respirations.

3 Note time elapsed since eating (at least one hour to prevent client discomfort or regurgitation).

4 Observe tenacity of secretions. Thick, tenacious secretions will require manual chest percussion and vibration as well as drainage.

5 Note any complicating conditions: hypertension, CHF, cerebral edema, abdominal distention, arrhythmias. Check with physician before performing chest physiotherapy.

PLANNING

GOALS

- Lungs cleared of retained secretions.
- Breath sounds clearer to auscultation; decreased *rales* and/or *rhonchi*.

Charting

- Number and times of breathing exercises
- Whether cough is productive or not
- Amount and quality of secretions expectorated
- Changes in pulse rate, depth of respirations, and color of client following exercise
- Client's acceptance of, participation in, and feelings about procedure

Rationale for Action

- To clear lungs of retained secretions
- To improve gas exchange in clients with chronic pulmonary disease
- To minimize ineffective coughing
- To prevent respiratory complications such as bronchopulmonary infections and atelectasis
- To prophylactically prevent complications during prolonged immobility

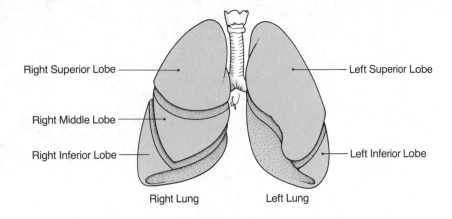

Right Superior Lobe

Right Middle Lobe

Right Inferior Lobe

Left Superior Lobe

Left Inferior Lobe

Right Lung   Left Lung

When performing PVD, place the client in positions which assist drainage of affected lobes of the lung.

- Shortness of breath reduced.
- Coughing more productive/effective.
- Respiratory rate decreased; ventilation and air exchange increased.
- Potential complications minimized.

EQUIPMENT

- Pillows for positioning
- Hospital bed that can be placed in reverse Trendelenburg (optional)
- Container for sputum

PREPARATION

- Establish the location of each lung segment. If the entire lung field is to undergo chest physiotherapy, the most affected lobe or segment (usually the lower or middle lobes) should be drained first.
- Protect client from falling by keeping siderails up when possible.
- If possible, arrange for privacy during procedure (client may be embarrassed and/or uncomfortable).
- Remain with client during entire procedure.
- Administer treatment every two to four hours.

INTERVENTION: Performing Percussion

1 Cover area to be percussed with gown or towel to prevent skin traumas.
2 Cup your hands and clap rhythmically, alternating hands over area to be drained. Each percussion should sound hollow and not cause redness of skin.
3 Relax wrist and elbows when percussing.
4 Percuss for three to five minutes over each segment.

INTERVENTION: Performing Postural Drainage

1 Loosen any binders or tight clothing.
2 Lower head of bed so that client's head is positioned in a 30° downward angle if not contraindicated.
3 Place sputum container and tissues within client's reach.

Nurse-Client Teaching

1 Prepare client by discussing preoperative aeration exercises.
2 Explain importance of practicing PVD exercises after an operation to counteract effects of hypoventilation and to prevent complications.
3 Demonstrate steps, allowing time for client to practice.
4 Instruct client, especially those with COPD, to perform diaphragmatic breathing with daily activities (sitting, walking) and to practice graded exercises to improve general physical fitness.

555

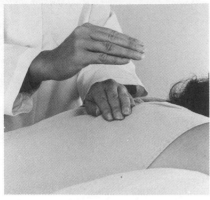

Cup your hands and use rhythmic motion when performing percussion.

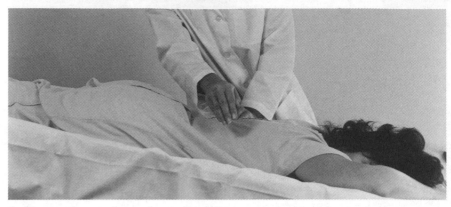

Position the client so that the "most affected" lobe is drained first, or place the client in Trendenburg's position to drain lower lobes first. Ensure that client is appropriately positioned to allow for drainage from all lobes.

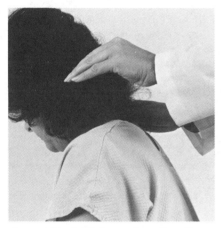

An upright, slightly forward position allows secretions to drain from the upper lobes.

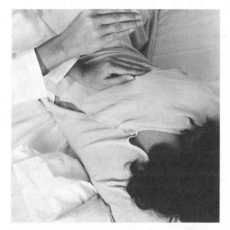

Position client on right side with head of bed raised slightly to facilitate drainage from posterior segment of left upper lobe. Position client on left side to drain right upper lobe.

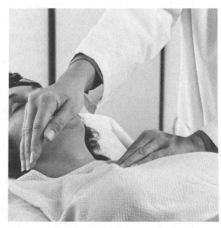

Raise head of bed slightly and percuss client's anterior upper lobes to facilitate drainage.

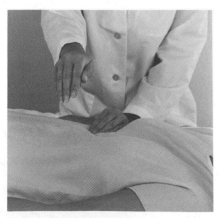

To drain the anterior base of the lobes, place client in supine position and percuss chest bilaterally, avoiding the center of the chest over the stomach.

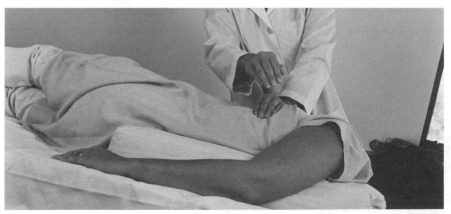

To drain the lateral segments of the lower lobes, place the client in a side-lying position with foot of bed elevated slightly.

4 Tell client to remain in position from 5–15 minutes to allow secretions to drain. (Amount of time will vary, depending on client's need and tolerance.)
5 Instruct client to make short, rapid-fire coughs to expectorate secretions.
6 Ask client to maintain deep abdominal breathing to help ventilate the lungs. (Client should deep breathe and cough between each position change.)
7 Assist client to slowly return to normal position.
8 Offer oral hygiene with mouthwash.
9 Discard container and/or send sputum specimens to lab, if ordered.
10 Remain with client and observe client's condition.

INTERVENTION: Performing Vibration

1 Instruct client to breathe deeply and exhale slowly.
2 Place your hands flat over area to be drained, keeping your arms and shoulders straight.
3 As client exhales, vibrate by quickly contracting and relaxing your arms and shoulders for ten seconds.
4 Vibrate for several minutes, depending on viscosity of secretions and client's tolerance.

EVALUATION

EXPECTED OUTCOMES

1 Lungs cleared of retained secretions. If the large bronchiole is blocked by a mucous plug, follow these alternative nursing actions:
   ANA: Attempt to dislodge plug by percussion and vibration.
   ANA: Attempt suctioning to dislodge plug.
   ANA: Notify physician if client becomes severely dyspneic and/or cyanotic. Bronchoscopy may be necessary to remove plug.
2 Breath sounds clearer to auscultation. Decreased rales and/or rhonchi. If not, follow these alternative nursing actions:
   ANA: Perform percussion and vibration again, after allowing time for client to rest.
   ANA: Suction oral-naso pharynx.
3 Shortness of breath reduced. If client is unable to breathe deeply and cough by himself, follow these alternative nursing actions:
   ANA: Medicate for pain if it is preventing the client from deep breathing and coughing.
   ANA: Obtain suction equipment immediately, especially if coughing ability is limited.
   ANA: Give assistance with incentive spirometer to induce coughing.
   ANA: Prepare for endotracheal or nasal intubation, if severe.
   ANA: Prepare for placement of intratracheal deseret where saline is injected.
4 Coughing more productive/effective. If not or if client has severe episodes of coughing, follow these alternative nursing actions:
   ANA: Client may need an expectorant or cough suppressant to decrease coughing spasm.

557

ANA: Raise client's head until coughing subsides.

ANA: If coughing continues, assess for blocked bronchiole.

5 Potential complications minimized. (Refer to Unexpected Outcomes below.)

UNEXPECTED OUTCOMES

1 Client experiences vertigo or syncope during postural drainage.

ANA: Modify position so that client's head is not as low, especially if client is elderly or very weak.

ANA: Employ mechanical means, such as suctioning, to remove secretions.

2 Client is unable to assume extreme head-down position for postural drainage.

ANA: Use all positions but modify degree of Trendelenburg's position so that the client's head is slightly lower than chest.

ANA: Turn client on side with pillow support to facilitate bronchiole drainage.

3 Client coughs and vomits with every PVD treatment.

ANA: Give treatments immediately before the meal.

ANA: Obtain physician's order for antiemetic before every treatment.

ACTION: PROVIDING ORAL, TRACHEAL, AND ENDOTRACHEAL SUCTIONING

ASSESSMENT

1 Determine need for suctioning.
   a Decreased or absent cough reflex.
   b Semi or comatose client.
   c Thick, tenacious mucus.
   d Debilitated, weak client.
   e Impaired pulmonary function.
2 Observe vital signs for increases in pulse and respiration and for changes in skin color.
3 Auscultate for adventitious sounds to evaluate lung field.
4 Assess respiratory status for tachypnea, shortness of breath, noisy respirations, and restlessness.
5 Determine level of consciousness to assess hypoxia. (To determine level of consciousness, see Neurological Assessment.)

PLANNING

GOALS

- Secretions removed.
- Increased respiratory ventilation.
- Clear breath sounds; no adventitious sounds auscultated.
- Decreased respiratory rate.
- Increased tissue oxygenation/pink color.

Charting

- Quantity and character of sputum
- Rate, depth of respiration, and pulse
- Any unusual symptoms following procedure, i.e., vertigo
- Client's physical tolerance, including strength and stamina to complete procedure
- Client's acceptance of and willingness to participate in procedure
- Lung sounds before and after PVD

Rationale for Action

- To provide patent airway
- To increase oxygenation and gaseous exchange
- To prevent respiratory complications due to accumulation of fluid in the lungs

Turn suction machine on and to appropriate setting before beginning procedure.

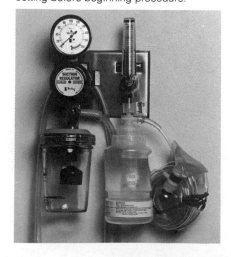

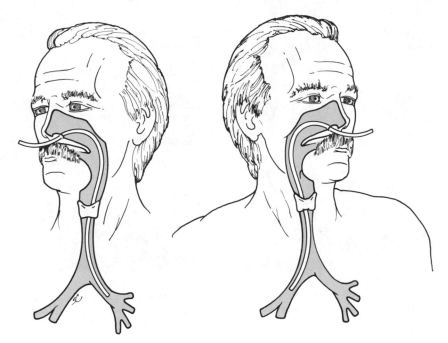

Suction the right and left main bronchus by turning the client's head in the opposite direction of the bronchus being suctioned.

EQUIPMENT

- Portable suction machine or wall suction with Y connector
- Disposable suction catheter (size 5 for infants, size 8–10 for children, and to size 18 for adults). Use size that is half the diameter of tube or nares to be suctioned
- Sterile gloves
- Container with sterile saline
- Bottle of sterile saline, labeled with date and time opened (opened bottles should be discarded after 24 hours)
- Receptacle for used equipment
- Bulb syringe for newborn

PREPARATION

- Wash your hands before starting procedure.
- Select a catheter that is one-half the diameter of the client's nares.
- Open catheter package, leaving protective covering over catheter.
- Attach catheter to tubing on suction machine.

INTERVENTION: Performing Naso-Oral Suctioning
Using Separate Catheter and Glove

1 Explain procedure and rationale to client regardless of level of consciousness. Allocate time for client to express fears and concerns or clarify steps of procedure. Administer pain medication to client if ordered.
2 Place client in semi-Fowler's position. (Or use dorsal recumbent position, with client's head turned toward you.)

559

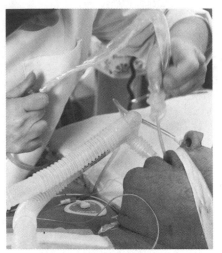

Suction nose and mouth before performing tracheal or endotracheal suction. This prevents pooled secretions from entering the lungs when the cuff balloon is deflated.

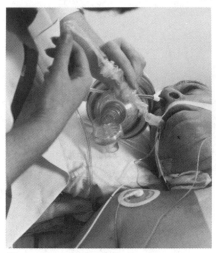

Change catheter between oral suction and endotracheal suction to maintain asepsis. Slide plastic protector back over catheter as it is inserted through endotracheal tube.

3 Put clean glove on the hand that will hold the sterile catheter unless otherwise dictated by hospital policy.

4 Turn on suction machine with ungloved hand. Set pressure of wall suction.

5 Lubricate catheter with sterile normal saline.

6 Instruct client to cough to mobilize secretions into pharynx, or if client is unable to cough, tickle back of throat with catheter.

7 Insert catheter 15 to 20 cm into nares. *Do not apply suction.* To introduce catheter into right and left main bronchi, turn client's head away from the bronchus to be suctioned. When using oropharyngeal route, insert catheter into mouth, using side or center approach.

8 Advance catheter as far as possible.

9 Begin suctioning by using a rotating motion as the catheter is withdrawn.

    a To provide suction, place your thumb over valve or Y connector on catheter.

    b To release pressure, remove your thumb from valve or Y connector.

10 If cough reflex is stimulated, withdraw catheter slightly to prevent excessive reflex stimulation.

11 Prevent removal of excessive oxygen by limiting suction to no more than 10 or 15 seconds at one time.

12 Rinse catheter in sterile saline, and repeat suctioning procedure in opposite nares.

13 Repeat procedure as necessary. If large amounts of secretions are present, allow at least three minutes between suctionings.

14 When procedure is completed, turn off suction machine.

Nursing Protocol

1 Introduce suction catheter without applying suction.

2 Apply suction while removing catheter.

3 Use rotating movement when withdrawing catheter.

4 Suction only 10–15 seconds.

15 Dispose of glove.
16 Dispose of catheter, or if catheter is to be used again, rinse it thoroughly in sterile saline and place it in receptacle as outlined in hospital policy. Replace catheter every eight hours or as directed by hospital policy.
17 Offer oral hygiene.
18 Place client in comfortable position.
19 Assess lung sounds.
20 Wash your hands.
21 Empty suction bottle at the end of every shift.

INTERVENTION: Performing Naso-Oral Suctioning Using Catheter and Sleeve

1 Review Preparing for Suctioning on page 559.
2 Explain procedure and rationale to client.
3 Place client in semi-Fowler's position. (Or place in dorsal recumbent position, with client's head turned towards you.)
4 Take container for normal saline out of package.
5 Pour 30 to 50 cc sterile saline in receptacle. Slide back protective covering over catheter.
6 Turn on suctioning machine with ungloved hand. Set pressure of wall unit according to chart.
7 Lubricate catheter tip with saline.
8 Continue to slide back protective covering over catheter as you insert catheter in nose or mouth.
9 Insert catheter 15 to 20 cm for naso-oral suctioning. *Do not apply suction.*
10 Advance catheter as far as possible.
11 Begin suctioning by using a rotating motion as the catheter is withdrawn.
    a To provide suction, place your thumb over valve or Y connector on catheter.
    b To release pressure, remove your thumb from valve or Y connector.
12 Withdraw catheter slightly if client begins to cough.
13 Limit suction to 10 or 15 seconds at one time to prevent removal of excessive oxygen.
14 Rinse catheter in sterile saline, and repeat suctioning procedure in opposite nares.
15 Repeat procedure as necessary. If large amounts of secretions are present, allow at least three minutes between suctionings.
16 When procedure is completed, turn off suction machine.
17 Dispose of glove.
18 Dispose of catheter after each use.
19 Offer oral hygiene.
20 Place client in comfortable position.
21 Assess lung sounds.
22 Wash your hands.
23 Empty suction bottle at the end of every shift.

Suction Catheters
Disposable plastic or rubber French catheters.
  Adults: 12 – 18 French
  Children: 8 – 10 French
  Infants: 5 – 8 French

Suction Machines
Wall Unit
  Adults: 120 – 150 mm Hg
  Children: 80 – 120 mm Hg
  Infants: 60 – 100 mm Hg
Portable Unit
  Adults: 5 – 10 cm Hg
  Children: 0 – 5 cm Hg
Portable units may be calibrated in inches or pounds of pressure

Clinical Alert
Do not suction clients who exhibit signs of laryngo or bronchospasm, as this could lead to occlusion of airway.

INTERVENTION: Performing Tracheostomy Suctioning

1　Complete nasopharyngeal or oropharyngeal suctioning.
2　Prepare sterile syringe with 2 to 10 cc sterile normal saline for tracheal lavage when applicable. (Amount is determined by hospital protocol.)
3　Change catheter and glove or obtain new catheter and sleeve package.
4　Suction client no more than 10 seconds at a time using sterile technique with tracheal cuff inflated.
5　Hyperinflate lungs on adult with ambu or Laerdahl bag at 100% oxygen.
6　Rinse catheter and deflate cuff. If using separate catheter and glove for suctioning, use ungloved hand to deflate cuff.
7　Instill prescribed amount of sterile normal saline slowly into tracheal tube. If feasible, ask client to take a deep breath while instilling saline. Allow solution to remain in bronchus for several seconds if possible; then complete suctioning procedure. (The cough reflex will be stimulated when the bronchus is reached with catheter.)
8　Inflate tracheal cuff again and hyperinflate lungs with ambu or Laerdahl bag and 100% oxygen.
9　Position client for comfort.
10　Assess breath sounds.
11　Wash your hands.
12　Empty suction bottle at the end of every shift.

INTERVENTION: Performing Sterile Suctioning for Client on Ventilator

1　Complete naso-oral suctioning before beginning endotracheal or tracheostomy suctioning, especially if tube has an inflated cuff.
2　If there is no cuff, then suction endotracheal or tracheostomy tube first. (This requires no change in catheter since first a sterile area then an unsterile area is being suctioned.)
3　Begin suctioning, deflating cuff after each attempt.
4　Take client off ventilator.
　a　Keep tube cuff inflated, and suction using sterile technique.
　b　Instill sterile NS, then oxygenate with ambu or Laerdahl bag at 100% oxygen for two to three breaths, gradually increasing the force of each breath.
5　Change catheter between suctioning.
6　Repeat procedure until both bronchi are suctioned. (The amount of time the cuff can be deflated will depend on the client's tolerance and whether a mechanical ventilator is being used.)
7　Inflate cuff again and place client on ventilator after suctioning.
8　Position client for comfort.
9　Wash your hands.

INTERVENTION: Using a Manual Resuscitator

1　Evaluate type of equipment needed, i.e., ambu or Laerdahl bag with mask or trach adapter.

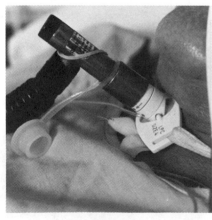

When taking the client off respirator for suctioning, place the plastic cup over the trach adapter.

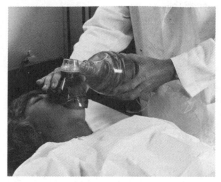

When using a manual resuscitator bag, form a tight seal by placing the apex of the mask over the nose and the base of mask between the lips and chin. (Laerdahl bag pictured here.)

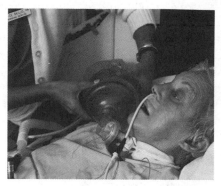

The manual resuscitator bag can be used with clients who have trach tubes in place by adding a trach adapter to the bag in place of the face mask.

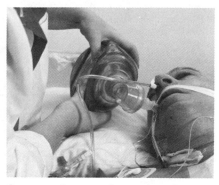

Compress the manual resuscitator bag every five seconds for an adult client.

2 Gather equipment.

3 Connect mask or trach adapter, oxygen tubing, and oxygen flow meter (reservoir) to bag.

4 Turn on oxygen flow meter to 15 l/minute.

5 When using a mask, hyperextend client's neck and place the apex of the mask over the nose. Place the base of the mask between the lower lip and chin. You may have to open client's mouth by pressing down on the chin.

6 When using a trach adapter, attach the universal adapter to the bag. Attach the adapter to the client's endotracheal or tracheostomy tube.

7 Compress the ambu or Laerdahl bag every five seconds for an apneic adult and every three seconds for an apneic infant.

8 If the client is able to breathe spontaneously, give the breaths in synchrony with his or her breaths. When using the bag to hyperinflate the lungs following suctioning, compress the bag three to five times each time you suction.

9 To keep the airway open when using a mask, seal the mask tightly by pressing down on the mask with the thumb and index finger of one hand and lifting up the client's mandible with your remaining fingers.

10 Observe the client's chest rise and fall with each compression to ensure adequate ventilation.

11 Observe for possible gastric distention with continued use of the bag.

INTERVENTION: Suctioning Infants with Bulb Syringe

1 Identify infant by checking arm band.

2 Place infant in supine position.

3 Squeeze air from bulb of syringe.

4 Insert tip of syringe into infant's mouth, then external nares. (It is important to suction mouth first, as delicate receptors in nose may be stimulated and cause infant to inhale mucus.)

563

5 Release bulb and remove from mouth or nares.
6 Squeeze bulb to expel secretions into basin or gauze.
7 Repeat steps 3 to 6 until mouth and nares are clear of secretions.
8 Rinse the syringe by immersing tip in water, expanding bulb, and squeezing bulb to expel water.
9 Reposition infant on side to promote drainage of secretions or on abdomen with head turned to one side.

EVALUATION

EXPECTED OUTCOMES

1 Secretions removed. *If not*, follow these alternative nursing actions:
ANA: Hydrate client to liquefy secretions.
ANA: Administer bronchodilators via IPPB or hand nebulizers to liquefy secretions.
ANA: Instill sterile NS and repeat suctioning procedure.
2 Increased respiratory ventilation with increased tissue oxygenation. *If not*, follow these alternative nursing actions:
ANA: If client needs frequent suctioning, ensure adequate hyper-oxygenation via ambu or Laerdahl bag between each suctioning procedure.
ANA: Assess for splinting when pain interferes with ventilation.
ANA: Obtain order for oxygen via nasal cannula.
3 Clear breath sounds; no adventitious sounds auscultated. *If not*, follow these alternative nursing actions:
ANA: Wait three to five minutes; repeat intervention if large amounts of secretion are still present.
ANA: Increase hydration if secretions are thick and tenacious.

UNEXPECTED OUTCOMES

1 Obstruction in nares.
ANA: Remove catheter from the nares, and insert into the other nares. (Deviated septum is more frequently found on left side of nose.)
ANA: Nasal or oral airway can be inserted and used to suction.
ANA: If both nares are obstructed, discontinue procedure and notify physician.
2 Irritation from frequent nasopharyngeal suctioning.
ANA: Obtain order and insert decongestive nose drops to decrease irritation.
ANA: Provide frequent care of nares.
3 Hypoxia may occur if incorrect techniques are used for suctioning.
ANA: Observe for signs of increased restlessness, shortness of breath, yawning and/or cyanosis while suctioning.
ANA: Limit suctioning time to no more than 15 seconds.
ANA: Ensure that catheter is half the diameter of the tube or nares.
ANA: Suction once, then reapply oxygen for a couple of minutes before continuing suctioning.

ANA: Hyperinflate lungs with oxygen, using ambu or Laerdahl bag and 100% oxygen.

ANA: Administer oxygen as ordered by physician.

4 Excessive secretions that require frequent suctioning are present.

ANA: After suctioning, attach new suction catheter to tubing on suction machine so that you have a catheter available in case of an emergency.

ANA: Oxygenate with ambu or Laerdahl bag connected to oxygen outflow meter at 100%. This procedure will allow you to suction more frequently.

ANA: Ascertain by assessment if other problems such as pulmonary edema or CHF are present.

5 Bleeding from nose or mouth.

ANA: Use smaller size catheter to prevent irritation.

ANA: Place client in semi-Fowler's position to prevent aspiration of blood.

ANA: Prevent irritation to mucous membrane by applying suction after inserting catheter and by keeping suction pressure low.

ANA: Administer oral hygiene and/or care of nares to prevent infection of mucous membranes.

ANA: Suction in different area of mouth or nose if area is excoriated.

6 Cuff leaks or breaks, which is suspected if client can talk or if liquids are suctioned from tracheostomy tube.

ANA: Notify physician of possible leak or TE fistula.

ANA: Follow orders for instillation of methylene blue.

ANA: Notify respiratory therapist to alter settings on respirator to compensate for leak.

7 Cardiac arrhythmias occur during suctioning due to decreased oxygenation.

ANA: Administer 100% oxygen.

ANA: Do not repeat suctioning for at least three to five minutes.

ANA: Monitor ECG strip for alterations in rhythm.

ANA: Monitor vital signs for changes.

ANA: Notify physician.

8 Wheezing sounds occur following suctioning due to laryngospasm.

ANA: Do not repeat suctioning.

ANA: Administer oxygen with mist.

ANA: Place client in semi-Fowler's position to assist in lung expansion.

9 After suctioning intubated client he or she still sounds congested.

ANA: Allow rest period before suctioning again.

ANA: Instill normal saline (2 to 5 cc) through endotracheal or tracheostomy tube.

ANA: Hyperinflate lungs with 100% oxygen using an ambu or Laerdahl bag.

ANA: Suction client following suctioning protocol.

10 Suctioning equipment is non-functioning.

ANA: Examine suction equipment to determine if it is securely attached to wall outlet or plugged into electrical outlet.

ANA: Check that suction equipment is turned on.

Charting

- Size of catheter (or put on Kardex) and technique
- Amount, color, and consistency of secretions
- Changes in breath sounds
- Respiratory rate
- Unanticipated complications and client's response to complications
- Client's tolerance and adaptive pattern to procedure
- Number of times client was suctioned
- Intake

ANA: If "hissing" sound is present, check that seal is around the top of the bottle.

ANA: Observe that connections between catheter and suction equipment are secure and tight without evidence of catheter or tube kinking.

ACTION: COLLECTING SPUTUM

ASSESSMENT

Rationale for Action
- To aid in diagnosis of disease process
- To identify predominant organisms, if respiratory disease is present.

1 Obtain diagnosis indicating advisability of having client cough. (With eye surgery and hernia repair, coughing should be inhibited.)
2 Assess client's ability to cough up specimen. Suction equipment may be necessary.
3 Determine the degree of pain the client can tolerate. You may need to assist client while obtaining a specimen.
4 Assess client's understanding of procedure so sputum and not saliva is obtained.

PLANNING

GOALS

▶ Sputum may be collected for culture by expectoration, nasotracheal or orotracheal suction, or transtracheal aspiration.

- Adequate sputum specimen obtained for laboratory examination.
- Client's respiratory status maintained during and after procedure.

EQUIPMENT

- Sterile container and cover for specimen
- Label for specimen
- Small plastic bag for delivery of specimen to laboratory
- Tissues
- Laboratory requisition slip

ADDITIONAL EQUIPMENT

For Mechanical Sputum Trap
- Suction machine
- Sterile catheter and glove
- Sterile saline
- Sterile sputum trap
- Culture tube

For Transtracheal Aspiration
- No. 14 needle with polyethylene tubing or small intracatheter (IV catheter)
- Sterile saline and 3–5 cc syringe
- Betadine or skin cleansing solution dictated by hospital policy
- Xylocaine injection

INTERVENTION: Obtaining Sputum Specimen (Non-Mechanical)

1 Explain procedure and rationale to client.
2 Have client rinse mouth before coughing to remove any oral contaminants.
3 Tell client to take several deep breaths and to cough up sputum (not saliva) directly into sterile container.
4 Obtain 1 – 2 tablespoons of sputum in container; close and seal lid.
5 If client is inhibited by pain, assist client by placing the palms of your hands or a rolled pillow around the incision area. Wrapping a sheet around chest or abdomen will also provide support for body walls during coughing.
6 Evaluate client's status after procedure.
7 Deliver sputum to the laboratory within 30 minutes after collection.
8 If client is receiving any respiratory treatment (IPPB or PVD), it is best to obtain specimen during treatment.

INTERVENTION: Collecting Sputum Using Lukin's Trap

1 Set up suction apparatus.
2 Attach sputum trap according to directions. (Procedure is the same as for naso-oral suctioning.)
3 Place your thumb on top of sputum trap to monitor; remove your thumb and provide intermittent suction, lifting thumb at intervals until specimen is collected.
4 Suction no more than 15 seconds at a time.
5 Turn off wall suction.
6 Send specimen that was collected in trap to laboratory. (In many hospitals suction tube is also sent to the lab with specimen.)
7 Place client in a comfortable position.

INTERVENTION: Collecting Sputum by Transtracheal Aspiration

1 Position by hyperextending client's neck and placing a pillow under shoulders.
2 Cleanse cricothyroid area of neck with Betadine solution.
3 Physician will anesthetize area with Xylocaine.
4 Physician will insert 14-gauge needle into cricothyroid area, thread polyethylene tubing through needle, withdraw needle, and leave tubing in place.
5 Attach syringe (3 – 5 cc) with 1 – 2 cc sterile saline into polyethylene tubing.
6 Inject saline into polyethylene tubing to initiate coughing response.
7 To obtain specimen, immediately pull back on barrel of syringe.
8 Withdraw catheter and apply pressure over puncture site.
9 Place sputum secretions in sterile container, label container, and send it to laboratory.

567

EVALUATION

EXPECTED OUTCOMES

1 Adequate sputum specimen obtained for laboratory examination. *If not*, follow these alternative nursing actions:

ANA: Leave instructions with client to notify you after obtaining a specimen.

ANA: Attempt procedure early in the morning when mucus has collected during the night and is more easily expectorated.

ANA: If appropriate, request an order for PVD to mobilize secretions. Then obtain specimen.

ANA: Use ultrasonic nebulization.

ANA: Institute mechanical tracheal aspiration technique.

ANA: Suction client's trachea to obtain specimen.

2 Client's respiratory status maintained during and after procedure. *If not*, follow these alternative nursing actions:

ANA: Give 100% oxygen via ambu bag before and at intervals during suctioning procedure.

ANA: Prepare for endotracheal intubation.

UNEXPECTED OUTCOMES

1 Pain inhibits client from coughing.

ANA: If diagnosis permits, support painful area with rolled pillows or tight sheet so that external pressure equals internal pressure, thus minimizing pain and discomfort.

ANA: Before beginning procedure, ask client to take several deep breaths. These breaths may trigger the cough reflex and aerate the lungs.

ANA: Give client pain medication 15 – 30 minutes before obtaining the specimen.

2 Client develops coughing spasms during procedure.

ANA: Press your third finger lightly over the client's trachea in the cricoid hollow. This pressure releases the nerve that innervates the coughing reflex.

ANA: Obtain an order for nebulization.

Charting

- Amount, color, and consistency of sputum
- Mechanical sputum trap used for collection
- Method of transtracheal or bulb-syringe suctioning
- Client's toleration of procedure

ACTION: ADMINISTERING OXYGEN THERAPY

ASSESSMENT

1 Check to see if client has a patent airway.
2 Assess client's vital signs.
3 Observe existence of PVC's if client is on monitor.
4 Observe client for any of the following signs. If these signs are evident, you may need to administer oxygen.
  a Tachycardia
  b Gasping and/or irregular respirations (dyspnea)
  c Restlessness
  d Flaring nostrils

Rationale for Action

- To provide FIO_2 (oxygen in higher concentration than exists in atmosphere) for hypoxic condition and to ensure adequate oxygenation.
- To return arterial pO_2 to normal range and to decrease work of ventilation.
- To avoid levels of FIO_2 which might produce toxicity or atelectasis.

    e Cyanosis
    f Substernal or intercostal retractions
    g Increased blood pressure followed by decreased blood pressure
    h Abnormal ABGs

PLANNING

GOALS

- Arterial pO_2 returns to normal range.
- Correction of hypoxic condition so that client is adequately oxygenated.
- Respiration returns to normal rate.
- Increased comfort and breathing efficiency for clients with chronic lung disease.

EQUIPMENT

- Source of oxygen supply: steel cylinder (oxygen tank) or wall oxygen with regulator and humidifier attached
- Regulator: flowmeter (regulates gas flow in liters/minutes) and cylinder contents' gauge
- Humidifier filled with sterile distilled water to indicated level

ADDITIONAL EQUIPMENT

For Nasal Catheter
- No. 8–10F for children, No. 10–12F for women, and No. 12–14F for men
  Water-soluble lubricating jelly for nasal catheter
  Adhesive tape
  Flashlight and tongue depressor
  Glass of water

For Nasal Cannula and Prongs
- This equipment is easily tolerated by most clients. It is also simpler than a mask, but provides less humidification. The FIO_2 will vary depending on the flow.
FIO_2: 24–28%	Flow:	1–2 liters
FIO_2: 30–35%	Flow:	3–4 liters
FIO_2: 38–44%	Flow:	5–6 liters

For Nasal Catheter
- This catheter is less comfortable than a cannula and is used infrequently.
FIO_2: 30%	Flow:	4–8 liters
- Size: No. 8–10F for children, No. 10–12F for women, and No. 12–14F for men.

For Face Mask Without Reservoir Bag
- This equipment requires fairly high flows to prevent rebreathing of carbon dioxide. Accurate FIO_2 is difficult to estimate.
FIO_2: 35–45%	Flow:	8–12 liters
FIO_2: 45–55%		
FIO_2: 55–65%		

▶ Arterial blood gases are the best method for determining the need for oxygen and for assessing the effectiveness of oxygen therapy and acid-base balance.

▶ Conditions Requiring Oxygen Therapy
1 Atmospheric hypoxia: oxygen therapy will correct depressed level of oxygen.
2 Hypoventilation hypoxia: 100% oxygen will yield five times more oxygen into the alveoli than normal air.

▶ Conditions Where Oxygen Therapy Is Not Corrective
1 Hypoxia caused by anemia, carbon monoxide poisoning, or abnormality of hemoglobin transport.
2 Inadequate tissue use of oxygen (cyanide poisoning).
3 Chronic obstructive lung disease requires that oxygen be used with caution since oxygen could suppress respiratory drive and result in respiratory arrest.

Symptoms of Hypoxia

Early symptoms
Restlessness
Headache
Visual disturbances
Slight confusion
Hyperventilation
Tachycardia
Hypertension
Dyspnea

Advanced symptoms
Hypotension
Bradycardia
Metabolic acidosis (production of lactic acid)
Cyanosis

Chronic hypoxia
Polycythemia
Clubbing of fingers and toes
Thrombosis

For Mask with Reservoir Bag
- The reservoir allows higher FIO_2 to be delivered. At flows of less than 6 L/min, the risk of rebreathing carbon dioxide increases.

  FIO_2: 50–60%   Flow: 6 liters
  FIO_2: 60–70%   Flow: 7 liters
  FIO_2: 70–100%   Flow: 8–10 liters
- Two types are available:

  Partial rebreathing mask: No inspiratory valve so that the beginning portion of exhaled air returns to the bag and mixes with the inspired air. Ports are present so that expired air escapes.

  Nonrebreather: Valve is present which closes during expiration so that any exhaled air is forced through the expiratory valve on the face piece.

For Venturi Mask
- This mask allows a fixed or predicted FIO_2 to be delivered. It is utilized effectively on clients with COPD when accurate FIO_2 is necessary for proper treatment. Carbon dioxide buildup is kept at a minimum.

  FIO_2: 24%   Flow: 2–4 liters
  FIO_2: 28%   Flow: 4–6 liters
  FIO_2: 35%   Flow: 6–8 liters

For Face Tent
- This tent is well tolerated by clients but is sometimes difficult to keep in place. It is convenient for providing humidification with compressed air in conjunction with nasal prongs.

  FIO_2: 35–50%   Flow: 8–10 liters

For Oxygen Tent
- An oxygen tent is useful for high concentration of oxygen (50–60%) and for circulation of moist air around the client. It will provide low-to-moderate concentration of oxygen in a temperature-controlled environment.

- An oxygen tent is also useful for clients who fear suffocation or experience claustrophobia. It allows clients to move freely but may produce feelings of isolation.

  FIO_2: 50–60%   Flow: 10+ liters

For Oxygen Hood
- This is a hood that fits over a child's head to provide warm humidified oxygen at high concentrations. It is useful because it includes an oxygen limiter to prevent oxygen concentration from exceeding 40%, thus reducing the hazard of retrolental fibroplasia.

  FIO_2: 28–40%   Flow: 5–8 liters
  FIO_2: 40–85%   Flow: 8–12 liters

  Less than 5 liters flow may lead to carbon dioxide narcosis.

For Croupette

- A croupette is used with premature infants to provide oxygen and to maintain temperature. It is also useful for a child who requires oxygen and/or high humidification. The unit prevents chilling in an atmosphere of aerated mist.

  FIO_2: 28–40%   Flow: 10 liters
  FIO_2: 40–50%   Flow: 10–15 liters

INTERVENTION: Monitoring Oxygen Administration

1 Check physician's order in chart for type of therapy, use of catheter or cannula, and desired liter flow.
2 Refer to following interventions for specific steps of oxygen administration according to method ordered.
3 Place client in semi- or high-Fowler's position to ensure adequate lung expansion.
4 Turn and reposition client frequently to prevent skin decubiti.
5 Encourage deep breathing and coughing exercises unless directed otherwise.
6 Ensure adequate hydration, especially if secretions are thick and tenacious.
7 Check equipment frequently to ensure functioning of oxygen flow, humidifier, and temperature.
8 Assess client's progress by frequently checking vital signs, color, and level of consciousness.
9 Remain with clients who are frightened or anxious until they feel secure.

INTERVENTION: Using an Oxygen Cylinder

1 Place oxygen cylinder in secure, upright position.
2 Check tag to determine amount of oxygen in the tank. Tag should say Full.
3 Slowly turn hand knob on cylinder clockwise to crack tank.
4 Attach regulator to valve outlet.
5 Attach top of humidifier to oxygen flowmeter.
6 Slowly open handwheel and adjust flowmeter to prescribed liters/minute.
7 Change sign on oxygen cylinder to read In Use.

INTERVENTION: Using an Oxygen Analyzer

1 Calibrate analyzer with room atmosphere prior to each reading.
2 Open tubing to the air, and compress two full times to fill analyzer.
3 Depress button. Analyzer should read 20% on room air. Adjust dial as necessary to obtain this reading.
4 Place tubing close to client's nose.
5 Compress bulb 3–6 times, depress button, and read findings.
6 Based on reading, adjust oxygen flow.
7 Check analyzer with 100% oxygen at least one time per day.

Clinical Alert

Oxygen is used very conservatively on anyone with chronic lung disease because high levels of oxygen will knock out carbon dioxide center and lead to respiratory arrest.

Clinical Alert:

Oxygen toxicity: This condition may result if high FIO_2 is delivered to the client over a long period of time (48 hours). The clinical picture of this condition resembles that of pulmonary edema where the pulmonary capillaries and lung tissue are destroyed.

▶ **Safety Precautions**
- Set up No Smoking and Oxygen in Use signs at the site of administration and at the door.
- Remove matches and lighters from bedside.
- Disconnect all electrical equipment.
- Remove all volatile materials except solutions and equipment to be used during intervention.
- Make sure that all electrical monitoring equipment is properly grounded.
- Locate fire extinguishers.

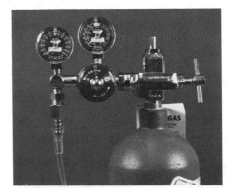

After the regulator and flow meter have been attached, crack the cylinder to clear dust out of the line. Turn knob on the right side counter clockwise until you hear a loud rush of air. Quickly turn knob off to close oxygen flow.

▶ An *oxygen analyzer* is used to measure the amount of oxygen delivered to the client.

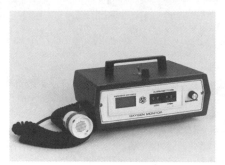

One type of oxygen analyzer.

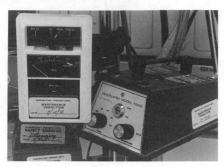

An oxygen analyzer used for in-line respirator oxygen checks.

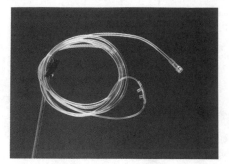

Nasal cannula or prongs deliver up to 44% oxygen with flow rate of 5-6 liters/min.

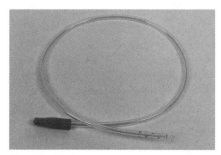

Nasal catheters are used less frequently than other oxygen delivery systems. This system can deliver no more than 45% oxygen.

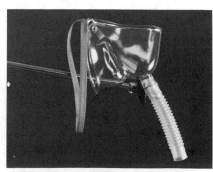

The oxygen face tent delivers an unpredictable oxygen flow rate, but does provide high humidity. The face tent is frequently used when a client cannot tolerate having the face mask over nose and mouth.

INTERVENTION: Using a Nasal Cannula

1 Explain the purpose and procedures of oxygen therapy to client.
2 Place tips of cannula no more than 1.25 cm into client's nares.
3 Fasten tubing to pillow and bed sheets if bedrest is maintained.
4 Adjust flow of oxygen. Should be limited to six liters/minute for nasal prongs. (There is variable oxygen concentration since atmospheric air mixes with prescribed oxygen concentration.)
5 Monitor vital signs and assess client's condition frequently.
6 Change equipment (tubing, catheter, cannula) daily.

INTERVENTION: Using a Nasal Catheter

1 Assemble necessary equipment for insertion of catheter.
2 Attach catheter to connecting tubing. Attach humidifier to flowmeter then to wall outlet or oxygen tank after cracking tank.
3 Turn on oxygen to three liters/minute, and test oxygen flow by inserting tip of catheter into a glass of water.
4 Lubricate tip of catheter with water-soluble lubricant.
5 Position client with neck hyperextended.
6 Start flow of oxygen at three liters/minute.
7 Slowly insert catheter no more than 12.7 cm into nares.
8 Examine placement (entrance to oropharynx) by depressing client's tongue with tongue blade and observing throat with the aid of a flashlight.
9 Adjust flow rate to the liters ordered. (Flow should be limited to five liters/minute.)
10 Secure catheter to bridge of client's nose with tape.
11 Attach connecting tube to bed with enough slack for free movement.
12 Observe for distention by palpating epigastrium.
13 Remain with client until client feels secure and is not coughing or gagging.
14 Insert a new catheter in the opposite nare every eight hours.

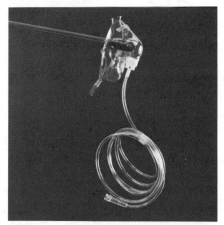
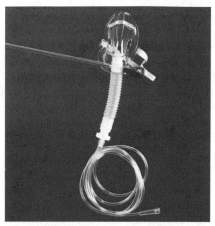
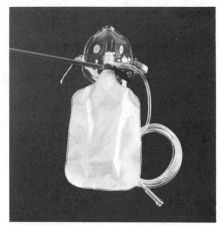

The face mask without reservoir bag delivers high oxygen concentration. Ensure that the mask fits snugly over mouth and nose to prevent oxygen loss.

The Venturi-type mask is used when an exact amount of oxygen must be delivered, as in the case of oxygen administered to clients with COPD.

Inflate bag with oxygen before placing the rebreather bag on client.

INTERVENTION: Using an Oxygen Face Mask

1   Check size of face mask to make sure it fits client.
2   Explain procedure and rationale for administration of oxygen to client.
3   Turn on oxygen flow to number of liters prescribed. If reservoir bag is attached, partially inflate it with oxygen.
4   Place client in semi- or high-Fowler's position.
5   Fit mask to client's face from nose downward during expiration. A tight fit prevents oxygen from escaping around eyes or nose. If reservoir bag is attached, oxygen flow must be at a level to prevent bag from collapsing.
6   Place elastic band around client's head.
7   Attach tubing to pillows and bedclothes, keeping tubing free of kinks.
8   Stay with client until client feels at ease with mask. Some clients may be afraid of suffocating.
9   Assess client's condition by checking vital signs and respiratory process.
10 Change mask and tubing daily, and apply skin care to face.
11 Observe for any change in client's condition.
12 Check equipment frequently. If humidifier is attached, check water level.
13 Obtain physician's order for a nasal cannula during meals.

▶ Three types of masks
● Oxygen mask
● Oxygen mask with partial rebreathing bag
● Venturi mask used to control low oxygen concentrations

INTERVENTION: Using a Pediatric Oxygen Mask

1   Choose a mask that will fit the child. The mask should cover child's mouth and nose, but not eyes.

2 Place mask so that it fits tightly.
3 Secure mask with elastic strap.
4 Adjust oxygen concentration as ordered. Venturi mask delivers 24–35% concentration.
5 Remove mask at frequent intervals for skin care if child's condition is stable and provided no ABGs are scheduled within one hour.
6 Observe child frequently for complications.

▶ Clients tend to feel isolated in oxygen tents. Talking to them frequently and assuring them that they are not alone is therapeutic.

INTERVENTION: Using an Oxygen Tent

1 Secure tent and place at head of bed with control knobs on opposite side.
2 Connect regulator into oxygen source.
3 Plug in machine.
4 Set up humidifier and check to make sure that water level (tray at back of machine) is adequate.
5 Adjust temperature control to 19–22° C (68–70° F).
6 Set circulation dial between high and low.
7 Turn on oxygen flow, and flush with high liter rate, or press flush button for one minute until desired concentration.
8 Position canopy one-half to one-third over length of bed.
9 Tuck all sides of canopy into mattress, and use draw sheet to secure seal over thighs.
10 Regulate flowmeter to 12–15 (minimum of 10) liters/minute so that carbon dioxide is removed.
11 Give client a special call button that can be attached to bed. (Electrical call bells can be an electrical hazard.)
12 Test oxygen concentration with oxygen analyzer every four hours.

Turn on oxygen supply or compressed air and mist before placing child in oxygen tent.

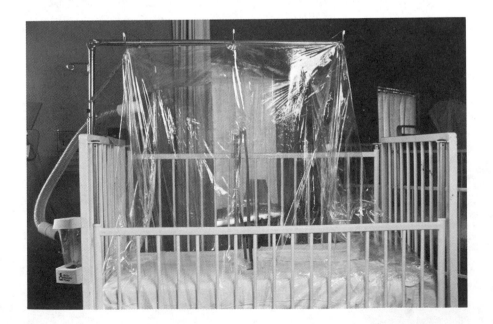

13 During procedure, open tent as infrequently as possible.
14 Flood tent with oxygen after tent has been opened.
15 If client complains of coldness, furnish additional clothing, wrap client's head and shoulders, or adjust the temperature of the tent.
16 Check equipment every four hours for liter flow, temperature, amount of water in humidifier, and oxygen in tank. Oxygen vent should remain unobstructed.
17 Observe client's progress by making a general check of his status every hour and by assessing his vital signs every four hours.

INTERVENTION: Using a Pediatric Oxygen Tent

1 Follow steps 1–4 for using an oxygen tent.
2 Select a tent that will deliver the desired concentration of oxygen to the child.
3 Pad the frame that supports the canopy.
4 Turn on the oxygen to desired concentration (30–50%), and maintain temperature at 17.8–21.1° C (64–70° F).
5 Secure the canopy by tucking in all sides and maintaining closure whenever possible.
6 Analyze and record tent atmosphere, and check child's vital signs every two hours.
7 Leave crib sides up for safety.
8 Select toys that are washable, do not produce static electricity, and are appropriate to the child's age.
9 Place on cardiac or apnea monitor.
10 Keep child warm and check dampness of clothes. Change as necessary.

INTERVENTION: Using a Croupette

1 Follow general steps above for administration of oxygen in a tent. A croupette can be connected to wall oxygen.
2 Secure oxygen tent and regulate according to prescribed orders, with or without oxygen. The croupette may be operated with compressed air when only high humidity is required.
3 Fill a receptacle in back of the croupette with ice if cool mist is ordered.
4 Check child frequently for signs of chilling or need for suctioning.
5 Complete postural drainage if secretions need to be drained.
6 Supply additional clothing or change clothing during the procedure if child is receiving high humidity.
7 Remove child from mist as frequently as possible to prevent maceration of skin.

INTERVENTION: Using an Oxygen Hood with Pediatric Clients

1 Place hood around child's head and attach tubing to oxygen supply. (Hood may be used alone or with isolette.)
2 Infants may be cared for through portholes or lid to avoid affecting oxygen level.

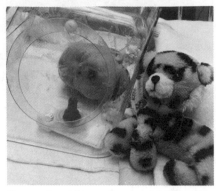

Oxygen hood lid can be opened to provide nursing care to infant without disturbing oxygen concentration.

3 Maintain oxygen levels at 40–50% and check amount of moisture that can accumulate inside hood.

4 Measure oxygen concentration as you would in isolette.

5 Observe usual oxygen administration precautions.

EVALUATION

EXPECTED OUTCOMES

1 Arterial pO_2 returns to normal range, and correction of hypoxic condition results. *If not*, follow these alternative nursing actions:
ANA: Immediately report vital signs and symptoms to physician.
ANA: Immediately assess blood gases to check efficiency of oxygen therapy and to determine if respiratory drive is suppressed from retained carbon dioxide.
ANA: Check oxygen equipment (regulator, liters/minute, oxygen tank, tubing, and connectors). Use oxygen analyzer to measure concentration of oxygen delivered to client.
ANA: Support client with mechanical ventilator if $PaCO_2$ is elevated and/or if client indicates rapid deterioration.

2 Increased comfort and breathing efficiency for clients with chronic lung disease. *If not*, follow these alternative nursing actions:
ANA: Observe for signs of carbon dioxide narcosis. Oxygen is used very conservatively on anyone with chronic lung disease.

UNEXPECTED OUTCOMES

1 Breathing passage is blocked.
ANA: If conscious, the client can usually tell you what he or she is experiencing and cough up mucus. Encourage coughing; suction if necessary.
ANA: If client is unconscious, be alert for wet gurgling respirations, which indicate need for suctioning. Suction frequently.
ANA: Utilize Sim's position so that secretions can run out of client's mouth.

2 Abnormal signs and symptoms: changes in blood pressure, tachycardia, increased respirations, cloudy consciousness, and abnormal color.
ANA: Determine if acute acidosis and/or carbon dioxide narcosis is present. These conditions can occur if hypoxic drive is removed by the administration of high oxygen concentration.
a Check blood gases.
b Check oxygen equipment and use oxygen analyzer to measure oxygen concentration.
c Reduce oxygen concentration.
ANA: Carbon dioxide retainers may require controlled low oxygen concentration method. Change oxygen therapy from cannula/catheter to Venturi mask.

3 Oxygen toxicity: pulmonary oxygen toxicity.
ANA: Reduce oxygen concentration to less than 50%.

4 Atelectasis.

ANA: Lower the oxygen concentration as ordered.

ANA: Encourage deep breathing, coughing, frequent position changes, and ambulation if possible. Avoid constrictive dressings and use sedatives carefully.

ANA: IPPB, postural drainage, and suctioning may be ordered.

ANA: Check breath sounds. (They are decreased with this condition.)

5 Tachypnea.

ANA: Check oxygen concentration immediately since inadequate flow rates may be causing the problem.

ANA: Increase flow rate, and monitor with oxygen analyzer.

ANA: Monitor vital signs and client's discomforts as pulmonary embolus may be cause.

ANA: Check client's breathing pattern and/or suction apparatus as mucous plug may be cause.

6 Retrolental fibroplasia.

ANA: Make sure that the premature infant receives no more than 40% oxygen unless infant suffers from sustained tachypnea or respiratory distress syndrome.

ANA: If higher concentrations of oxygen are used, maintain and monitor the oxygen so that the range is 50 to 70 mm Hg in radial artery.

7 Infection.

ANA: Change humidifier every 24 hours.

ANA: Keep water at appropriate level in humidifier.

ACTION: INTUBATING CLIENT WITH ORAL AIRWAY

ASSESSMENT

1 Assess client's level of consciousness.
2 Observe client's respiratory status. Note shortness of breath, severe dyspnea, tachypnea, or tachycardia.
3 Note quality and quantity of secretions.
4 Check to see if all lung lobes are ventilated adequately.
5 Note presence of rhonchi, rales, or wheezes.
6 Determine if gag and swallowing reflex are absent.
7 Assess client's use of accessory muscles for breathing.
8 Observe client's ability to control tongue.
9 Listen to cough for signs of weakness.
10 Listen to chest for signs of right ventricular failure.

PLANNING

GOALS

- Patent airway maintained in emergency situation.
- Route established for mechanical ventilation in either short-term or long-term therapy.

Rationale for Action

Oropharyngeal or Nasopharyngeal Intubation

- To provide patent airway in an emergency situation.
- To provide patent airway when physician is not available.

Endotracheal Intubation

- To provide patent airway for surgical interventions.
- To provide route for short-term mechanical ventilation.
- To facilitate removal of pulmonary secretions.
- To provide cardiopulmonary rest after cardiovascular surgery.
- To relieve carbon dioxide retention in clients with chronic pulmonary disease.
- To treat acute respiratory failure.
- To prevent aspiration.

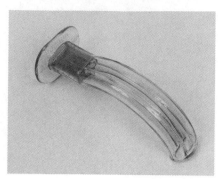

Insert oral airway by turning it sideways. Slide it along the buccal mucosa until flange end touches lips, then turn airway in place.

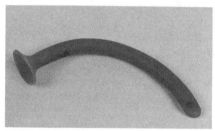

Insert the bevel of the nasopharyngeal airway facing the nasal septum.

- Secretions easily suctioned so that pulmonary complications can be treated or prevented.
- Lungs aerated more easily.

EQUIPMENT

- Oropharyngeal or nasopharyngeal tube
- Tongue depressor
- Water-soluble lubricant for nasopharyngeal airway

ADDITIONAL EQUIPMENT

For Endotracheal Intubation
- Oral or nasal endotracheal tube (size of tube determined by client's needs, physician's orders, and type of intervention) may be rubber or plastic with cuff or no cuff
- Topical and local anesthetic agents: usually 4% xylocaine spray for tongue, gums, and pharynx; 10% cocaine hydrochloride for nares
- Laryngoscope with several blade sizes
- Water-soluble lubricant
- McGill forceps
- 2.5-cm micropore tape
- Disposable plastic syringes (5–10 cc) for cuff inflation
- Manual resuscitation bag: ambu or Hope
- Mechanical ventilator if needed
- Suction equipment with Yankauer suction tip or suction catheter

INTERVENTION: Using an Oropharyngeal Airway

1 Select appropriate size airway.
2 Wash your hands.
3 Open client's mouth with tongue depressor. You may need to hyperextend client's neck to insert tube.
4 Turn airway sideways and slide it along buccal mucosa until the flange on the end touches the lips.
5 Turn airway so that the curve fits over the tongue. It will extend from the lips to the pharynx, displacing the tongue anteriorly.
6 Tape airway in position, if necessary.
7 On an uncooperative client, turn airway upside down, and once the flange on the end touches the lips, turn the airway as described.

INTERVENTION: Using a Nasopharyngeal Airway

1 Select appropriate size tube.
2 Wash your hands.
3 Lubricate entire length of tube.
4 Insert tube gently through one nares. If obstructed, try other nares.
5 Tape tube in position if necessary.

INTERVENTION: Assisting with Endotracheal Intubation

1 Explain procedure and rationale to client or to family.
2 Assemble all equipment.
3 Wash your hands.
4 Check laryngoscope light. (Extra batteries and bulbs should be available.)
5 Inspect tracheal cuff for intactness by inflating cuff.
6 Lubricate tube.
7 Make sure that all necessary mechanical devices are plugged in and operational.
8 Place client in supine position with head and neck hyperextended and a pillow under shoulders.

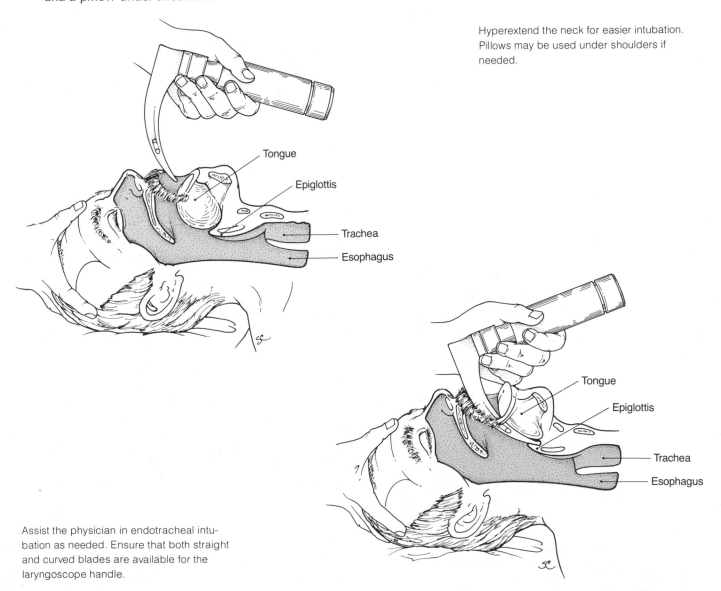

Hyperextend the neck for easier intubation. Pillows may be used under shoulders if needed.

Assist the physician in endotracheal intubation as needed. Ensure that both straight and curved blades are available for the laryngoscope handle.

9 Restrain client's hands if necessary.
10 Suction and oxygenate client before beginning procedure.
11 Explain procedures as you proceed to reduce client's anxiety.
12 Mark tube at level of client's mouth, and tape securely with micropore tape so that tube will not slip. Insert oral airway or bite block if tube is positioned orally. (Benzoin may be applied before taping to secure tape.)
13 After intubation is completed, inflate cuff and place client on ventilator or administer humidity and/or oxygen with T-piece.
14 Assess lung fields for ventilation and aeration.
15 Prepare client for chest x-ray to assess tube placement.
16 Place client in semi-Fowler's or Fowler's position to increase ventilation.
17 Place call bell within client's reach.
18 Discard disposable equipment.
19 Clean and return nondisposable equipment to designated place.

EVALUATION

EXPECTED OUTCOMES

1 Patent airway maintained in emergency situation. *If not*, follow these alternative nursing actions:

For airway obstructed by mucous plug:
ANA: Suction aggressively and instill 5–10 cc normal saline into tube to help liquefy plug.
ANA: If plug causes severe respiratory distress, call physician to remove tube and to insert new tube.
ANA: If client is arrested and physician not at bedside, remove tube and begin CPR.
ANA: Hydrate client to keep secretions thin so that suctioning will be more efficient.
ANA: Apply chest physiotherapy to mobilize secretions.
ANA: Apply artificial humidification to tracheal bronchial tree to prevent thick secretions.

For airway obstructed by kinking of endotracheal tube:
ANA: Avoid flexing client's head.
ANA: Support ventilator tubing to prevent kinking.
ANA: To prevent clamping down on tube, place bite blocks or oral airway in client's mouth.
2 Route established for mechanical ventilation in either short-term or long-term therapy. *If not*, follow these alternative nursing actions:
ANA: Refer to steps 1 to 3 in section following Unexpected Outcomes.
3 Secretions easily suctioned so that pulmonary complications can be treated or prevented. *If not*, follow these alternative nursing actions:
ANA: Instill 5–10 cc NS into tube to liquefy secretions.
ANA: Hydrate client to keep secretions thin.
ANA: Apply chest physiotherapy to mobilize secretions.

4 Work of breathing reduced. *If not*, follow these alternative nursing actions:

ANA: Check for obstruction in respiratory system (i.e., mucous plug).

ANA: Assess for bilateral breath sounds and symmetry of chest movement.

ANA: If in doubt, request order for x-ray to ascertain exact placement of tube.

UNEXPECTED OUTCOMES

1 Pharyngeal airway cannot be inserted.

ANA: Change size of tube.

ANA: Relubricate nasopharyngeal airway and attempt to reinsert.

ANA: Hyperextend client's neck.

ANA: Insert tube at different angle.

2 Laryngospasm on intubation of endotracheal tube.

ANA: Provide humidity to prevent edema.

ANA: If not severe, remove tube and wait a few minutes.

ANA: If severe, give client a muscle relaxant such as succinylcholine chloride. You also may need to perform an emergency cricothyrotomy. Physician's orders are required for this ANA.

ANA: If severe and causing respiratory distress, you may need to perform a tracheostomy.

3 Inaccurate placement of endotracheal tube into right main bronchus.

ANA: Obtain order for chest x-ray to ascertain exact placement of tube.

ANA: Pull back slightly on tube, and assess for ventilation of left lung field.

4 Inaccurate tube placement into pharynx which bypasses larynx so that air is instilled into GI tract. Stomach becomes distended.

ANA: Assess lung fields. Remove tube if aeration poor and abdomen is getting more distended.

ANA: Insert NG tube or Salem-sump after tube placement.

5 Laryngeal damage due to prolonged endotracheal intubation.

ANA: Decompress cuff five minutes every hour unless contraindicated. (There is controversy that this procedure is effective.)

ANA: Listen to trachea. Inflate cuff until there is a slight hissing sound at the peak of inspiration. You may also inflate cuff and remove ½–1 cc of air when you do not hear any leak. Cuff pressure should not exceed 20 mm Hg.

ANA: Tell the physician how long the client has been intubated, and discuss the possible need for a tracheostomy.

6 Bradycardia from vagal stimulation during tube insertion.

ANA: Administer atropine sulfate IM or IV to increase heart rate.

7 Accidental extubation.

ANA: Call physician immediately. Obtain laryngoscope, blades, and extra endotracheal tubes.

ANA: Observe the marking on the tube every 2–4 hours to ensure tube placement and to prevent accidental extubation.

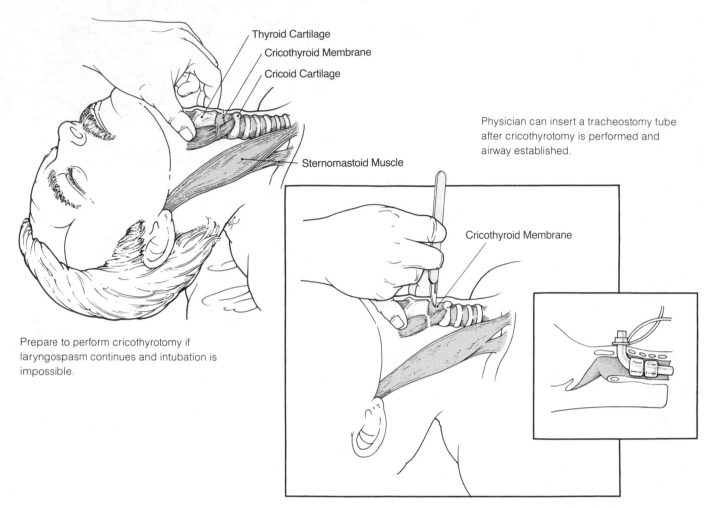

Thyroid Cartilage

Cricothyroid Membrane

Cricoid Cartilage

Sternomastoid Muscle

Physician can insert a tracheostomy tube after cricothyrotomy is performed and airway established.

Cricothyroid Membrane

Prepare to perform cricothyrotomy if laryngospasm continues and intubation is impossible.

Charting
- Clinical manifestations and need for intubation
- Size and type of tracheal tube inserted
- Name of physician performing procedure
- Client's tolerance of procedure
- Amount, color, and consistency of secretions
- Respiratory status before and after procedure
- Any equipment attached to tracheal tube, type of ventilator, and percent oxygen

ANA: Have two people change tape of endotracheal tube every 24 hours.

ANA: Have face mask and manual resuscitator bag at bedside.

8 Vomiting during endotracheal tube intubation.

ANA: If client's condition is unstable, vomiting must be prevented.

ANA: Prevent aspiration by quickly turning client on side.

ANA: Suction orally or have client rinse mouth.

ANA: If possible, wait a few minutes before attempting procedure again.

ANA: Have NG or Salem-sump ready for insertion. (Insertion is usually done after intubation.)

9 Infection.

ANA: Assess for vital sign changes, particularly increased temperature.

ANA: Assess secretions for consistency and color. Report unusual findings to physician.

ANA: Culture sputum for identification of specific organisms before instituting antibiotic therapy.

ACTION: INTUBATING CLIENT WITH TRACHEOSTOMY

ASSESSMENT

1. To intervene into an emergency situation effectively when client's life is at stake.
2. Determine need for tracheostomy as compared to less intrusive methods of providing patent airway.
3. Assess client's level of consciousness to determine client's ability to understand explanation and instructions.
4. Observe client's respiratory status: shortness of breath, severe dyspnea, tachypnea, or tachycardia.
5. Note presence of rhonchi, rales, or wheezes.

PLANNING

GOALS

- Artificial airway provided when upper airway is obstructed.
- Anatomic dead space decreased in clients with chronic obstructive disease.
- Route established for long-term ventilatory assistance.
- Secretions easily suctioned.
- Pulmonary toilet with hyperinflation of lungs accomplished, and effective treatment for atelectasis or other pulmonary complications.

EQUIPMENT

- Sterile tracheostomy tray
- Betadine solution for cleansing skin
- Xylocaine for local anesthesia
- Sterile tracheal tube with obturator, sized for client
- Sterile gloves
- Suction equipment
- Manual resuscitator bag

Rationale for Action

- To provide route for long-term mechanical ventilation (as necessary with pulmonary edema or lung surgery).
- To provide patent airway.
- To eliminate 150 cc physiological dead space in respiratory tree for clients with chronic obstructive disease.
- To facilitate removal of pulmonary secretions.
- To increase respirations if client is unconscious or has respiratory paresis.

▶ *To prevent infections during intubation:*
- Maintain sterile technique during intubation and suctioning.
- Maintain good handwashing technique.
- Administer good oral care every four hours.
- If client is on ventilator, do not drain condensed water from tubing into lungs.
- Change ventilatory equipment every 24 hours.
- Change sterile water in humidifier every eight hours.

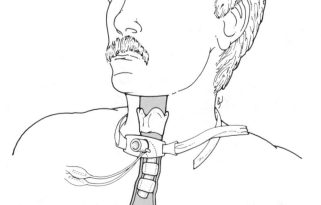

Anatomical placement of tracheostomy tube.

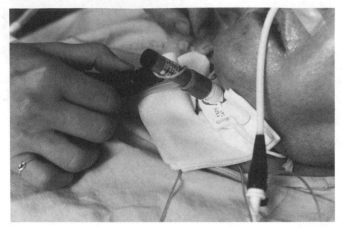

Tie trach ties at side of client's neck for comfort.

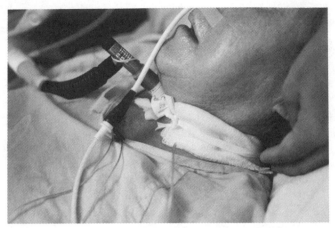

Place 4 × 4 under trach tie to prevent tie from cutting into skin. The knot should not be tied close to flange as seen in the photograph.

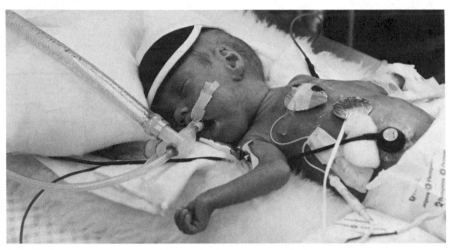

After the trach tube is inserted, it is attached to the mechanical ventilator.

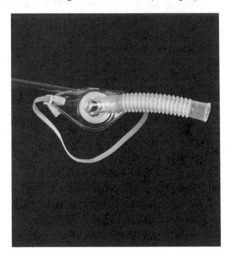

Clients requiring tracheostomy tubes, but who are not on ventilators, need a tracheostomy mask attached to the trach tube to supply mist and/or oxygen.

- Mechanical ventilator
- T-piece, mask, tubing, and oxygen flow meter if necessary
- Humidifier

PREPARATION

- Assemble all necessary equipment.
- Wash your hands.

INTERVENTION: Assisting with Tracheostomy Intubation

1 Explain procedure and rationale to client and/or relatives.
2 If not an emergency situation, obtain permit from client or other legally responsible individual prior to tracheostomy.

3 Set up tracheostomy tray where sterile field may be maintained; open tray when physician is ready.
4 Open sterile gloves.
5 Assist physician by pouring Betadine solution into sterile containers on tray. To maintain sterile technique, xylocaine is usually held by the nurse while the physician draws it out of vial.
6 Restrain client if necessary.
7 If client is alert, explain procedure as it is being done.
8 Have suction equipment ready when tracheal tube is inserted.
9 Suction when tube is inserted. If necessary, suction when tube is in place.
10 Secure tracheal ties (two people are needed: one for holding tracheostomy tube and the other to secure ties).
   a Turn end of twill tape back on itself 5 cm.
   b Make 2.5-cm cut horizontally in tape.
   c Thread one end of tape through flange of tracheal tube.
   d Pull other end of tape over flange and through slot in the tape.
   e Repeat for other side of flange.
   f Tie two ends of tape to side of client's neck to secure tracheal tube in place.
   g For children, pull tape through each side, doubling it, and tie all pieces in the back of the neck.
   h To ensure ties are not too tight, insert one finger between neck and tape before securing and knotting ties.
11 Attach tracheal tube with an adapter to mechanical ventilator or to humidification system.
12 Cleanse tracheal opening with applicator sticks and hydrogen peroxide and/or normal saline to remove blood from site. (This is a clean procedure; gloves may or may not be worn, depending on hospital policy.)
13 Apply antibiotic ointment if hospital policy allows.
14 Apply sterile tracheal dressing around tracheal opening under tube.

EVALUATION

EXPECTED OUTCOMES

1 Artificial airway inserted due to upper airway obstruction. *If not*, follow these alternative nursing actions:
   ANA: Obtain smaller size tracheostomy tube or change type of tubes (i.e., use rubber instead of plastic).
   ANA: Hyperextend neck more.
   ANA: Have CPR cart available for immediate use.
   ANA: Auscultate all lung fields to assess degree of ventilation.
2 Established route for long-term ventilatory assistance. *If not*, follow these alternative nursing actions:
   ANA: Check Unexpected Outcomes on following pages.
3 Secretions easily suctioned. *If not*, follow these alternative nursing actions:
   ANA: Change suction catheter size.

ANA: Provide warm, humidified air through ventilator, tracheostomy mask, or T-piece.

ANA: Before suctioning, instill 5–10 cc sterile normal saline (not bacteriostatic) into tracheal tube to liquefy and mobilize secretions. Allow saline to remain in tube for a few seconds, or ventilate 5–6 times with ambu bag before suctioning again.

4   Pulmonary toilet with hyperinflation of lungs is accomplished, and treatment for atelectasis or other pulmonary complications is effective. *If not*, follow these alternative nursing actions:

ANA: Check Unexpected Outcomes, steps 1–4, in oxygen section.

UNEXPECTED OUTCOMES

1   Client begins choking while tracheal tube is inserted.

ANA: Suction through tracheal opening or through nose.

ANA: If possible, prevent choking by premedicating client with muscle relaxant.

2   Inaccurate placement of tube in prebronchial tissue.

ANA: Auscultate all lung fields at least every four hours to ensure ventilation.

ANA: Observe for signs of surgical emphysema or cardiopulmonary collapse.

ANA: Obtain physician's order for x-ray to verify tube placement.

ANA: Replace tube with different size.

3   Accidental extubation. (Usually occurs within first five days or during suctioning when cuff is deflated.)

ANA: Have emergency equipment at bedside.

a   Sterile tracheal set of same size and style

b   Ties and syringes for inflating cuff

c   Tracheal dilator, scissors, and hemostats

d   Sterile gloves and dressings

ANA: Insert old tube if new one not available to preserve patent airway.

ANA: Immediately insert tracheal dilator into stoma to preserve airway.

ANA: Suction stoma, if there is time. Then reinsert new tracheal tube, secure with tapes, and establish ventilation. Oxygenating with ambu bag is desirable, especially if any signs of respiratory distress are present.

4   Sudden overventilation resulting in rapid reduction of pCO_2. May occur if client is on mechanical ventilator.

ANA: Ventilate client adequately prior to intubation to prevent build-up of carbon dioxide.

5   Hemorrhage from tracheostomy site.

ANA: Apply pressure if hemorrhage site accessible.

ANA: Have physician cauterize bleeding vessels.

ANA: Take client to operating room for exploration of site and ligation of bleeding vessel if physician orders surgery.

6   Obstructed tracheostomy.

ANA: If no physician available, follow these procedures:

Clinical Alert

If there is no time to get a new tube in an emergency situation, just insert old one. The critical objective is to get airway open.

a Deflate cuff.

b Cut tracheostomy ties.

c Remove tube.

d Insert tracheal dilator (if at bedside).

e Establish airway. (You may need to suction through tracheal stoma although this is contraindicated if tracheostomy is new.)

f Insert new tube and reestablish ventilation.

7 Bleeding into innominate artery from erosion of tube.

ANA: Call physician immediately and hyperinflate cuff to tamponade the bleeding. (Client may need endotracheal intubation and immediate surgery to suture site of erosion.)

ANA: Start IV and give Pitressin immediately if ordered.

Charting

- Clinical manifestations indicating need for intubation
- Specific reason for intubation
- Size and type of inserted endotracheal, nasopharyngeal, or oropharyngeal tube
- Preoxygenation if completed
- Type and quantity of secretions
- Client's tolerance of procedure
- Type of ventilator connected to tube

ACTION: CARING FOR CLIENT WITH TRACHEOSTOMY

ASSESSMENT

1 Note dried or moist secretions surrounding cannula or on tracheal dressing.

2 Note excessive expectoration of secretions.

3 Assess result of routine tracheal care to determine if routine care is adequate for this client.

4 Observe client's ability to sustain respiratory function by ability to breathe through normal airway.

5 Assess respiratory status: breath sounds, respiratory rate, use of accessory muscles for breathing while tracheal tube is plugged.

6 Assess for labored breathing, flaring of nares, retractions, and color of nail beds.

Rationale for Action

- To prevent airway obstruction by liquefying and mobilizing secretions.
- To prevent infections of tracheal site.
- To improve respiratory function so that client can breathe normally, without artificial support.

PLANNING

GOALS

- Tracheal site and pulmonary system free of infection.
- Secretions easily liquefied and mobilized with saline instillations.
- Secretions easily suctioned.
- Client adequately ventilated and calm after tube removed.

EQUIPMENT

- Tracheal dressing tray
- Sterile gloves if required by hospital policy
- Suction equipment
- Complete tracheal tube set for emergency use
- Interchangeable inner cannula of same size if available or No. 4 entire set
- Hydrogen peroxide
- Sterile NS
- Pipe cleaners

▶ Metal tracheal tubes usually have inner cannulas that need to be cleaned. Some plastic or rubber tubes have removable inner cannulas. If tube has inflatable cuff, cuff must be deflated before removing inner cannula.

ADDITIONAL EQUIPMENT

For Instillation of Normal Saline
- Sterile normal saline (not bacteriostatic)
- Sterile 10 cc syringe with needle
- Sterile suction catheter and glove
- Suction machine
- Resuscitation bag
- Tracheostomy plug

PREPARATION

- Assemble equipment.
- Make sure suction equipment and additional tracheal tubes are available.

INTERVENTION: Cleaning Inner Cannula

1. Explain procedure and rationale to client.
2. Put on gloves if required by hospital policy.
3. Suction before cleaning tracheal tube.
4. Unlock the inner cannula by turning the lock to the left about 90°. Secure the outer cannula of the neck plate with your left index finger and thumb.
5. Gently pull the inner cannula slightly upward and out towards you.
6. Wash cannula thoroughly with cool, sterile water, saline, or hydrogen peroxide to remove secretions. (Tapwater may be used if hospital policy allows.)

Illustration depicts how inner cannula fits onto outer cannula. When cleaning, outer cannula is not removed.

Step 1: Unlock inner cannula and remove for cleaning.

Step 2: After cleaning replace inner cannula.

Step 3: Gently slip the inner cannula in place by inserting it at an angle.

Step 4: Turn lock to the right to secure the tube in place.

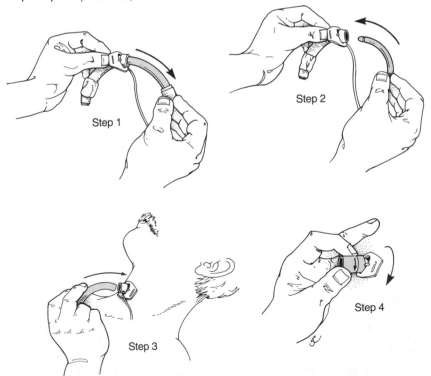

7   To remove dried-on secretions, cleanse the lumen and outer surface of the cannula with pipe cleaners moistened with hydrogen
peroxide. (Some hospitals use sterile normal saline.)

8   Soak the cannula in a hydrogen-peroxide filled sterile bowl to further remove dried secretions.

9   Rinse cannula thoroughly with sterile water or saline.

10   Dry tube

11   Replace the inner cannula carefully by grasping the outer flange of
the cannula with your left hand as you insert the cannula.

12   Lock the inner cannula by turning the lock to the right so that it is in
an upright position.

13   Cleanse around the incision site with applicator sticks soaked in
normal saline and/or hydrogen peroxide (one-half strength).

14   Apply antibiotic ointment around incision site if ordered.

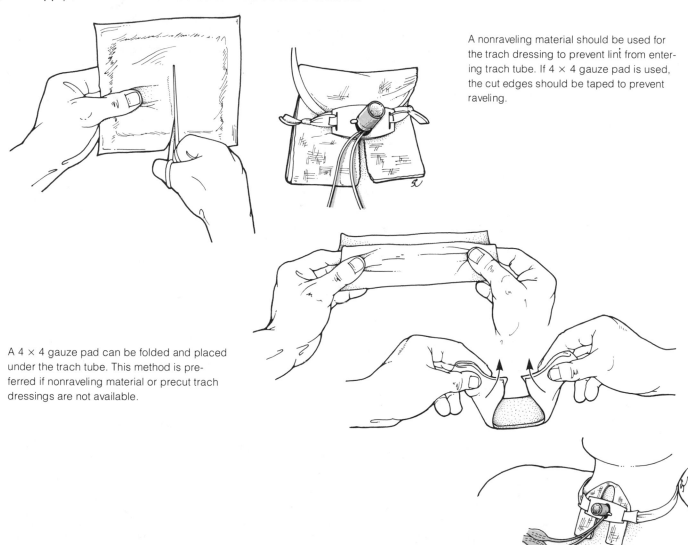

A nonraveling material should be used for
the trach dressing to prevent lint from entering trach tube. If 4 × 4 gauze pad is used,
the cut edges should be taped to prevent
raveling.

A 4 × 4 gauze pad can be folded and placed
under the trach tube. This method is preferred if nonraveling material or precut trach
dressings are not available.

15 Apply trach dressing around insertion site, and change tracheal ties if needed.
16 If tracheal ties are to be changed, ask another person to hold the tracheal tube in place while you change the ties. This procedure prevents accidental extubation if the client coughs.
17 Make client comfortable.
18 Discard soiled dressings, tapes, and cleaning equipment.

INTERVENTION: Instilling Normal Saline

1 Attach sterile catheter to suction machine tubing.
2 Draw up prescribed amount of normal saline (usually 3–5 cc) in syringe.
3 Remove needle from syringe.
4 Turn on oxygen supply to resuscitation bag.
5 Turn on suction equipment.
6 Remove needle before injecting saline into tube.
7 Instill prescribed amount of normal saline into tracheostomy or endotracheal tube with ungloved hand.
8 Give client 3–5 breaths with resuscitation bag if client can tolerate this procedure.
9 Put on sterile glove and begin deep suctioning. Client may be hyperventilated with resuscitator bag after suctioning.
10 Turn off oxygen for resuscitator bag.
11 Discard used equipment.
12 Make client comfortable.

INTERVENTION: Plugging Tracheostomy

1 Suction nasopharynx.
2 Change suction catheters, and suction trachea.
3 Deflate tracheal cuff; suction again if necessary.
4 Place tracheal plug in either the inner cannula or outer cannula with inner cannula removed.
5 Observe client for respiratory distress.

EVALUATION

EXPECTED OUTCOMES

1 Client adequately ventilated with no evidence of respiratory distress. *If not*, follow these alternative nursing actions:
  ANA: If respiratory distress is caused from excessive mucus, remove plug and suction. Then notify physician.
  ANA: Remove plug if you observe any changes in client's vital signs, especially increased respiratory rate.
2 Secretions easily liquefied and mobilized with saline instillations. Secretions easily suctioned. *If not*, follow these alternative nursing actions:

ANA: Check to make sure humidification system is functioning properly.

ANA: Wait 15 minutes, then repeat procedure with 5–10 cc normal saline.

ANA: Repeat saline instillations every hour.

UNEXPECTED OUTCOMES

1 Accidental extubation.

ANA: Have second tracheal set available. (Follow the directions on page 584 for insertion.)

2 Excessive secretions and coughing while inner cannula is cleansed.

ANA: Suction before removing inner cannula.

ANA: Suction lumen if necessary, while soaking inner cannula.

3 Inner cannula dislodged.

ANA: Insert extra cannula from emergency set if cannulas are interchangeable. If not, insert new tracheal set.

ANA: If cannula is metal, send it to CSR for autoclaving. If cannula is disposable, discard in trash. If plastic, soak in hydrogen peroxide for one hour, then rinse in sterile NS.

Charting

- Location of plug: outer or inner cannula
- Baseline vital signs before procedure
- Respiratory status during procedure
- Vital signs, any indications of cyanosis or respiratory distress
- Amount of normal saline instilled into tracheal tube
- Hyperventilation of lungs if ventilator utilized
- Inner cannula cleansed with H_2O_2, saline, and replaced
- Color and consistency of secretions
- Unusual reactions by client

ACTION: REMOVING ARTIFICIAL AIRWAY (ENDOTRACHEAL OR TRACHEOSTOMY)

ASSESSMENT

1 Determine the amount and consistency of secretions (should be minimal).
2 Assess client's ability to handle secretions.
3 Assess client's respiratory status. Respirations should be unlabored, all lobes aerated, and lungs clear to auscultation.
4 Check to see if client can breathe for several hours without ventilatory assistance.
5 Note if client's gag and swallowing reflexes are intact.

Rationale for Action

- To remove artificial airway when it is no longer required.
- To assess client's ability to handle his or her own secretions.
- To evaluate client's respiratory status without ventilatory assistance.

PLANNING

GOALS

- Adequate ventilation and sustained respiration without the use of a mechanical ventilator.
- Minimal amount of pulmonary secretions.
- Gag and swallowing reflex present.

EQUIPMENT

- Tissues
- Receptacle for disposable items
- Oxygen cannula or mask if ordered

INTERVENTION: Removing an Artificial Airway

1 Wash your hands.
2 Explain procedure and rationale to client.
3 Suction through tube.
4 Preoxygenate with manual resuscitation bag.
5 Suction oropharynx.
6 Deflate cuff.
7 Remove tube quickly. (This will prevent gagging if removing an endotracheal tube.)
8 Cleanse nares or tracheal site, and allow client to clear airway by coughing and/or blowing nose.
9 Apply oxygen cannula and mask if ordered.
10 Place 4×4 sterile dressing over tracheal opening.
11 Observe client for respiratory difficulty.
12 Provide oral hygiene.
13 Discard disposable equipment.
14 Clean and return reusable equipment to proper area.

EVALUATION

EXPECTED OUTCOMES

1 Adequate ventilation and sustained respiration without the use of a mechanical ventilator. *If not*, follow these alternative nursing actions:
ANA: Assess presence and degree of respiratory distress.
ANA: Assess need for immediate intervention.
ANA: Notify physician for reintubation.
2 Minimal amount of pulmonary secretions. *If not*, follow these alternative nursing actions:
ANA: Notify physician that pulmonary secretions are not decreased. Airway should not be removed.
ANA: Assess respiratory status, and if labored, suction more frequently through tube.
3 Gag and swallowing reflex present. *If not*, follow these alternative nursing actions:
ANA: Notify physician for reintubation for artificial airway.
ANA: Have suction and airway equipment available for immediate use.

UNEXPECTED OUTCOMES

1 Sore throat and hoarseness.
ANA: Provide humidification via mist mask.
ANA: Give client throat lozenges.
2 Laryngeal edema.
ANA: Give client humidification with mist mask.
ANA: Assess for inspiratory stridor, and if client in respiratory distress, notify physician immediately for reintubation.
ANA: Administer local steroids and/or vasoconstrictors to reduce edema.

Charting

1 Tube removed
2 Respiratory status, i.e., color, respiratory rate, adventitious breath sounds, and signs of respiratory distress
3 Method of oxygenation or humidification and flow rate if ordered

ACTION: INFLATING AND DEFLATING TRACHEOSTOMY OR ENDOTRACHEAL CUFF

ASSESSMENT

1   Listen for audible hissing sounds indicating an air leak.
2   Check to see if pilot balloon is deflated.
3   Assess client's ability to make sounds.

Rationale for Action
● To prevent aspiration while feeding
● To prevent tracheal damage
● To prevent tracheal ulcerations and necrosis

PLANNING

GOALS

● Client can eat without aspirating food while tracheostomy cuff is inflated.
● Tracheal necrosis prevented.
● Lungs adequately ventilated by mechanical ventilation.

EQUIPMENT

● 10 cc syringe
● Hemostat with padded rubber tubing on ends for some tracheal tubes

INTERVENTION: Deflating Tracheal Cuff

1   Suction airway before deflating cuff.
2   Attach 10 cc syringe to distal end of inflatable cuff, making sure seal is tight.
3   Slowly withdraw 5 cc of air. Amount of air withdrawn is determined by type of cuff used and whether minimal air leak is utilized.
4   Keep syringe attached to end of cuff.
5   Suction if cough reflex stimulated.
6   Keep cuff deflated five minutes if client can tolerate.

INTERVENTION: Inflating Cuff

1   Suction airway before inflating cuff.
2   If syringe is not already attached, attach 10 cc syringe to distal end of inflatable cuff, making sure seal is tight.
3   Inflate prescribed amount of air to create leak-free system. Cuff is inflated correctly when you cannot hear the client's voice or any air movement from nose or mouth.
4   Remove syringe and apply rubber-tipped forceps to maintain air in cuff, depending on the type of tube used.
5   If cuff has two balloons, alternately inflate them every hour.

EVALUATION

EXPECTED OUTCOMES

1   Client can eat without aspirating food while tracheostomy cuff is inflated. *If not*, follow these alternative nursing actions:
    Feed intravenously if ordered.

Check pillow port for pressure level to determine balloon inflation. When pillow port feels taut this indicates it is distended and the balloon is inflated.

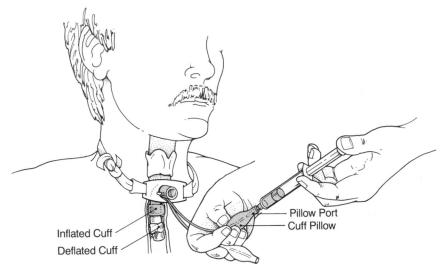

Inflated Cuff
Deflated Cuff
Pillow Port
Cuff Pillow

2 Tracheal necrosis prevented. *If not*, follow these alternative nursing actions:

ANA: Keep cuff pressure below 20 mm Hg. Utilize minimum air leak and compensate with respirator adjustment. Withdraw ½–1 cc air after obtaining leak-free system.

ANA: Deflate cuff five minutes every hour.

UNEXPECTED OUTCOMES

1 Balloon ruptures and herniates over the end of the tube.

ANA: Replace tube immediately.

ANA: Assess client for respiratory dysfunction. A portion of the cuff may have been aspirated.

2 Client is unable to tolerate cuff deflating for prescribed five minutes.

ANA: Release cuff for as long a time as client can tolerate.

ANA: May hyperinflate lungs with manual resuscitator while cuff deflated.

Charting
- Tracheal cuff release time
- Amount of air used for cuff inflation
- Changes in respiratory status during deflation/inflation
- Amount, color, and consistency of secretions suctioned

Rationale for Action
- To evacuate air or a combination of air and serosanguineous fluid from the intrapleural space
- To reestablish negative pressure after an intrathoracic procedure
- To provide continued suction that functions as a safeguard against pneumothorax
- To facilitate drainage of accumulated fluid within the thoracic cavity after open heart surgery

ACTION: CARING FOR CLIENT WITH CHEST TUBES

ASSESSMENT

1 Monitor client's respiratory status while tubes inserted.
2 Check to see that all connections between the water-seal system and the client are securely taped.
3 Check patency of chest tubes.
4 Note if mediastinal shift present.
5 Auscultate breath sounds.
6 Observe for bilateral chest expansion.
7 Note chest drainage as ordered.

PLANNING

GOALS

- Closed water-seal drainage system maintained until client's lung is reexpanded and air or serosanguineous fluid is removed from pleural space.
- Normal respiratory function restored.

EQUIPMENT

- Chest-tube insertion tray with appropriate chest-tube size
- Tape or wire for connectors
- Suction source
- Lotion or alcohol wipes for chest-tube stripping or a mechanical chest-tube stripper
- Rubber-tipped hemostats (carmalts) for clamping air leak
- Tape for drainage bottle markings

- The waterseal mechanism operates on the principle of negative pressure. (The pressure in the chest cavity is lower than the pressure of atmosphere, which causes air to rush into the chest cavity when an injury, such as a stab wound, occurs.)
- When the chest has been opened, a vacuum must be applied to chest to re-establish negative pressure.
- Water acts as a seal and keeps the air from being drawn back into the pleural space.
- An open-drainage system would allow air to be sucked back into the chest cavity and collapse the lungs.

INTERVENTION: Assisting Physician with Chest-Tube Insertion

1 Assemble chest-tube insertion tray, sterile gloves, chest tubes, and water-seal drainage.
2 Plug system water-seal drainage equipment into outlet.
3 Place client in a semirecumbent position to allow air to rise to the apex of the pleural space.
4 Open equipment tray and prepare tray as needed.
5 Following chest tube insertion, connect chest tube to water-seal drainage equipment.
6 Turn suction control to low suction.
7 Secure connection sites with wire or tape.
8 Observe for possible air leaks or excessive suction in the system.

Tape all connections to prevent accidental interruption of the water-seal drainage system.

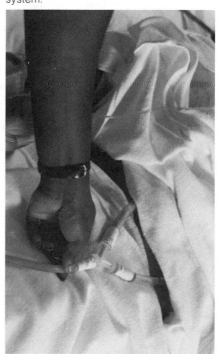

INTERVENTION: Establishing a Closed System

1 Attach tubes to water-seal suction so that closed system is maintained after insertion of chest tubes.
2 Tape all connectors to ensure airtight seals.
3 Make sure that all stoppers in bottles fit tightly if bottle suction is used.
4 Check tubing to make sure fluid does not collect, as this prevents suction from being exerted.
5 Provide a straight line of tubing from bed to collection system to prevent pooling of fluid.
6 Keep collection system below level of chest-tube insertion site so that fluid flows downward.
7 Make sure that tubing is free and not coiled. Do not use pins or restrain tubing.

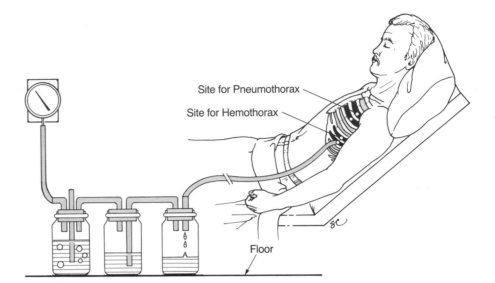

Provide a straight line of tubing from chest tube to collection system. Keep collection system below level of chest tube insertion site (on the floor).

Site for Pneumothorax

Site for Hemothorax

Floor

INTERVENTION: Maintaining a Closed System

1   Safety Monitoring.
   a   Monitor tubes for air leaks, which may cause the client's lung to collapse.
   b   If air leaks occur, clamp off tube momentarily (if you have orders to do so) and inform physician immediately.
   c   Keep rubber-tipped hemostats (carmalts) at client's bedside so that if ordered, the tube can be clamped off nearest to chest insertion site. Place clamps facing in opposite directions.
   d   Obtain a chest x-ray to identify the correct placement of chest tubes.
2   Maintaining Pressure.
   a   Keep suction bottles of Pleur-evac system below level of bed.
   b   Keep suction control pressure where ordered. (Make sure that bubbling is not excessive in the control bottle.)
   c   Maintain water level in water-seal bottle.
3   Maintaining Chest Tube Patency.
   a   Milk chest tubes every 30 to 60 minutes.
   b   Milk away from client toward the drainage receptacle (Pleur-evac or bottles).
   c   Pinch tubing close to the chest with one hand as you milk the tube with your other hand. Continue going down tube in this method until you come to the drainage receptacle. (You may use a Lundy roller for this procedure. If you do, use the roller with caution.)
   d   Use lotion or alcohol wipes to make stripping easier.

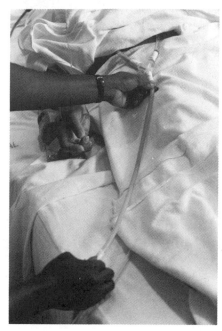
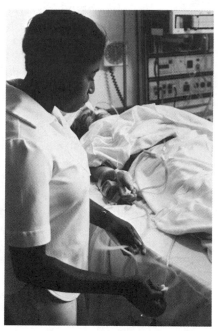

Maintain chest tube patency by milking the tubes every 30 to 60 minutes. For better friction when milking the tube use alcohol wipe.

Start milking from the chest tube connection site and milk the tube until you reach the collection system.

4 Record Intake and Output.
   a With Pleur-evac suction equipment, visually measure and mark level of chest drainage as ordered. (System holds up to 2800 to 3000 cc drainage.) Change equipment only when the drainage chamber is full.
   b With two- or three-bottle suction, estimate drainage and mark bottle. Change drainage bottle only when full.
5 Assess Client's Status.
   a Instruct client to deep breathe and cough at frequent intervals.
   b Tell the client to change positions frequently.
   c Observe and report any unusual respiratory signs/symptoms: rapid, shallow breathing, cyanosis, pressure in chest, or hemorrhage.

EVALUATION

EXPECTED OUTCOMES

1 Closed water-seal drainage system maintained until client's lung is reexpanded and air or serosanguineous fluid is removed from pleural space. *If not*, follow these alternative nursing actions:

597

If air leaks occur at the insertion site and/or in tubing:

ANA: Apply Vaseline gauze around opening at insertion site.

ANA: Secure all connections with tape.

ANA: Clamp tubing (if not tension pneumothorax); turn suction motor off; ask physician for orders.

If client's lung remains unexpanded:

ANA: Check client's chest x-ray to determine if chest tubes are inserted correctly. Notify physician of findings.

ANA: Observe water-seal suction system for proper functioning.

ANA: Check pressure level on suction apparatus.

2 Normal respiratory function restored. *If not*, follow these alternative nursing actions:

ANA: Continue monitoring chest tube and water-seal suction system for possible problems.

ANA: Position in Fowler's position to assist in lung expansion.

ANA: Strip chest tubes every two hours to ensure clot removal and to maintain normal pressure within the system.

UNEXPECTED OUTCOME

Chest tube becomes dislodged.

ANA: Apply pressure over insertion site with the palm of your hand or any available material, e.g., sheet, dressings. Notify physician.

ANA: When sterile pressure dressing is obtained, instruct client to exhale. Then compress the opening and provide tight seal with dressing.

ANA: Observe for signs of respiratory distress: symmetry of chest, respiratory rate, changes in color, or level of consciousness.

ANA: Observe for mediastinal shift to unaffected side from tension buildup.

ACTION: MONITORING WATER-SEAL CHEST DRAINAGE

ASSESSMENT

1 Assess client's respiratory rate, rhythm, and breath sounds for signs of respiratory distress.
2 Check to make sure all connections on tubing are airtight and the suction control is connected.
3 Examine system to see if it is set up and functioning properly.
4 Identify any malfunctions in system, i.e., air leaks, negative pressure, or obstructions.

PLANNING

GOALS

- Closed water-seal chest drainage maintained, drainage evacuated, and lung reexpanded
- Negative pressure reestablished and lung reexpanded

Charting

- Size of chest tubes inserted
- Level of pressure ordered
- Client's tolerance of procedure
- Vital signs
- Breath sounds
- Amount, color, and character of drainage
- Chest expansion: symmetrical or asymmetrical

Rationale for Action

- To remove air and serosanguineous fluid from pleural space so that reexpansion of lung may occur
- To maintain closed system

Mediastinal Shift: The sternum is shifted to unaffected side of the chest, e.g., if right-sided pneumothorax, the sternum is shifted to the left side.

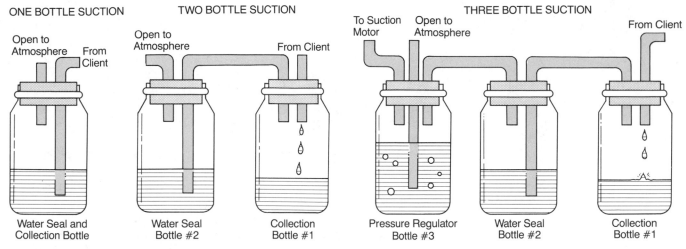

ONE BOTTLE SUCTION

Open to Atmosphere   From Client

Water Seal and Collection Bottle

TWO BOTTLE SUCTION

Open to Atmosphere   From Client

Water Seal Bottle #2   Collection Bottle #1

THREE BOTTLE SUCTION

To Suction Motor   Open to Atmosphere   From Client

Pressure Regulator Bottle #3   Water Seal Bottle #2   Collection Bottle #1

One bottle system is used for lung reinflation. Two bottle system is not connected to mechanical suction device. Three bottle system is used for clients who require chest drainage.

EQUIPMENT

- Appropriate water-seal bottle or disposable unit system for closed chest drainage
- Suction source
- Tape and plastic cables or wires for connectors
- Two hemostats

INTERVENTION: Monitoring Closed Water-Seal Drainage (Three-Bottle System)

1 Examine the control bottle (bottle #3) to check the depth to which the third, longer tube is submerged in the water. This depth determines the pressure in the drainage system—usually 10 to 20 cm negative water pressure.

2 Regulate the wall suction to maintain continuous suctioning.
   a To increase suctioning, increase the depth to which the third, longer tube in the control bottle is submerged.
   b To decrease negative pressure, decrease the depth to which the third, longer tube is submerged.
   c Constant bubbling in the control bottle indicates the desired pressure level has been reached.

3 Examine the water-seal bottle (bottle #2).
   a Make sure the long tube is covered with water to maintain the water seal.
   b Check the water level in this bottle to prevent changes in the amount of negative pressure the client receives.
   c Tape all connections between the water seal and the client to prevent air leaks. You may also band taped connections with wire or plastic cable as an extra precaution against air leaks.

Three bottle suction is frequently attached to the Emerson suction machine when wall suction is not available.

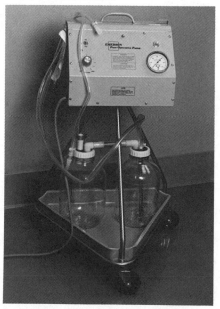

4　Monitor the water-seal bottle for air leaks in the system. These leaks can be identified by constant bubbling in the water-seal bottle.

5　If air leaks occur, clamp tubing close to client's chest (if you have standing orders to do so) and notify physician immediately.

6　Examine the collection bottle (bottle #1) to make sure it is not constantly bubbling indicating an air leak.

7　Observe and record the drainage level on the collection bottle as ordered:

　　a　Every hour immediately after surgery, or if there is a large amount of drainage.

　　b　At least every eight hours while chest tube is inserted; mark the time on the drainage bottle every shift.

8　Whenever the suction motor is off, keep the drainage system open to the atmosphere by detaching the tubing from the motor to provide a vent.

INTERVENTION: Setting Up Disposable Water-Seal Suction

1　Gather the Pleur-evac, suction equipment if not wall suction, rubber extension tubing.

2　Unwrap the Pleur-evac.

3　Hang the Pleur-evac on its disposable floor stand.

4　Remove the plastic connector on the short tube that is attached to the water-seal chamber.

5　Remove the plunger from the large 50 to 60 cc Asepto syringe. Attach the barrel of the syringe to the short rubber tube.

6　Pour sterile water into the barrel of the syringe.

7　Fill the water-seal chamber to the 2-cm level.

The Pleur-evac and Argyle are disposable water-seal suction containers. Fill the suction control chamber and water-seal chamber with sterile water before attaching to external suction source and client.

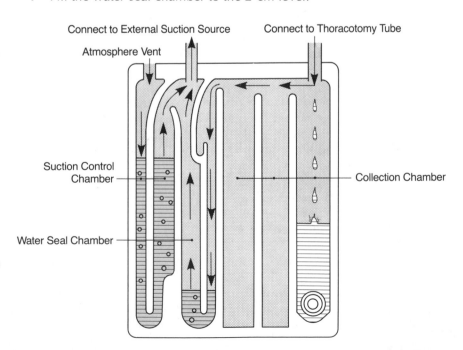

Connect to External Suction Source
Connect to Thoracotomy Tube
Atmosphere Vent
Suction Control Chamber
Collection Chamber
Water Seal Chamber

8   Remove the plastic plug from the vent to the suction control chamber.

9   Attach the syringe barrel to the vent. Pour sterile water into the chamber. (The tip of the syringe fits into the top of the chamber vent. There is no rubber tubing attached.)

10 Fill the suction control chamber to the 20-cm level.

11 Insert the plastic plug into the vent.

12 After the physician has inserted chest tubes, remove the long tube adapter from the collection chamber and attach it to the chest tubes.

13 Tape or wire the connector sites.

14 Attach short rubber tube on the water-seal suction to the suction machine (wall or portable) using an adapter connection piece.

15 Turn suction device on slowly until bubbling occurs in the suction control chamber.

16 Monitor water levels daily in both the water-seal chamber and the suction control chamber. Refill to level with sterile water as needed.

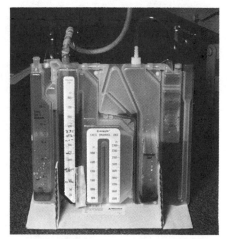

Mark the drainage on the collection chamber at least every eight hours.

INTERVENTION: Monitoring for Disposable Water-Seal Suction

1   Monitor the collection chamber for chest drainage every fifteen minutes immediately after surgery and every hour for first 24 hours and then as ordered by the physician. Record the results.

2   Mark the drainage on the collection chamber every shift. Place a line at the top level of fluid and place the time on the chamber.

3   Observe the suction control chamber for excessive suction as evidenced by excessive bubbling in the chamber. (Suction control set on low suction.)

4   Observe the water-seal chamber; there should be no air bubbles present if chest tubes are inserted for drainage. Bubbles will be present if the lung is being reinflated. When the lung is inflated, the bubbles will cease.

5   Check that all connections are secured with wire or tape.

6   Check that there are no kinks or dependent loops in the extension tubing.

7   Observe and strip chest tubes for drainage and possible clots at least every 15 minutes immediately after surgery and every hour until discontinued.

Monitor disposable water-seal system frequently for air leaks and correct fluid level in water-seal and control chambers. Add sterile water to keep chamber level.

INTERVENTION: Obtaining Chest Drainage Specimen

1   Obtain 18- or 20-gauge needle with 10 cc syringe.

2   Swab self-sealing diaphragm on back of the collection chamber with Betadine swab.

3   Insert needle into diaphragm.

4   Withdraw specified amount of drainage.

5   Place needle protector on needle, label specimen with name, hospital number, and source from where specimen was collected.

6   Fill out requisition form and send to lab with specimen.

601

EVALUATION

1 Closed chest drainage maintained, drainage evacuated, and lung reexpanded. *If not*, follow these alternative nursing actions:
ANA: Observe suction control bottle to ensure adequate system pressure being maintained.
ANA: Strip chest tubes to ensure patency of chest tube.
ANA: Ensure all connections are tight to prevent air leaks.
ANA: Observe that ordered amount of water is in suction control bottte to ensure adequate pressure in the system.

2 Negative pressure reestablished and lung reexpanded. *If not*, follow these alternative nursing actions:
ANA: Continue to monitor for problems in the system and correct immediately.
ANA: Assess and record breath sounds at least every four hours.
ANA: Notify physician of any unusual findings with breath sounds.

UNEXPECTED OUTCOMES

1 Air leak indicated by bubbling in water-seal bottle.
ANA: Check for specific leak area by clamping chest tube (if physician's orders allow) between water-seal bottle and client.
- If water-seal bottle continues to bubble, the leak is in the tubing.
- If water-seal bottle stops bubbling, the leak is in the client's chest tube at the site of the insertion.
ANA: Secure all connections with tape or wire.
ANA: Change tubing if necessary. (Obtain physician's order.)
ANA: Apply sterile Vaseline gauze and pressure dressing around chest-tube insertion site.

2 Control bottle not bubbling.
ANA: Pressure is too low. Check gauge to walled suction for proper amount.

3 Chest tube becomes disconnected from water-seal drainage system at any one of the connection sites.
ANA: Observe for signs of respiratory distress due to potential pneumothorax.
ANA: Replace the extension tubing leading from the chest tube with sterile tubing as infection can occur from contamination of the lumen.
ANA: Turn suction source down before clamping chest tube to prevent rapid increase in intrapleural pressure when clamps removed.
ANA: Clamp chest tube near catheter insertion site while replacing extension tubes to prevent pneumothorax from atmospheric air entering intrapleural space during inspiration.
ANA: Unclamp chest tube as soon as extension tubing replaced to prevent tension pneumothorax.
ANA: Reset suction pressure. Observe force of bubbles in suction control compartment to prevent suction from being too great.

ANA: Tape or wire new extension connection sites to prevent disconnection.

4 Chest tubes become obstructed by a clot, kink in the chest tube, or pressure on the chest tube.

ANA: Observe for respiratory distress especially if suction is being used to reexpand the lung.

ANA: Observe entire system for kinks in tubing. Loop the tubing on bed. Do not secure with tape. Loop rubber band around the chest tube and put safety pin through rubber band and then pin to linen. Allow sufficient slack.

ANA: Observe tubing for signs of clot, decreased flow of fluid through tube, visualization of clotted material in tube.

ANA: Milk chest tubes several times to force clot out into drainage bottle.

5 Suction source for water-seal drainage malfunctions due to defect in suction pump, wall plug outlet, or disconnection of suction tube.

ANA: Open up the distal end of the chest tube by disconnecting the suction tube to prevent back pressure.

ANA: Observe for decreased flow of fluid through chest tube.

ANA: Monitor respiratory rate, rhythm, and chest excursion for signs of respiratory distress.

6 Loose connection on rubber stopper caps (bottle suction) or suction tubes.

ANA: Check each suction tube connection site for looseness and tighten each site.

ANA: Push rubber stopper caps down into bottles.

ANA: Push rubber tubing down securely on stopper caps.

Charting

- Drainage—amount, color, presence of clots
- Any abnormalities in the system and treatment of abnormalities
- Respiratory status, including rate, rhythm, and breath sounds
- Frequency of chest-tube milking

ACTION: MAINTAINING MECHANICAL VENTILATION

ASSESSMENT

1 Complete a respiratory physical assessment to assist in determining the need for mechanical ventilation (auscultation, palpation, percussion).

2 Identify if need for mechanical ventilation is present. Criteria for non-COPD clients:
   a Vital capacity is less than 15 ml/kg of body weight.
   b Inspiratory pressure is less than -25 cm H_2O.
   c $PaCO_2$ is below 30 mm Hg or above 50 mm Hg.
   d Alveolar-arterial oxygen difference (A-a Δ pO_2) is greater than 350 mm Hg on 100 percent oxygen.
   e Pulmonary shunt is greater than 30 percent.
   f Deadspace-tidal volume (V_D-V_T) ratio is greater than 60 percent.
   g PaO_2 is less than 60 mm Hg on an FIO_2 of 1.0.

3 Observe for trend of respiratory values (trend is more important than isolated measurements).

Rationale for Action

- To maintain physiological functioning in:
  respiratory center failure (brainstem injury or narcotic overdose)
  neuromuscular diseases (myasthenia gravis)
  musculoskeletal disorders (flail chest)
  pulmonary disorders (adult respiratory distress syndrome)
- To maintain cardiopulmonary functioning in cardiopulmonary arrest
- To maintain acid-base balance of the body

PLANNING

GOALS

- Adequate respiratory function is maintained for clients with altered respirations.
- Acid-base balance is improved in altered respiratory states.

EQUIPMENT

- Specific ventilator ordered, i.e. Bennett MA-I, Bennett PR 2, etc.
- Handheld resuscitator connected to oxygen flowmeter (ambu or Laerdahl bag)
- Sterile suction supplies
- Ventilator flowsheet

INTERVENTION: Placing Client on a Ventilator

1 Double check the ventilator settings against those ordered by the physician.
2 Plug the machine in and turn it on.
3 Familiarize yourself with location of alarm systems on the ventilator and turn on all alarm systems.
4 Connect the ventilator tubing to client's endotracheal tube or tracheostomy tube.
5 Monitor client's pulse and blood pressure every five minutes until stable.
6 Obtain arterial blood gases 15 minutes after ventilation is established.

INTERVENTION: Managing Client on Mechanical Ventilation

1 Monitor ventilator settings and delivered values every hour: tidal volume, inspiratory pressure, peak pressure, rate, FIO₂, I:E ratio, in addition to PEEP or IMV when ordered.
2 Check thermometer every hour in inspiratory tubing line. Maintain temperature of inspired air between 32° C and 35° C.
3 Check humidifier fluid level every eight hours and refill as necessary.
4 Record intake, output, and daily weights. Positive pressure ventilation may cause a positive water balance due to humidification of inspired air.
5 Suspend ventilator tubing from an IV hook or support it on a pillow to reduce traction on the endotracheal or tracheostomy tube.
6 Change ventilator tubing every 24 hours.
7 Check vital signs every hour and auscultate lungs.
8 Observe and listen for possible cuff leaks around tracheostomy or endotracheal tubes.
9 Empty accumulated water in the ventilator tubing as needed. (Disconnect the tubing, stretch it to release water trapped in the corrugated areas, and drain the water into a basin or trap in tubing.) Do not drain water back into the humidifier because this action increases the risk of infection.

▶ **Initial Ventilator Settings**

- Tidal volume of 10 ml/kg (High tidal volumes help prevent atelectasis.)
- Respiratory rate of 10 to 15 per minute
- Inspiratory pressure of 25 cm H₂O
- Inspiratory-expiratory (I:E) rate 1:2 (I:E ratio should be set at less than 1:1 to prevent air trapping in the lungs.)
- Pressure pop-off setting of 50 cm H₂O
- FIO₂ of 0.4 to 1.0

▶ "Mechanical ventilators" is the correct term for artificial breathing machines because they can achieve gas exchange only in the lungs.

▶ **Clinical Alert**
Positive pressure ventilation may decrease venous return and cardiac output.

▶ Compliance is determined by $\dfrac{TV}{PIP}$

where TV = tidal volume
PIP = peak inspiratory pressure

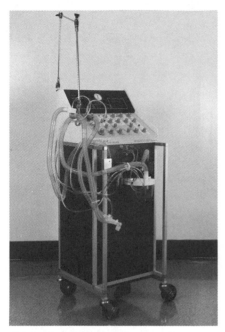

Adult volume respirator.

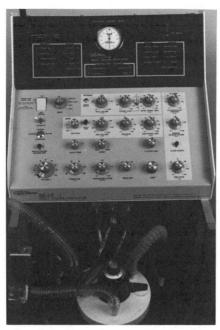

Check all ventilator settings with physician's orders before placing client on ventilator.

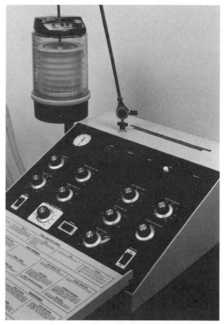

Identify location of alarm systems and what these alarms mean when they are triggered.

10 Provide client with a method of communication, such as a "magic slate."

11 Test the nasogastric drainage pH every hour and administer antacids to maintain the pH above 5. Stress ulcers are frequently associated with mechanical ventilation.

12 Test the nasogastric drainage and fecal matter daily for occult blood.

13 Assess lung compliance frequently; lung compliance falls before changes are evident in blood gas analysis or clinical manifestations.

14 Implement methods of stress reduction, such as careful explanation of procedures even if client appears comatose.

15 Keep ventilator alarms *ON*.

16 "Sigh" the client six to eight times an hour to prevent atelectasis. (Use the sigh button if the ventilator has one, or ventilate the client manually, using a volume larger than the ventilator set tidal volume.)

▶ Criteria for assisted ventilation in neonates
pO_2 less than 40 on 100% oxygen
pH less than 7
pCO_2 greater than 70 to 75
Criteria for assisted ventilation in infants
pO_2 less than 55 to 60
pH less than 7.25
pCO_2 greater than 60

EVALUATION

EXPECTED OUTCOMES

1 Adequate respiratory function is maintained. *If not*, follow these alternative nursing actions:
ANA: Auscultate lungs to determine if air flow through the lungs is adequate.
ANA: Auscultate lungs to identify presence of adventitious lung sounds.

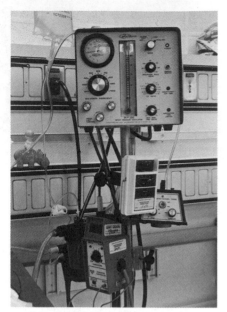

Examples of equipment that monitor ventilator settings, oxygen percentage, humidification and temperature, CPAP and PEEP, IPPB, IMV.

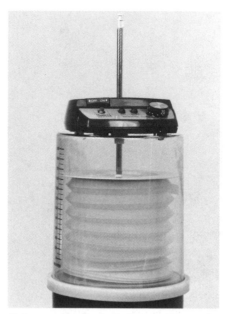

Bellows spirometer includes an alarm to alert nursing staff when adequate tidal volume is not achieved.

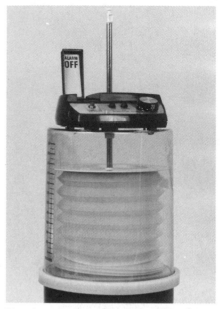

The alarm should always be on. When the alarm is off a red "alarm off" plate is easily observed for safety check.

ANA: Suction lungs frequently to increase pulmonary ventilation.

ANA: Assess that the ventilator is set at the proper settings and that the system is functioning properly.

ANA: Observe for possible leak in cuff if pressure settings are not maintained.

2 Arterial blood gas values are improved. *If not*, follow these alternative nursing actions:

ANA: Auscultate lungs for adventitious lung sounds and suction as needed.

ANA: Obtain order to "sigh" client, if not already doing so.

ANA: Assess if client is ventilated adequately via the respirator.

UNEXPECTED OUTCOMES

1 Client breathes out of synchronization with the ventilator.

ANA: Check arterial blood gases; as anxiety increases, struggling occurs, which is a common sign of hypoxemia.

ANA: Remove client from the ventilator, and hand ventilate at a rate faster than the machine (to blow off carbon dioxide and diminish client's ventilatory drive). Slowly decrease rate until it is the same as the ventilator setting. Place client back on the ventilator, while reassuring and coaching client to breathe in synchronization with ventilator.

ANA: If problem persists and arterial blood gas values and ventilator settings are adequate, consult with physician about the use of sedation or neuromuscular blocking agents to paralyze client.

ANA: Remove client from the ventilator, and hand ventilate with ambu or Laerdahl bag connected to 100 percent oxygen.

ANA: Request therapist or physician to recheck accuracy of settings.

2 Sudden respiratory distress, cyanosis, distended neck veins, or a possible tracheal shift.

ANA: Immediately remove client from ventilator and hand ventilate.

ANA: Immediately notify physician as these are signs of a tension pneumothorax.

ANA: If physician is not immediately available and you are trained in performing emergency chest decompression, insert a large bore (15 gauge) needle in the second intercostal space.

ANA: Prepare equipment and client for chest tube insertion.

ANA: Assist the physician with chest tube insertion.

3 Blood gas alterations, decreased compliance, and diminished breath sounds.

ANA: Suction client more frequently as these are signs of atelectasis.

ANA: Implement program of chest physical therapy. Provide percussion, vibration, drainage, deep breathing/sighing, and suctioning at least every two hours.

ANA: Turn client frequently.

ANA: "Yawn" client several times an hour to reopen atelectatic alveoli, hyperinflate lungs with a brief pause at the end of inspiration mimicking a normal yawn.

4 Symptoms of dyspnea, burning chest pain on inspiration, decreasing PaO_2, and dry cough, indicating oxygen toxicity.

ANA: Prevent oxygen toxicity by returning FIO_2 to specified setting after increasing it to 1.0 for oxygenation pre and post-suctioning or for determination A-a Δ pO_2 difference.

ANA: Obtain physician's order to reduce the FIO_2 as quickly as possible. (The danger of oxygen toxicity is increased with prolonged use of FIO_2 over 0.5.)

ANA: Check FIO_2 settings hourly.

5 Rales, edema, weight gain, and pulmonary edema, indicating fluid imbalance.

ANA: Notify physician for orders to slow IV rates.

ANA: Administer diuretics.

ANA: Apply rotating tourniquets.

6 Pressure alarm is activated.

ANA: Check for kinks or obstructions in tubing and take corrective measures.

ANA: Suction client for possible mucus obstruction.

ANA: Obtain order for and administer bronchodilators.

ANA: Assess for pneumothorax.

ANA: If unable to find cause for alarm, remove client from the ventilator and hand ventilate while respirator is checked for malfunction.

7 Volume alarm is activated.

ANA: Check if inspiratory phase is shortened due to pressure being reached earlier than normal. Tidal volume is decreased when this occurs.

607

ANA: Check for disconnected tubing.

ANA: Check for loose connections and tighten them if present.

ANA: Check whether the plug has been pulled out of the wall socket.

ANA: Check the volume indicator stick on the ventilator bellows. In some models, the arm that supports the ventilator tubing may become jostled and obstruct the movement of the stick. If so, readjust the arm so the bellows can move freely.

ANA: Deflate and reinflate the airway cuff to detect a cuff leak.

ANA: If unable to identify and relieve the cause immediately, disconnect the ventilator tubing, hand ventilate the client, and summon help.

8 Fever, elevated white blood cell count, or changed odor or color of respiratory secretions.

ANA: Send sputum specimen for culture and sensitivity.

ANA: Administer antibiotics as ordered.

ANA: Examine suctioning technique for breaks in aseptic technique.

9 Subcutaneous or mediastinal emphysema, as manifested by puffy tissues that crackle on palpation, or a crunching sound with each heartbeat when the heart is auscultated.

ANA: Notify physician.

ANA: If ordered, assist with chest tube insertion.

ANA: If chest tube already in place, switch to a drainage system with an air leak indicator.

ANA: If ordered, assist physician with expelling air from tissues by placing needles or drains in tissues and "milking" the tissues toward you.

ANA: Observe client closely for development of respiratory distress due to tracheal compression.

Charting

- Type of ventilator used
- Ventilator settings
- Time mechanical ventilation started
- Any problems with ventilator and actions taken
- Results of suctioning, i.e., amount of secretions obtained and color and odor of secretions
- Tidal volume obtained, sighing volume if indicated

ACTION: WEANING CLIENT FROM VENTILATOR

ASSESSMENT

1 Measure vital signs, inspiratory pressure, vital capacity, and arterial blood gases.

2 Evaluate client parameters indicating readiness for weaning.

   a PaO_2 of 70 mm Hg or better on an FIO_2 of 0.5 or less.

   b   PEEP 5 cm or less, if used.

   c   Vital capacity of 15 ml/kg or better.

   d   Inspiratory pressure of -25 cm H_2O or better.

   e   A-a Δ pO_2 difference less than 350 mm Hg on 100 percent oxygen.

   f   Shunt less than 30 percent.

   g   Respiratory rate between 12 to 20 breaths per minute.

   h   Blood pressure and pulse stable.

3 Note current ECG pattern as a baseline.

4 Review the physician's order regarding details of weaning.

Rationale for Action

- To identify clients who are capable of maintaining respirations without the use of mechanical ventilators
- To reestablish normal breathing patterns for clients on mechanical ventilators

PLANNING

GOALS

- Laboratory parameters indicate client is ready for weaning.
- Client is able to maintain respiratory status without mechanical ventilation.
- Arterial blood gases maintained within normal range for client.

EQUIPMENT

- Heated humidified oxygen source with wide bore tubing
- T-piece adaptor
- Suctioning supplies
- Arterial blood gas sampling supplies

INTERVENTION: Taking Client off Ventilator

1 Explain the discontinuation process to client. Reassure client that you will watch closely and, if necessary, discontinue weaning and attempt later.
2 Suction client. Hyperinflate client's lungs with 100 percent oxygen before and after suctioning.
3 Maintain inflated endotracheal or tracheostomy cuff during weaning.
4 If physician orders cuff deflated during weaning, suction secretions that have accumulated above the cuff as follows:
   a Provide positive pressure to end of tube with a hand-held resuscitation bag and 100 percent oxygen.
   b Place tip of suction catheter in the posterior pharynx.
   c Deflate cuff and apply suction to catheter. The positive pressure will blow the secretions into the pharynx, where they can be suctioned out.
   d Hyperinflate lungs with 100 percent oxygen for 3 to 5 breaths.
5 Elevate head of the bed to facilitate diaphragmatic excursion.
6 Connect T-piece to wide bore oxygen tubing leading to the source of warm, humidified oxygen.
7 Set oxygen concentration as ordered by physician, usually 0.10 higher than the ventilator FIO_2 the client has been receiving.
8 Remove ventilator tubing from airway and connect airway to the T-piece.
9 Cover end of ventilator tubing with sterile gauze.
10 Monitor vital signs every 5 minutes until stable.
11 Observe for vital sign changes, apprehension, diaphoresis, and dysrhythmias. (A mild increase in blood pressure, pulse, and respiratory rate is normal. Mild-to-moderate anxiety is also normal.)
12 Measure arterial blood gases fifteen minutes after initiating weaning.
13 Proceed with weaning procedure. Length of the weaning is ordered by physician.

With client on ventilator a short time
a Continuous weaning may be ordered.
b Leave client on the T-piece.
c Obtain vital signs hourly.
d Monitor arterial blood gases every four hours.
e If client tolerates weaning well for two to six hours, weaning may be discontinued and the artificial airway may be removed.
With client on prolonged ventilation
a Gradual weaning may be ordered.
b Following intermittent weaning time period, remove T-piece and place client back on ventilator.
c Obtain vital signs hourly.
d Monitor arterial blood gases every four hours.
e Extend weaning periods 15 to 30 minutes each time until client is able to tolerate several hours on the T-piece.
f Remove the artificial airway.
14 Following weaning, measure vital signs, vital capacity, inspiratory pressure, and arterial blood gases.

EVALUATION

EXPECTED OUTCOMES

1 Laboratory parameters indicate client is ready for weaning. *If not*, follow these alternative nursing actions:
   ANA: Continue mechanical ventilation as ordered.
   ANA: If ventilation settings do not improve client's respiratory status, notify physician for change in orders.
   ANA: Attempt to use T-piece and 40 percent oxygen for longer time periods each hour until laboratory parameters are reached.
   ANA: Assess client for possible respiratory complications that may be interfering with the weaning process.
2 Client able to maintain respiratory status without mechanical ventilation. *If not*, follow these alternative nursing actions:
   ANA: Continue use of ventilator.
   ANA: If client has been extubated, prepare equipment and client for intubation and placement on a ventilator.
   ANA: If respiratory distress occurs with unintubated client, ventilate with ambu or Laerdahl bag, using a face mask.
3 Arterial blood gases (ABGs) maintained within normal range. *If not*, follow these alternative nursing actions:
   ANA: Notify physician of abnormal ABGs and obtain order for alteration in ventilation, i.e., increased percent of oxygen, added dead space, etc.
   ANA: Maintain mechanical ventilation. Do not attempt to wean or extubate client.
   ANA: Suction client frequently if secretions are thick and/or copious in amount.
   ANA: If severe acidosis occurs, obtain order for increasing the respiratory rate to blow off carbon dioxide, or administer sodium bicarbonate to buffer acidotic state.

UNEXPECTED OUTCOMES

1 Decreased level of consciousness, dyspnea, severe anxiety, or severe fatigue.

ANA: Obtain arterial blood gases.

ANA: Place client back on ventilator.

2 Unstable vital signs, development of premature beats on ECG, or ST segment depression.

ANA: Place client back on ventilator.

ANA: Monitor vital signs q 15 minutes and obtain blood gases to determine oxygen concentration.

3 Client unable to be weaned because of emotionally-induced anxiety.

ANA: Reassess that anxiety is emotionally based by measuring physical parameters. Anxiety is a common early sign of hypoxia.

ANA: Provide increased reassurance to client.

ANA: Consult with physician about weaning with intermittent mandatory ventilation (IMV). The IMV allows brief rest periods, decreases fatigue, and facilitates psychological adaptation. Since client is usually unaware of exact rate adjustments, weaning with IMV is less emotionally traumatic than weaning with a T-piece.

▶ Intermittent mandatory ventilation (IMV) delivers a specific number of breaths, in addition to client's spontaneous breaths.

Charting

- Preweaning vital signs, vital capacity, inspiratory pressure, and blood gas values
- Method of weaning
- FIO$_2$
- Time weaning started
- Vital signs, blood gases, and physical signs and symptoms during weaning period
- Time weaning terminated and reason

ACTION: PROVIDING POSITIVE END EXPIRATORY PRESSURE (PEEP)

ASSESSMENT

1 Assess client for presence of risk factors for acute respiratory distress syndrome: massive trauma, massive fat embolism, aspiration pneumonia, and other disorders characterized by abnormal gas distribution (due to airway or alveolar closure) and pulmonary interstitial edema.

2 Assess client for indications for PEEP:

a Inability to maintain arterial pO$_2$ of at least 70 mm Hg on 50 percent oxygen during continuous mechanical ventilation.

b Failure of other methods to reduce pulmonary shunt, e.g., treatment of cardiac failure or pneumonia.

c Normovolemia. (Normal state of blood volume.)

3 Check physician's orders regarding amount and duration of PEEP. Usual range is 5 to 15 cm H$_2$O. (20 to 35 cm H$_2$O have been used.)

4 Assess vital signs and measure arterial blood gases and hemodynamic pressures (CVP and pulmonary artery wedge pressure).

PLANNING

GOALS

- Oxygenation of tissue is improved and pO$_2$ is maintained at 80 to 100 mm Hg on low oxygen concentration.
- Pulmonary pathology is reduced.
- Functional residual capacity and compliance are increased.

Rationale for Action

- To assist in keeping the alveoli open on expiration, thereby reducing shunt, increasing functional residual capacity (FRC), and improving compliance
- To assist in surfactant regeneration
- To improve oxygenation without prolonged use of high oxygenation concentrations
- To maintain respiratory function in adult respiratory distress syndrome (ARDS)

611

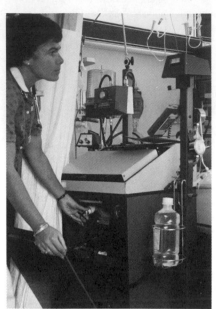

PEEP and CPAP settings are checked hourly to ensure accuracy of treatment.

EQUIPMENT

- Mechanical ventilator with built-in PEEP device or
- Mechanical ventilator without PEEP
- Connecting tubing attached to ventilator expiratory port
- Cylinder containing water, under which the end of the connecting tubing is submerged.

INTERVENTION: Maintaining Mechanical Ventilation with PEEP

1 Notify respiratory therapist of order for PEEP.
2 Briefly explain procedure to client.
3 Gradually increase PEEP to specified level while monitoring respiratory and cardiovascular status.
4 Monitor vital signs every 15 minutes × 4 and then hourly. Transient hypotension is common with PEEP.
5 Check blood gases 15 to 30 minutes after stabilization and adjust PEEP accordingly.
6 Check inspiratory pressure and PEEP setting dial hourly on ventilators with built-in PEEP. On other setups, check inspiratory pressure and level of water column hourly.
7 Check exhalation port tubing hourly for kinks or other obstructions.
8 Monitor blood gases every two to four hours.
9 Inspect, palpate, and auscultate chest hourly to detect subcutaneous emphysema, or pneumothorax development.
10 Monitor cardiac outputs hourly if Swan-Ganz catheter is in place and PEEP is more than 5 cm H_2O. (May see fall in cardiac output.)
11 As condition improves, lower PEEP pressure.

INTERVENTION: Providing Hand Ventilation with PEEP

1 Identify need for hand ventilation, i.e., mechanical ventilator failure or client transport.
2 Start oxygen flow through handheld ventilating device.
3 Attach expiratory resistance, for example PEEP valve.
4 Disconnect ventilator tubing from airway at end of inspiration.
5 Attach handheld ventilator to airway during expiration.
6 Watch chest and provide breaths in synchrony with client's inspirations (if any) or at rate of 10 to 12/minute.

EVALUATION

EXPECTED OUTCOMES

1 Oxygenation of tissues is improved and pO_2 is maintained at 80 to 100 mm Hg. *If not*, follow these alternative nursing actions:
ANA: Continue delivery of PEEP at ordered prescribed volume. If this is not affective, obtain an order for increased volume.
ANA: Do not attempt to wean client off PEEP until parameters are maintained or improved.

2 Pulmonary pathology is reduced. *If not*, follow these alternative nursing actions:

ANA: Continue with PEEP.

ANA: Evaluate other treatment modalities for effectiveness.

ANA: Monitor drug therapy, such as antibiotic or diuretic and cardiotonic for effectiveness.

ANA: Evaluate the results of respiratory toilet and monitor amount, type, and consistency of secretions.

UNEXPECTED OUTCOMES

1 Significant decrease in cardiac output.

ANA: Anticipate that clients with decreased sympathetic reserve may have difficulty adjusting to increased intrathoracic pressure. Examples are clients who are elderly, hypovolemic, or on sympatholytic medications.

ANA: If cardiac output falls abruptly, or severely decreases, terminate PEEP trial and notify physician.

2 Pneumothorax occurs.

ANA: Discontinue PEEP and take client off ventilator; hand ventilate with ambu or Laerdahl bag and 100 percent oxygen.

ANA: Notify physician and prepare to assist with chest tube insertion.

ANA: If tension pneumothorax occurs, assist with emergency chest decompression with large-bore needle, three-way stopcock, and large syringe.

Charting Content

- Pre-PEEP assessment including presence of risk factors
- Time of trials on PEEP and levels of PEEP used, with client's responses
- Volume of PEEP on which client is stabilized
- Arterial blood gas values
- CVP and/or PAWP readings
- Results of lung and cardiac auscultation

ACTION: PROVIDING CONTINUOUS POSITIVE AIRWAY PRESSURE (CPAP)

ASSESSMENT

1 Review physician's order for amount and duration of CPAP.
2 Obtain baseline vital signs, blood gas values, and hemodynamic pressures if CVP and Swan-Ganz lines are in place.
3 Auscultate heart and lung sounds for baseline data.

PLANNING

GOALS

- Oxygenation to tissues is improved.
- Pulmonary pathology is decreased.

EQUIPMENT

- Clear face mask with straps
- Inspiratory and expiratory tubing with one-way valves
- Oxygen source
- Oxygen-air mixer

Rationale for Action

- To improve oxygenation for clients who are able to spontaneously ventilate without the use of mechanical ventilation
- To establish a resistance to expiration to maintain the airway under constant positive pressure
- To enable clients to avoid mechanical ventilation when pulmonary dysfunction is acute and reversible

▶ Do not use an opaque mask. To minimize aspiration, you need to be able to see if the client vomits into the mask.

613

- Reservoir bag
- Humidification warming device
- CPAP device with safety pop-off (PEEP valve, cylinder containing water)
- Pressure gauge

INTERVENTION: Initiating CPAP

1 Notify respiratory therapist of physician's order.
2 Briefly explain procedure to client and family.
3 Start flow of warm, humidified oxygen through CPAP system.
4 Strap facemask on client to form tight seal.
5 Connect CPAP device to expiratory tubing.
6 Slowly increase expiratory resistance to level specified by physician. CPAP is usually not delivered at more than 10 cm of H_2O.
7 Reassure client, especially if dyspneic, that CPAP will help to ease his or her underlying condition.
8 Instruct client to breathe slowly and deeply. Clients may panic due to mask over nose and mouth. In addition, there is the increased work of breathing caused by CPAP.
9 Monitor vital signs, blood gases, and pulmonary artery wedge pressures.

INTERVENTION: Maintaining CPAP

1 Monitor respiratory and cardiovascular status hourly as CPAP may precipitate acute respiratory failure. This may be due to CO_2 retention from fatigue, or cardiac failure due to increased intrathoracic pressure.
2 Observe frequently for air leaks in system, especially around mask.
3 Check pressure gauge frequently.
4 Observe for abdominal distention due to air swallowing.
5 Interrupt CPAP every 2 hours and provide warm, humidified oxygen via face tent for ten minutes.
   a During this time, check respiratory and cardiovascular status to aid in determining resolution of pulmonary disorder.
   b Clean and dry face. Lotion may be applied to reddened areas.
   c Provide time to eat and talk in addition to relieving pressure on face.
6 Reapply CPAP.
7 Change the tubing every 48 hours to minimize infection.
8 Provide communication method such as a "magic slate" for client while mask is in place.

EVALUATION

EXPECTED OUTCOMES

1 Oxygenation is improved to the tissues. *If not*, follow these alternative nursing actions:

ANA: Monitor blood gases and pulmonary artery wedge pressures. If they remain abnormal even with treatment, notify physician for possible orders for mechanical ventilation and PEEP.

ANA: Continue to use CPAP and instruct client to breathe slowly and deeply. Anxiety decreases the client's ability to utilize oxygen.

2 Pulmonary pathology is decreased. *If not*, follow these alternative nursing actions:

ANA: Ensure adequate pulmonary toilet is being done in addition to CPAP with clients who have increased secretions.

ANA: Monitor effects of drug therapy for cardiac or pulmonary disorders.

ANA: Assess client's need for mechanical ventilation with PEEP.

UNEXPECTED OUTCOMES

1 Client complains of nausea.

ANA: Immediately remove mask and supply oxygen via face tent while assessing cause of nausea.

ANA: Insert nasogastric tube to remove air and fluid from stomach.

ANA: If impending vomiting, place client in supine position with head turned to side or place client on side to minimize risk of aspiration.

2 Client complains of fatigue, increasing dyspnea or coma, or apnea occur.

ANA: Assist physician with intubation and mechanical ventilation.

3 Pneumothorax occurs.

ANA: Discontinue CPAP and bag the client with an ambu or Laerdahl bag if necessary. Use 100 percent oxygen with bagging.

ANA: Notify physician and prepare to assist with chest tube insertion.

ANA: If tension pneumothorax occurs, assist with emergency chest decompression.

Charting
- Pressure volume of CPAP utilized
- Client's ability to tolerate CPAP
- Findings of cardiac and respiratory assessment
- Vital signs
- Complications that occurred and specific treatment
- Blood gas values and pulmonary artery wedge pressures

ACTION: PROVIDING INTERMITTENT POSITIVE PRESSURE BREATHING (IPPB)

ASSESSMENT

1 Evaluate client's need for IPPB.
2 Evaluate arterial blood gases, sputum cultures, and chest x-rays.
3 Review the physician's IPPB order for settings, length of treatment, and medications to be used.
4 Assess client's lung sounds before and after each treatment.
5 Observe consistency, amount and color of expectorated sputum.
6 Assess need for additional physiotherapy to improve respiratory function.

Rationale for Action
- To deliver aerosol medications
- To decrease the work of breathing
- To promote a better ventilation/perfusion ratio by increasing bronchodilatation and alveolar ventilation
- To prevent or treat atelectasis
- To loosen secretions
- To decrease pulmonary edema

615

PLANNING

GOALS

- Increased expectoration of secretions.
- Decreased work of breathing.
- Improved blood gas values.
- Lung sounds improved.
- Aerosol medications administered into deep air passages.

EQUIPMENT

- IPPB machine (Bennett or Bird) or pressure-preset ventilator
- Ventilator tubing
- Nebulizer and manifold
- Mouthpiece
- Nose piece (optional)
- Power source (oxygen, compressed air, or electricity, depending on the machine)
- Tidal volume spirometer

INTERVENTION: Setting Up the Puritan-Bennett PR 2

1   Notify respiratory therapy department regarding the order for IPPB therapy.
2   Gather equipment if nursing performs this activity in your facility. The PR 2 can be used as an IPPB machine or a pressure-preset ventilator.

Clinical Alert

Do not use oxygen as the power source for clients with COPD.

▶ IPPB is contraindicated in any condition predisposing to pneumothorax (such as bullous emphysema), in some cardiovascular disorders, and for clients unable to cooperate.

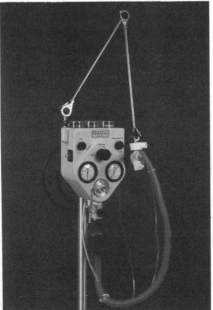

Bennett PR-2 respirator is most commonly used for IPPB treatments.

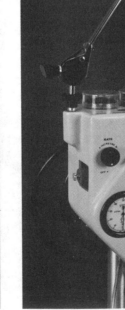

Check all the settings on the Bennett respirator before each IPPB treatment.

3 Connect pressure hose to wall oxygen outlet or compressed air.
4 Attach tubing to the machine.
5 Unscrew the nebulizer cup.
6 Place medication or distilled water in the cup and replace it.
7 Adjust the air mix knob: pull it out to give 100 percent oxygen and push it in to administer an air mix.
8 Set the pressure: turn the pressure control knob (in the middle front of the machine) clockwise until the right-hand pressure control gauge reads the ordered pressure.
9 Check that the peak flow knob is completely open (at the maximal counterclockwise position). Do not adjust peak flow without checking with a therapist or physician.
10 Turn the ventilation rate off. This dial is turned on only for use of the PR 2 in controlled ventilation.
11 Remove the nebulizer from the manifold. Remove the dust cap and lift the drum pin.
12 Adjust the inspiration nebulization knob until a fine mist appears. Lower the drum pin and replace the dust cap.
13 Replace the nebulizer in the manifold.
14 Set the sensitivity control to off by turning the knob clockwise.

INTERVENTION: Setting Up the Bird Mark 7

1 Notify respiratory therapy department regarding the order for IPPB therapy.
2 Gather equipment if nursing performs this activity in your facility. The Bird can be used as an IPPB machine or as a pressure-preset ventilator.
3 Attach tubing to the machine.
4 Hold the nebulizer unit with the cap uppermost. Remove the cap, instill the medication or distilled water, and replace the cap.
5 Adjust the air mix. Push the knob in for 100 percent oxygen and pull it out for an air mix. The positioning of this knob for 100 percent oxygen is the exact opposite of that for the Bennett PR 2.
6 Connect the pressure hose to the oxygen outlet.
7 Set the pressure, using the pressure control on the right side of the machine. The usual initial setting is 15 cm.
8 Turn off the dial marked "expiratory time for apnea."
9 Set the sensitivity to 15. The sensitivity control is on the left side of the machine.
10 Set the flow rate dial (on the right side of the machine) to 15 cm. This turns the machine on.

INTERVENTION: Administering a Nebulized Treatment

1 Explain rationale for treatment.
2 Complete client teaching.
3 Administer pain medication about 30 minutes before treatment if client has postsurgical chest or abdominal pain.

Nurse-Client Teaching

1 Explain the rationale for the treatment in understandable terms.
2 Place client in high-Fowler's position. Place client on side of bed in sitting position with feet on floor, or have client sit in chair.
3 Instruct client on the following:
   a Keep lips closed tightly around the mouthpiece.
   b Breathe only through mouth.
   c Breathe slowly.
   d To trigger the machine, breathe in slightly. Then relax and let the machine complete the breath while client expands lower chest and abdomen.
   e Hold breath briefly at the end of each inspiration.
   f Exhale normally, around the mouthpiece.

4 Post a ''No Smoking'' sign and alert visitors and other clients in the room not to smoke.
5 Check client's pulse rate before, during, and after treatment.
6 Begin treatment by placing nose clip on client and having client inhale through the machine.
7 Provide instruction until client has mastered the correct technique.
8 Gradually increase pressure until client is receiving the ordered pressure.
   a On the Puritan-Bennett PR 2, turn the pressure control knob until the left-hand delivered pressure gauge reads the ordered pressure.
   b On the Puritan-Bennett AP 5, turn the pressure control knob until the pressure gauge shows the ordered pressure at the end of inspiration.
   c On the Bird, turn the pressure control until the gauge on the front of the machine shows the ordered pressure.
9 Observe the chest for full expansion.
10 Encourage periodic coughing to remove secretions.
11 Tap the nebulizer cup periodically to move moisture to the bottom. Continue treatment until the nebulizer is empty, usually about 20 minutes. If the nebulizer becomes empty before the end of the prescribed treatment period, add distilled water.
12 Check pulse, blood pressure, and respiratory rate at the end of treatment.
13 Assist client to a comfortable position.
14 Remind client of the value of the treatment and give positive reinforcement for cooperation.

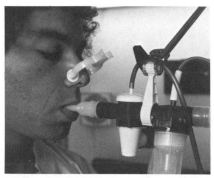

Place nose clip on the client, instruct client to inhale through mouthpiece and observe that the nebulizer emits a fine mist during the treatment.

Ensure that client is receiving an adequate tidal volume. The tidal volume can be measured while giving the IPPB treatment.

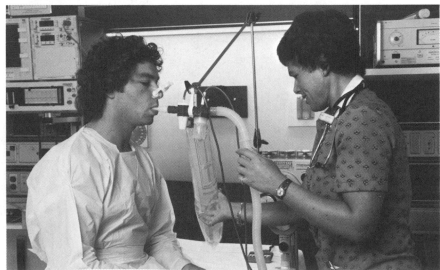

The Misty Nebulizer with Tee adapter is a new type of nebulizer.

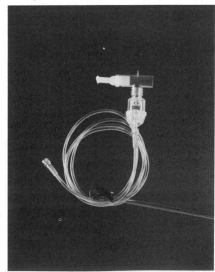

EVALUATION

1 Increased expectoration of secretions. *If not*, follow these alternative nursing actions:
   ANA: Check that the nebulizer is expelling a fine mist.
   ANA: Notify physician for medication order change to a drug that lowers surface tension of sputum, thereby facilitating expectoration.
   ANA: Encourage deep breathing and coughing between IPPB treatments.
   ANA: Obtain order for PVD.
2 Decreased work of breathing. *If not*, follow these alternative nursing actions:
   ANA: Ensure that client is positioned in Fowler's or at least semi-Fowler's position to facilitate breathing.
   ANA: Have client expectorate mucus. If unable to cough productively, suction client.
   ANA: Evaluate need for additional treatments or potential need for assisted mechanical ventilation.
   ANA: Use relaxation techniques if client is anxious.
3 Improved blood gas values. *If not*, follow these alternative nursing actions:
   ANA: Promote client's ability to deep breathe and cough by placing in Fowler's position and splinting client while client is deep breathing and coughing.
   ANA: Provide suctioning at least every two hours if client is unable to expectorate by him or herself.
   ANA: Evaluate client's need for continuous mechanical ventilation.
   ANA: Notify physician of assessment findings.
4 Lung sounds improved. *If not*, follow these alternative nursing actions:
   ANA: Monitor lung sounds before and after each treatment.
   ANA: Identify area of lung that contains adventitious sounds, and administer PVD to the specific area.
   ANA: Obtain order to change medications or increase number of treatments.
5 Aerosol medications administered into deep air passages. *If not*, follow these alternative nursing actions:
   ANA: Monitor client's ability to inhale deeply, thereby ensuring penetration of medications into deep passages.
   ANA: Observe for air leaks around nose and mouth, which would prevent medications from reaching deep passages.
   ANA: Place client in semi- or high-Fowler's position.

UNEXPECTED OUTCOMES

1 Persistent breathing through nose during treatment.
   ANA: Instruct the client to use only mouth breathing.
   ANA: Apply a nose clip if not already being used to occlude the nose.

2 Pulse rate increased 20 or more beats per minute.

ANA: Evaluate cause; the most common causes are anxiety, decreased venous return, and drug reactions.

ANA: Reassure the anxious client.

ANA: Discontinue treatment and consult with physician.

3 Vertigo and tingling of extremities (symptoms of respiratory alkalosis secondary to hyperventilation).

ANA: Reduce rate of breathing.

4 Inability to trigger the machine at the usual sensitivity setting.

ANA: On the PR 2, increase sensitivity by turning the sensitivity knob to the left. On the Bird, increase sensitivity by pushing the sensitivity control lever toward the back of the machine (toward a lower number).

5 Pressure setting reached too quickly.

ANA: Check tubing for kinks.

ANA: Encourage client to cough.

ANA: Suction client if client is unable to expectorate secretions.

ANA: Instruct client not to resist the airflow or blow back into the machine.

ANA: Decrease the flow rate (and the pressure) in the Bird.

6 Machine will not cycle off.

ANA: Check for leak in tubing.

ANA: Check for leak around mask, mouthpiece, or tracheostomy tube.

ANA: Increase the flow rate (and the pressure) in the Bird.

7 Chest does not expand fully even though set pressure is reached.

ANA: Check for kinks in tubing.

ANA: Increase inspiratory pressure slowly to a maximum of 25.

ANA: If more than 25 cm of pressure are needed, obtain a physician's order specifying maximum pressure.

8 Development of pneumothorax.

ANA: Terminate treatment and notify physician.

ANA: Assist with chest tube insertion if indicated.

9 COPD client becomes lethargic, and respiratory rate slows (signs of suppression of the hypoxic drive to breathe).

ANA: If physician has ordered oxygen during IPPB, ensure that the air-oxygen mix is correct.

ANA: Terminate treatment and consult physician.

ANA: If respiratory arrest occurs, ventilate client mouth-to-mouth or with a handheld resuscitator.

ANA: Use compressed air rather than oxygen in future treatments.

ANA: Switch to a unit powered by electricity, such as the Puritan-Bennett AP 5.

Charting
- Medication and dose
- Type of machine used for IPPB
- Settings used on IPPB machine
- Duration of treatment
- Amount, consistency, and color of secretions obtained
- Client's tolerance for treatment

SUPPLEMENT

RESPIRATORY CONDITIONS

atelectasis: This condition may be caused by a mucous plug closing a bronchus. Atelectasis can also occur when nitrogen is washed out of the lungs because a high FIO_2 has been delivered to the client. Symptoms of atelectasis include dyspnea, chest pain, cyanosis, and sweating.

chylothorax: Milky chyle that has entered pleural space from the thoracic duct.

hemothorax: Blood in pleural space as a result of severed blood vessels.

pneumothorax: The presence of air or gas in the intrathoracic space; results in lung collapse.

pyothorax: Exudate in pleural space.

retrolental fibroplasia: A condition marked by the presence of opaque tissue behind the lens, which can lead to blindness. Condition is usually caused by elevated arterial levels of oxygen in premature infants.

spontaneous pneumothorax: Develops from air leaks in pulmonary alveoli or from erosion by a disease process through the pulmonary pleura.

tension pneumothorax: Massive lung collapse and shift of the mediastinum resulting from extensive accumulation of air in the intrapleural space.

RESPIRATORY PRESSURES

A   At inspiration the intraalveolar pressure is more negative than the atmospheric pressure.

B   At expiration the intraalveolar is more positive, thereby pressing the air out of the lungs.

C   A negative pressure exists in the intrapleural space and aids in keeping the visceral pleura of the lungs against the parietal pleura of the chest wall. Lung space enlarges as the chest wall expands.

D   Recoil tendency of the lungs is due to the elastic fibers in the lungs and the surfactant.

LUNG VOLUMES

A   Vital capacity (VC) — volume of air that is able to be expelled following a maximum inspiration.

B   Tidal volume — amount of air normally inspired.

C   Reserve volume (RV) — volume of air remaining in the lungs at the end of maximum expiration.

D   Inspiratory reserve volume (IRV) — volume of air that can be inspired above the tidal volume.

E   Inspiratory capacity (IC) — volume of air with maximum inspiration; comprises tidal volume and inspiratory reserve volume.

F   Expiratory reserve volume (ERV) — volume of air that can be expelled following a resting expiration.

CHAPTER 17
Alterations in Circulation

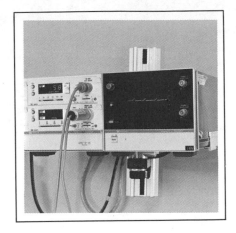

This chapter presents the conceptual basis for alterations in circulation and their nursing management. It includes planned nursing intervention and skills necessary to promote circulation and to preserve the integrity of the circulatory system if nursing and/or medical procedures become necessary. A brief anatomical review with physiological considerations provides an introduction to the cardiovascular system.

ANATOMY AND PHYSIOLOGY OF THE CIRCULATORY SYSTEM

The heart is a three-layered, four-chambered vessel, approximately the size of an adult fist. It weighs close to 600 grams in the normal adult. A thick, fibrous sheath, called the pericardium, surrounds about two-thirds of the heart's surface. Most of the mass lies in the heart's middle layer — the myocardium, or cardiac muscle. The endocardium, a thin, inner layer, lines the four chambers.

In considering the heart's chambers, imagine two major pump systems. The right and left atria contract in one phase, and the right and left ventricles contract in the successive phase. The tricuspid, pulmonary, mitral, and aortic valves are the four flow regulators for the chambers.

Three properties of cardiac muscle best illustrate the heart's specialization. Automaticity physiologically differentiates heart muscle from all other muscle tissue. The other two properties — conductivity and contractility — characterize all muscle; however, a cardiac contraction is normally all or none, as opposed to partial contractions in other muscles.

The heart serves as a pump to maintain blood flow and blood pressure. Adequate blood flow perfuses the lungs for oxygenation. Blood pressure is a driving force for that flow and is normally highest during ventricular contractions. The heart pumps 4 to 7 liters of blood per minute. This constitutes a normal cardiac output, formulated by multiplying contraction volume times ventricular rate.

When the heart maintains a safe blood pressure and blood flow, it is in a state of compensation, regardless of cardiac output. If the heart cannot maintain a safe blood pressure and blood flow, it is in a state of decompensation. Three cardiac reserves allow for compensation: inotropic reserve, increased venous filling pressure, and chronotropic reserve.

Inotropic reserve is under the control of sympathetic nerve stimulation. Adrenergic drugs, as well as some others, exert an inotropic effect by increasing the force of the cardiac contraction and therefore stroke volume. Cardiac output will also increase with additional filling pressure in the atria. Starling's Law of the Heart summarizes the relationship by stating that an increased filling pressure causes an increased force of contraction within the elastic limits of the heart. Finally, chronotropic reserve refers to increased cardiac output. Atropine-like drugs exert a chronotropic effect by increasing the heart rate.

Blood vessels, together with the heart, form a closed circulatory system unless there is damage or abnormalities that result in leakage. When the ventricles contract, blood leaves the right ventricle through the pulmonic valve into the pulmonary artery. Blood is now in the pulmonary circulation for oxygenation of the red blood cells or erythrocytes. This occurs due to a specialized "heme complex," constituting the erythrocyte's molecular structure. After gas exchanges occur at the cellular

Blood flow pattern through right and left side of the heart.

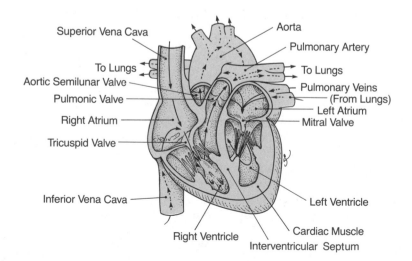

Superior Vena Cava

Aorta

Pulmonary Artery

To Lungs

To Lungs

Aortic Semilunar Valve

Pulmonic Valve

Pulmonary Veins (From Lungs)

Left Atrium

Right Atrium

Mitral Valve

Tricuspid Valve

Inferior Vena Cava

Left Ventricle

Right Ventricle

Cardiac Muscle

Interventricular Septum

level, the blood is returned to the left atrium through four pulmonary veins. This is normally the most oxygenated blood in the human body.

On the left side of the heart during a ventricular contraction, blood travels through the aortic valve out of the left ventricle into the ascending aorta. Five percent, or 200 to 250 ml, of this blood enters coronary circulation for oxygenation and waste removal from the cardiac tissue. Fifteen percent, or 750 to 850 ml, travels to the brain and twenty-five percent, or 1400 to 1600 ml, goes to the kidneys, and the same amount to other viscera. The extremities and skin normally receive thirty percent of the circulating volume.

Arteries carry blood from the heart throughout the body unless obstructed or severed. The largest subdivision is the aorta and the smallest subdivision is the arteriole. Similar to the heart, arteries have three layers: endothelium, involuntary muscle, and connective tissue. Capillaries join the arterial system to the venous system and are a single cell layer in thickness. The thinness allows gas, nutrient, and waste exchanges to occur throughout the body. Blood enters the venous system from the capillary beds for eventual return to the right side of the heart via the superior and inferior venae cavae.

PATHOLOGY OF THE CIRCULATORY SYSTEM

There are many ways to taxonomize disorders of the heart, arteries, and veins. Endocarditis, myocarditis, and pericarditis classify cardiac problems according to inflammation of a particular heart layer. Another classification is congenital heart disease, such as tetralogy of Fallot and transposition of the great vessels. For the purpose of this chapter alterations of circulation are divided into hemorrhage, shock, pump failure, ischemia, thrombosis, and embolism.

Hemorrhage Hemorrhage results when trauma or disease causes leakage in the closed circulatory system. Damage to the heart or arteries usually constitute the greatest danger because of the high pressures and large volumes. Normally, when a blood vessel is ruptured or severed, compensatory mechanisms protect the body from significant blood loss. The wall of the injured vessel contracts immediately. A platelet plug forms at the site, and intrinsic/extrinsic blood clotting occurs. New connective tissue penetrates the clot for permanent closure. Interventions for clients who are hemorrhaging are based on one of these compensatory mechanisms.

To prevent, correct, or compensate for hemorrhage, the nurse must assess the client. He or she identifies the nature of the bleeding as external and/or internal and establishes baseline data, which includes blood pressure and vital signs. A determination is made whether or not the body's response is adaptive, excessive, or deficient. Immediately a nursing diagnosis is formulated and interventions are planned. The first concern is to minimize the client's stress since sympathetic stimulation of the heart increases heart rate (chronotropic effect) and force of contraction (inotropic effect). Interventions for hemorrhage involve restricting activity, elevating involved body areas above the heart if possible, applying direct pressure, and replacing lost fluid volume. A tourniquet is generally used as a last resort. It is placed proximal to the site of the hemorrhage with the knowledge that the extremity may be sacrificed.

Shock Unchecked hemorrhage eventually leads to hypovolemic or hemorrhagic shock, a serious state with a poor prognosis. Peripheral resistance is of great significance. In hemorrhagic shock, high peripheral resistance is secondary to pronounced peripheral vasoconstriction in the initial stage. Due to the loss of blood volume it becomes very difficult to start an intravenous line in a superficial vein. Vasoconstrictors, such as Levophed, are undesirable since they cause a further decline in tissue perfusion. Successful recognition and early treatment of hemorrhagic shock depends heavily upon sophisticated monitoring devices, the nature of the fluid for volume replacement, and the use of blood components instead of whole blood. Intervention centers on establishing one or more intravenous lines for fluid replacement, drug administration, and blood component therapy. Careful monitoring of peripheral pulses, blood pressure, central venous pressure, and even more sophisticated hemodynamic parameters, such as pulmonary arterial wedge pressures, is desirable.

The use of pressure devices, such as the antigravity suit (G-suit), the Jobst extremity pump, and inflatable splints are helpful adjuncts in treating clients in hemorrhagic shock. These devices provide pneumatic compression for immobilizing the client, controlling bleeding, and counteracting hypotension by maintaining venous pressure.

Pump Failure Heart failure results from any condition that reduces the ability of the heart to pump blood. The heart is no longer in a state of compensation, and cardiac output will fall. Cardiac arrhythmias and congestion are the most common types of pump failure.

Effective cardiac contraction depends upon correctly timed depolarization of cardiac cells, that is achieved in normal sinus rhythm. When a dysrhythmia (abnormal rhythm) occurs, the ideal timing of depolarization is disrupted, and pump failure can occur particularly when the dysrhythmia interferes with proper filling and emptying of the ventricles. This problem occurs when the client experiences ventricular fibrillation or tachycardia.

Heart failure has three successive phases of variable duration. The first phase is pathologic cardiac overloading due to excessive pressures, too much fluid, and/or myocardial tissue loss. The second phase of failure is cardiovascular compensatory response, such as dilatation and reflex responses. Finally, the heart fails to compensate, producing a wide variety of signs (objective data base) and symptoms (subjective data base).

Heart failure should not be confused with circulatory overload, a condition in which cardiac output is adequate but blood volume and/or venous return is excessive. Excessive infusion of IV fluids in too short a period of time results in circulatory overload.

Pulmonary edema, the most common result of pump failure, is a life threatening condition. Pulmonary edema is a disorder in which alveoli fill with fluid. It produces severe abnormalities in gas exchange and can lead to death if not treated immediately. There are several disorders that can cause pulmonary edema, all of which produce a high hydrostatic pressure in the pulmonary capillaries. Right ventricular output into the pulmonary capillaries depends in part on the volume of venous return to the heart.

Interventions for treating pump failure and pulmonary edema focus on correcting the arrhythmias and removing excess body fluid. One way to restore ideal timing is to terminate the dysrhythmia by delivering an electrical countershock. This countershock causes simultaneous depolarization of the entire myocardium. It thus interrupts the dysrhythmia, allowing the sinoatrial node to resume control of the sequence and coordination of depolarization. Two types of electrical countershock are used — defibrillation, and cardioversion.

Defibrillation is an emergency procedure in which the maximum dose of electricity possible is delivered, and the timing of the shock is not synchronized with ventricular depolarization.

Cardioversion is an elective procedure. An electrical countershock is synchronized with ventricular depolarization for the purpose of converting a pathological cardiac rhythm to normal sinus rhythm. Cardioversion is contraindicated in rhythms due to digitalis toxicity, because of the danger of inducing lethal ventricular dysrhythmias.

Interventions to reduce congestion include drug therapy and the temporary use of rotating tourniquets. Drug therapy is long term therapy for treating and preventing pump failure as a result of fluid overload. Drugs most often used are digitalis p.o. or IV, Lasix IV, and potassium chloride IV.

Application of tourniquets to extremities retards venous flow, thereby decreasing right ventricular output into the pulmonary vascular tree. The lessened pressure in the capillaries reduces the transudation of fluid into the alveoli and improves gas exchange. The use of rotating tourniquets causes a temporary reduction in circulating blood volume, "buying time" while morphine, digitalis, and diuretics take effect to lower pulmonary vascular pressure.

Ischemia Ischemia is a circulatory condition in which blood supply to a body part or region is reduced to a critical level. Relative ischemia occurs with hypotension or the inability to meet increased metabolic demands. Absolute ischemia is usually a sudden, complete occlusion of a blood vessel resulting in tissue necrosis. Leaving a tourniquet on an extremity for more than 15 minutes may cause tissue necrosis. Other causes of ischemia include Raynaud's disease, Buerger's disease, thromboembolism, mechanical obstruction, arteriosclerosis, and atherosclerosis. Atherosclerosis is currently under study in relation to hypertension, cigarette smoking, genetic factors, obesity, physical activity, hypercholesterolemia, and emotional stress. The actual cause of coronary athero-sclerotic disease (CAD) remains a mystery, and the incidence in the United States continues to increase.

Thrombosis and Embolism Blood clot formation within the circulatory system causes thrombi. Endothelial injury, decreased blood flow, and changes in blood constituency lead to blood clot formation and there-fore thrombosis. If veins are inflamed, the condition is termed thrombo-phlebitis. This phlebitis is usually of bacterial origin with the thrombi firmly attached in the lower extremities. Thrombophlebitis should be differentiated from phlebothrombosis or thrombus in a vein.

A dislodged, or migrating, thrombus becomes an embolus. Embolism is the process of impaction somewhere within the circulatory system and may be solid, liquid, or air. Liquid emboli are usually injected intraven-ously by accident such as during a hyperalimentation procedure (TPN). Similarly, air emboli occur when air is not removed from intravenous or arterial lines before infusion of solutions.

Elastic hosiery (TED, Jobst, and others) is used to prevent venous stasis, avoid thrombus formation and subsequent emboli. The hosiery produces compression of peripheral leg veins. This pressure forces the venous blood into deeper, larger leg veins for a more rapid return to the heart.

INTERVENTIONS IN ALTERED CIRCULATION

Assessment of Altered Circulation Alterations in circulation are indicated by a variety of signs and symptoms. The nurse should not overlook the behavioral manifestations or the more physical signs and symptoms. Systematic client evaluation considers whether or not there is a signif-icant blood loss. If bleeding exists, external and/or internal sites must be identified. Special attention is given to the family history for disease con-ditions of the heart, vessels, liver, spleen, kidneys, brain, lungs, and co-agulation mechanisms. Baseline data is gathered for vital signs and arte-rial blood pressures. The color, temperature and condition of the skin are closely noted. Cyanosis is differentiated as peripheral versus central. Weakness and fatigue is significant, as well as physical discomforts such as pain, pressure, or numbness. Abnormalities of superficial veins often indicate obstruction and/or pooling. Impaired renal function, especially related to output, is closely considered. Edema is differentiated as de-pendent versus generalized. Special observations include such findings as clubbing of the fingers, petechiae, and calf tenderness with dorsiflex-ion of the foot (positive Homan's sign). Information obtained from the drug history and present medications the client is taking may affect the diagnosis and therefore the nursing intervention. Trauma victims re-quire especially close inspection since more overt signs and symptoms may not appear until days later. Table 1 illustrates an assessment of a hemorrhaging client.

TABLE 1 ASSESSMENT GUIDE FOR A HEMORRHAGING CLIENT

1 Observable bleeding from skin, mucous membranes. Check under the person, clothing, dressings, casts.
2 Observable bleeding into the skin, mucous membranes. Check for petechiae, ecchymosis, hematomas, purpura.
3 Observable bleeding from body orifice. Check for epistaxis, hematemesis, hemoptysis.
4 Observable bleeding from tubes. Check T-tubes, endotracheal tubes, suction drainage, urinary catheters.
5 Generalized signs and symptoms of bleeding.
   a Low blood pressure (systolic below 90 mm Hg and diastolic below 50 mm Hg).
   b Progressive drop in blood pressure.
   c Rapid, weak pulses or absence of pulses.
   d Clammy skin and central cyanosis.
   e Deep, rapid respirations (above 24/minute).
   f Low body temperature (one or more degrees below 98.6° F, or 37° C, for oral temperature).
   g Reduced urine output (less than 30 ml per hour).
   h Behavioral changes.
   i Syncope and visual disturbance.
   j Loss of consciousness.
6 Localized signs and symptoms of bleeding.
   a Painful, swollen, tender, or hot joints.
   b Soft, spongy uterus high in abdominal cavity during postpartum period.
   c Pupillary and visual changes, behavioral shifts, tinnitus, vertigo, breathing pattern shifts, loss of consciousness following head injury.

Planning and Intervention Once an initial assessment of a client for alterations in circulation has been made, the nurse develops a prioritized problem list for planning and intervention. Nurses monitor circulatory status with a variety of sophisticated tools. Again, however, the most valuable approach is direct observation of the client. Blood pressure measurements are usually noninvasive, taken with a blood pressure cuff, stethoscope, and sphygmomanometer. The central venous line and the Swan-Ganz catheter for pulmonary arterial pressures (PAP and PAWP) are invasive methods used under certain conditions.

Interventions for circulatory problems cover numerous therapeutic modalities, but usually fall into three broad categories: inputs, outputs, and pressure/supports. Inputs include arterial lines, venous lines, drug regimens, transfusions, blood component therapies, etc. Outputs include suctioning with specialized equipment like hemovacs and procedures like thoracentesis. Pressure/supports include dressings, bandages, digital compression, tourniquets, and cardiopulmonary resuscitation. This chapter outlines some of the most common skills required in the management of circulatory problems.

In coping with alterations in circulation, nursing care should be directed toward promoting, maintaining, or regaining the best possible cardiopulmonary function. Nursing process provides the basic structure for problem solving. The design for nursing action is to assess the situation and client for stressors. The client should be interviewed if possible, observed, and examined to identify actual and/or potential circulatory problems. The client's responses will be appropriate, deficient, or excessive, and interventions should be planned accordingly. The nurse reduces stress, supports adaptive behaviors, replaces deficiencies, modifies or removes excessive responses, and prevents injury and complications. The nurse should always evaluate her actions and modify the interventions as indicated.

GUIDELINES FOR MANAGING CLIENTS

The rapid loss of more than 25 to 30 percent of the total blood volume leads to death.

- Controlling hemorrhage with use of direct pressure, pressure dressings, or tourniquets is an early emergency treatment.
- Completing an accurate assessment to determine cause and extent of the bleeding is required to provide optimal client care.
- Elevating an affected extremity decreases arterial blood supply to the area and promotes venous return.

Early identification of the signs of cardiac pump failure leads to prompt and effective treatment.

- If left untreated, ventricular arrhythmias and some atrial arrhythmias can lead to low cardiac output and pump failure.
- A direct relationship exists between the speed and regularity of the sinoatrial (SA) node generating electrical impulses and the rate and rhythm of cardiac contractions.
- Pulmonary edema leads to severe pulmonary congestion and increased pulmonary hydrostatic pressure if not treated promptly.
- Rotating tourniquets is a palliative procedure for treating pulmonary edema.
- Drug therapy is the most effective treatment for long term care of clients with congestive heart failure who experience pulmonary edema.

Cardiopulmonary resuscitation is usually not effective in preventing brain damage unless initiated within four minutes of an arrest.

- For an unwitnessed arrest, call for assistance and begin CPR immediately.
- Continue administering CPR until the code team arrives or a physician instructs you to stop.
- According to the Heart Association, a precordial thump is used only for a witnessed arrest and for clients on a monitor.

Being apprised of the location of the crash cart, its contents, and knowledge of emergency drugs assists the nurse in providing quick and competent care to clients in arrest situations.

- Crash carts should be kept in uncluttered, easily accessible areas of the hospital.

- Nurses need to be familiar with the contents in each drawer to quickly find emergency equipment.
- A competent knowledge of emergency drugs assists the nurse in determining the protocol for drug administration in arrest situations.

ACTION: CONTROLLING BLEEDING

ASSESSMENT

1 Observe the amount of bleeding.
2 Assess the source of bleeding.
3 Assess the extent of the wound.
4 Identify familial history of bleeding disorders.
5 Obtain baseline vital signs and arterial blood pressure readings.
6 Observe color, temperature, and condition of the skin.
7 Evaluate medications taken routinely by client.

PLANNING

GOALS

- Bleeding is detected early.
- Client's loss of blood is minimized.
- Pressure points are identified and utilized, and bleeding is controlled.
- Pressure dressings are applied and bleeding is controlled.
- Wound edges are approximated.
- Collateral circulation is minimally inhibited.

EQUIPMENT

- Towel
- 4 × 4 gauze pad
- Sterile dressings — number and size depends on wound
- Sterile gloves
- Cleansing solution
- Tape

INTERVENTION: Using Digital Pressure to Control Bleeding

1 Identify the closest artery proximal to the bleeding site.
2 Apply direct pressure to artery using your fingers.
3 Raise the affected limb above the level of the heart about 30 degrees.
4 Maintain direct pressure for at least five minutes.
5 Do not remove pressure before five minutes as clot formation has not had an opportunity to stabilize.
6 If towels or 4 × 4 gauze pads are available, apply direct pressure to site if wound does not contain glass particles.
7 When bleeding has subsided, proceed to clean and dress the wound.

Rationale for Action

- To stop bleeding or hemorrhage before large blood loss occurs
- To provide pressure as an assist (adjunct) to stop bleeding
- To minimize capillary seepage, hematoma, and serum accumulation

631

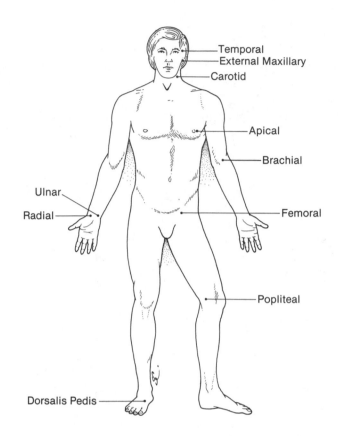

Temporal
External Maxillary
Carotid

Apical

Brachial

Ulnar
Radial

Femoral

Popliteal

Dorsalis Pedis

Apply direct pressure to artery proximal to bleeding site.

8 To control nose bleeds, place client in sitting position, with head tilted forward. Pinch nose for five minutes. Apply ice pack to assist in vasoconstriction.

INTERVENTION: Using Pressure Dressing to Control Bleeding

1 Check physician's order if needed or indicated.
2 Assemble necessary supplies according to extent of wound.
3 If time permits, explain procedure to client, and provide light and privacy.
4 Wash your hands thoroughly if time permits.
5 Set up sterile field and prepare cleansing solution if time permits.
6 Put on sterile gloves. If alone, place sterile glove on dominant hand leaving other hand free to work with unsterile supplies.
7 Cleanse wound and apply dressing.
8 To provide an occlusive dressing, place tape over entire dressing. Do not completely circle an extremity or the body so that collateral blood flow is maintained.
9 Place all soiled materials in red plastic bag.
10 Wash your hands thoroughly.

11 Monitor vital signs and observe for signs of shock.
12 Position client for comfort.
13 Elevate extremity to prevent bleeding.
14 Monitor frequently for signs of bleeding and hematoma. Hematomas feel spongy even under bandages.

EVALUATION

EXPECTED OUTCOMES

1 Early detection of bleeding occurs and loss of blood minimized. *If not*, follow these alternative nursing actions:
ANA: Continue to apply pressure and elevate extremity.
ANA: Place client in shock position, supine with feet and head slightly elevated.
ANA: Start IV and infuse with normal saline solution.
ANA: Obtain orders for and draw type and cross match for blood replacement.
ANA: Monitor vital signs frequently.
ANA: If bleeding is from large vessel and/or wound, obtain suture material for physician and assist in wound closure.
2 Pressure dressing is applied and bleeding controlled. *If not*, follow these alternative nursing actions:
ANA: Assess wound area frequently to observe amount of drainage.
ANA: Position extremity above level of heart.
ANA: Reapply a dressing that is more occlusive and provides more pressure.
ANA: If bleeding continues, notify physician and be prepared to assist with wound closure.
ANA: Monitor vital signs to assess for shock.
3 Collateral circulation is minimally inhibited. *If not*, follow these alternative nursing actions:
ANA: Assess peripheral pulses to determine adequacy of blood flow.
ANA: If peripheral blood flow is impeded, remove pressure dressing and apply a new one that is not as tight.
ANA: If bleeding is uncontrolled with new dressing, notify physician and be prepared to assist with wound closure.

UNEXPECTED OUTCOMES

1 Even with direct pressure and application of pressure dressing, bleeding continues.
ANA: Ensure IV placement and fluid administration to maintain intravascular compartment.
ANA: Notify physician and be prepared to send client to surgery for wound closure.
ANA: Prepare client psychologically for operative procedure.
ANA: Monitor closely for signs of shock.

ANA: Aid with placing of tourniquets proximal to the site of the hemorrhage to control bleeding.

ANA: Blood pressure cuffs may be used to control bleeding. Inflated blood pressure cuffs with aneroid sphygmomanometers make excellent tourniquets due to ongoing pressure control.

ANA: When using tourniquets, release the pressure every fifteen minutes in order to not compromise the extremity.

ANA: Other pressure devices include the antigravity suit (G-suit), the Jobst extremity pump, and inflatable splints. They provide circumferential pneumatic compression for immobilization, control of bleeding, and counteraction of hypotension by maintaining venous pressure.

2 Wound edges do not approximate.

ANA: Notify physician.

ANA: Be prepared to assist with wound closure or to send client to surgery.

3 Glass particles are evident in wound.

ANA: Irrigate wound profusely with sterile saline solution.

ANA: If large amount of glass or if glass is difficult to extract, notify physician and be prepared to send client to surgery for wound cleansing and debridement.

ANA: Do not apply direct pressure or pressure dressing to wound containing glass.

Charting

- Size, location, condition of wound
- Color, odor, amount of drainage
- Type and number of dressings used
- Approximate amount of blood loss
- Condition of dressing when changed, i.e., soaked with drainage, etc.

ACTION: RESTORING CIRCULATORY FUNCTION

ASSESSMENT

1 Evaluate client's overall physical condition, particularly client's cardiovascular status.

2 Assess baseline vital signs before procedures are initiated.

3 Determine if client is at risk for pooling of blood in extremities. Conditions that require use of elastic stockings are leg varicosities, thrombophlebitis, lymphedema, orthostatic hypotension, immediate postcast removal, postoperative venous ligation or stripping, and venous insufficiencies due to muscular inactivity.

4 Assess lungs for signs of pulmonary edema — rales or rhonchi.

5 Assess for peripheral edema by palpating pulses and observing color and temperature as well as fluid accumulation.

6 Evaluate ECG, serum potassium levels, and blood gas values before cardioversion is attempted.

7 Before defibrillating, confirm absence of carotid pulses if client is in ventricular tachycardia or ventricular fibrillation.

8 Evaluate outcomes of procedures to determine if alternate interventions are needed.

Rationale for Action

- To prevent venous stasis
- To prevent thrombus formation and subsequent emboli
- To temporarily reduce venous return to the heart through use of rotating tourniquets
- To improve oxygenation in pulmonary edema
- To terminate ventricular tachycardia or fibrillation accompanied by unresponsiveness or hypotension (systolic blood pressure below 90 mm Hg) with defibrillation
- To terminate supraventricular tachycardia or atrial arrhythmias with cardioversion

PLANNING

GOALS

- Elastic hose remain wrinkle-free, and pressure is evenly distributed.
- Pulmonary vascular pressure is lowered through use of rotating tourniquets and medications.
- No evidence of respiratory distress following use of rotating tourniquets.
- Peripheral pulses are present throughout use of rotating tourniquets.
- Ventricular tachycardia is terminated with defibrillation.
- Supraventricular tachycardia and ventricular tachycardia (in which consciousness is maintained) are terminated with cardioversion.
- Defibrillation converts ventricular fibrillation or tachycardia to normal sinus rhythm.

EQUIPMENT

FOR ELASTIC HOSIERY

- Tape measure
- Specific type of hosiery, e.g., below-the-knee or above-the-knee
- Talcum powder

FOR ROTATING TOURNIQUET

- Automatic rotating tourniquet machine: four separate blood pressure cuffs; or four soft rubber, 5-cm (2 inch) wide tourniquets
- Diagram and chart for tourniquet rotation pattern

FOR CARDIOVERSION

- Cardioverter (defibrillator unit with synchronizer switch)
- Paddles — anteroposterior or anterolateral
- ECG monitor and recorder
- 12-lead ECG machine
- Conductive paste or saline gauze pads
- Emergency cart and equipment
- IV solution of 5 percent dextrose in water, administration set, and medium-gauge IV needle or catheter

FOR DEFIBRILLATION

- Defibrillator
- "Quick look" paddles or ECG monitor
- ECG recorder
- Defibrillator paddles of correct size (adult or pediatric)
- Conductive paste, saline gauze pads, or defibrillator pads
- Emergency cart and equipment

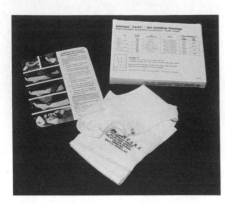

Elastic hosiery (also called Jobst or Ted hosiery) are used to prevent pooling of blood in the extremities and to promote venous return.

INTERVENTION: Applying Elastic Hosiery

1 Identify specific reason client is in need of elastic stockings.
2 Check physician's order for type and specifications. Below-the-knee type is the most common.
3 Gather supplies, identify client, and explain procedure.
4 Wash your hands, and provide for client's privacy and comfort.
5 Apply drape as top linens are removed. Bathe, dry, and powder client's legs.
6 Position client in dorsal recumbent position, and elevate bed to working height.
7 Measure client for size.
   a For below-the-knee stockings, measure from the Achilles tendon to the popliteal fold, and measure the midcalf circumference.
   b For high stockings, measure midcalf and midthigh circumference to determine size. Length is determined by measuring the distance from gluteal furrow to bottom of the heel.
8 Compare your measurements to manufacturer's chart to obtain correct hose size.
9 Powder client's heel and foot.
10 Invert foot of stocking back to heel area.
11 Holding both sides of hose at inverted foot area, pull hose over toes and ease gently toward top of foot.
12 Gather top of hose down to heel area, and with curving motion, cover heel and then pull hose up the leg.
13 Reposition client and wash your hands.
14 Observe extremities for edema above level of hose.
15 Remove hose two to three times daily for 30 minutes.
16 Hose can be washed in mild detergent and warm water as needed.

INTERVENTION: Applying Automatic Rotating Tourniquets

1 Check the physician's order.
2 Explain the procedure to client. Alert client that extremities may be temporarily swollen and discolored during treatment.
3 Place client in high-Fowler's position.
4 Obtain baseline blood pressure.
5 Assess quality of peripheral pulses and color and temperature of each limb.
6 Mark pulse locations with a pen for future reference.
7 Note extremities in which IV lines are present.
8 Apply the cuffs as proximal or close to the trunk as possible.
9 Connect the air tubes of the cuffs to the valves on the machine.
10 Adjust the cuff release timer to cycle length ordered by physician.
11 Set cuff pressure by using the pressure control valve. Select a cuff pressure 10 mm above the client's diastolic pressure.
12 Activate the alarm system which indicates air leak or failure of rotation.

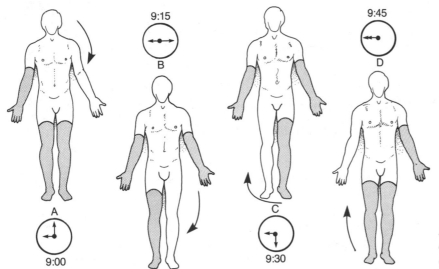

Apply tourniquets or cuffs high up on limbs close to trunk. Rotate cuff pressure in clockwise pattern every fifteen minutes.

13 Open cuff valves one at a time while observing client for shock.
14 Check that the cuffs are inflating and deflating properly. The machine will cycle the cuff inflations automatically.
15 Check blood pressure and pulse every 15 to 30 minutes. To check blood pressure, close valve when cuff deflated. Disconnect cuff from machine and attach it to a sphygmomanometer. After you have measured the blood pressure, reconnect the cuff to the machine and open the valve.
16 When physician orders procedure terminated, wait until each cuff deflates in sequence; then close the valve.
17 Leave cuffs deflated in place for a few minutes in case it is necessary to reinstitute the rotating tourniquets.
18 Monitor vital signs, lung sounds, and heart sounds immediately after tourniquets are discontinued and then as ordered.

INTERVENTION: Applying Manual Rotating Tourniquets

1 Review physician's order.
2 Explain procedure and position client in high-Fowler's position.
3 Apply blood pressure cuffs or wide rubber tourniquets to three limbs as close to the trunk as possible. The client will be more comfortable if the rubber tourniquets are placed over soft pads.
4 If using cuffs, inflate them to a pressure just 10 mm above the diastolic pressure.
5 Palpate peripheral pulses. Lower cuff pressure or loosen rubber tourniquets if pulses are not palpable.
6 Remove one tourniquet and apply another one on the previously unoccluded limb every 15 minutes.
7 Measure blood pressure every 15 to 30 minutes.

Clinical Alert

Do not deflate all the cuffs at once, since the sudden return of fluid to the circulation is likely to precipitate another episode of pulmonary edema.

Clinical Alert

Never leave a limb occluded by a tourniquet for more than 15 minutes.

8   Check pulses, color, and temperature of the extremities every hour.
9   Chart the sequence of cuff or tourniquet rotation meticulously.
10 To remove the tourniquets, remove one tourniquet every 15 minutes, following the rotation sequence.

INTERVENTION: Preparing Client for Cardioversion

1   Discontinue digitalis 48 hours or more before cardioversion, as ordered by physician.
2   Withhold food and fluids for 6 to 12 hours before cardioversion.
3   Determine client's understanding of procedure and instruct in areas where needed.
4   Obtain consent form.
5   Remove dentures.
6   Have client void before procedure.
7   Administer prophylactic atropine or quinidine if ordered.
8   Obtain baseline 12-lead ECG and label it "preconversion."
9   Place emergency cart in room or immediately outside.
10 Verify that emergency drugs are prepared and available on a "standby" basis. Emergency drugs are atropine, isoproterenol infusion, lidocaine bolus, and lidocaine infusion.

INTERVENTION: Assisting with Cardioversion

1   Review cardioversion orders and check that equipment is functioning properly.
2   Obtain baseline assessment values for vital signs and ECG rhythms.
3   Review serum electrolyte values, particularly potassium level as hypokalemia may increase risk of dysrhythmias after cardioversion.
4   Review arterial blood gas values to detect hypoxemia and acid-base imbalances.
5   Transport client to area of hospital where cardioversion will be performed.
6   Place client in supine position.
7   Establish IV line and administer fluids at "keep open" rate.
8   Administer oxygen if needed or part of protocol.
9   Connect client to ECG monitor.
10 Check monitor pattern for size and clarity of pattern.
11 Plug cardioverter in and turn power switch on.
12 Turn synchronizer switch on.
13 Test synchronization by pushing manual synchronization button and noting spike (indication of electrical stimulus) on the R wave downslope or during the S wave of the ECG.
14 Turn off oxygen. Failure to turn off oxygen can cause a fire if electrical arcing occurs.
15 Disconnect client from all electrical equipment except ECG monitor and cardioverter.
16 Administer sedative as ordered by physician, usually IV diazepam.

17 Apply conductive paste to surface of paddles or place saline pads on chest at anticipated paddle placement sites. If using anterolateral paddles, make sure that there is no perspiration between the two paddle sites.

18 Charge machine to level specified by physician, usually 25 to 50 joules to start.

▶ 1 joule = 1 watt second.

19 Place paddles on chest.

  a Anterolateral paddles are placed as in defibrillation, one over the second intercostal space to the right of the sternum and the other over the fifth intercostal space in the left midclavicular line.

  b Anteroposterior paddles are placed with the flat paddle posteriorly between the scapulae and the hand-held paddle over the fifth intercostal space in the left midclavicular line.

20 Observe ECG rhythm on monitor.

21 Start ECG recorder.

22 Note whether the synchronization indicator is superimposed on the R waves of ECG.

23 Give command to "stand clear," and stand clear yourself.

24 The physician will simultaneously depress discharge buttons on paddles and keep them depressed until the countershock is delivered. The shock may not occur instantly, since the machine will wait until the next appropriate point in the ECG to discharge.

Clinical Alert
If spike appears on T wave, do not use machine as it is not synchronizing.

25 Observe the postcardioversion rhythm.

26 Provide postcardioversion care:

  a Evaluate vital signs, ECG, level of consciousness, peripheral pulses, and neurological vital signs every 15 minutes until stable, and then routinely.

  b Administer oxygen as ordered.

  c Monitor ECG continuously for at least two hours.

  d Obtain 12-lead ECG and label it "postconversion."

  e Keep client under observation for 12 to 24 hours. Transient hypotension and minor dysrhythmias are common. Thromboemboli to the lungs or systemic circulation may occur, especially if the client has been in long-standing atrial fibrillation.

INTERVENTION: Defibrillating Client

1 Verify need for defibrillation:
  a Palpate for carotid pulse.
  b Assess level of consciousness.
  c Look at monitor screen.

2 Plan sequence of activities according to type of arrest, availability of equipment, and availability of assistants.

  a In monitored arrest with defibrillator, defibrillate immediately.

  b In monitored arrest without defibrillator, give precordial thump and start basic CPR if thump is unsuccessful in restoring heart rhythm. Send assistant for defibrillator.

▶ Defibrillation is not indicated in ventricular standstill, because depolarizations are absent in standstill.

▶ If client is not on a monitor, apply "quick-look" paddles to chest if immediately available, while someone else is instituting CPR.

639

c In unmonitored arrest, start basic CPR. Send assistant for emergency cart and defibrillator.

3 Plug defibrillator in electrical outlet unless defibrillator is battery-operated.

4 Make sure defibrillator paddles are appropriate size; change if necessary.

5 Turn off electrical equipment attached to client, e.g., 12-lead ECG machine, temporary pacemaker, to prevent damage to equipment.

6 Prepare conductive medium by one of the following methods:

  a Place thin layer of conductive paste on paddles.

  b Place saline pads on chest at anticipated sites of paddle placement.

  c Apply adhesive-backed defibrillator pads to chest at anticipated paddle sites.

7 Activate defibrillator.

  a Turn defibrillator on.

  b Dial the appropriate energy charge as ordered by the physician. The charge varies according to defibrillator model and client size. Typical setting is 200 to 300 joules of delivered energy for an adult. Make sure synchronizer switch is off. Press charge button.

8 Defibrillate the client.

  a Place paddles on chest so that current flows across the axis of the cardiac muscle mass.

  b Avoid dressings, ECG electrodes, cables, and permanent pacemaker generators.

  c Ideally, place one paddle at the second intercostal space, right side of the sternum, and the other paddle at the fifth intercostal space, midclavicular line.

  d Protect yourself and others from accidental shock. Give the command "stand clear." Visually check that no one, including yourself, is in contact with the client, bed, IV lines, or cables.

Remove paddles from unit and charge defibrillator to prepare for defibrillating client.

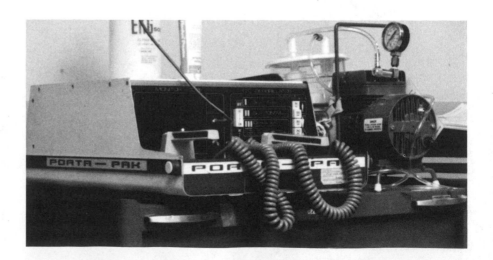

e Look at the monitor to see whether the cardiac rhythm has changed. If not, press both buttons on the defibrillator handles simultaneously.

9 Check the ECG and the carotid pulse to determine the effect of defibrillation.

10 Continue to monitor client and place on life-support measures if needed.

11 Transport client to the intensive care unit if not already there.

EVALUATION

EXPECTED OUTCOMES

1 Hose remains wrinkle-free and pressure is evenly distributed. *If not*, follow these alternative nursing actions:
   ANA: Remeasure leg to determine that hosiery size is correct.
   ANA: Elevate extremity to increase venous return.

2 Pulmonary edema is relieved following use of rotating tourniquets. *If not*, follow these alternative nursing actions:
   ANA: Reinstitute rotating tourniquet therapy.
   ANA: Reassess drug therapy being used in addition to tourniquets.
   ANA: Keep client in high-Fowler's position.
   ANA: Assess lung and heart sounds frequently.
   ANA: Monitor vital signs frequently.
   ANA: Measure CVP readings frequently, if CVP catheter is in place.
   ANA: Monitor blood gas values frequently.

3 Peripheral pulses are present throughout use of rotating tourniquet. *If not*, follow these alternative nursing actions:
   ANA: Palpate peripheral pulses at least every 15 minutes.
   ANA: Observe color of extremities frequently.
   ANA: Release cuff pressure until pulse is palpable.
   ANA: Monitor blood pressure readings more frequently to obtain changes in pressure early.

4 Supraventricular tachycardias or ventricular tachycardias are terminated with cardioversion. *If not*, follow these alternative nursing actions:
   ANA: Increase energy dose in increments of 50 to 100 joules as ordered by physician.
   ANA: Terminate the procedure, and reschedule cardioversion for next day.

5 Termination of fibrillation or tachycardia occurs with defibrillation. *If not*, follow these alternative nursing actions:
   ANA: Administer sodium bicarbonate IV to correct for acidosis.
   ANA: Repeat defibrillation immediately at 200 to 300 joules. If still unsuccessful, continue basic life support with supplemental oxygen. Then assist with administration of IV epinephrine (to convert fine

fibrillation to coarse fibrillation, which is easier to terminate electrically) and IV sodium bicarbonate. Then defibrillate a third time with a maximum of 360 joules of delivered energy.

ANA: Assist with administration of antidysrhythmic drugs.

ANA: Continue advanced life-support measures until condition reverses.

6 Normal sinus rhythm and presence of carotid pulse occur within 10 seconds. *If not,* follow these alternative nursing actions:

ANA: Identify and treat the existing arrhythmia.

ANA: Continue with CPR.

ANA: Initiate drug therapy if client goes into ventricular standstill.

ANA: Prepare for pacemaker insertion if needed.

ANA: Continue to defibrillate client and monitor drug therapy.

ANA: Follow steps in administering advanced CPR.

UNEXPECTED OUTCOMES

Charting

For Elastic Hose
- Size and type of elastic hose applied
- Condition of skin
- Presence of pulses
- Edema formation below or above hose
- Time and length of time hose removed

For Elastic Hosiery

1 Elastic hosiery is not available.

ANA: Use elastic (Ace) bandages. Anchor bandages on top of the foot and in front of the leg using metal clips or tape. Overlap should be one-third of bandage width; for a 10-cm width each turn overlaps by 3.3 cm.

ANA: Assess that elastic bandages are tight enough for support but do not obstruct arterial flow.

ANA: While making each turn, place a finger between the bandage and skin to prevent bandage from becoming too tight.

2 Below-the-knee stockings do not fold over at top.

ANA: Remeasure client's leg from heel to popliteal fold.

ANA: If hosiery is not available in proper size, apply Ace bandages or contact physician for thigh-high hosiery order.

Charting

For Rotating Tourniquets
- Time rotating tourniquets applied
- Presence of peripheral pulses
- Color and condition of extremities
- Rotation pattern
- Client's response to procedure
- Time procedure discontinued and client's response

For Rotating Tourniquets

1 On initial assessment, limb is ischemic, infected, or being used for IV infusion.

ANA: Do not apply tourniquet on that limb.

ANA: Rotate tourniquet application among remaining limbs.

2 Shock develops with rotating tourniquet therapy.

ANA: Notify physician, and remove tourniquets as per prescribed procedure.

3 Client is moved before therapy is terminated.

ANA: Close all four valves, keeping three cuffs inflated; or, if manual tourniquets, leave three tourniquets in place. Transfer client to stretcher and reopen valves if automatic unit is being used. Continue rotation pattern.

For Cardioversion

1 On preconversion assessment there is elevation of serum digitalis level.

   ANA: Notify physician and cancel cardioversion if ordered.

   ANA: If ordered, proceed with cardioversion but use very low-energy levels and do not increase if any sign of ventricular irritability occurs.

2 Ventricular premature beats or ventricular tachycardia after cardioversion.

   ANA: Implement medical orders, usually IV bolus of lidocaine followed by IV infusion of lidocaine.

3 Ventricular fibrillation occurs.

   ANA: Immediately turn off synchronizer switch. Increase energy setting to maximal level and defibrillate.

4 Asystole occurs.

   ANA: Immediately institute artificial ventilation and circulation.

   ANA: Assist physician in advanced cardiac life-support measures.

For Defibrillation

1 On initial assessment, carotid pulse and consciousness are present, although monitor shows pattern of ventricular fibrillation.

   ANA: Check electrodes for firm contact with body and wires, and check cables for intactness and tight connections as findings indicate electrical artifact. Tighten or replace electrodes, wires, and cables if necessary.

   ANA: Reassure client that a false alarm occurred and that staff responded just as promptly as they would in a real emergency.

2 Failure of defibrillator to discharge.

   ANA: Check that defibrillator is plugged in.

   ANA: Check that unit is turned on.

   ANA: Make sure synchronizer switch is off.

3 Electrical arc across chest when paddle buttons are depressed.

   ANA: Wipe off any conductive paste or perspiration between the paddle sites, and defibrillate again.

   ANA: When client is resuscitated, consult physician about use of steroid creams on chest burns.

   ANA: If fire ensues from arcing, implement emergency fire control procedures.

4 After defibrillation, rhythm changes to standstill. Presence of rhythm appears on monitor but carotid pulse is absent (electromechanical dissociation).

   ANA: Institute artificial ventilation and closed-chest massage.

   ANA: If electrical mechanical dysfunction, start CPR and administer calcium as ordered by physician to improve excitation-contraction coupling.

   ANA: Turn off main switch on unit.

   ANA: Do not hold paddles in air. Do not put paddles together and depress firing buttons.

Charting

For Cardioversion

- Preconversion rhythm
- Preconversion client preparation
- Time of cardioversion attempts
- Energy dose for each attempt
- Postconversion rhythm
- Postconversion problems, if any
- Drugs administered

Charting

For Defibrillation

- Time of arrest or discovery
- Type of arrest (respiratory first or full cardiorespiratory)
- Predefibrillation rhythm
- Number of defibrillation attempts and dose of energy for each
- Postdofibrillation rhythm
- Other resuscitative measures
- Time resuscitation discontinued
- Outcome of resuscitation
- Drugs administered

643

Rationale for Action

- To provide adequate oxygenation of lungs through mechanical support
- To provide oxygenated blood to vital organs
- To support the client via mechanical ventilation or mouth-to-mouth ventilation until other equipment is available

▶ Head board or foot board of most hospital beds can be removed and used as a cardiac board.

ASSESSMENT

1 Assess the responsibilities of personnel involved in an arrest situation.
2 Identify location of resuscitation equipment.
3 Identify the location of the emergency cart, nearest defibrillator/monitor (if none on cart), and 12-lead ECG machine.
4 Identify procedure for activation of cardiac arrest team.

PLANNING

GOALS

- Basic life support measures are established within three minutes of arrest.
- Emergency measures are performed according to established protocol.
- Client is adequately oxygenated by use of mechanical adjuncts.

EQUIPMENT

- Cardiac board
- Crash cart with equipment

INTERVENTION: Maintaining the Emergency Cart

1 Gather emergency equipment in advance.
2 Place equipment in a logical order on the emergency cart.
3 Familiarize personnel with cart layout so equipment can be retrieved promptly.
4 Time ability to locate items against predetermined standards.
5 Check the completeness of the cart at least once a shift or as determined by hospital policy.
6 Keep cart in an open area; determine that access to the cart is unimpeded.

INTERVENTION: Using the Emergency Cart

1 Assess and evaluate condition of contents of cart.
2 Observe the expiration date on drugs.
3 Practice retrieving and setting up items from the cart (in anticipation of resuscitation measures) in mock situations.
   a Airway equipment
   b Ventilation equipment
   c Circulatory equipment:
     Monitor and defibrillator
     IV lines
     Emergency drugs

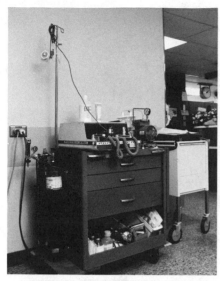

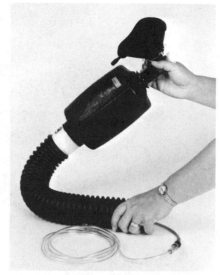

Self-contained emergency cart with defibrillator unit placed on the top for easy access. Some carts include an ECG monitor and readout.

Hope resuscitator bag is often found on emergency carts. Ventilation can be started by staff members before code team arrives.

4   Restock the cart promptly and return it to its usual location following an emergency, or obtain a fully stocked cart from central supply.
5   Fill out charge slips for items used from the cart.

INTERVENTION: Administering Cardiopulmonary Resuscitation (CPR)

1   Take the following measures if you suspect unconsciousness:
   a   Call out for help.
   b   Quickly approach client.
   c   Check responsiveness. Shake shoulders. Shout, "Are you OK?"
   d   Obtain proper position. Place victim flat on firm surface and position yourself next to victim at approximately the same level.
2   Take the following measures if you suspect airway obstruction from food or some other foreign body.
   a   Tilt head: hyperextend neck with chin forward.
   b   Remember that one attempt to ventilate will not be successful if airway is obstructed.
   c   If not successful, reposition head and attempt to ventilate.
   d   Deliver four back blows.
   e   Deliver four abdominal thrusts.
   f   Finger probe for obstruction.
   g   Repeat steps until foreign body is removed.
3   Ensure open airway in adult client:
   a   Use head-tilt method.
   b   Use jaw-thrust or chin-lift method if neck injury is even remotely possible.

CPR Protocol

1   Shake and shout.
2   Open airway.
3   Look, listen, and feel for breathing.
4   Call code.
5   Ventilate client with four quick breaths.
6   Check carotid pulse for 5 to 10 seconds.
7   Initiate CPR at 15 cardiac compressions to two ventilations.
8   Check for carotid pulse after one minute. If absent, continue CPR.

645

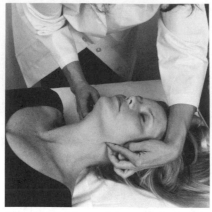

Hyperextend the neck to open airway. Jaw-thrust method should be used if neck injury is suspected.

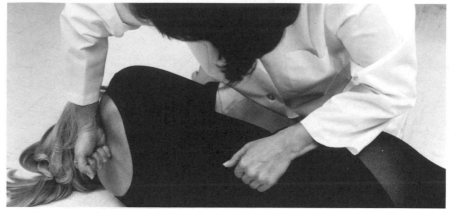

Expel foreign objects from airway and deliver four back blows with client placed on side.

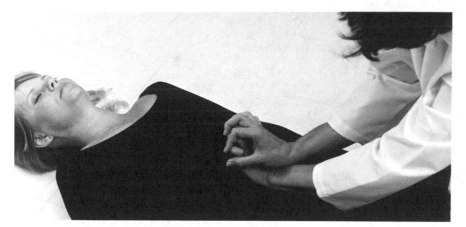

Deliver four abdominal thrusts quickly following the back blows.

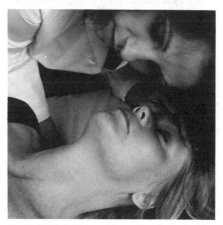

Begin CPR by looking, listening, and feeling for client's breath.

4 Evaluate respiratory function:
  a Maintain an open airway and observe for respiratory activity.
  b Put your ear down near client's mouth.
  c Look for chest movement.
  d Feel for air flow against your cheek.
  e Listen for exhalation of breath.
5 Prepare to ventilate if no respirations are present.
  a Replace victim's dentures (necessary to form tight seal).
  b Pinch off nostrils.
  c Fit mouth-to-mouth seal.
6 Administer four quick, full breaths.
  a Give breaths as fast as you can.
  b Between breaths, release seal for exhalation.

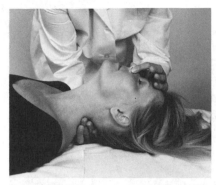

Hyperextend neck and pinch off nostrils in preparation for delivery of artificial ventilation.

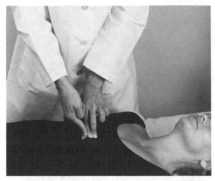

Measure two fingerbreadths above xiphoid each time heel of the hand is placed in preparation for delivering compressions.

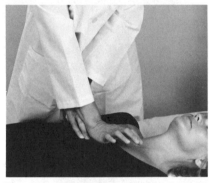

Keep fingers in position when placing heel of hand down on sternum.

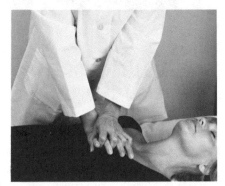

Do not take hands off chest surface between compressions to prevent injury to ribs and/or lungs.

  c Take fresh breath; do not allow complete deflation of lungs (stairstep volume).
  d Maintain position next to client.
  e Provide 800 cc minimum tidal volume per breath.
7 Feel for carotid or femoral pulse and palpate one side with two fingers for five seconds.
8 If pulse is absent, begin CPR.
  a Position hands midline, lower half of sternum, two fingers above xiphoid.
  b Place heel of one hand on sternum and other hand superimposed on top of first hand.
  c Interlace fingers and extend fingers off rib cage.
  d Administer compressions at a rate of 60 to 80 per minute. Compress chest 3.8 to 5 cm (1½ to 2 inches).
  e Count compressions: one-and-two-and, etc.
  f Release pressure between compressions for cardiac refilling but do not take heel of hand off chest.

Protocol for Precordial Thump
USED ONLY ON ADULTS MONITORED BY ECG.
1 Strike midline, lower half of sternum, two fingerbreadths above xiphoid process.
2 Administer single sharp blow from 20 to 30 cm (8 to 12 inches) above sternum.
3 Use fleshy side of fist.
4 Evaluate effectiveness immediately on ECG and confirm with pulse, or proceed with CPR as indicated.

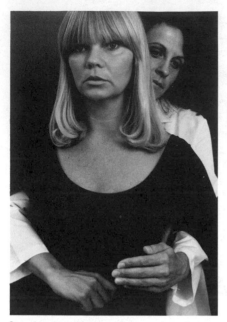

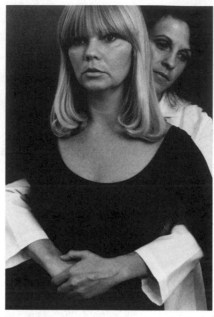

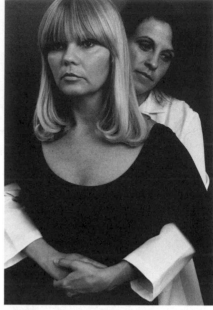

Stand behind choking client, make a fist and place it between the xiphoid and umbilicus.

Place second hand over fist for secure grasp.

Quickly thrust your hands backward, toward you and upward to expel the foreign object.

Protocol for Heimlich Maneuver

1   Assess choking client for pale color progressing to cyanosis.
2   Be familiar with choking signs. Ask client to hold hand on neck if choking.
3   Stand behind client. Place your arms around the client's waist.
4   Make a fist with one hand. Place other hand over the fist.
5   Position hands halfway between xiphoid process and umbilicus. (Client will probably fall over your arms.)
6   Press your fist into client's abdomen.
7   Using a rotating motion of the hands, forcefully thrust your hands in an upward direction to assist in expelling the foreign body.
8   Repeat measures until foreign body is expelled.

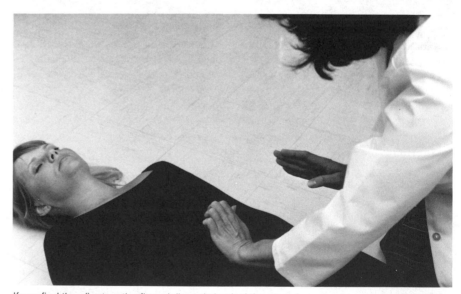

If you find the client on the floor deliver abdominal thrusts to force foreign object out of airway.

The Heimlich Maneuver

Heimlich maneuver is used when client has foreign body occlusion. The maneuver uses residual air in the lungs to push foreign body out. This is an alternative intervention for airway obstruction.

9 Continue CPR at the following rate:
   a Lone rescuer: 15:2 for adults.
   b Two rescuers: 5:1 for adults.
10 If help arrives, follow this protocol for changing roles.
   a Compressor: sets pace (one, one thousand, two, one thousand, three, one thousand, four, one thousand, breath).
   b Compressor: observes for need and institutes change.
   c Compressor: states, "Change on five next time."
   d Rescuer giving breaths: gets into position to give compression after giving the breath.
   e Rescuer giving compressions: moves to victim's head after fifth compression and counts pulse for five seconds.
   f If no pulse, rescuer checking pulse states, "No pulse, start CPR," and gives a breath, and CPR is begun again.
11 As CPR continues, follow this protocol:
   a Check major pulse after one minute of CPR.
   Equal to 4 sets of 15:2 by one rescuer.
   Equal to 12 sets of 5:1 by two rescuers.
   b Check major pulse every four to five minutes thereafter.
   c Check pupil every four to five minutes (optional if a third trained person is present) — not always a conclusive indicator.
   d Observe for abdominal distention (all age groups).
   If evident, reposition airway and reduce force of ventilation.
   Maintain a volume sufficient to elevate ribs.
   e Ventilator: check carotid pulse frequently between breaths to evaluate perfusion.
   f Ventilator: observe each breath for effectiveness.
   g If respiratory arrest only, check major pulse after each minute (12 breaths) to ensure continuation of cardiac function.
12 Terminate CPR under the following conditions:
   a The resuscitation was successful.
   Spontaneous return of vital functions.
   Assisted life support measures initiated.
   b Client is transfered to emergency vehicle or code team arrives.
   c Client is pronounced dead by physician.
   d Rescuer is exhausted and cannot continue.

INTERVENTION: Administering CPR to Infant or Small Child

1 If you suspect cardiac or respiratory arrest, follow these steps:
   a Call for help.
   b Check responsiveness by shaking child, slapping bottom of feet or rubbing chest to elicit a cry.
   c Place child on your lap, over your arm, or on a firm surface.
2 If foreign body aspiration is suspected, follow steps for CPR.
3 Clear airway by lowering child's head, turning to side, and sweeping mouth with your little finger.

4   If unable to clear airway with sweeping motion, place child in airway position (chin forward with neck slightly extended). This position usually pulls the tongue from the back of the throat and opens the airway.

5   Place rolled towel under shoulders to maintain chin in a jutting-out position, without causing hyperextension of the neck.

6   Evaluate respiratory function by following these steps:
    a   Place cheek next to child's mouth and nose.
    b   Observe for chest movement.
    c   Feel for air flow against cheek.
    d   Listen for exhalation.

7   For absent respirations, begin artificial ventilation.
    a   Maintain open airway.
    b   Form tight seal by encircling nose and mouth of child.
    c   Maintain tight seal.

8   Administer four quick breaths.
    a   Give breaths as fast as you can.
    b   Fill cheeks with air and use short puffing breaths. Do not use full breaths for children.
    c   Between breaths, release seal for exhalation, and turn your head to side.
    d   Take fresh breath; do not allow complete deflation of lungs (stairstep volume).
    e   Maintain position.

9   Do not release the child when giving ventilations; just turn your head to side.

10 Administer ventilations at 20 per minute for children under one year of age, and at 15 per minute for children over one year of age.

11 Continue ventilations until child is intubated or ambu bag is available.

12 For cardiopulmonary arrest, follow these steps:
    a   Follow procedure for initiating artificial ventilation.
    b   After administering four quick breaths, check for presence of pulse by placing two fingers over cardiac area on chest (between nipple line).
    c   Begin cardiac compression.

13 For infants to one year of age:
    a   Place two fingers at midsternum or midline of chest.
    b   Alternate method: grasp both hands behind the infant's back for support and overlap your thumbs at midsternum.

14 For children one to four years of age, use the heel of one hand at the junction of the middle and lower third of the sternum.

15 For children over four years of age, use two hands over the lower third of the sternum.

16 Remember that compression depth for children is half that of the adult victim.

17 Do not take fingers or heel off skin between compressions.

18 Perform cardiac compression and ventilate at the rate of one breath to five compressions.

a For infants under six months, administer compression 100 times per minute.

b For infants over six months, administer compression 80 times per minute.

19 Follow usual steps in CPR for single rescuer.

20 Continue CPR until code team arrives or you are instructed to stop by a physician.

INTERVENTION: Administering Advanced Life Support Measures

FIRST PERSON TO DISCOVER ARREST

1 Note time. (Activate elapsed time clock if available.)

2 Call for help by utilizing one of the following options:
  a Push emergency buzzer if one in room.
  b Call out "code blue" or another emergency phrase.
  c Use bedside telephone to alert hospital operator.
  d Send visitor or other person to summon assistance.

2 Begin basic cardiac life support procedure.

SECOND PERSON IN ROOM—DESIGNATED AIRWAY NURSE

1 Alert staff to situation and call resuscitation team if not already done.

2 Bring emergency cart to bedside.

3 Place cardiac arrest board under client's back.

4 Ventilate client with self-inflating bag.

5 Connect bag to 100 percent oxygen via wall oxygen outlet or portable oxygen tank.

6 Offer to change positions with person doing the cardiac compressions. Make change smoothly and swiftly following designated protocol for CPR.

THIRD PERSON—DESIGNATED CIRCULATION NURSE

1 Bring ECG machine and defibrillator to bedside and connect ECG leads to client.

2 Obtain ECG pattern by either:
  a Checking "quick-look" paddles on monitor/defibrillator unit.
  b Placing chest electrodes and connecting them to monitor.
  c Placing limb electrodes and connecting them to 12-lead ECG machine.

3 Defibrillate client if pattern is ventricular fibrillation and you are authorized to do so.

4 Prepare emergency medications and administer per standing orders if authorized to do so.
  a Sodium bicarbonate
  b Epinephrine
  c Atropine
  d Lidocaine

5 Prepare heparinized syringe for arterial blood gas sample.

Nursing Protocol

1 First person notes time and calls for help.

2 Second person brings cart and notifies code team.

3 Third person brings necessary equipment and prepares medications.

4 Fourth person coordinates team effort.

Protocol for Advanced CPR

1 Intubation.

2 Oxygenation: provision of supplemental oxygen.

3 Ventilation: gas exchange through a patent airway.

4 Perfusion: delivery of blood to major organs and peripheral tissues.

FOURTH PERSON—DESIGNATED COORDINATOR

1 Establish IV line if not already in place before administering emergency drugs. Use a #18 IV angiocath and 5 percent dextrose in water unless arrest procedure specifies otherwise.
2 Establish a recording of interventions on resuscitation recording sheet.
3 Move visitors or other clients out of room if possible. If not, draw curtains, give a brief explanation of the emergency, and try to have someone remain with other occupants.
4 Establish crowd control and direct traffic.
5 Assign staff not involved in the resuscitation effort to continue care of other clients on the unit.
6 Assign one person to act as a runner, if a runner is not preassigned.
7 Continue to follow standardized procedures for codes until physician arrives and begins directing the code.

INTERVENTION: Providing Care Following Code

1 Remind physician to talk with family.
2 Wash client's face and hands and provide clean top sheet.
3 Escort family in to see client.
4 Arrange for transfer of client to intensive care unit or morgue, if necessary.
5 Provide one-to-one nursing care for client until ICU transfer is accomplished.
6 Update charting.
7 Restock emergency cart or obtain replacement cart.
8 Return all equipment to original location. Remember to recharge defibrillator.
9 Clean room.
10 Allow other clients to return to room.
11 Provide emotional support to staff members involved in resuscitation.
12 Participate in staff critique of resuscitation management.

EVALUATION

EXPECTED OUTCOMES

1 Basic life support measures established within three minutes after arrest. *If not*, follow these alternative nursing actions:
ANA: Continue CPR and begin advanced life support measures as indicated.
ANA: If staff reaction time or procedure for administering CPR is not clearly understood, encourage the institution to offer surprise practice resuscitations and participate in them to improve your skills.
2 Emergency measures performed according to established protocol. *If not*, follow these alternative nursing actions:

ANA: Identify areas for improvement by using a code critique form. Following each code, the members should review the critique and then make plans for altering procedure as indicated.

ANA: Have mandatory code classes for staff to ensure that the standard protocol is followed in each code situation.

3 Client is adequately oxygenated by use of mechanical adjuncts. *If not*, follow these alternative nursing actions:

ANA: Use manual resuscitator connected to 100 percent oxygen during CPR. It is very difficult to administer oxygen via ventilators during code situations.

ANA: If intubation and/or oxygenation is ineffective, you may need to prepare for a tracheostomy.

UNEXPECTED OUTCOMES

1 Equipment is missing from cart.

ANA: Immediately notify physician. If item is minor, ask if substitute can be used. If item is major, immediately obtain replacement from floor stock or nearby unit.

ANA: After emergency is over, notify charge nurse of possible breakdown in cart-checking procedure or pilferage.

ANA: Obtain missing item and place on cart. If any delay in obtaining item, tape warning notice to cart that item is missing.

ANA: Encourage the use of plastic emergency cart seals that visually indicate if the cart has been opened.

2 Additional useful equipment is not included on cart.

ANA: When emergency is over, explain rationale for including item to charge nurse and ask him or her to obtain necessary approval to add item to cart on a trial basis.

3 Inability to promptly locate equipment on cart.

ANA: During resuscitation, look for item in other drawers, or ask another nurse for assistance.

ANA: After resuscitation, suggest to charge nurse a more logical placement of item.

ANA: After resuscitation, practice quick retrieval of items.

4 Equipment is inaccessible or malfunctions.

ANA: Refer to ANAs under specific resuscitation procedures, e.g., defibrillation, hand-held resuscitation device, and emergency cart.

5 Choking client is found on floor. Heimlich maneuver cannot be performed in usual manner.

ANA: Perform alternate procedure.

Lie client flat on back.

Kneel over client with your head facing client's head and your legs on each side of the client's hips.

Make a fist with one hand. Place second hand over fist.

Place hands between client's xiphoid and umbilicus.

Make a forceful upward thrust with the heel of the fisted hand.

6 Inadequate individual staff performance of prioritized nursing actions.

ANA: Remain nonjudgmental while person regains control.

ANA: Offer assistance with improving skills or decision-making in high-stress situations.

7 Poor team coordination efforts.

ANA: Attend practice CPR drills.

ANA: Evaluate after every drill and assist in revising or reassigning personnel.

8 Client is revived but maintained on life-support system.

ANA: Continually reassess CPR protocol.

ANA: Prepare client for serial ECGs if brain hypoxia is suspected.

ANA: Reassess for developmental level.

ANA: Give custodial care if required.

9 Hysterical staff member blames self for unsuccessful resuscitation.

ANA: Provide secluded place in which to grieve.

ANA: Allow person to express feelings, but correct misconceptions and prevent fantasizing.

ANA: Use therapeutic touch to comfort person.

Charting

- Time of arrest
- Type of arrest
- Initial resuscitation efforts before arrival of team
- Resuscitation efforts after arrival of team
- Time of cessation of resuscitation efforts
- Outcome of resuscitation efforts
- Outcome of Heimlich maneuver

TERMINOLOGY

adrenergic drugs Drugs that act like epinephrine and increase the force of cardiac contraction

arrhythmia Irregular heart action caused by disturbances in discharge of cardiac impulses from the SA node or their transmission through conductile heart tissue.

automaticity Ability to initiate an electrical impulse without external stimuli.

cardiac output Cardiac output equals the heart rate (beats/minute) times the stroke volume (liters/minute).

cardioversion Procedure for delivering a countershock to the heart for the purpose of converting a pathological cardiac rhythm to normal sinus rhythm.

chronotropic reserve Refers to an increased cardiac output.

conduction system Composed of specialized tissue that allows rapid transmission of electrical impulses through the myocardium.

conductivity Ability to transmit electrical impulse.

contractility Ability of muscle to shorten with electrical stimulation.

contraction The heart muscle utilizes chemical energy to do the work of contraction — a shortening or increase in tension.

defibrillation Stopping fibrillation of the heart through the use of drugs or the discharge of electrical current.

depolarization The act of neutralizing polarity.

dysrhythmia   Abnormal heart beat or rhythm.

erythrocyte   A mature red blood cell or corpuscle.

excitability (irritability)   Ability to be stimulated.

Frank-Starling law   The more the heart is filled during diastole, within physiological limits, the greater the quantity of blood pumped into the aorta and pulmonary artery.

hydrostatic pressure   Pertains to a liquid in a state of equilibrium.

inotropic   Increases the myocardial force and contractility.

sinoatrial (SA) node   Main pacemaker of heart in which normal rhythmic self-excitatory impulse is generated.

stroke volume   Amount of blood ejected by the left ventricle at each beat.

tachycardia   Abnormal rapid heart beat — over 100 beats per minute.

taxonomy   Method of classifying heart disease.

ventricular fibrillation   Disorganized, rapid and ineffective ventricular depolarization.

APPENDIX
CONTENTS OF TYPICAL EMERGENCY CART

Top of cart
  ECG monitor with readout
  ECG electrodes and extra roll
    of recording paper
  Defibrillator
  Defibrillator paddles and
    conductive medium

First drawer
  Emergency medications
  IV additive labels

Second drawer
  Venipuncture supplies: steel
    needles, over-the-needle
    catheters, inside-the-needle
    catheters, short intra-
    catheters, macrodrop admin-
    istration sets, microdrop
    administration sets, extension
    tubing, stopcocks, syringes,
    tape, alcohol swabs, tour-
    niquets, tincture of benzoin,
    gauze pads

  Blood sampling supplies:
    venous blood tubes, arterial
    blood gas kits or glass
    syringes
  Spinal needles for intracardiac
    injections
  Scalpels with blades attached
  Alligator clips

Third drawer
  Oral airways
  Endotracheal tubes
  Laryngoscope handle, curved
    blades, straight blades, extra
    batteries, extra bulbs, stylet
  McGill forceps
  Tonsil suction
  Surgical lubricant
  Hand-held self-inflating resus-
    citation bag
  Oxygen masks, connecting
    tubing, flowmeter
  Suction catheters
  Nasogastric tubes

Bottom shelf
  Tracheostomy tray
  Cutdown tray and sutures
  IV solutions, armboards
  Portable suction device
  Pacemaker and electrodes

Back of cart
  Cardiac arrest board

Side of cart
  CVP catheters or long intracaths
  Emergency cart checklist
  Cardiac resuscitation recording
    sheet and clipboard

SELECTED EMERGENCY CART MEDICATIONS

DRUG	ACTIONS	INDICATIONS	DOSES	ADMINISTRATION	POSSIBLE COMPLICATIONS
Drugs to Control Heart Rate and Rhythm					
Lidocaine	Decreased automaticity Increased fibrillation threshold	Dangerous ventricular premature beats: Frequent Sequential Multifocal R wave close to preceding T wave Ventricular tachycardia Ventricular fibrillation	50 – 100 mg (1 mg/kg) every 3 – 5 minutes until rhythm suppressed or to maximum of 300 mg Followed by infusion of 1 – 4 mg/min Doses reduced in renal failure, liver failure, and decreased cardiac output	IV bolus IV infusion: prepared by mixing 1 gram in 250 ml 5% dextrose in H$_2$O (equal to concentration of 4 mg/ml). Administered with volumetric infusion pump	Slurred speech Drowsiness Altered level of consciousness Twitching Seizures Heart block
Bretylium tosylate	Increased fibrillation threshold Decreased defibrillation threshold	Ventricular fibrillation and ventricular tachycardia unresponsive to lidocaine and electrical shock	Ventricular fibrillation: 5 mg/kg initially. If unresponsive to repeated attempt at defibrillation, increased to 10 mg/kg every 15 – 30 minutes to maximum of 30 mg/kg Ventricular tachycardia: 5 – 10 mg/kg over 10 minute period, followed by infusion of 1 – 2 mg/minute	IV bolus, undiluted, and rapid IV infusion of 500 mg diluted to 50 ml	Severe hypotension Arrhythmias Severe nausea and vomiting with rapid infusion Potentiation of antihypotensive agents (pressor amines, sympathomimetics) Anginal pain
Atropine	Parasympathetic action: blockage of action of vagus nerve on heart, so increased heart rate	Severe sinus bradycardia Atrioventricular block with slow ventricular rate Asystole	Adult: 0.5 mg repeated every 5 minutes as necessary, up to total dose of 2 mg Pediatric: 0.01 – 0.03 mg/kg	IV bolus	Increased myocardial oxygen consumption (due to increased heart rate) Ventricular tachycardia or fibrillation
Isoproterenol	Beta-adrenergic stimulation	Decreased cardiac output Sinus bradycardia Atrioventricular block	Adult: 1 – 4 micrograms (15 – 60 microdrops) per minute Children: 0.1 micrograms/kg/minute to start	IV infusion: prepared by mixing 5 ml of 1:5000 solution in 250 ml 5% dextrose in H$_2$O (equal to concentration of 4 micrograms/ml). Administered with volumetric infusion pump	Tachycardia Hypotension

DRUG	ACTIONS	INDICATIONS	DOSES	ADMINISTRATION	POSSIBLE COMPLICATIONS
Drugs to Improve Cardiac Output and Blood Pressure					
Epinephrine	Alpha and beta-adrenergic stimulation: increased heart rate, contractility, blood pressure, myocardial oxygen consumption, and automaticity	Asystole Ventricular fibrillation refractory to defibrillation	Adult: 0.5 – 1.0 mg (5 – 10 ml of 1:10,000 solution) Repeat every 5 minutes Pediatric: 0.1 ml/kg of 1:10,000 solution	IV bolus (preferred); instillation into tracheobronchial tree via endotracheal tube; intracardiac only as last resort Dilute 1:1000 solution with 9 ml normal saline if prepared; 1:10,000 solution unavailable Do not mix in alkaline solution	Intracardiac route: cardiac tamponade; coronary artery laceration; intramyocardial injection; pneumothorax
Dopamine	Precursor of norepinephrine Alpha and beta-adrenergic stimulation (dose related) Dilatation of renal and mesenteric arteries (low doses)	Cardiogenic shock	Adult: 2 – 5 micrograms/kg/minute initially; then titrated to desired blood pressure up to 50 micrograms/kg/minute Children: 2 – 10 micrograms/kg/minute	IV infusion: prepared by mixing 5 ml (200 mg) in 250 ml 5% dextrose in H_2O (equal to concentration of 800 micrograms/ml). Administered with volumetric infusion pump	Premature heart beats Tachycardia Nausea and vomiting Angina Excessive vasoconstriction in high doses (over 20 micrograms/kg)
Dobutamine hydrochloride	Synthetic catecholamine	Cardiac pump failure unresponsive to other forms of therapy	2.5 – 10 micrograms/kg/minute	IV infusion	Tachycardias and premature ventricular beats, especially when rate exceeds 20 micrograms/kg/minute
Sodium nitroprusside	Direct peripheral vasodilatation, leading to afterload reduction, decreased ventricular filling, reduction of pulmonary congestion, and decreased myocardial consumption	Cardiac pump failure Hypertensive emergencies	0.5 – 10 micrograms/kg/minute	IV infusion. Light sensitive, so wrap bag with foil. Discard after 4 hours and replace with fresh solution. Administer with volumetric infusion pump	Hypotension Cyanide toxicity Tissue irritation with extravasation

DRUG	ACTIONS	INDICATIONS	DOSES	ADMINISTRATION	POSSIBLE COMPLICATIONS
Miscellaneous Drugs					
Sodium bicarbonate	Buffering of hydrogen ions	Metabolic acidosis Respiratory acidosis Ventricular fibrillation refractory to defibrillation	Adult: 1 mEq/kg initially, then no more than half of initial dose every 10 minutes. Whenever possible, determine dose according to blood gas values Pediatric: 1 – 2 mEq/ kg/dose	IV bolus Do not mix with epinephrine or calcium	Metabolic alkalosis Impaired release of oxygen to tissues Hypernatremia Hyperosmolality, bradycardia or heart block
Calcium gluconate, chloride, or gluceptate	Increased ventricular excitability Increased myocardial contractility	Asystole Decreased contractility Electromechanical dissociation	Calcium chloride: 10% solution Adult: 5 ml Pediatric: 25 mg/kg Calcium gluceptate 5 – 7 ml (adult dose) Calcium gluconate 10 – 15 ml of 10% solution (adult dose)	IV bolus (slow) Do not mix with bicarbonate	Rapid administration in still-beating heart: cardiac arrest Possible precipitation of digitalis toxicity in client receiving digitalis

LEVEL IV
Critical Alterations in Homeostasis

CHAPTER 18
Managing the Perioperative Client

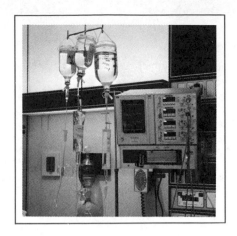

This chapter provides an overview of the care given to clients undergoing surgical intervention. Perioperative nursing includes care given to the surgical client during the preoperative, intraoperative, and postoperative stages.

Nurses are taking a more active role in the psychological and physiological preparation of the surgical client. In many areas of the country, nurses are instructing the preoperative client in stress reduction techniques, expectations for the postoperative period, as well as special postoperative equipment. In fact, many hospitals provide time for the operating room nurse to make postoperative visits to assess the client's evaluation of the surgical intervention.

PERIOPERATIVE STAGES

The first stage of the perioperative period is the preoperative stage. During this stage a thorough physical assessment of the client is completed. The nurse records all baseline data and reports any alteration from normal to the surgeon and/or anesthesiologist. Client teaching and interviewing are also completed during this period. The physical preparation of the client includes the preoperative shave, identifying the correct client in the operating room, and the preoperative scrub.

The intraoperative stage is the period of time from when the client undergoes the surgical procedure until the client is admitted to the re-

LEARNING OBJECTIVES

Define the word perioperative.

Discuss the nursing care focus in each of the three stages of the perioperative period.

Identify at least three factors that influence the surgical client's degree of stress.

State the primary purpose of providing preoperative care for clients.

Describe how preoperative teaching reduces the surgical client's stress.

List at least four safety measures implemented during the intraoperative stage.

Outline the essential postoperative nursing interventions completed in the recovery room and in the surgical unit.

Describe the parameters for discharging clients from the recovery room.

Discuss at least three major postoperative complications and nursing interventions to prevent and treat the complications.

Summarize the major categories of postoperative pain medications and describe the general side effects of each category.

659

covery room. During the intraoperative stage, nursing interventions are focused on the surgical scrub, positioning, and safety measures.

The postoperative stage can be divided into three segments. The immediate postoperative period includes the care given to the client in the recovery room and in the first few hours on the surgical floor. The intermediate period usually involves the care given during the course of surgical convalescence to the time of discharge. The third segment in the postoperative stage is discharge planning, teaching, and referral.

Besides nursing care, nursing management during the postoperative period centers around assessing the client's postoperative condition and monitoring for complications. It also includes client teaching, pain control, and psychological support of both the client and family.

In each phase of the client's perioperative experience — preoperative, intraoperative and postoperative — physiological and psychological elements will be affected by the threat of the surgical trauma, the actual trauma, and the response to the trauma. The predominance of each element varies in each operative phase.

PREOPERATIVE ANXIETY AND STRESS

Admission to the hospital and anticipation of surgery result in some degree of anxiety and/or stress. Stress is a physiological and psychological response to a stressor — a demand to adapt. Anxiety is a stress response to an existing stressor. The degree of anxiety and stress is dependent on many factors.

The client's proneness to react to anticipated stressors with high anxiety.

The number of stress-producing events that have occurred recently in the client's life or within the client's family.

The client's perceptions of the hospitalization and surgical experience.

The significance of the surgery to the client.

The number of unknowns that confront the client on admission.

The body responds physiologically to an actual or perceived threat. The hypothalamus controls a neurohormonal response. The heart rate is increased, and the heart contracts more forcefully. Blood volume is redistributed by vasoconstriction of the vessels in the skin, stomach, mesentery, and kidneys. Increased blood volume increases cardiac output. Increased blood flow to the skeletal muscles results in the muscles becoming tensed for action. The bronchi dilate, and the increased respiratory rate increases oxygenation. Mechanisms that provide energy include increased glucose release and decreased insulin production.

Behavioral responses to stress or anxiety can be adaptive or maladaptive. Adaptive behaviors are purposeful. The client adapts him or herself to a stressful situation by preparing to face it or by removing the threat. Maladaptive behaviors result from the inability to adapt to a stressful situation.

One of the objectives of providing preoperative care is to identify the level of stress present in the client. If nursing interventions can be planned that will reduce high anxiety levels, a safer intraoperative period will result. High levels of anxiety can prevent successful preoperative adaptation and can negatively influence postoperative recovery. Mild anxiety, on the other hand, increases alertness, increases the ability to learn, and increases the ability to assess and to adjust to one's environment. Mild anxiety also increases the ability to adjust to several simultaneous stressors. In the preoperative client this level of anxiety is adaptive in nature, while a high level is maladaptive. When levels of anxiety or stress become intolerably high, defense mechanisms are unconsciously implemented to reduce the distress by concealing, falsifying, or distorting reality.

Preoperative anxiety is increased by ambiguity, conflicting perceptions, misconceptions, fears of the unknown, and bombardment by many simultaneous stressors. Ambiguity occurs from uncertainty or vagueness concerning the hospital environment, preoperative procedures, intraoperative procedures, and/or postoperative events.

Conflicting perceptions occur when preconceived notions about the operative experience are different from those actually encountered. The client who thought that a herniorrhaphy would be a quick, safe cure can become quite anxious after the anesthesiologist informs him of potential complications.

Misconceptions arise when inaccurate information is given, when terminology used is not understood, and when events are not explained clearly. A client who is scheduled for bronchoscopy in the morning, and whose nurse silently places an n.p.o. sign over the bed, may believe that he is destined for the same hospital regimen as his roommate, who had a gastrectomy.

Stress responses are additive. An increasing number of stressors can eventually drain adaptive energy. The newly admitted surgical client who has been confronted with many stressors before admission will have increased vulnerability and is likely to respond with a higher stress as each new stressor is encountered.

Psychological preparation includes preoperative teaching of the client and the family as well as the administration of preoperative medications. Preoperative teaching prepares the client by explaining the events that will occur preoperatively and postoperatively. To be most effective, these explanations should include descriptions of sensory experiences as well as the procedure methodology. An informed client will experience less stress because the stressful situation will not be unfamiliar or unexpected. Preoperative teaching reduces stress by minimizing the client's fears—fears of the unknown, pain, anesthesia, and loss of control.

Postoperative complications can also be decreased by reducing stress levels. Prolonged high stress levels are associated with deficient immune systems, stress ulcers, hypertension, life-threatening arrhythmias, sodium and water retention, and congestive heart failure.

The need for frequent and high doses of analgesia is reduced when

TABLE 1 RESPONSES TO ANXIETY STATES

LOW ANXIETY	HIGH ANXIETY
Less prone to react with high anxiety to stressors	Prone to react with high anxiety to stressors
Few changes in personal situation in recent past	Many changes in personal situation in recent past
Perceives hospital and surgical experience as beneficial	Perceives hospital and surgical experience as threatening
Believes surgery will end chronic problem	Fears that surgery may lead to pain, disability, and possibly death
Regards admission procedures as friendly and supportive	Regards admission procedures as strange and frightening
Finds hospital conditions comfortable and the nursing staff supportive and informative	Finds hospital conditions unbearable and the nursing staff nonsupportive

stress levels are low and when clients are assured of pain relief when needed. Levels of stress closely correlate with levels of perceived pain. Reduction of stress reduces perceived pain. Anxiety levels are increased when the client envisions having to endure pain without relief. Assurance that medication is available and encouragement to utilize the medication for relief reduce anxiety significantly.

The client's degree of participation in recovery affects the complication rate. Effective pulmonary care significantly curtails the most frequent postoperative complication — atelectasis and pneumonia. The client's active and willing participation in deep breathing, coughing, use of incentive spirometers, and early ambulation will enhance a rapid recovery and thus shorten hospitalization.

The influence of the family can also affect the client's recovery. In many cases, the client's strongest support system is the family. To be an effective support system, the family must be informed. Also, the anxiety and/or stress of each family member must be within tolerable limits. Knowledge of the client's problems, type of surgery proposed, and recovery rate will allow the family to provide support. The knowledgeable family can reinforce preoperative teaching for each other and the client.

GUIDELINES FOR MANAGING CLIENTS

Conscientious preoperative care of clients prevents postoperative complications.
- Preparing the client psychologically reduces the client's stress level and helps to prevent postoperative complications.
- Completing the surgical scrub reduces microorganisms on the body surface and the possibility of wound infections postoperatively.

Scrupulous asepsis throughout the perioperative period reduces complications.
- Maintaining strict asepsis reduces cross contamination.
- Identifying breaks in sterile technique and taking appropriate action decrease the risk of postoperative complications.

Preoperative client-teaching increases the client's knowledge base.

- Reducing the client's fear of the unknown reduces the possibility of stress, a condition that can interfere with the client's postoperative course.
- Teaching coughing and deep breathing exercises, procedures for getting out of bed, and uses of specialized equipment enhance the client's cooperation postoperatively.

Appropriate nursing assessment and interventions during the preoperative and intraoperative stage prevent postoperative complications.

- Initiating exercises early in the postoperative period assists in preventing postoperative complications.
- Providing a continuous, comprehensive physical assessment assists in identifying early manifestations associated with postoperative complications.
- Encouraging early ambulation and self-care assist in promoting a sense of well-being and reduces postoperative complications.
- Assessing for and managing the client's pain can promote postoperative ambulation and self-care, decreasing the possibility of complications associated with immobility.

ACTION: IDENTIFYING STRESS IN PREOPERATIVE CLIENTS

ASSESSMENT

1 Identify if high level of stress exists.
  a Heart rate: rate increases 10 beats per minute over baseline during three observations.
  b Presence of palpitations.
  c Blood pressure: increases more than 10 mm Hg over baseline during three observations.
  d Respiratory rate: increases more than five per minute over baseline during three observations.
  e Vasoconstriction of cutaneous vessels: cool, pale fingers and toes; increased capillary filling time more than 3 seconds.
  f Vasoconstriction of renal vessels: decreased urine output compared to baseline and fluid intake.
  g Vasoconstriction of gastric and mesenteric vessels: anorexia, nausea, vomiting, abdominal distention with flatus, decreased bowel sounds, hyperactivity, diarrhea.
  h Increased muscle tensing: furrowed eyebrows, facial tics, clenched jaws, loud or high-pitched voice, stammering, rapid speech, elevated shoulders, clenched fists, urinary frequency. Client complains of tension or inability to relax.
  i Increased energy and preparedness: restlessness, easily startled, increased activity level.
2 Assess exaggerated anxiety and/or stress behaviors.
  a Hyperactivity: pacing, hand-wringing, lip or nail biting, finger-tapping, impatience, irritability, insomnia.

Rationale for Action

- To identify level of stress and/or anxiety present in preoperative clients
- To provide interventions that decrease stress levels and promote optimal preoperative behavioral and physiological responses
- To observe for use of defensive behaviors that mask a failure to adapt appropriately in stressful situations

b Disorganization of thought: repetitive speech, constant conversation, difficulty concentrating.
   c Increased sensitivity to environmental noise, light, temperature, activity.
3 Evaluate defensive behaviors.
   a Withdrawal: daydreaming, increased time in sleep, unwillingness to talk, disinterest.
   b Anger: resentment, aggressiveness, noncompliance, swearing, boasting, attempts to gain control and independence.
   c Denial: joking, carefree attitude, inappropriate laughter, refusal to discuss impending surgery.
4 Assess vulnerability of client due to number and significance of changes in life before admission.
5 Evaluate level of client knowledge and perceptions of the impending surgery and perioperative period.

PLANNING

GOALS

- Excessive preoperative anxiety and high stress level are prevented.
- Preoperative learning and ability to successfully adapt to surgery are enhanced.
- A smooth intraoperative and postoperative course is experienced.
- Postoperative complications are prevented.

INTERVENTION: Preventing Anxiety and Stress

1 Establish a trusting relationship.
2 Encourage ventilation of feelings.
3 Listen attentively.
4 Communicate acceptance of the client as an individual.
5 Plan care based on assessment of needs and vulnerability.
6 Give adequate information regarding hospital procedures.
   a Hospital environment, including sights, sounds, and equipment.
   b Hospital personnel and routine procedures: mealtimes, telephone usage, call light.
   c Ordered perioperative procedures: lab tests, diagnostic procedures (explain sensory experiences that will be encountered).
   d Scheduled time of surgery.
   e Hospital regulations: visiting hours, smoking.
   f Preoperative procedures: shave, n.p.o., medications, side rails, dentures, nail polish.
   g Anticipated postoperative events: recovery room, pain and pain medications, coughing and deep breathing exercises, dressings, IVs.

INTERVENTION: Reducing Anxiety and/or Stress

1 Establish a trusting relationship.
2 Encourage ventilation of feelings.

3 Use touch to communicate caring and genuine interest.
4 Avoid reassurance.
5 Utilize realistic outcomes.
6 Assist client in exploring effective coping methods to reduce anxiety and/or stress.
  a Ask the client or the family what method the client normally uses to successfully reduce stress.
  b Provide activity: walking, range of motion.
  c Instruct client in "bottle breathing": Have client imagine his or her chest is a large bottle that needs to be filled with air on inspiration and slowly emptied through pursed lips with exhalation. Breathing should be slow and deep over one to two minutes.
  d Provide a back rub to loosen tense muscles. (Physical relaxation will often lead to mental relaxation.)
  e Teach client relaxation techniques. One technique is to ask the client to picture a blue sky that is clear except for one white, fluffy cloud. Tell client to concentrate on this scene for ten minutes. This technique will often relax the mind and the body.
  f An alternative is to ask the client to picture a favorite place, e.g., a warm, sunny beach with sand and gentle surf.
7 As the client begins to relax, reinforce success. Assist client in recognizing client's strengths and progress.
8 Encourage self-awareness of increasing tension and immediate reversal of escalation.

INTERVENTION: Assisting the Client Using Denial

1 Establish a trusting relationship.
2 Encourage ventilation of feelings.
3 Use touch to communicate caring and genuine interest.
4 Do not attempt to enforce reality. The client is denying reality to prevent outright panic. Allow use of this defense.
5 Utilize techniques to reduce anxiety and/or stress to manageable proportions.
6 Attempt to determine the cause of the need for denial.
7 Listen for cues that indicate readiness to discuss the stressors causing the need for denial.
8 Seek additional information and collaboration from other members of the health team.

EVALUATION

EXPECTED OUTCOMES

1 Level of stress and/or anxiety in preoperative client is identified. *If not*, follow these alternative nursing actions:
   ANA: Reassess client for signs of stress and anxiety.
   ANA: Plan to spend more time with client so a therapeutic relationship can develop. With rapport established, client may be able to discuss fears and concerns.

ANA: Ask family members to validate client's stress level and suggest ways to assist client to reduce stress.

2 Nursing interventions are provided that decrease stress levels and promote optimal preoperative responses. *If not*, follow these alternative nursing actions:

ANA: Before interventions will be successful, it is important to identify specific stressors and the client's response patterns. Discuss with client the concept of stress, his feelings and the ways he usually handles stress.

ANA: Give client adequate information so he or she will know exactly what to expect pre- and postoperatively. Clear expectations reduce anxiety.

ANA: Introduce relaxation techniques and plan time with client to practice these stress reducing processes.

3 Denial, as a defense mechanism, is identified in the client. *If not*, follow these alternative nursing actions:

ANA: Review knowledge of defense mechanisms so you will be able to recognize denial and understand that the client is using it as a way of coping with a fearful reality. Allow use of this defense.

ANA: Provide opportunity and openings for client to express fears and concerns, as often talking about feelings reduces anxiety and fear.

UNEXPECTED OUTCOMES

1 Anxiety level escalates rapidly.

ANA: Maintain calm composure and speak in a soft, caring manner. Use touch to communicate caring and peacefulness.

ANA: Reinforce client's self-acceptance as an individual.

ANA: If unable to achieve success with stress reducing techniques, consider medication.

2 Client becomes angry or hostile.

ANA: Maintain calm composure.

ANA: Accept anger but place limits on how it may be expressed, i.e., destructive behavior. Understand that anger is usually the result of feeling helpless and powerless to change an intolerable situation.

ANA: Do not reward the behavior but explore other means of meeting client's needs.

ANA: Do not isolate client, but continue to respond to needs.

ANA: Consult and collaborate with other health team members to provide consistent client care.

3 Client becomes depressed because of overwhelming anxiety and feelings of helplessness or hopelessness.

ANA: Convey respect and belief that the client is worthwhile. Question the client's appraisal of reality and provide support while the client works through his or her feelings.

ANA: Provide positive feedback and recognition of strengths, progress, and improved self-esteem.

ANA: Consult and collaborate with other health team members to plan consistent nursing care.

Charting

- Observed and subjective indications of anxiety and/or stress levels
- Nursing interventions used to decrease stress and the results of the intervention
- Evaluation of intervention success in terms of physiologic and behavioral changes
- Plans for maintaining desired level of client comfort throughout perioperative course
- Client teaching presented
- Describe behaviors that indicate learning has occurred

ACTION: PROVIDING PREOPERATIVE TEACHING AND PSYCHOLOGICAL PREPARATION

ASSESSMENT

1 Assess the client's readiness to learn.
2 Assess the family's readiness to learn.
3 Assess the client's cognitive level to determine appropriate teaching strategy.

PLANNING

GOALS

- Client is provided with sufficient data in order to promote a sense of self-control during the postoperative period.
- Family is provided with pertinent data to promote a sense of well-being during the operative and postoperative period.
- Potential postoperative pain and complications associated with surgery are reduced.
- A stress-free environment for client and family teaching is provided.

EQUIPMENT

- Use of prepared teaching aids when available — audio-visual, film-strips, pamphlets, pictures, posters, programmed learning, slides, cassette tapes, overhead transparencies
- Quiet room for client and family where there will be no interruptions during the teaching program
- Collection of equipment that may be used for the client, e.g., IV bottle and tubing, Stryker frame, nasogastric tube, cardiac monitor and electrodes
- Visit by the client to the ICU

INTERVENTION: Providing Client Education

1 Provide preoperative information.
   a Blood work, ECG, urinalysis, chest x-ray.
   b Preoperative skin preparation.
   c Placement of nasogastric tube, Foley catheter, as indicated.
   d Enema or special bowel preparation as ordered.
   e Use of medications preoperatively and postoperatively.
   f Deep breathing and coughing exercises (use of spirometer or IPPB if indicated).
   g Leg exercises and antiembolic stockings.
   h Turning and moving in bed.
   i Reason for n.p.o. and when it begins.
   j Alterations in diet preoperatively or postoperatively.
   k Activities and preparation the morning of surgery.
   l Need for quiet environment after medications have been given.
   m Information usually provided by anesthesiologist and surgeon.
   n Tour and explanation of monitoring devices and special equipment in ICU if client is assigned there.

Rationale for Action

- To enhance a rapid recovery from surgery
- To reduce postoperative stress
- To reduce the dose and/or frequency of postoperative pain medications
- To reduce postoperative complications
- To decrease length of hospitalization
- To increase client participation in his or her postoperative recovery

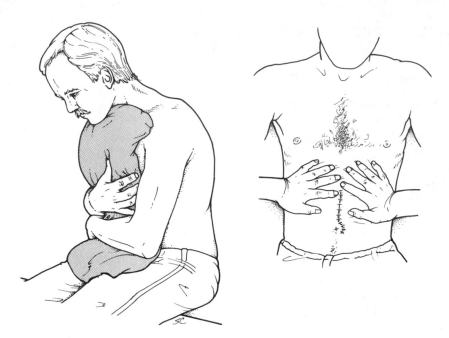

Instruct the client in deep breathing and coughing exercises preoperatively to enhance lung expansion postoperatively.

2 Provide intraoperative information.
  a Mode of transportation to operating room.
  b Discussion of procedure in preinduction room or operating room suite in relationship to anesthesia.
  c Reinforce physician's explanation of surgery.
  d Description of dressings, tubes, or equipment that will be used postoperatively.
  e Recovery room physical environment and procedures.
3 Provide postoperative information.
  a Assessment procedures.
  b Routine procedures of vital signs.
  c Deep breathing, turning, and coughing exercises.
  d IV therapy if indicated.
  e Irrigation of tubes when directed.
  f Catheter care.
  g Dietary alterations. .
  h Observation and changes of dressing.
  i Ambulation and/or restrictions in ambulation.
  j Medications.

INTERVENTION: Providing Family Teaching

1 Include information provided to client.
  a Visiting hours.
  b Where to wait during surgery.
  c Where the surgeon will meet with them, and when.
  d Where they can find bathrooms, telephones, and food and beverage service.
  e When they can see the client after surgery. Explain what the client will look like after surgery.

2 How to contact a spiritual/religious resource person.

3 How they can best get information regarding the client's condition while they are at home or in the hospital.

4 Whether they will be called if there is a change in the client's condition.

5 What to expect: client's behavior, which may be regressive; attitude which may be depressed and/or angry; physical condition, which may appear worse than it is, and post recovery period.

EVALUATION

EXPECTED OUTCOMES

1 Client provided with sufficient data to feel sense of self-control. *If not*, follow these alternative nursing actions:

ANA: Ask specific questions of client to ascertain where data is insufficient, unclear, or not clearly understood.

ANA: Repeat teaching area identified as not sufficient.

ANA: Explain content using different approach and vocabulary or provide additional information.

ANA: Use additional audio-visual equipment for explanations.

2 Family has sufficient data to cope during intraoperative and postoperative period. *If not*, follow these alternative nursing actions:

ANA: Evaluate content areas that remain unclear and then reinstruct.

ANA: Contact support group (clergy, human support services, client advocate, etc.) to assist family during the operative phase.

ANA: Take family on tour of facilities available to them during intraoperative phase.

3 Postoperative pain and complications are reduced. *If not*, follow these alternative nursing actions:

ANA: Notify physician of symptoms that indicate potential complications.

ANA: Increase deep breathing and coughing exercises to every hour if alterations in pulmonary function are noted.

ANA: Observe for signs of thrombophlebitis and report unusual findings.

ANA: When pain is not relieved by medications, utilize stress reduction techniques, and provide perceptual alterations; if these methods fail, you may request order for change in medication.

4 Stress-free environment is provided for client and family. *If not*, follow these alternative nursing actions:

ANA: Explore feelings and reasons for client's and/or family's stressful situation.

ANA: Explore ways most effective in reducing stress for client and family.

ANA: Provide stress reduction exercises.

UNEXPECTED OUTCOMES

1 Stress and/or anxiety is increased with preoperative teaching.

ANA: Determine which, if any, specific facet of the teaching is disturbing. Clarify misconceptions and inappropriate perceptions.

ANA: Utilize stress reduction techniques.

ANA: If anxiety and/or stress levels remain high, stop instruction since it will be ineffective. Resume instructions when client shows readiness to resume.

ANA: Enlist the help of the family or significant other to provide client teaching.

ANA: Leave pamphlets or educational materials for client and family to read.

ANA: Introduce client to another client who has had similar surgery.

2 Stress and/or anxiety is increased with visit from anesthesiologist or surgeon.

ANA: Determine which, if any, specific facets are disturbing the client. Clarify misconceptions and inappropriate perceptions.

ANA: Ask the physician to return to clarify misconceptions and erroneous perceptions.

ANA: Utilize realistic optimism in helping client deal with mortality and morbidity statistics, i.e., if there is a 5 percent risk, encourage the client to think in terms that 95 percent make a complete recovery and that he or she is more likely to be among the 95 percent. Do not give false reassurance.

ANA: Employ stress reducing techniques.

ANA: Resort to medications if ordered.

3 The family is *not* useful as a support system.

ANA: Ascertain if client has a friend who is supportive.

ANA: Ask the client if a priest, minister, or rabbi could act as a support.

ANA: Utilize the clinical nurse specialist's services.

ANA: If a staff nurse has developed a therapeutic relationship with the client, find out if the nurse can spend extra time with the client.

4 The family's anxiety increases until it is detrimental to the client.

ANA: Counsel the family using stress-reducing techniques.

ANA: Seek or have another member seek out a supportive friend or spiritual counselor.

ANA: Direct the family to a crisis intervention center or other supportive agency.

5 The evening hypnotic or sedative does not assist the client to sleep.

ANA: Employ stress-reducing techniques including back rub.

ANA: If not n.p.o., offer glass of warm milk. Milk contains tryptophan, an amino acid that promotes sleep.

ANA: Determine if there are specific concerns that you can alleviate.

ANA: Reduce environmental noise.

ANA: Administer a repeat dose of the medication if ordered.

6 The client complains of a sore throat, runny nose, and cough before the scheduled surgery.

ANA: Inform the surgeon and anesthesiologist.

7 You are not familiar with the postoperative routine for the particular surgery of your client.

ANA: Ask a nurse who is familiar with the postoperative procedure to complete client teaching.

Charting

- Document teaching on preoperative teaching check list
- Document areas of teaching that were completed on both Kardex and client chart
- Make notations of any area of teaching that needs to be reinforced or additional instruction that needs to be completed
- Describe indications that the client's and family's anxiety/stress levels are appropriate. Use objective and/or behavioral signs or quotations
- Return demonstrations of deep breathing, use of equipment, tour of critical care units etc.

ANA: Ask the surgeon to explain the postoperative routine either to the client or to you.

ANA: Call upon the clinical nurse specialist to talk with the client.

ANA: Seek advice from your head nurse or supervisor.

8 The client or family asks a question for which you do not have an answer.

ANA: State that you do not know the answer but will get the answer or send someone who does know the answer.

ANA: Ask someone who knows the answer, and pass the information on to the client or family immediately.

ANA: Look up the answer and have the answer available to other nurses who may be asked the same question.

ACTION: PREPARING CLIENT FOR SURGERY

ASSESSMENT

1 Assess type of surgical procedure to be carried out and extent of data base needed.
2 Evaluate the ability of the client to provide accurate data base information.
3 Assess level of anxiety present that may interfere in the transmission of information at the moment.
4 Identify the appropriate physical care needed for the specific surgical intervention.
5 Check for potential complications postoperatively.
6 Identify clients at risk for surgery.
7 Assess special needs for the surgical shave.
   a Evaluate need for special permits for shaving, such as the head for neurosurgical clients, extremities for orthopedic clients, or children.
   b Assess need for special soap or antiseptic scrub prior to shave.
   c Evaluate need for sterile drape following shave.
   d Check if a policy exists in the hospital for disposing or handling of scalp hair.
   e Assess area before shaving for unusual cuts, abrasions, or markings and report findings to physician.

PLANNING

GOALS

- Client's physical or emotional deviations that could interfere with safe intraoperative or postoperative care are identified.
- Baseline data is obtained and compared with postoperative clinical findings to determine alterations.
- Chronic problems or allergies that could affect postoperative nursing care are documented.

Rationale for Action

- To assist with monitoring the client's progress through the operative experience
- To identify deviations from the client's usual baseline data that may occur as a result of anxiety or stress of admission, preoperative events, diagnostic procedures, the surgical trauma, postoperative complications, responses to and side effects of drugs
- To distinguish perioperative changes from chronic physical changes that were present on admission
- To identify pertinent data for the nursing care plan that may affect the postoperative period, such as the presence of arthritic changes in the neck or back, allergies, or chronic use of prescribed and/or nonprescription drugs
- To provide appropriate preoperative physical care to enable the client to have a safe intraoperative and postoperative period

▶ Preoperative nursing responsibilities:
1 Gather baseline data.
2 Assess client's anxiety or stress.
3 Initiate interventions to prevent or reduce anxiety or stress.
4 Prepare client physically and psychologically for surgery.
5 Start postoperative planning.

671

- Information for developing an individualized nursing care plan is obtained.
- Safe intraoperative and postoperative period is ensured when explicit preoperative care is given.
- Surgical shave is completed correctly without cuts.

EQUIPMENT

- Tools for completing a physical assessment
- Specific equipment needed to provide physical care such as enema equipment, nasogastric tube, Foley catheter
- Preoperative check list
- Chart for documenting findings
- Spirometers or pillows for teaching deep breathing exercises

ADDITIONAL EQUIPMENT

For Preoperative Shave
- Absorbent pad
- Bath blanket or drape
- Scissors
- Disposable prep kit (if available)
- If kit not available
  Sterile safety razor and blades
  Two sterile bowls
  4 × 4 gauze pads
  Emesis basin
  Applicator sticks
  Cleansing solution
  Sterile water
  Sterile gloves

INTERVENTION: Obtaining Baseline Data

1 Establish rapport with the client.
2 Explain why you are going to take a nursing history and perform a physical examination.
3 While taking a nursing history, observe the client's emotional status, color, skin condition, hair condition, and posture.
4 Ask about allergies to drugs or food.
5 Complete a physical examination.
6 Take and record vital signs and weight of client.
7 Check if client wears dentures, hearing aid, or glasses, or has an artificial eye.
8 Ensure that the laboratory tests, ECG, and x-rays have been ordered.
9 Review the results of the laboratory studies, ECG, and x-rays. Notify physician of abnormal findings.
10 Identify areas where client teaching is needed and complete the instruction.

COMMUNITY HOSPITAL

AUTHORIZATION FOR AND CONSENT TO SURGERY, ADMINISTRATION OF ANESTHETICS, SPECIAL DIAGNOSTIC OR THERAPEUTIC PROCEDURES

Date _____ Time _____

Your admitting physician is _____, M. D.

Your surgeon is _____, M. D.

1. The hospital staff and facilities assist your physicians and surgeons in the performance of various surgical operations and other diagnostic and therapeutic procedures. These surgical operations and special diagnostic or therapeutic procedures all may involve calculated risks of complications, injury or even death, from both known and unknown causes and no warranty or guarantee has been made as to result or cure. Except in a case of emergency or exceptional circumstances, these operations and procedures are not performed upon clients unless and until the client has had an opportunity to discuss them with his/her physician. Each client has the right to consent to or refuse any proposed operation or special procedure (based upon the description or explanation received).

2. Your physicians and surgeons have determined that the operations or special procedures listed below may be beneficial in the diagnosis or treatment of your condition. Upon your authorization and consent, the operations or special procedures will be performed by your physicians and surgeons and their staff. The persons in attendance for the purpose of administering anesthesia or performing other specialized professional services, such as radiology, pathology and the like, are not the agents, servants or employees of the hospital or your physician or surgeon, but are independent contractors performing specialized services on your behalf and, as such, are your agents, servants, or employees. Any tissue or member severed in any operation will be disposed of in the discretion of the pathologist, except _____ and those body parts specified as donor organs.

3. Your signature opposite the operations or special procedures listed below constitutes your acknowledgement (a) that you have read and agreed to the foregoing, (b) that the operations or special procedures have been adequately explained to you by your attending physicians or surgeons and that you have all of the information that you desire, and (c) that you authorize and consent to the performance of the operations or special procedures.

Operation or Procedure

_____

_____

Signature _____   Signature _____
                       Client   Witness

(If client is a minor or unable to sign, complete the following): Client is a minor, is unable to sign because

_____

_____   _____
          Father   Guardian

_____   _____
          Mother   Other person and relationship

The exact surgical procedure is written on the surgical permit. Client signs permit only after the physician has explained the procedure and the possible complications.

SURGICAL CHECK LIST

Unit Check List   PLEASE PRINT

1. Surgical Procedure scheduled: _____

   _____ Rt. _____ Lt. _____
                                                      (circle)

2. Consent for surgery _____
                        Yes or No

3. Consent for Sterilization or Special Procedure _____
                                                   Yes or No

4. Consultation _____
                Yes or No

5. Surgical Prep done by _____
                              (Signature)

6. History and Physical _____
                        Yes or No

7. Urinalysis _____ CBC _____ Type & Xmatch _____
              Yes or No   Yes or No   Yes or No

8. Chest X-ray _____ EKG _____
               Yes or No   Yes or No

9. List allergies (if none, state "none") _____

10. Allergy Band _____
                 Yes or No

11. TPR _____ BP _____

12. Voided _____ Time _____ Retention Cath. _____
                                                               Yes or No

13. Pre-op medication and times _____

14. Condition after pre-op medication: _____ awake   asleep   drowsy
                                                     (circle)

15. Prosthesis:	None	Removed	Disposition	Left In
a. Bridge				
b. Partial				
c. Plates				
d. Artificial limbs				
e. Artificial eyes				
f. Contact lenses				
g. Hearing aid				
h. Pacemaker				
i. Hairpieces, Hairpins, Eyelashes				

16. Valuables	Removed Yes or No	Disposition, if yes
a. Rings		
b. Watch		
c. Medal and chain		
d. Glasses		
e. Radio		
f. Wallet		
g. Other		

17. Identification band checked with chart _____
                                            Yes or No

    Signature _____ R.N.

Operating Room Check List

Check	Comment
1.	
2.	
3.	
4.	
5.	
6.	
7.	
8.	
9.	
10.	
11.	
12.	
13.	
14.	
15.	
a.	
b.	
c.	
d.	
e.	
f.	
g.	
h.	
i.	
16.	
17.	

Signature _____
                    Circulating Nurse

POSTOPERATIVE

Sponge Count _____

Needle Count _____

Drains Left In _____

Catheter In _____

Scrub Nurse _____

Signature _____
                    Circulating Nurse

The preoperative check list must be completed prior to client transfer to the operating room.

INTERVENTION: Providing Safety Measures for Surgical Clients

1 Ensure all lab work (CBC, UA, Hgb, Hct) has been drawn and reports are on chart.
2 Make sure physician's history and physical examination is documented on chart.
3 Check to see that chest x-ray report is on chart.
4 Ensure ECG report is included on chart for clients over forty years of age who are scheduled for major surgery.
5 Obtain signed operative and sterilization permit when needed.
6 Document preoperative client teaching.
7 Complete preoperative checklist.

INTERVENTION: Shaving the Surgical Client

1 Refer to physician's orders for specific operative site or area to be shaved. If orders do not state preference for site, refer to procedure manual for appropriate area to be shaved, based on surgical procedure.
2 Gather equipment.
3 Explain procedure to client and provide privacy.
4 Adjust light to ensure good visualization.
5 Wash your hands.
6 Position client for maximum comfort and prep site exposure.
7 Drape client for comfort and to prevent undue exposure.
8 Protect bed with absorbent pad.
9 Arrange shaving equipment for your convenience.
10 Cut long hair with scissors.
11 Dispose of cut hair.
12 Put on sterile gloves.
13 Apply cleansing solution with 4 × 4 gauze pads.
14 Begin at incision site and, with light friction, make ever-widening circles, moving outward from the center to the most distant line of prep area.
15 Discard soiled sponges frequently.
16 Using sharp razor, shave hair moving away from incision site. With free hand, stretch skin taut and shave, following the hair growth pattern and using firm, steady strokes.
17 Change blade as often as necessary. Avoid nicking the skin. Report if skin is nicked.
18 When all hair has been removed, re-scrub area as above. Scrub area for at least two to five minutes. Orthopedic surgery may require a ten-minute scrub.
19 Rinse shaved area with warm water and blot dry with 4 × 4 gauze pads.
20 Assist client to put on clean gown.
21 Remove and dispose of equipment.
22 Position the client for comfort.

▶ Wound infection and poor wound healing are caused by contamination of wound during surgery and decreased client resistance.

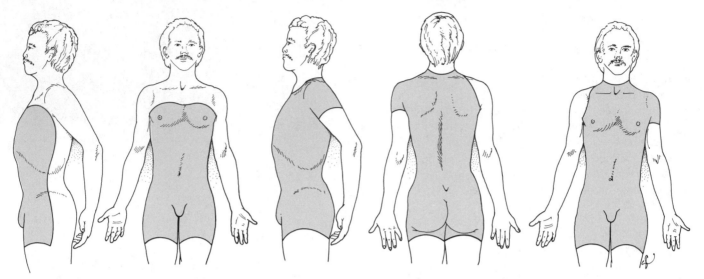

Illustrated is the area shaved for abdominal surgeries such as appendectomy and hernia repair. The upper thigh areas do not necessarily need to be shaved for cholecystectomy, gastrectomy, or bowel resections.

Illustrated are the areas shaved for thoracotomy and upper abdominal surgeries. Back view indicates the area included when lateral thoracotomy incision is used.

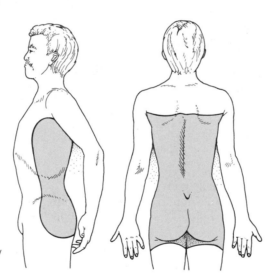

Illustrated are shaved areas for laminectomy and renal surgery.

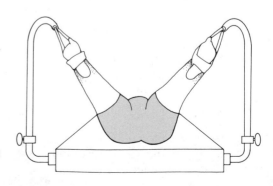

The area shaved for gynecological and genito-urinary surgery.

INTERVENTION: Preparing the Client for Surgery

1 Notify surgeon and anesthesiologist for orders regarding administration, dosage or restriction of anticoagulants, antiarrhythmics, insulin, digitalis, Inderal, or steroids being taken by the client.
2 Obtain orders for preoperative medications and information to be contained on preoperative permit.
3 Administer enema if ordered.
4 Assess for proper completion of skin prep and shave.
5 Observe for signs of cold or upper respiratory infection.
6 Keep n.p.o. for 8 to 10 hours preoperatively.
7 Provide adequate hydration.
8 Remove hair pieces and dentures.
9 Place surgical cap on client's head.
10 Remove contact lenses and glasses.
11 Remove earrings, necklaces, medals, watch, rings (ring may be taped on).
12 Remove lipstick and nail polish.
13 Insert Foley catheter if ordered.
14 Take and record vital signs.
15 Assess chart for presence of operative permit, blood and urine reports, time and amount of last voiding, time and dose of preoperative medication given, and completion of preoperative check list.
16 Provide preoperative showers with bacteriostatic soap.
17 Administer preoperative medications.
18 Place side rails in UP position following administration of medications.
19 Darken room and provide quiet environment following administration of medications.
20 Check client's name band with transporter from operating room.

INTERVENTION: Administering Preoperative Medications

1 Complete preoperative check list that includes assessing vital signs.
2 Follow procedure for administration of intramuscular injections.
3 Have the client void before the preoperative medications are administered.
4 Record time and amount of void.
5 Explain the purpose of the medication to the client.
6 Warn the client that the injection may sting or burn.
7 Administer medication.
8 Raise side rails.
9 Explain why the client should not get out of bed after the medications have been given.
10 Place the call light within reach and encourage the client to use it.
11 Ask if there are any questions or assistance you can offer before leaving the room.
12 Give the client the estimated time of surgery.

▶ **Preoperative Medications: Type and Action**

Hypnotic or opiate—given night before surgery
   Decreases anxiety
   Promotes good night's sleep
Hypnotic or opiate—preoperative medication
   Decreases anxiety
   Allows smooth anesthetic induction
   Provides amnesia for immediate perioperative period
Anticholinergic—preoperative medication
   Decreases secretion
   Counteracts vagal effects during anesthesia

EVALUATION

EXPECTED OUTCOMES

1   Client's physical and/or emotional deviations from normal are identified preoperatively. *If not*, follow these alternative nursing actions:

ANA: Notify a clergy or support person in the hospital to visit the client.

ANA: Be a good listener and pick up cues as to the cause of client's concerns.

ANA: Assist the client in expressing fears. Offer explanations and clarification where needed.

ANA: Notify physician if client expresses an inordinate amount of fear or seems severely distressed. Surgery may be cancelled.

2   Preoperative baseline data is obtained. *If not*, follow these alternative nursing actions:

ANA: Be sure temperature, pulse, respiration, blood pressure, and lab results are on the chart before the client leaves the unit. This baseline data is required before the client is taken to the operating room.

ANA: Read the physician's history and physical to detect any abnormalities that could interfere with the postoperative stage if you have not been able to complete a physical examination.

ANA: Ask the client and/or family for specific information related to the client's condition.

3   Explicit preoperative care is provided to ensure a safe intraoperative and postoperative course. *If not*, follow these alternative nursing actions:

ANA: If adequate preoperative care was not given, inform both the surgeon and anesthesiologist because anesthetic induction may be difficult to attain.

ANA: Be prepared to have a more anxious client postoperatively.

ANA: Be prepared to administer more pain medication and provide more assistance with stress reduction.

4   Surgical shave is completed correctly and without cuts. *If not*, follow these alternative nursing actions:

ANA: Check procedure manual for appropriate area to be shaved.

ANA: Report cuts to physician so the need to postpone surgery can be evaluated and specific treatment for lacerations ordered.

UNEXPECTED OUTCOMES

1   Laboratory values or results of ECG or x-ray come back with abnormal findings.

ANA: Evaluate accuracy of test results. If extremely abnormal, ask laboratory to recheck the specimen.

ANA: If client has been n.p.o., identify if the client had eaten prior to the tests.

ANA: Notify physician of abnormal findings.

2   Factors that can affect the postoperative course are identified during the physical examination, i.e., arthritic changes in client's back, history of thrombophlebitis, etc.

▶ Surgery is contraindicated for clients who are severely anxious. These clients frequently have major postoperative complications. Death has occurred in some cases.

ANA: Place information on client's care plan and develop individualized interventions with the client's assistance.

ANA: Write a note on client's chart and alert the operating room and recovery room staff of the findings so that they can assess for the problems.

3 Client refuses to go to operating room without dentures.

ANA: Explain to client that dentures are likely to be lost, broken, or inadvertently pushed to back of mouth if not removed.

ANA: If client refuses to remove dentures, alert anesthesiologist that dentures are in place.

4 Client unable to void before surgery.

ANA: Run water so client can hear trickling sound to stimulate voiding.

ANA: Place ammonia or oil of wintergreen on a cotton ball in urinal or bedpan.

ACTION: CARING FOR THE INTRAOPERATIVE CLIENT

ASSESSMENT

1 Assess correct operative position for client.
2 Evaluate completeness of preoperative checklist information.
3 Identify time and amount of preoperative medication administered.
4 Identify the stage of anesthesia the client is going through.
5 Assess areas for potentially unsafe situations during the operative procedure.

PLANNING

GOALS

- Client is positioned on operating table for optimal exposure of surgical site.
- Client progresses through induction of anesthesia without complications.
- Client is free of circulatory or nervous complications due to malposition on operating room table.
- Safety measures are carried out throughout operative procedure.

EQUIPMENT

- Operating room table
- Restraints
- Blanket or drape

INTERVENTION: Positioning the Operative Client

1 Assess surgical procedure to be performed.
2 Identify individual surgeon's preference for position.

Charting

- Pertinent findings from nursing history and physical examination
- Physical findings that could alter postoperative nursing measures
- Safety measures carried out preoperatively
- Completion of preoperative shave and area involved
- Completed operative checklist
- Solution used and length of time of scrub
- Witness physician's explanation of potential surgical complications
- Physical care completed prior to surgery
- Preoperative medications given and effects of medications
- Time and method of transportation to operating room

Rationale for Action

- To position the client for optimal exposure of surgical site
- To prevent complications associated with circulation or nervous impairment while positioned on the operating table
- To identify the stages of anesthesia induction

Operative Positions

- Dorsal recumbent: open heart and abdominal surgery.
- Trendelenburg's: lower abdominal and pelvic surgery.
- Lithotomy: perineal, rectal, and vaginal surgery.
- Sims': kidney and thoracotomy surgery.
- Jackknife: anal surgery.
- Prone with head and feet lowered: spinal surgery.

3 Assess client's skin and tissue turgor to preserve intact skin.

4 Assess number of personnel needed to transfer client to operating table.

5 Explain move to operating table and position client on table according to procedure.

6 Protect client from injury.

    a Use padded straps.

    b Pad bony prominences to prevent nerve and tissue damage.

    c Prevent dangling of extremities over sides of table without support.

    d Use care moving client to and from the operating table.

    e Be certain body does not rest on arm, hand, or fingers.

7 Avoid undue exposure to preserve client's sense of modesty.

8 Position client for adequate chest expansion and circulation.

    a Avoid placing straps across chest.

    b Place straps across extremities in manner that prevents occlusion of circulation.

9 Prevent chilling of client by placing warm blanket or drape over client.

Six positions commonly used for surgical procedures.

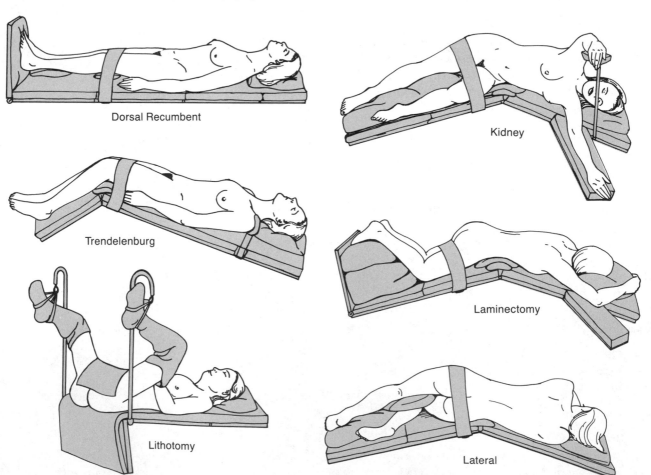

Dorsal Recumbent

Trendelenburg

Lithotomy

Kidney

Laminectomy

Lateral

INTERVENTION: Understanding the Principles of Anesthesia

1 Be familiar with the principles of general anesthesia.
   a Balanced anesthesia (combination of two or more drugs) is used to decrease side effects and complications of anesthetic agents.
   b Goals of general anesthesia.
      Analgesia.
      Unconsciousness.
      Skeletal muscle relaxation.
   c Classifications of general anesthesia.
      Potent anesthesia (halothane, ether, chloroform): Capable of achieving all three goals of general anesthesia but with severe side effects.

      Nonpotent anesthesia (nitrous oxide): If given in large dose, can achieve all three goals of general anesthesia but produces toxicity. When given in smaller doses, lacks analgesia or skeletal muscle relaxation.

      Basal anesthesia (thiopental, Pentothal): Ultra short-acting barbiturate so high doses needed for prolonged deep anesthesia, which can lead to respiratory depression. Used for induction — effects are rapid, allowing for less inhalation anesthesia.

      Dissociative anesthesia (ketamine HCl and Innovar): Used with nitrous oxide and oxygen for short anesthesia. Client is awake but unaware of what is actually happening. Useful for burn dressings.

2 Be familiar with the principles of topical anesthetics.
   a Poorly absorbed through skin but usually rapid through mucous membranes (mouth, GI tract, etc.).
   b Systemic toxicity is rare but local reactions common, especially if used for long periods of time on clients allergic to chemicals.
   c Used for hemorrhoids, episiotomy, nipple erosion, and minor cuts and burns.
   d Used on eye procedures extensively — removing foreign bodies and tonometry.
   e Types of local anesthesia.
      Infiltrated local anesthesia (or field block): Anesthesia directly applied to surgical area. Drug is injected into bloodstream. Can have systemic effects if injected into highly vascular area.

      Regional anesthetics (central nerve blocks): Types — spinal, caudal, saddle, epidural. Precautions for spinal and epidural anesthesia: position client with head and shoulder elevated (prevents diffusion of anesthesia to the intercostal muscles which could produce respiratory distress). Epidural (continuous anesthesia used in O.B.): make sure catheter is securely fastened to prevent it from slipping out.

3 Know the action and principles of preoperative drugs.
   a General actions.
      Decreases secretions of mouth and respiratory tract.
      Depresses vagal reflexes — slows heart and prevents complications with excitation during intubation.

Anesthetic Agents

1 Anesthesia produces insensitivity to pain or sensation.
2 Dangers associated with anesthesia depend on overall condition of client. High risk if associated cardiovascular, renal, or respiratory conditions. High risk for unborn fetus and mother. High risk if stomach full (chance of vomiting and aspiration).
3 Types of anesthesia. General—administered IV or by inhalation. Produces loss of consciousness and decreases reflex movement. Local—applied topically or injected regionally. Client is alert, but pain and sensation are decreased in surgical area.

681

Produces drowsiness and relieves anxiety.

Allows anesthesia to be induced more smoothly and in smaller amounts.

b Types of drugs.

Barbiturates.

Intermediate-acting barbiturate at bedtime (Seconal or Nembutal).

Short-acting barbiturate one hour preoperatively (decreases blood pressure and pulse and relieves anxiety).

Belladonna alkaloids.

General action.

Decreases salivary and bronchial secretions.

Allows inhalation anesthetics to be administered more easily.

Prevents postoperative complications such as aspiration pneumonia.

Scopolamine is used in conjunction with morphine or Demerol to to produce amnesic block.

Atropine blocks the vagus nerve response of decreased heart rate, which can occur as a reaction to some inhalation anesthetics.

Nonnarcotic analgesic (Stadol)

General actions.

Stadol used as component of balanced anesthesia.

Given IM.

Does not cause dependence or respiratory depression with increased dose.

Contraindicated in narcotic addiction.

Side effects.

Sedation, lethargy.

Headache, vertigo.

Nervousness, palpitations, diplopia.

Nausea, dry mouth.

INTERVENTION: Monitoring for Safety During Operative Procedure

1 Identify appropriate client by checking name band and chart.
2 Check that operative permit is signed for appropriate surgical intervention.
3 Ensure that preoperative lab work is completed and results are within normal range.
4 Check that preoperative check list is completed and no problems are identified that could lead to potential complications.
5 Observe shaved area for cuts or unusual markings.
6 Check operative permit for exact procedure to be done and position client in appropriate position.
7 Secure client on operating table with restraints to prevent injury of the client during the operative procedure.
8 Complete a surgical scrub maintaining principles of asepsis.
9 Monitor for breaks in sterile technique during operative procedure.

10 Monitor client during surgical procedure to identify potential complications.

EVALUATION

EXPECTED OUTCOMES

1 Client progresses through the induction of anesthesia without complications. *If not*, follow these alternative nursing actions:

ANA: Be prepared to assist with resuscitation measures. Unnecessary and loud noises during induction can cause the client to become overexcited and pass into the fourth (and dangerous) stage of anesthesia.

2 Safety measures are maintained throughout the operative procedure. *If not*, follow these alternative nursing actions:

ANA: If instruments become contaminated, remove them from the surgical field immediately and replace them.

ANA: If personnel contaminate themselves unknowingly, the circulating nurse needs to call attention to it and have them regown.

ANA: Make sure the grounding device is secured to the client's body so that the client will not experience electrical shock during the surgical procedure.

ANA: Make sure that straps are secured at all times to prevent alterations in client's position during the operative procedure.

3 Nurse's knowledge of anesthetic agents is sufficient to allow for safe observation during the operative period. *If not*, follow these alternative nursing actions:

ANA: Review all new anesthetic agents to ensure that your knowledge base is sufficient to detect abnormal client reactions during the operative period.

ANA: Attend in-service classes on anesthetic agents to expand your knowledge base.

ANA: Check with the surgeon or another nurse if client's clinical manifestations seem abnormal.

UNEXPECTED OUTCOMES

1 Preoperative medications were not given on time.

ANA: Anesthesiologist must be notified so he or she can change the amount of anesthesia to provide sufficient medications. Preoperative medications are included as part of the balanced anesthesia planned for the client.

ANA: If this is a persistent problem within the hospital arrange for a nursing audit to be completed to determine the reasons.

ANA: Reinforce the need for prompt administration of medications with nursing personnel.

2 Preoperative medications appear to be ineffective.

ANA: Notify anesthesiologist so he or she can adjust the inhalation anesthesia during induction.

ANA: Provide alternative nursing actions to reduce stress or anxiety and therefore increase the effectiveness of the medications.

Charting
- Identaband checked
- Preoperative check list checked
- Safety measures taken before and during operative procedure
- Effects of anesthesia
- Untoward effects of anesthesia
- Length of time of surgical procedure
- Needle, sponge, and instrument count

- To provide safe, effective nursing care in the immediate postoperative period
- To identify the parameters for discharging the client from the recovery room
- To be aware of the common postoperative drugs for pain control

▶ Clients at risk for postoperative infection:
- Uncontrolled diabetes
- Renal failure
- Obesity
- Receiving corticosteroids
- Receiving immunosuppressive agents
- Prolonged antibiotic therapy
- Protein and/or ascorbic acid deficiencies
- Marked dehydration and hypovolemia
- Decreased cardiac output
- Edema and fluid and electrolyte imbalances
- Anemia
- Preoperative infection

ACTION: PROVIDING POSTOPERATIVE CARE

ASSESSMENT

1. Assess for patent airway.
2. Assess need for oxygen.
3. Check gag reflex, especially in recovery room.
4. Observe for adverse signs of general anesthesia or spinal anesthesia.
5. Assess vital signs.
6. Evaluate client's temperature for heat control.
7. Observe dressings and surgical drains.
8. Assess IVs for type and amount of fluid to be infused.
9. Observe color and amount of urine.
10. Observe client's overall condition.

PLANNING

GOALS

- Client experiences an uneventful postoperative course.
- Postoperative complications are identified rapidly and appropriate interventions instituted.
- Client is discharged from recovery room at appropriate time.
- Postoperative pain is relieved promptly.

EQUIPMENT

For Recovery Room
- Blood pressure sphygmomanometer
- Stethoscope
- Oxygen nasal cannula or mask
- IV pole
- Special equipment depending on type of procedure, i.e., wall suction for chest tubes or nasogastric tubes

ADDITIONAL EQUIPMENT

For Surgical Unit
- Surgical bed
- Absorbent pads
- Warm blankets
- IV pole
- Oxygen source, tubing, and equipment
- Emesis basin and tissues
- Sphygmomanometer and stethoscope
- Thermometer (rectal or oral)
- Nurses' notes
- Intake and output record
- Special equipment depending on type of surgery

INTERVENTION: Providing Recovery Room Care

1. Assess for patent airway. Leave airway in place until gag reflex returns.
2. Administer oxygen by mask or nasal cannula at 6 l/min.
3. Position client for adequate ventilation. Side-lying position is best if not contraindicated.
4. Observe for adverse signs of general anesthesia or spinal anesthesia.
   a. Level of consciousness.
   b. Movement of limbs.
5. Monitor vital signs every 10 to 15 minutes. Vital signs are sometimes difficult to obtain due to hypothermia. Movement from operating room table to guerney can alter vital signs significantly, especially with cardiovascular clients.
   a. Pulse: check rate, quality, and rhythm.
   b. Blood pressure: check pulse pressure and quality as well as systolic and diastolic pressure.
   c. Respiration: check rate, rhythm, depth, and type of respiration (abdominal breathing, nasal flaring).
6. Maintain temperature (operating room is usually cold) — apply warm blankets.
7. Monitor IV fluids.
   a. Check type and amount of solution being administered.
   b. Adjust correct flow rate.
   c. Check IV site for signs of infiltration.
8. Check blood transfusion.
   a. Client's name and identification number.
   b. Blood type and blood bank number.
   c. Expiration date.
   d. Time transfusion started.
   e. Amount in bag upon arrival in recovery room.
   f. Color and consistency of blood.
9. Measure urine output hourly for major surgical procedures and before leaving recovery room for minor surgical procedures.
10. Monitor surgical dressings hourly.
    a. Mark any drainage on dressings and note time by drawing a line around the drainage.
    b. Note color and amount of drainage on dressings and in drainage tubes.
    c. Check that dressing is secure.
    d. Reinforce dressings as needed.
11. Check skin for warmth, color, and moisture.
12. Check nailbeds and mucous membranes for color and blanching; report if cyanotic.
13. Observe for return of reflexes.
14. Administer medications.
    a. Begin routine drugs and administer all STAT drugs.
    b. Pain medications are usually administered sparingly and in smaller amounts. Usual route is intravenous.

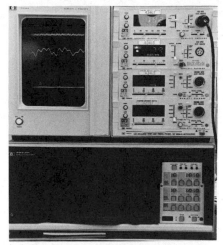

Check vital signs every 10 to 15 minutes. Placing clients on monitors in the recovery room promotes early detection of alterations.

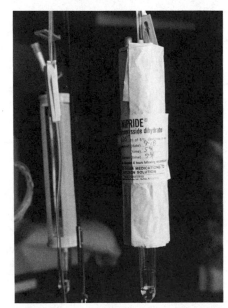

Administer all "Stat" drugs such as Nipride and begin routine medications in the recovery room.

685

INTERVENTION: Discharging Client from Recovery Room

1 Be sure vital signs are stable and within normal limits for at least one hour.
2 See if client is awake and reflexes are present (gag and cough reflex). Check for movement and sensation in limbs of clients with spinal anesthesia.
3 Take oral airway out (if not out already). Observe for cyanosis.
4 Be sure dressings are intact and there is no excessive drainage.
5 Ensure all drains are functioning.
6 Record amount of remaining IV fluid and amount absorbed. Check for IV patency.
7 Record amount of urine in drainage bag and empty bag.
8 Record all medications administered in recovery room.
9 Cleanse client as needed: change gown and wash off excess surgical scrub solution.
10 Call anesthesiologist for order to discharge client from recovery room.
11 Recovery room nurse accompanies client to nursing unit.
12 Give report to unit nurse.
  a Type of operative procedure.
  b Length of operation.
  c Length of time in recovery room.
  d Vital signs, condition of dressings, condition of IV, and amount and type of IV fluids infused.

INTERVENTION: Completing Postoperative Care on Surgical Unit

1 Assess for patent airway; administer oxygen as necessary.
2 Assess vital signs: usual orders are q15 minutes until stable; then q½ hour × 2; qhour × 4; then q4 hours for 24–48 hours.
3 Check IV site and patency frequently.
4 Observe and record urine output.
5 Assess intake and output.
6 Observe skin color and moisture.
7 Position client for comfort and maximum airway ventilation.
8 Turn every two hours and p.r.n.
9 Give back care at least every four hours.
10 Encourage coughing and deep breathing every two hours (may use IPPB or blow bottles).
11 Keep client comfortable with medications.
12 Check dressings and drainage tubes every two to four hours; if abnormal amount of drainage, check more frequently.
13 Give oral hygiene at least every four hours; if nasogastric tube, nasal oxygen, or endotracheal tube is inserted, give oral hygiene every two hours.
14 Bathe client when temperature can be maintained (bathing removes the antiseptic solution and stimulates circulation).

15 Keep client warm and avoid chilling, but do not increase temperature above normal.

    a Increased temperature increases metabolic rate and need for oxygen.

    b Excessive perspiration causes fluid and electrolyte loss.

16 Irrigate nasogastric tube every two hours and p.r.n. with normal saline to keep patent and to prevent electrolyte imbalance.

17 Maintain dietary intake: type of diet depends on type and extent of surgical procedure.

    a Minor surgical conditions: client may drink or eat as soon as he or she is awake and desires food or drink.

    b Major surgical conditions.

        n.p.o. until bowel sounds return.

        Clear liquid advanced to full liquid as tolerated.

        Soft diet advanced to full diet within three to five days (depending on type of surgery and physician's preference).

18 Place client on bedpan two to four hours postoperatively if catheter not inserted.

19 Start activity as tolerated and dictated by surgical procedure. Most clients are dangled within first 24 hours.

20 Monitor for postoperative complications. See Postoperative Complications chart.

INTERVENTION: Administering Postoperative Medications

1 Evaluate client's need for pain relief.

2 Provide nonmedication measures for relief of pain such as relaxation techniques, back care, client positioning.

3 Identify the pharmacological action of the medication.

4 Review the general side effects of the medication.

    a Drowsiness.

    b Euphoria.

    c Sleep.

    d Respiratory depression.

    e Nausea and vomiting.

5 Administer medications at three to four hour intervals for first 24 to 48 hours for better action and pain relief. Assess for pain relief.

6 Know the action of opiates.

    a Morphine sulfate — potent analgesic.

        Specific side effects: miosis (pinpoint pupils) and bradycardia.

        Usual dosage: 1/4 to 1/6 gr IM q3 – 4 hours p.r.n.

    b Dilaudid — potent analgesic.

        Specific side effects: hypotension, constipation, euphoria.

        Usual dosage: 2 – 4 mg p.o., IM or IV q4 – 6 hours.

    c Numorphan — potent analgesic.

        Specific side effects: urinary retention, ileus, euphoria.

        Usual dosage: 1 – 1.5 mg IM or sub q 4 – 6 hours; 0.5 mg IV q4 – 6 hours.

d Codeine sulfate — mild analgesic.

Specific side effect: constipation.

Usual dosage 30 – 60 mg q3 – 4 hours sub q.

7 Know the action of synthetic opiate-like drugs.

a Demerol (meperidine) — potent analgesic.

Specific side effects: miosis or mydriasis (dilatation of pupils), hypotension, and tachycardia.

Usual dosage: 25 – 100 mg q3 – 4 hours IM.

b Talwin (pentazocine) — potent analgesic.

Specific side effects: gastrointestinal disturbances, vertigo, headache, and euphoria.

Usual dosage: 50 mg oral tablets q3 – 4 hours; 30 mg IM q3 – 4 hours p.r.n.

8 Understand the action of nonnarcotic pain relievers.

a Salicylates (aspirin).

Decrease pain perception without causing drowsiness or euphoria. Act at point of origin of pain impulses.

Side effects:

Gastrointestinal irritation (give client milk and crackers).

Gastrointestinal bleeding.

Increased bleeding time (watch if client is on anticoagulants).

Hypersensitivity reactions to aspirin.

Tinnitus indicates toxic level reached.

Thrombocytopenia can occur with overdose (especially in children).

Usual dosage: 300 – 600 mg q3 – 4 hours, orally or rectally.

b Nonsalicylate analgesics (acetaminophen).

Action similar to aspirin.

Side effects: hemolytic anemia and kidney damage.

Usual dosage: 325 – 650 mg q3 – 4 hours orally.

c Nonsteroid antiinflammatory (Zomax).

Action: Analgesic and antipyretic for moderate to severe pain.

Side effects: nausea, gastrointestinal distress, vertigo, drowsiness, rash.

Usual dosage: 100 mg q4 – 6 hours.

9 Know the action of antiemetics.

a Pharmacological action.

Reduces the hyperactive reflex of the stomach.

Makes the chemoreceptor trigger zone of medulla less sensitive to nerve impulses passing through this center to the vomiting center.

b General side effects.

Drowsiness.

Dry mouth.

Nervous system effects.

c Compazine (phenothiazine).

Specific side effects: amenorrhea, hypotension, and vertigo.

Normal dosage: 5 – 10 mg q3 – 4 hours IM.

d Phenergan (phenothiazine).
  Specific side effects: dryness of mouth and blurred vision.
  Normal dosage: 12.5 – 50 mg q4 hours p.r.n.
e Dramamine (nonphenothiazine).
  Specific side effect: drowsiness.
  Normal dosage: 50 mg IM q3 – 4 hours.
f Tigan (nonphenothiazine).
  Specific side effects (rare): hypotension and skin rashes.
  Normal dosage: 200 mg (2 cc) t.i.d. or q.i.d. IM.

EVALUATION

EXPECTED OUTCOMES

1 Client experiences an uneventful postoperative course. *If not*, follow these alternative nursing actions:
  ANA: If client experiences untoward effects, complete a physical assessment and plan nursing interventions based on findings of assessment.
  ANA: Prevent postoperative complications by having client deep breathe, cough, turn, perform leg exercises and ambulate as early as possible.
  ANA: Continually assess for possible postoperative complications to identify condition early and perform appropriate interventions.
2 Client is discharged from recovery room at appropriate time. *If not*, follow these alternative nursing actions:
  ANA: If client is discharged when still under effects of anesthesia, speak to nursing personnel about parameters for discharge.
  ANA: Assign skilled personnel to care for client postoperatively if discharged early from recovery room due to high census.
  ANA: Follow established discharge criteria to ensure that clients are not discharged too early from recovery room.
  ANA: If clients continue to be discharged too early from recovery room go over discharge policy and parameters with all personnel.
3 Postoperative pain is relieved promptly. *If not*, follow these alternative nursing actions:
  ANA: Assess if adjunct measures such as relaxation techniques and back care have been used to reduce pain. If not, use these in conjunction with medications.
  ANA: Evaluate effects of medication and determine if drug is ineffective in pain control.
  ANA: Ask physician for change in medication orders when medication is not effective.

UNEXPECTED OUTCOMES

See Postoperative Complications chart.

Charting
- Assessment findings
- Effects of anesthesia
- Fluid replacement—type and amount of solution
- Condition of dressings and drains
- Intake and output
- Vital signs
- Complications
- Preventive nursing measures
- Client's activity level
- Clinical manifestations indicating pain
- Type and amount of pain medication administered
- Site of injection
- Any side effects observed
- Whether or not pain relieved

689

POTENTIAL COMPLICATION	CLIENTS AT RISK	INDICATIVE FINDINGS

Atelectasis: collapse of alveoli; may be diffuse and involve a segment or lobe, or lung
 	
Potential Onset:
First 48 hours
	All with general anesthesia
	Special risk clients:
	Smokers
	Chronic bronchitis
	Emphysema
	Obesity
	Elderly
	Upper abdominal surgery
	Chest surgery
	Abdominal distention
		Fever to 102° F
		Tachycardia
		Restlessness
		Tachypnea 24–30 min
		Altered breath sounds
		    Dullness to percussion
		    Diminished or absent breath sounds
		    Rales
		ABGs: decreased PaO_2

Pneumonia: inflammatory process in which alveoli are filled with exudate
 	
Potential onset:
First 36 to 48 hours.
	Clients with unresolved atelectasis
	Following aspiration
	Smoker
	Elderly
	Chronic bronchitis
	Emphysema
	Heart failure
	Debilitated
	Alcoholic
	Immobile
	Cough suppressant medications
	Respiratory depressant medications
		Client complains of dyspnea; tachycardia; increasing temperature; productive cough and increasing amount of sputum becoming tenacious, rusty, or purulent
		Tactile fremitus
		Dullness to percussion
		Bronchial breath sounds
		Increased wet rales or rhonchi
		Voice sounds present
		    Bronchophony
		      Egophony
		        Whispered pectoriloquy
		ABGs: decreased PaO_2

Gastric distension: accumulation of swallowed air and gastric juices in presence of ileus *Potential onset:* First 24 to 36 hours.	All surgical clients	Increased abdominal circumference (measured) Client's complaining of fullness and/or "gas pains" Tympanic abdominal percussion sounds
Ileus: failure of peristalsis *Potential onset:* First 24 to 36 hours.	All surgical clients Stress response to surgical trauma	No bowel sounds or fewer than 5/min. (normal: 5–35 clicks or gurgles/min.)

PREVENTION	INTERVENTION	CHARTING

Preoperative: have client practice turning, coughing, and deep breathing
Discuss importance of exercises
Postoperative clients at risk:
    Turn q30 min.
    Deep breathe and cough
Other clients:
Initiate turning and deep breathing exercises q1–2 hrs.
Ambulate as soon as possible
Medicate to reduce pain, splinting, and resistance to treatment
	Increase effectiveness of pulmonary toilet
	Administer supplemental oxygen as ordered
	Monitor response to treatment
	Monitor for onset of pneumonia
	If entire lobe of lung is involved, prepare for bronchoscopy to remove plug
		Signs and symptoms noted
		Location of abnormal chest findings
		Frequency of nursing treatment
		Client's response to treatment
		Oxygen: method of administration in liters per min.
		Sputum: character, color, and amount in teaspoons or cc
		Changes in chest findings in response to treatment

Provide vigorous treatment of atelectasis Prevent aspiration	Turn, cough, and deep breathe q1 hr. May need to stimulate cough with nasotracheal suctioning Send sputum for culture and sensitivity Administer antibiotic as ordered Frequent mouth care for comfort Administer oxygen as ordered Increase fluid intake Administer antipyretic as ordered Monitor for response to treatment	Frequency of nursing treatment Client's response to treatment Resolution or lack of resolution of auscultated findings Sputum character and amount Fluid intake Frequency of spontaneous cough
Encourage client to avoid air swallowing	Provide frequent turning to move air and secretions Have client sit up in chair or ambulate if appropriate Insert nasogastric tube and connect to low suction Monitor abdominal circumference by measuring q1 hr. Monitor for return of bowel sounds Monitor for passage of flatus Insert rectal tube	Measurement of changes in abdominal girth Client's complaints Presence/absence of bowel sounds Presence/absence of flatus Nursing treatment Client's response to treatment
None	Monitor for return of normal bowel sounds Offer only sips of water until return of bowel sounds Monitor for distention Monitor for passage of flatus signaling return of peristalsis	Presence/absence of bowel sounds Presence/absence of distention Results obtained from client's ingestion of water Presence/absence of nausea or vomiting Presence/absence of flatus

POTENTIAL COMPLICATION	CLIENTS AT RISK	INDICATIVE FINDINGS
Paralytic ileus: paralysis of intestinal peristalsis *Potential onset:* First three to four days	Intraperitoneal surgery Peritonitis Kidney surgery Decreased cardiac output Pneumonia Electrolyte imbalance Wound infection	No bowel sounds Abdominal distention No passage of flatus Nasogastric drainage green to yellow, 1–2 liters in 24 hrs.
Intestinal obstruction: adhesions, trap or kink in segment of intestine *Potential onset:* Third to fifth day	Abdominal surgery	No postoperative bowel movement Abdominal distention Client complains of periodic sharp, colicky pains Hyperactive bowel sounds Abdominal tenderness Nasogastric drainage: dark brown or black The lower the obstruction the more gradual the onset
Wound infection *Potential onset:* Streptococcal: 24 to 48 hrs. after contamination Staphylococcus gram-negative rods, etc.: five to seven days postoperatively	*Slow to heal:* Obese Diabetic *Poor nutrition:* Debilitated Elderly Ulcerative colitis *Poor circulation:* Elderly Hypovolemic Heart failure *Lack of oxygen to wound:* Vasoconstriction Severe anemia Depressed immunity Cancer Renal failure Preoperative steroid therapy Prolonged complex surgery (stress response leading to increased ACTH) Malnutrition Elderly At risk for transmission Proximity of another client with infection Transmission by hands of personnel	Initial inflammation: 36–48 hrs. Wound tender, swollen, warm, increased redness Increasing heart rate Increasing temperature Increasing or recurring serous drainage There may be no local signs if infection is deep

PREVENTION	INTERVENTION	CHARTING
None Maintain electrolyte balance Maintain cardiac output Prevent pneumonia Prevent wound infection Provide early ambulation	Same as for gastric distention Maintain nasogastric suction until peristalsis returns Monitor for intestinal obstruction	Character, color and quantity of nasogastric drainage Measurement of changes in abdominal girth Client's complaints Presence/absence of bowel sounds Presence/absence of flatus Nursing treatment Client's response to treatment
None	Identify condition early Report to physician immediately Reduce client anxiety Maintain patent nasogastric tube Never give laxative or purgative if obstruction is suspected Prepare for insertion of intestinal tube (Miller-Abbott, Canton, or Harris) Prepare for surgery if necessary	Signs and symptoms that led to physician notification Actions for client support and anxiety reduction Client's response to nursing intervention
Maintain nutrition Maintain good circulation Maintain normal blood volume Provide nonrestrictive dressings, casts, etc. Provide frequent turning Have client sit up in chair or ambulate as soon as possible Maintain PaO_2 Treat atelectasis Prevent pulmonary complications Monitor ABGs if necessary Prevent severe anemia: replace lost RBCs Increase attention to prevention for clients with depressed immunity *Prevent transmission:* Practice effective handwashing Practice aseptic technique in wound care Separate postoperative from infected clients Maintain dry dressings Use special caution for a new wound, easily contaminated	Maintain nutrition Maintain oxygenation Maintain circulation and blood volume Maintain pulmonary toilet Send wound drainage specimen for culture and sensitivity Administer antibiotics as ordered Cleanse wound or irrigate as ordered Monitor for systemic response to infection, fever, malaise, headache, anorexia, nausea Treat symptoms	Description of appearance of wound in measurable terms: define redness in cm squared; define drainage in cc's Description of tissue surrounding wound Condition of dressing Client's complaints of wound discomfort Type of dressing used Nursing interventions Cleansing and dressing of wound Method of irrigation and fluid used Client comfort measures Presence/absence of systemic signs and symptoms Client's response to therapy

POTENTIAL COMPLICATION	CLIENTS AT RISK	INDICATIVE FINDINGS
Urinary tract infection *Potential onset:* Third to fifth day or 48 hrs. after removal of catheter	*Decreased resistance:* History of bladder distention History of urinary retention Previous urinary tract infection History of prostatic hypertrophy History of catheterization Diabetic Debilitated Immobile	Dysuria Frequency Urgency High fever: up to 104° F with fewer systemic toxic symptoms than would be expected Change in urine odor Pus in urine Sediment May be asymptomatic
Thrombophlebitis: inflammation of vein with clot formation *Potential onset:* Seventh to fourteenth day	*Abnormal vein walls:* Varicose veins Previous thrombophlebitis Trauma to vein wall Tight strap on operating room table Surgery on hips or in pelvis Age more than 60 (arteriosclerosis) *Venous stasis:* Immobility Casts, restrictive dressings Constant Fowler's position Prolonged dependent lower extremities Knee-gatch elevated Pillows under knees Pillows under calves Obesity Abdominal distention Shock Heart failure *Hypercoagulability:* Surgical stress response Stress and anxiety Infection Anesthesia Decreased circulation Hypovolemia Malignant neoplasms Postpartum Oral contraceptives	*Superficial vein thrombophlebitis:* Pain, redness, tenderness, and induration along course of vein Palpable "cord" corresponding to course of vein History of trauma including IV site *Deep small-vein thrombophlebitis:* Increased muscle turgor and tenderness over affected vein Deep muscle tenderness Most frequent site: vessels at calf Affected limb warm to touch with occasional swelling Client complains of tightness or stiffness in affected leg Positive Homan's sign (dorsiflexion of foot leads to calf pain) Fever rarely more than 101°F *Major deep-vein thrombophlebitis:* No superficial signs of inflammation Homan's sign unreliable *Femoral vein thrombosis:* Pain and tenderness in distal thigh and popliteal region. Swelling extends to level of knee *Iliofemoral vein:* Often massive swelling, pain and tenderness of entire lower extremity Cyanosis of extremity when dependent Superficial veins sometimes visibly dilated Circumference differential more than 15 mm in males and more than 12 mm in females; most reliable for diagnosis

PREVENTION	INTERVENTION	CHARTING
Maintain sterile technique with catheterization and catheter removal Provide competent indwelling catheter care Encourage early ambulation to decrease retention and stasis	Encourage fluid intake; cranberry juice to decrease urine pH Increase activity to enhance bladder emptying Encourage voiding q2 hrs. while awake Send specimen for culture and sensitivity Administer antibiotic as ordered Monitor for residual urine of more than 100 cc	Signs and symptoms that led to notification of physician Nursing interventions Client's response to nursing intervention and medical therapy

Avoid injury to vein wall:
Use care when strapping to operating room table
Avoid IVs in lower extremities
Pad side rails for restless, convulsive, and/or combative client
Avoid restraints
 	
Avoid venous stasis:
Encourage early ambulation
Provide feet and leg exercises: 10 min. q1–2 hr. while in bed
Increase frequency of exercise for client at risk
Prevent client's sitting with legs in dependent position
Place pillow between legs while client is lying on side to prevent pressure from upper leg on lower
Provide deep breathing exercise
Provide active and passive range of motion
Prevent restrictive dressings, casts, and positions
Increase velocity of blood flow:
  No standing
  Steady IV flow
  Antiembolic stockings (controversial)
Decrease hypercoagulability:
  Provide adequate hydration
  Prevent infections
  Maintain circulation
  Decrease stress/anxiety
	Superficial vein thrombophlebitis:
	Treat symptoms
	Analgesic
	Local heat
	Continue ambulation unless accompanied by deep venous involvement
	Monitor for progression toward saphenafemoral junction (may need ligation)
	
	Deep vein thrombophlebitis:
	Provide adequate bed rest
	Elevate foot of bed with 6–8" blocks
	Administer warm moist compresses to relieve venospasm and help resolve inflammation
	Administer and monitor:
	  Heparin therapy
	  Fibrinolytic therapy
	Monitor for pulmonary embolism
		Signs and symptoms that led to physician notification
		Nursing actions
		Client's response to therapy

POTENTIAL COMPLICATION	CLIENTS AT RISK	INDICATIVE FINDINGS
Pulmonary embolism: foreign object has migrated to branch of pulmonary artery *Potential onset:* Seventh to tenth day *Massive embolism:* Pulmonary hypertension, dyspnea, right heart failure, shock, ABGs: decreased PaO_2, increased $PaCO_2$	Superficial vein thrombosis: rare Deep vein thrombosis: 40 to 60 percent Air emboli: intraperitoneal surgery Fat emboli: long bone fracture, split sternum	Only 10 percent recognized clinically Pain sharp and stabbing, occurs with breathing; localized (right lower lobe most frequent) Increased respiratory rate Increased heart rate Restlessness
Pulmonary infarction: necrosis of lung tissue due to occlusion of blood supply (less than 10 percent develop) *Potential onset:* 2 to 72 hrs. after arterial obstruction	Pulmonary embolism	Hemoptysis Cough Fever 101° to 102°F Pleural friction rub Pleuritic pain

PREVENTION	INTERVENTION	CHARTING
Provide range of motion Encourage early ambulation Prevent thrombophlebitis Do not massage a potential or suspected thrombophlebitic area	Administer oxygen to relieve hypoxia Reduce anxiety Position client on left side with head dependent to prevent air embolus Prevent recurrent embolization; prepare for fibrinolysis; prepare for anticoagulation Prepare for x-ray, angiography, and/or ventilation/perfusion scan	Signs and symptoms that led to physician notification Nursing actions Client's response to therapy
None	Describe indicative findings to physician Institute relaxation techniques to decrease client's anxiety Administer oxygen Support and comfort client	Signs and symptoms that led to physician notification Nursing interventions Client's response to treatment

CHAPTER 19
Monitoring for Alterations in Homeostasis

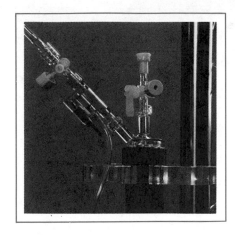

This chapter presents a conceptual framework for interventions used in the diagnosis and maintenance of homeostasis during lifethreatening conditions. Provision for competent care during critical periods requires a knowledge of monitoring techniques. Working with monitors and providing client care at the same time can be a challenging experience for the nurse.

Although monitors have been utilized in hospitals for many years, they are becoming more complex and technical. Often it is totally the nurse's responsibility to initiate the procedure, evaluate the data, and be prepared to intervene if anything adverse happens. Because of this responsibility, the nurse must become proficient in monitoring skills.

Essentially, monitoring techniques allow for rapid documentation of the pathophysiology of the major systems and the confirmation of the efficacy of treatment. The monitoring modalities presented in this section can be easily learned and assimilated into clinical practice.

MONITORING SKILLS

In the clinical setting nurses are constantly faced with new equipment, new techniques, and better and more sophisticated methods. To keep pace in the area of technological advancement can be a monumental task, one that tries the nurse's energy, patience, and abilities. The

LEARNING OBJECTIVES

Differentiate between a normal and abnormal ECG pattern.

Identify a normal arterial waveform depicted on an oscilloscope.

Explain what hemodynamic information is obtained when the client has a Swan-Ganz catheter inserted.

Describe the relationship between the ECG and the intraaortic waveform patterns.

Describe the hemodynamic alterations that occur when the intraaortic balloon pump deflates early or late in the balloon pumping cycle.

Compare and contrast nursing interventions for clients on peritoneal dialysis and hemodialysis.

Describe maternal and fetal parameters which can be identified through fetal monitoring devices.

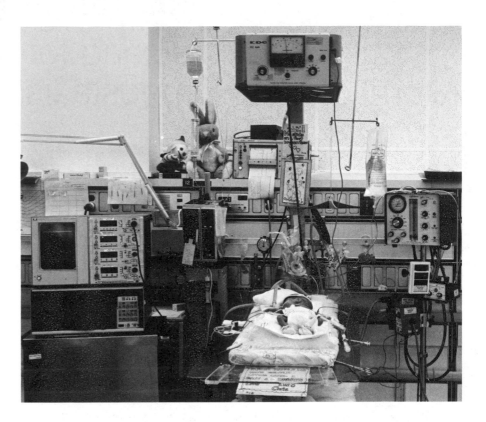

Sophisticated monitoring techniques are utilized for improved client care.

nurse's role in assessment, planning, intervention, and evaluation is based in part on the nurse's familiarity with monitoring data. Ability to integrate that data with other physiologic parameters is essential to providing excellent nursing care. Monitoring is a method of providing additional data, which does not obviate the need for quality care based on the nursing process. In fact, it is important that monitors do not become more important than the client. The first objective, then, is to care for the client, not tend the monitor.

One of the ways to achieve both goals, the mastery over monitoring procedures and the attainment of high-quality client care, is to become familiar with the technical equipment so that it no longer causes anxiety and uncertainty. Once this level of understanding is realized, the focus can be on the client, not the monitoring equipment.

ELECTROCARDIOGRAM (ECG)

Utilizing monitoring devices to measure cardiac function provides important indices of the overall condition of the client. The electrocardiogram is a noninvasive test that is a graphic recording of the electrical activity of the heart reflected by changes in electrical potential at the skin surface. The purpose of this monitoring device is to determine types and extent of heart damage, cardiac irregularities, and electrolyte imbalances.

The four functional properties of the myocardium include excitability, automaticity, contractility, and conductivity. Excitation waves produced from the myocardial cells are recorded as electrical phenomena. This activity is detected on the skin surface because body fluids are an excellent conductor of electricity. Electrodes placed on the skin surface record voltage and intervals of electrical activity over time as a result of depolarization and repolarization. This recording provides a continuous picture of the electrical activity of the heart.

The P wave represents atrial depolarization, the electrical activity associated with the original impulse from the SA node and its spread throughout the atria. P waves should always be present and precede the QRS complex. They should also be upright in leads II, III, and AVF. The PR interval — atrial depolarization and atrial systole — is the period of time from the beginning of the P wave to the beginning of the QRS complex. A normal PR interval should be no longer than 0.12 to 0.2 seconds. The PR interval represents the conduction time that occurs as the impulse traverses the atria and AV node. The QRS complex consists of an initial downward deflection (Q wave), a sharp upward spike (R wave), and a final downward deflection (S wave). The entire complex represents depolarization of the ventricular muscle. The activity normally takes less than 0.12 seconds. The T wave represents the recovery phase, or repolarization, following contraction.

The electrocardiographic recording of the ECG has a characteristic appearance of waveforms. Letters have been chosen arbitrarily to represent each of the particular aspects of the graphic record. The electrical activity of the heart is recorded on ECG paper, where each small block is 1 mm tall and .04 seconds wide and each large block is 5 mm tall and .20 seconds wide (5 small blocks equal 1 large block). Voltage is shown by the horizontal lines and time by the vertical lines. The heart rate may be calculated in a number of ways. One way is to count the number of cycles (usually represented by QRS complexes) in a six second strip and multiply that number by 10. Another method is to divide the number of small blocks between R waves into 1500 to obtain the ventricular rate,

It is important to determine the configuration and location of the wave pattern to interpret an ECG.

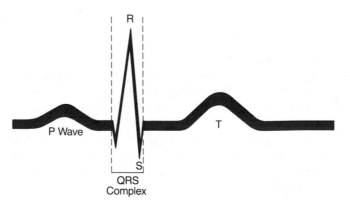

R

P Wave

S

T

QRS
Complex

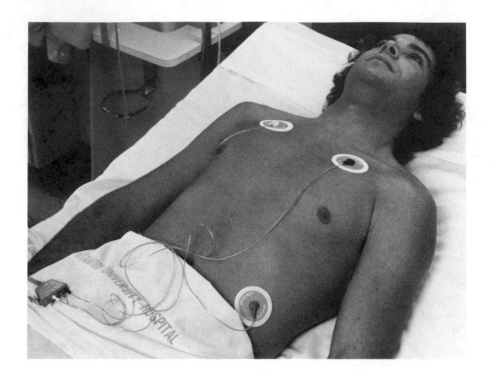

Sites for ECG lead placement when using three bipolar leads.

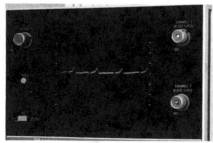

ECG pattern on monitor electrically transmitted from the bipolar leads placed on the client.

and to divide the number of small blocks between P waves into 1500 to obtain the atrial rate.

In general, continuous monitoring of the ECG requires only three bipolar leads (as opposed to the twelve bipolar leads for diagnosis). The most frequent sites are right arm, left arm (ground), and the left leg.

The cardiac monitor, it must be remembered, is only a machine and has no inherent ability to assess or make decisions from a data base. In fact, the ECG monitor is never used in diagnosis; its role is simply to monitor heart function as a preventative measure for cardiac complications. Decisions or diagnosis are based on a variety of observational, hemodynamic, and monitoring parameters.

ARTERIAL BLOOD GASES

Arterial blood gas analysis is important clinical data. The blood gas studies assist in determining the respiratory or metabolic acid-base status of the client and reveal the lung capacity to provide oxygen. The measurements serve as a guide to altering or validating treatment modalities.

Blood gases are measured on arterial rather than venous blood because arterial blood is representative of the total body, not just a single extremity. In addition, arterial blood provides information on how well the lungs are functioning.

The parameters of arterial blood gases that are important for the nurse to understand are listed below. pH normal value is 7.4; normal range is 7.35 to 7.45. This is a measure of the acidity or alkalinity level in the blood. Blood contains a certain amount of normal acid and is represented by the hydrogen ion (H^+) concentration. Acid in the form of lactic acid and ketoacids is produced by the breakdown of food and proteins. The largest source of acid in our body is H_2CO_3, and for each hydrogen ion that is excreted by the kidney, one HCO_3^- ion is reabsorbed by the blood. The lungs, in a normal state, excrete 99 percent of the acid in the body, and the kidneys excrete the remaining 1 percent. Acidosis produces acidemia, an acid condition of the blood evidenced by a pH below 7.4. Alkalosis produces alkalemia, an alkaline condition of the blood evidenced by a pH above 7.4. Pathological processes that can produce acidosis or alkalosis are shown in Table 1.

The $PaCO_2$ normal value is 40 mm Hg. $PaCO_2$ is the partial pressure of gas in arterial blood. CO_2 is an acid waste product of the cells excreted by the lungs. This parameter is measured by the tension exerted when CO_2 goes into the bloodstream and dissolves to form H_2CO_3. This value tells how well the lungs are eliminating CO_2 at the alveolar level. In alveolar hyperventilatory conditions (respiratory alkalosis), CO_2 is blown off rapidly to a value of less than 40 mm Hg. Since CO_2 is an acid, an alkalotic state results. In alveolar ventilatory failure (respiratory acidosis), found with cardiac arrest, CO_2 is retained to a value above 40 mm Hg resulting in an acidotic state.

HCO_3^- (normal value is 24 mEq/l; normal range is 22 to 26 mEq/l) is a bicarbonate base that evaluates the metabolic parameters of kidney function. The kidneys normally excrete hydrogen and conserve and regulate the HCO_3^- derived from the H_2CO_3 in the blood. Bicarbonate levels greater than 24 mEq/l indicate a metabolic alkalosis, while levels less than 24 mEq/l indicate a metabolic acidosis.

pO_2 (normal value is 80 to 100 mm Hg) is the partial pressure of oxygen in the blood. pO_2 is a direct reflection of hypoxemia. pO_2 levels of less than 80 mm Hg indicate mild hypoxemia while levels of less than 60 mm Hg indicate moderate hypoxemia. To correctly interpret this value, it is necessary to know the FIO_2 (fraction of inspired oxygen) the client is receiving. Room air is 21 percent and ventilators and masks usually deliver at least 40 percent.

Base excess (normal range is −2 to +2 mEq/l) provides information regarding metabolic imbalances and the degree of acidity or alkalinity. It is

TABLE 1

ACIDOSIS	ALKALOSIS
Hypoventilation	Hyperventilation
COPD	Anxiety
Cardiac Arrest	Pulmonary Embolus
Narcotic or Barbiturate Overdose	Mechanical Ventilatory Assistance
Diabetic Ketoacidosis	Diuretics

ACID-BASE IMBALANCES

RESPIRATORY ACIDOSIS			COMPENSATION
pH:	decreased	<7.40	7.40
pCO₂:	increased	>40	
HCO₃⁻:	normal	24	↑ >24

RESPIRATORY ALKALOSIS			COMPENSATION
pH:	increased	>7.40	7.40
pCO₂:	decreased	<40	
HCO₃⁻:	normal	24	↓ <24

METABOLIC ACIDOSIS			COMPENSATION
pH:	decreased	<7.40	7.40
HCO₃⁻:	decreased	<24	
BE:	decreased	<0	
pCO₂:	normal	40	↓ <40

BE (base excess): reflection of HCO₃⁻:

METABOLIC ALKALOSIS			COMPENSATION
pH:	increased	>7.40	7.40
HCO₃⁻:	increased	>24	
BE:	increased	>0	
pCO₂:	normal	40	↑ >40

calculated by determining the amount of buffer base above or below the blood level. If HCO_3^- increases, the base excess increases too; conversely, when HCO_3^- decreases, a base deficit occurs.

ARTERIAL LINES

Arterial lines, an invasive device, measure systolic, diastolic, and mean arterial pressures. This is a direct blood pressure measurement as opposed to the indirect measure obtained with a sphygmomanometer and stethoscope. This method of evaluating cardiac output and peripheral resistance is determined indirectly by arterial blood pressure measured in the cuff of the sphygmomanometer. The values reflect the arterial blood pressure which rises to a maximum value during ventricular systole (systolic pressure) and falls to its minimum value during diastole (diastolic pressure). Indirect measurements are most useful when cardiac output and peripheral resistance is normal. During critical situations, when there are changes in cardiac hemodynamics, direct measurements are more accurate. Human factors, such as the nurse's skill and auditory ability, as well as the condition of the stethoscope, may lead to imprecision.

Invasive arterial pressure measurement permits early detection of alterations in hemodynamic status in clients who have low cardiac output, excessive vasoconstriction, or an unstable condition. Arterial lines are also indicated for surgical clients, for clients on mechanical ventilators, and for clients who require vasodilator or vasopressor drugs and frequent arterial blood gas studies.

Continuous direct monitoring of intra-arterial blood pressure is possible with an arterial catheter attached via a pressure transducer to an arterial monitor, where continuous arterial waveforms are seen on an oscilloscope and numerical pressures are observed on a digital readout. Deviations from the client's normal range can be immediately detected and appropriate therapy can be instituted without delay.

In addition to systolic and diastolic pressures, the intra-arterial catheter is used to determine mean arterial pressure. Mean arterial pressure is not an arithmetic average of systolic and diastolic pressure. Rather, it is a measure of the total area located under the arterial pressure curve divided by the concurrent time period. A representative formula is:

$$\frac{\text{systolic pressure} + \text{diastolic pressure}}{3} \times 2 = \text{mean arterial pressure}.$$

Since diastole lasts longer than systole, the mean pressure is generally closer to diastole in value. It can be approximated by adding one-third of the pulse pressure (difference between the systolic and diastolic pressures) to the diastolic pressure. The pressure curve represents the pressure waveforms.

Arterial catheter insertion sites commonly include the brachial, radial, or femoral arteries. The radial artery, although more distal to the left ventricle, is the vessel chosen most often for cannulation. In order to preserve the patency of the intra-arterial catheter, a continuous flush mechanism identical to that for the Swan-Ganz catheter is used.

Normally, pressures determined by the indirect method are slightly lower than direct arterial pressure. Significant variations should be checked by recalibrating the machine and by periodically checking cuff pressures.

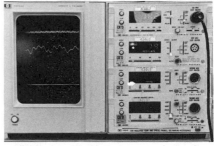

Arterial waveform on monitor depicts direct monitoring of intra-arterial blood pressure via an arterial catheter.

ACTION: MEASURING CARDIOVASCULAR FUNCTION

ASSESSMENT

1   Determine preexisting cardiac disease and/or electrocardiographic abnormalities.
2   Determine client's level of understanding and cooperation with procedures.
3   Determine client's level of fear or anxiety about diagnosis or procedures.
4   Using the following criteria, select artery for drawing arterial blood gases:
    a   Adequate collateral blood flow.
    b   Palpable.
    c   Accessible.
5   Evaluate preceding arterial blood gas values to use as a baseline.
6   Palpate for presence of peripheral pulses distal to catheter insertion site when an arterial line is inserted.

Rationale for Action
- To directly assess data related to systolic, diastolic, and mean pressures
- To provide essential information regarding impending shock states, low cardiac output, or vasoconstriction
- To provide immediate access to arterial blood gas samples
- To assess the adequacy of oxygenation
- To assess the adequacy of alveolar ventilation
- To evaluate acid-base balance
- To evaluate effectiveness of ventilatory treatment modalities

7 Observe the mean arterial pressure on the monitor.
8 Measure the systolic and diastolic pressure reading on the monitor.
9 Observe for trends in arterial pressure readings.
10 Evaluate the patency of the arterial catheter.
11 Assess catheter insertion site for signs of infection or bleeding.
12 Determine pressure in flush bag. (Pressure should be 300 mm Hg.)

PLANNING

GOALS

- Data is collected, and signs of impending shock or vasoconstrictive states are identified.
- Arterial catheter remains patent.
- Arterial blood samples are obtained.
- Fear, anxiety, and discomfort are minimized.
- ECG pattern is clearly displayed on oscilloscope.
- Abnormal heart rate or rhythm is detected by ECG monitoring.
- Potentially dangerous rhythms are identified and treated accordingly.

EQUIPMENT

For ECG Monitoring
- Electrodes
- Electrode jelly (if not prejelled)
- Cardiac monitor and cable
- Alcohol wipes or acetone pledges
- Razor
- Wash cloth; or 4 × 4s, soap, and towel

For Arterial Line Placement
- Arterial catheter with introducer
- Intravenous solution (usually 500 cc D$_5$W)
- Heparin (4 to 5 units per cc of IV solution)
- One 5 cc syringe
- Pressure infusion bag
- IV tubing with microdrip
- Three-way stopcocks
- Pressure transducer
- Valve device for system flush (e.g., Sorenson Intraflo)
- Pressure monitor
- IV pole
- Sterile gloves
- Sterile towels
- Skin antiseptic solution (povidone-iodine)
- Sterile 4 × 4 gauze pads
- Lidocaine 1 to 2 percent
- Syringe with #18- and #25-gauge needle for topical anesthetic
- Alcohol wipes

- Antiseptic ointment
- Tape
- Cutdown tray

For Drawing Blood from Arterial Line
- Specimen label
- Container with ice
- Two 5-cc syringes
- Cork for needle

For Drawing Arterial Blood
- 5 to 10 cc glass syringes
- Heparin, 1000 units per cc
- 20-gauge needle
- 22-gauge needle
- Alcohol wipes
- Container with ice
- Rubber stopper or rubber cap for syringe
- Label
- Sterile 2 × 2s
- Elastoplast

INTERVENTION: Monitoring Cardiovascular Function with the Electrocardiogram (ECG)

1 Explain rationale for procedure to client.
2 Verbally reassure client.
3 Turn monitor power switch on.
4 Attach cable to monitor.
5 Cleanse electrode placement site as needed.
   a Shave chest sites if necessary, since hair interferes with conductivity.
   b Cleanse site well with alcohol or acetone to remove dead skin and oils, which may affect conductivity.
   c Allow site to dry well, or dry with 4 × 4s.
6 Determine the lead placement that will give the best ECG pattern.
   a Lead II:
   Positive (+) lead — left side of chest, lowest palpable rib, midclavicular.
   Negative (−) lead — right shoulder region below clavicular hollow.
   Ground (G) lead — left shoulder, below clavicular hollow opposite negative lead.

    b Lead MCL₁ (Modified Chest Lead):
Positive (+) lead — right
sternal border, lowest
palpable rib.
Negative (−) lead — left
shoulder, below clavicular
hollow.
Ground (G) lead — right
shoulder, below clavicular
hollow — opposite negative
lead.

    c Other leads such as Lead I and MCL₆ can also be useful in specific situations.

7 Apply electrodes.

    a Peel off paper backing on electrode. Check that sponge pad in center of electrode is moist with conductive jelly. Place electrode on skin with adhesive side down.

    b Apply electrodes in areas where there will not be excessive movement.

    c Place near but not directly on bone surfaces; however, if client is overly obese, electrodes may have to be placed on the bones, since a large amount of adipose tissue results in a poor image on the oscilloscope.

ECG pattern depicted from Lead I placement.

Lead I

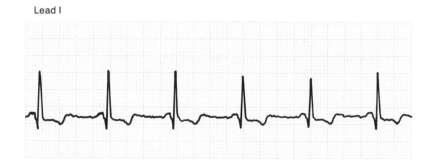

ECG pattern depicted from Lead II placement.

Lead II

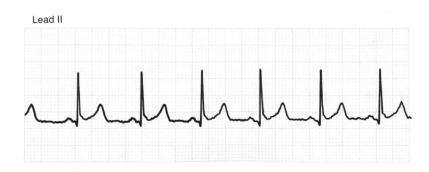

8 Attach the electrodes to the monitor cable using the lead wires. The client end of the cable is coded to facilitate connection with the electrodes. Common codes are — (neg), + (pos) and G (ground) or RA, LA, and LL or color codes. Be sure that the positive lead wire is connected to the electrode in the positive position, the negative lead wire to the electrode in the negative position, and the ground lead wire to the electrode in the ground position.

9 Set high and low alarm limits on the monitor.

10 Turn alarm buttons to "on."

INTERVENTION: Interpreting an ECG Strip

1 Determine heart rate by calculating atrial rate (P-P) interval) and ventricular rate (R-R interval). Normal pulse is 60 to 100.

2 Determine regularity of rhythm (atrial and ventricular). Check if complexes look alike and are equally spaced.

3 Measure P-R interval to determine conduction time in atria and AV junction (0.16 to 0.20 seconds).

4 Measure QRS duration to determine ventricular conduction (0.04 to 0.12 sec.). There are six complexes.

5 Measure Q-T interval (rate of 70 in one minute occurring 0.36 seconds apart).

▶ **Heart Rate Calculation**

1 Count the number of cardiac cycles (QRS complexes) in a six-second strip and multiply that number by ten to obtain the pulse.

2 Count the number of small boxes between R waves. Divide that number into 1500. The quotient is the ventricular rate.

3 Count the number of small boxes between P waves. Divide that number into 1500. The quotient is the atrial rate.

MCL₁

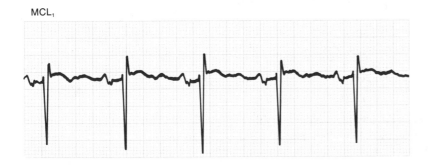

ECG pattern depicted from MCL₁ placement.

Artifact

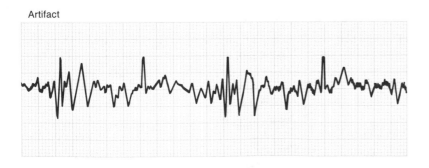

ECG pattern shows artifact. Assess lead placement and ECG system interference.

709

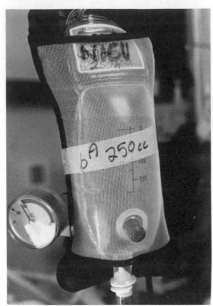

Heparin is added to IV solution and IV bag is placed in pressure infusion bag.

6 Check configuration and placement of P waves, QRS complex, ST segment, and T wave.
7 Summarize findings to obtain interpretation.
8 Document interpretation of findings and place ECG strip in client's chart.

INTERVENTION: Monitoring Cardiovascular Function with Arterial Lines

1 Explain rationale for procedure to client.
2 Gather equipment.
3 Wash your hands.
4 Add heparin to the D_5W solution and label bag with medication and date (commonly 1 unit heparin/1 cc fluid).
5 Connect IV tubing to solution bag.
6 Insert IV bag into pressure infusion bag and inflate bag to a pressure of 300 mm Hg.
7 Prepare and assemble the pressurized monitoring system (transducer, flush system device, and stopcocks), following the manufacturer's instructions.
8 Level, calibrate, and balance the transducer at the level of the client's right atrium (fourth intercostal space, midaxillary line).
9 Assist the physician as needed.

Physician's Actions

a Skin is prepped with povidone-iodine solution.
b Lidocaine vial is cleansed with alcohol wipe.
c Physician dons sterile gloves.
d Sterile drape is placed over arterial site.
e Physician aspirates lidocaine with #18-gauge needle, changes needle, and injects client's skin with #25-gauge needle.
f Percutaneous or cutdown insertion is made at radial or brachial artery site, and arterial catheter is inserted.
g Physician advances catheter in artery.

10 Observe for pulsating bright-red blood spurting retrograde to ensure catheter position.
11 Attach catheter to pressure monitoring system tubing, and flush system by pulling for three seconds on red pigtail of Sorenson Intraflo device.
12 Observe oscilloscope for arterial waveform tracing.
13 Apply sterile antiseptic ointment, sterile dressings, and tape.
14 Reassure client during arterial catheter insertion.
15 Determine pressure reading following catheter insertion.
   a Calibrate and balance transducer at appropriate intervals to maintain continuity. Transducer to be calibrated at level of right atrium.
   b Determine systolic, diastolic, or mean pressures by selecting the appropriate position on the pressure monitor.

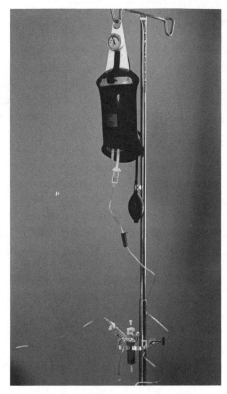

Pressurized monitoring system for maintaining a patent arterial line.

Arterial Line - Normal Waveform

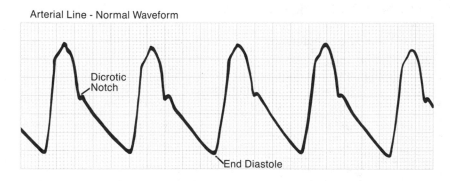

Dicrotic
Notch

End Diastole

Normal arterial blood pressure waveform. The dicrotic notch indicates aortic valve closure.

Arterial Line - Flattened Waveform

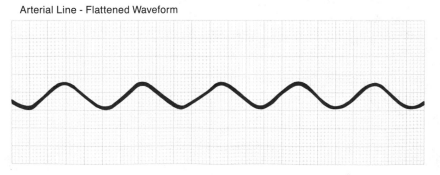

Flattened arterial waveform indicates damping. Damping results from an obstruction in the arterial line or from the transducer which may require balancing.

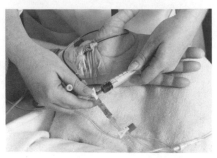

Before obtaining blood sample, take protective cap off three-way stopcock. Attach sterile syringe to port of stopcock and withdraw 5 cc of blood.

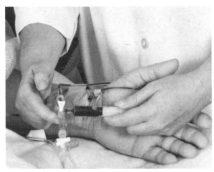

Discard first blood sample, which is part blood and part heparinized saline. Attach a sterile 5 cc heparinized syringe and obtain the arterial blood sample.

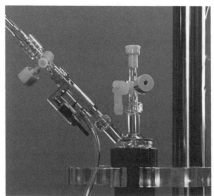

Flush the arterial line by pulling back on the pigtail of the Sorenson Intraflo.

▶ Do not draw blood from a limb with an external AV shunt or internal fistula.

c Observe waveform at eye level for sharp upstroke, peak, and dicrotic notch.
d Flush line.
e Record readings as often as ordered and report as necessary.

INTERVENTION: Withdrawing Arterial Blood Samples from the Arterial Line

1 Turn off stopcock to IV solution.
2 Remove protective cap from open port on a three-way stopcock.
3 Attach sterile syringe to open port of three-way stopcock.
4 Aspirate to 5 cc of blood.
5 Turn stopcock midway between open port and IV tubing to prevent escape of blood or introduction of IV solution. Discard syringe.
6 Attach a second sterile 5-cc syringe preflushed with 1 cc heparin and aspirate arterial blood sample. Remove all air bubbles from syringe and cap because air bubbles alter laboratory values.
7 Place blood specimen in container of ice. Label specimen.
8 Close stopcock to open port to reestablish solution flow between IV bag and client.
9 Flush arterial catheter using pigtail of Sorenson Intraflo.
10 Replace protective cap on open port.

INTERVENTION: Drawing Arterial Blood Samples for ABGs

1 Wash your hands thoroughly.
2 Attach label with client's name, hospital number, and room number to syringe.
3 Fill plastic bag or emesis basin with shaved ice.
4 Attach 20-gauge needle to syringe.
5 Cleanse heparin vial with alcohol wipe.
6 Withdraw 1 cc heparin, 1000 units per cc.
7 Withdraw plunger to coat barrel of syringe with heparin.
8 Expel air and heparin, leaving 0.1 cc of heparin in syringe.
9 Remove #20-gauge needle from the syringe and replace it with a #22-gauge needle.
10 Expel remaining heparin from syringe. Recap needle.
11 Explain procedure to the client. Include a brief but clear description of what, why, and how the procedure will be done.
12 Position client's arm in a well-lighted area, and select the artery to be punctured.
13 Choose an artery without a surrounding hematoma or obvious circulatory difficulty.
14 Perform Allen test to ascertain distal peripheral perfusion.
15 Position extremity in a stable comfortable position.
16 Cut three pieces of tape 9 cm long.
17 Open sterile 2 × 2s and place on table.
18 Palpate the linear course of the artery.

19 Cleanse the puncture site with an alcohol wipe. Begin at the center of the puncture site and clean in a circular motion toward the periphery.
20 Remove cap from the needle.
21 Continue to palpate the artery. Anchor the artery between two fingers without contaminating the puncture site.
22 Insert the needle with the bevel in the up position. Using a 45- to 90-degree angle, penetrate the skin and move the needle down to the artery. Observe for a spontaneous backflow of bright-red pulsating blood into the syringe.
23 Fill syringe with at least 5 cc of arterial blood.
24 Withdraw needle gently and immediately apply digital pressure over the puncture site with sterile 2 × 2s. Keep pressure on the puncture site for at least five minutes. It may be necessary for you to have another nurse perform this while you complete the remainder of the procedure.
25 Hold needle and syringe upright maintaining a firm hold on the plunger, and thrust the needle through a sterile alcohol wipe.
26 Expel all air and gas bubbles from syringe.
27 Remove alcohol wipe and insert needle into rubber stopper or remove needle and place cap on syringe.
28 Gently rotate syringe to prevent blood from clotting.
29 Place blood specimen in a plastic bag filled with shaved ice, or in an empty plastic bag and place in emesis basin filled with shaved ice.
30 Send specimen immediately to the laboratory. Include the following information with the specimen:
  a Time sample was drawn.
  b Whether client is receiving oxygen.
    If client is on a ventilator, include the FIO_2 setting and tidal volume.
    If client is receiving oxygen by mask or cannula, include the liter flow per minute.
    If client is not receiving oxygen, state "room air."
  c The client's temperature.
  d The client's respiratory rate.
31 Check the puncture site for continued bleeding, and apply Elastoplast tape to site.
32 Reposition client for comfort.
33 Wash your hands.
34 Recheck puncture site for bleeding.

EVALUATION

EXPECTED OUTCOMES

1 ECG pattern is clearly displayed on oscilloscope. *If not,* follow these alternative nursing actions:
ANA: Ensure that electrodes are applied in correct position and are securely attached.

Clinical Alert

Allen's test. The purpose of the Allen's test is to assess the blood supply to the client's hand to determine how well the radial and ulnar arteries are functioning before an arterial line is inserted.
1 Compress both arteries at the client's wrist for about one minute.
2 Instruct the client to clench and unclench fists several times. This should cause blanching in the hand and palm.
3 Release pressure on the ulnar artery and have client open hand.
4 Observe how quickly the palm returns to normal color. If normal color does not return within 5 seconds, there may be occlusion, poor cardiac output, or poor capillary refill.
5 Repeat procedure with the radial artery. If both arteries are not functioning well, report to physician. If the ulnar artery cannot support distal peripheral perfusion, choose another site for arterial line insertion.

▶ It may be necessary to gently aspirate on the plunger to obtain the sample.

ANA: Observe for electrical interference resulting in a 60-cycle interference on oscilloscope.

ANA: Observe for excessive client activity resulting in artifact display on oscilloscope.

2   Data is collected and signs of impending shock or vasoconstriction are identified. *If not*, follow these alternative nursing actions:

ANA: Evaluate patency of arterial catheter if abnormal findings are detected.

ANA: Assess for malfunction of arterial line system.

ANA: Prepare for insertion of new arterial catheter if unable to re-establish normal pressures.

3   Arterial catheter remains patent. *If not*, follow these alternative nursing actions:

ANA: Assess insertion site for signs of hemorrhage or infection.

ANA: Attempt to aspirate blood from the arterial line using a syringe. If blood can be aspirated, then flush the arterial line using the flush bag and the Sorenson Intraflo.

ANA: If unable to flush arterial catheter, remove catheter and apply direct pressure over artery for five to ten minutes. Apply Elastoplast tape over artery.

4   Arterial blood samples are obtained using existing arterial line. *If not*, follow these alternative nursing actions:

ANA: Release pressure on syringe, allow spasm of artery to stop, and then attempt to aspirate blood with gentle pressure.

ANA: If unable to obtain blood sample, check that catheter is in artery (observe waveform on oscilloscope). If catheter is malfunctioning, attempt to aspirate blood from the catheter. If blood is aspirated, flush the catheter using the flush bag and the Sorenson Intraflo. Then, try to obtain the sample again. If blood cannot be aspirated, remove the arterial catheter and draw the blood sample directly from another artery.

5   Arterial blood sample obtained with arterial puncture. *If not*, follow these alternative nursing actions:

ANA: Attempt another puncture in same artery using new equipment.

ANA: Choose another puncture site.

ANA: If unable to obtain sample with a second puncture site, notify physician. An arterial catheter may need to be inserted.

UNEXPECTED OUTCOMES

1   Electrical interference continues after lead wires and cable connections are secured.

ANA: Check all other electrical equipment in the immediate environment.

ANA: If excessive electrical equipment is used, the electrical bed may need to be changed to a non-electrical bed.

ANA: Check for proper grounding of monitor.

ANA: Check all connections. Ensure that cable that goes to client is pinned to client's gown to prevent disturbance of electrodes.

ANA: Change electrodes and cable; sometimes poor conduction results in 60-cycle interference.

ANA: Check that monitor is in calibration.

2 Skin irritation occurs with use of electrodes.

ANA: Remove electrodes, cleanse site, and reapply electrodes on new site.

3 Chaotic rhythm appears on oscilloscope.

ANA: Check client's other assessment parameters to determine if clinical changes have occurred.

ANA: Check electrode contact on skin, and ensure that wires are in contact with cable.

ANA: Determine activity level of client.

4 Safety alarms on monitor continue to sound.

ANA: Check for loose electrodes.

ANA: Observe activity level of client.

ANA: Check that alarm parameters on monitor are not set too close to client's pulse.

ANA: Check position of client.

ANA: Reposition electrodes, avoiding large muscle masses or bone.

5 Client demonstrates increasing anxiety regarding diagnosis, alarms, or arrhythmias.

ANA: Elaborate on rationale and necessity for procedure. Answer client's questions accurately and promptly.

ANA: Reassure client by frequently checking to determine that electrodes have not become loose.

ANA: Demonstrate competence and confidence while caring for the client.

ANA: Check monitor immediately when alarm goes off.

6 Electrodes conduct poorly on diaphoretic client.

ANA: Clean skin sites as usual, apply benzoin to the skin, and let dry and apply electrodes.

ANA: Clean skin sites as usual, apply spray deodorant to the skin, allow skin to dry, and apply electrodes.

7 Wires do not stay attached to electrodes because client is restless.

ANA: Place paper tape over wires and electrodes.

8 Asystole occurs.

ANA: Before beginning CPR, check client's LOC and electrodes, wires, and cables.

ANA: If the client has an arterial line, check for an arterial waveform in the absence of an ECG waveform.

9 Absence of collateral or distal peripheral perfusion when performing Allen test (negative Allen test).

ANA: Choose brachial artery.

ANA: Choose femoral artery.

ANA: Notify physician.

ANA: Anticipate intra-arterial line catheter insertion.

Charting

ECG

- Lead used in monitoring: I, II, MCL_1
- Arrhythmias noted during routine monitoring and treatment initiated
- Client attitude toward procedure
- Health teaching completed
- Heart rate and rhythm
- When physician was notified of abnormal findings
- Rhythm strip on admission and at least one strip every shift.

Arterial Line

- Size of arterial catheter inserted
- Technique used to insert catheter
- Pressure readings
- Unexpected outcomes and appropriate interventions
- Client's response and tolerance of the procedure
- Condition of extremity in which catheter is inserted
- Presence of peripheral pulses
- Appearance of catheter insertion site

Arterial Blood Gases

- Date and time sample was withdrawn and sent to laboratory
- Puncture site selected
- Difficulty or complications of puncture
- Record client's temperature, respiratory rate, FIO_2, tidal volume, mask or cannula oxygen liter flow
- Condition of puncture site and extremity

10   Artery not located immediately upon puncture.

ANA: Gently probe area keeping needle tip under skin.

ANA: Withdraw needle and apply digital pressure.

ANA: Attempt another arterial stick using new equipment.

11   Blood ceases to flow while puncture is being performed.

ANA: Advance needle further into artery and slowly withdraw until complete specimen is obtained.

12   Specimen appears dark.

ANA: Suspect a venipuncture: apply digital pressure and attempt another puncture using new equipment.

ANA: If blood flow is pulsatile, the blood may be arterial with poor oxygenation.

13   Blood does not pulsate in syringe during puncture.

ANA: Suspect a venipuncture: apply digital pressure and attempt another puncture using new equipment.

14   Hematoma occurs at insertion site.

ANA: Compress puncture site for an additional five minutes.

15   Thrombus forms at catheter insertion site.

ANA: Palpate extremity distal to insertion site to assess blood flow.

ANA: Insert syringe into stopcock and attempt to aspirate thrombus.

ANA: Prepare for removal of catheter if unable to aspirate thrombus.

ANA: Apply direct pressure over artery and apply Elastoplast tape.

16   Diminished or absent distal peripheral perfusion.

ANA: Check periphery for changes in color, warmth, movement, and pain resulting from thrombus occlusion.

ANA: Prepare for removal of catheter.

17   Infection or inflammation at insertion site.

ANA: Cleanse site and change dressings every 24 hours using strict aseptic technique to prevent infection.

ANA: Change tubing every 24 hours using sterile technique.

ANA: Flush open port after aspirating blood to prevent build-up of old blood.

ANA: Cover open port on stopcock to maintain asepsis.

ANA: Prepare for catheter removal if infection occurs.

18   Hematoma or hemorrhage at insertion site.

ANA: Apply direct pressure over artery while you check for leaks in the system. Check all stopcocks and see if catheter is inserted in artery as far as it should be.

ANA: Remove catheter if oozing or hemorrhage continues.

19   Damped pressures observed on oscilloscope.

ANA: Check for beginning thrombus formation by aspirating blood through stopcock and then flushing system.

ANA: Check for presence of air in system.

ANA: Check that there is 300 mm Hg pressure in pressure bag.

ANA: Assure secure fit of all stopcocks and connections.

ANA: Change position of extremity in which catheter is placed.

ANA: Be sure to flush arterial line thoroughly after arterial blood samples are obtained.

20 Air in system.

ANA: Change equipment if air cannot be withdrawn from system.

ANA: Flush air through external port; do not allow air to travel through the artery.

ANA: Check puncture site for delayed hematoma.

ANA: Check distal circulation for thrombus formation (cool, pale skin and absent or diminished pulses).

21 Inability to obtain any blood from port.

ANA: Reposition catheter and arm, gently pulling back on plunger.

ANA: If necessary, remove dressing and check if any pressure was applied at the site.

ANA: Notify physician, who may need to remove sutures and reposition catheter.

SWAN-GANZ HEMODYNAMIC MONITORING

The Swan-Ganz catheter measures the pulmonary artery pressure (PAP) as well as the pulmonary artery wedge pressure (PAWP), a direct reflection of left ventricular pressure. It is a balloon tipped catheter that is inserted percutaneously or through a cutdown and threaded through the right atrium, the tricuspid valve, the right ventricle, and the pulmonary valve to the pulmonary artery. When inflated, the catheter inhibits blood flow by wedging in a small pulmonary capillary, thereby allowing left heart pressure to be reflected backward on the tip. This pressure, called the pulmonary artery wedge pressure, is transmitted through the catheter to a transducer. The transducer converts the pressure waves to an electronic representation viewed on an oscilloscope. After obtaining the pressure, the balloon is deflated, allowing the catheter to float back to the pulmonary artery. Even though the catheter is in the pulmonary artery, the blood is venous.

The catheter is used to obtain a precise indication of the function and hemodynamics of the left heart so that early detection and treatment of cardiopulmonary changes can be promoted. Reduction of cardiac func-

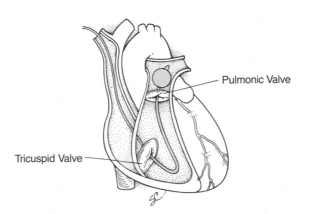

Anatomical placement of Swan-Ganz catheter.

Pulmonic Valve

Tricuspid Valve

Normal Pressures

Right Atrial (RA):   2–12 mm Hg

Right Ventricle (RV): $\dfrac{25}{5}$ mm Hg

Pulmonary Artery (PA): $\dfrac{25}{10}$ mm Hg

PA mean: 15 mm Hg

Left Atrial (LA) mean: 5–12 mm Hg

Left Ventricle (LV): $\dfrac{130}{5-12}$ mm Hg

Aorta: $\dfrac{130}{80}$

tion is manifested primarily by two hemodynamic abnormalities: decreased cardiac output and increased left ventricular end diastolic pressure. The Swan-Ganz catheter measures the left ventricular filling pressure by directly measuring pulmonary artery and pulmonary artery wedge pressures. At the end of diastole (filling), the mitral valve is open, and the left atrium, left ventricle, and pulmonary vasculature momentarily act as a single chamber. Since the normal pressures of each of the chambers and vessels are known, changes in pressures of the pulmonary artery indicate changes in the left ventricular end diastolic pressure (LVEDP). This could indicate changes in a client's circulatory status (fluid balance), vascular tone, and the heart's pumping action.

The pulmonary artery wedge (PAW) or pulmonary capillary wedge (PCW) pressures are measured by inflating the balloon, which results in a reflection of backward pressure from the cardiovascular system on the catheter tip. The pulmonary capillary wedge pressure reflects left ventricular pressure. Left ventricular pressure indicates important data regarding cardiac output. The advantage of Swan-Ganz catheter readings over central venous pressure readings is that central venous pressures do not measure left ventricular function until hemodynamic changes are reflected back through the pulmonary system, right ventricle and right atrium. Neither do central venous pressure readings reveal data regarding cardiac output or left heart pressure.

ACTION: MONITORING CARDIOVASCULAR FUNCTION WITH A SWAN-GANZ CATHETER

Rationale for Action

- To indirectly assess left ventricular end-diastolic pressure (LVEDP) in the absence of mitral valve disease
- To provide essential information regarding shock syndromes and intravascular fluid volumes
- To obtain samples of mixed venous blood (mixed due to blood from systemic and coronary sinuses)
- To administer intravenous solutions and determine response to fluid therapy
- To measure cardiac output
- To assess data related to central venous pressure
- To determine need for additional drug therapy

ASSESSMENT

1 Determine baseline vital signs.
2 Obtain a 12-lead electrocardiogram.
3 Observe for presence of edema or thrombi distal and proximal to insertion site.
4 Determine client's level of fear or anxiety regarding procedure.
5 Evaluate pressure waveforms and readings for accuracy.
6 Evaluate if transducer, oscilloscope, and monitor are balanced and calibrated.

PLANNING

GOALS

- Diagnosis of cardiac or pulmonary disease is established, and medical management is instituted.
- Intravascular volume status is determined.
- Catheter line remains patent.
- Client remains free of anxiety or discomfort.
- Pulse waveforms and readings are within normal limits.

EQUIPMENT

- Swan-Ganz flow-directed catheter (size 5 or 7 French)
- Catheter introducer (size 7 or 8 French depending on catheter size)
- Intravenous solution (usually 500 cc D₅W)
- Heparin (1 to 2 units per cc of IV solution)
- Tuberculin syringe
- Pressure infusion bag
- IV tubing
- Pressure monitor
- Transducer
- Valve device for system flush (i.e., Sorenson Intraflo)
- High-pressure tubing
- Three-way stopcocks
- IV pole
- CVP solution using triple lumen catheter
- 12 to 16 gauge intracatheter
- Sterile gloves
- Sterile towels
- Skin antiseptic solution (povidone-iodine)
- Razor
- Sterile 4 × 4s
- Sterile basin and sterile irrigating solution
- Lidocaine 1 to 2 percent
- Syringe with #18- and #25-gauge needle for topical anesthetic
- Alcohol wipes
- Antiseptic ointment
- Tape
- Suture with attached needle
- Sterile needle holder or clamp
- Cutdown tray, sterile gown, mask, and cap
- Defibrillator
- Emergency cart
- Xylocaine bolus for arrhythmias (50 to 100 mg)

INTERVENTION: Inserting a Swan-Ganz Catheter

1 Explain rationale for procedure to client.
2 Heparinize the IV solution with heparin and label the contents. Many hospitals require the removal of all air from bag by withdrawing the air with a 10- to 20-cc syringe because air in the line gives inaccurate readings.
3 Connect IV tubing to fluid bag.
4 Place prepared IV solution in pressure bag and inflate to 300 mm Hg pressure.
5 Prepare and assemble the pressurized monitoring system (transducer, system flush device, and stopcocks) following the manufacturer's instructions.
6 Place client in a horizontal position.

▶ Rise in client's pulmonary artery wedge pressure may indicate
- Left ventricular failure
- Fluid overload
- Pulmonary hypertension
- Mitral stenosis
- Mitral insufficiency

Normal PAWP is 8 to 12 mm Hg

Swan-Ganz catheter or pulmonary artery catheter. The syringe is attached to the part used for balloon inflation. The proximal lumen is attached to the pressure line which measures arterial venous pressure.

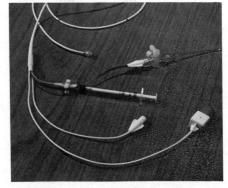

7   Calibrate and balance the transducer according to manufacturer's instructions. The transducer must be at the level of the client's right atrium (fourth intercostal space at the midaxillary line).

8   Shave and scrub the skin with antiseptic solution.

9   Open sterile gloves for physician.

10 Open drape for physician.

11 Continuously monitor the client's ECG throughout the insertion of the catheter.

12 Cleanse lidocaine vial with alcohol wipe.

13 Fill all lumens with the flush solution.

14 Catheter is attached to the pressure monitoring system.

Physician's Actions

a   Physician dons sterile mask, cap, gown, and gloves. Catheter is tested for air leaks by inflating the balloon with 0.8 cc of air for #5 French and 1.0 to 1.5 cc of air for #7 French catheter while balloon is submerged in a sterile basin filled with sterile irrigating solution.

b   Physician aspirates lidocaine with 18-gauge needle, changes needles, and injects skin with 25-gauge needle. Physician performs cutdown or percutaneous insertion. (The most frequent site chosen is the subclavian vein; however, the jugular may also be selected.)

c   Catheter is advanced with balloon deflated or partially inflated until the correct right atrial waveform and pressure appears on the monitor.

d   The balloon is now fully inflated to assist in the catheter's flow through the tricuspid valve into the right ventricle.

15 The catheter is attached to the pressure monitoring system.

16 The catheter is flushed to prevent air embolism. Pull on the red pigtail of the intraflow device.

17 After catheter is advanced, record right atrial pressure.

18 Observe for larger pressure waveform indicating catheter's presence in the right ventricle.

19 Record right ventricular pressure and observe for dysrhythmias (PVC's).

20 Inflate balloon with 0.5 cc of air to assist with the catheter's passage into the pulmonary artery.

21 Observe monitor for higher diastolic pressure waveform.

22 Inflate balloon fully or until a change is seen in the waveform. (Inflation assists passage of catheter into a distal pulmonary capillary.)

23 Record pressure.

24 Deflate balloon by removing tuberculin syringe and allowing air to escape.

25 Determine balloon deflation by observing pulmonary artery waveform tracing.

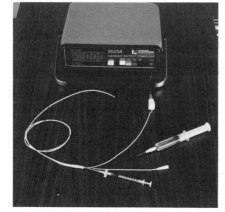

The Swan-Ganz catheter measures cardiac output by connecting the thermistor outlet of the catheter to the cardiac output computer.

▶ In some hospitals carbon dioxide, which is 20 times more soluble in blood than it is in air, is used to inflate the balloon to prevent air from entering the artery.

26 Repeat steps to ensure that catheter is wedging and deflating properly.

27 Replace empty syringe in place on balloon port.

28 Flush line.

29 After the physician secures the catheter with sutures, apply sterile antiseptic ointment and occlusive dressing to site.

30 Reassure and position client as needed.

31 Ensure placement by chest x-ray if fluoroscopy has not been used during insertion.

INTERVENTION: Obtaining Pressure Readings

1 Calibrate transducer every four hours to maintain accurate readings. (Transducer is placed at right atrial level.)

2 Place client in horizontal position.

3 Change monitor switch to determine pulmonary artery systolic, pulmonary artery diastolic and pulmonary artery mean pressures. Use the "mean" designation when determining the pulmonary artery wedge pressure. All pulmonary artery pressure readings are taken from the distal lumen of the Swan-Ganz catheter while the right atrial pressures are taken from the proximal lumen.

4 Remove syringe from balloon port.

5 Inject 0.8 to 1.5 cc air into balloon depending on size of catheter. The waveform on the monitor should change from pulmonary artery to pulmonary artery wedge pressure. Inflate *only* until a change is seen from the pulmonary artery waveform to the wedge position.

6 Balloon should not be inflated for longer than 30 seconds. Deflate balloon once the pulmonary artery wedge pressure reading is obtained.

7 If client is on ventilatory assistance, ensure that readings are taken with the client consistently on or off the ventilator. If client is on a respirator, slightly higher readings will be obtained. If client is taken off the ventilator return client to ventilator when readings are completed. If client is left on a ventilator, take readings at end of expiration, before next inspiration.

8 Flush line.

9 Record readings as often as ordered and report unusual findings to physician.

10 Reposition client in a comfortable position.

11 Change dressings daily and observe for infection at site of catheter insertion.

INTERVENTION: Balancing the Transducer

1 Open transducer dome. Use upright arm for balancing port.

2 Position top of balancing port (not the transducer) at level of right atrium.

3 Maintain balancing port at the proper level throughout monitoring.

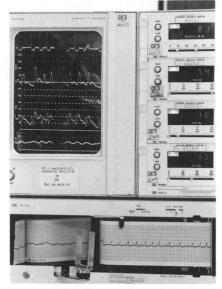

The third line on the oscilloscope indicates pulmonary artery pressure wave pattern.

▶ Pressure waveforms are similar to ventricular tachycardia or ventricular fibrillation patterns on the oscilloscope.

721

Waveform changes depicted on the monitor as the Swan-Ganz catheter traverses through the heart.

Right Atrial (RA) Pressure

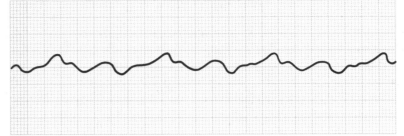

(a) Catheter in right atrium.

Right Ventricular (RV) Pressure

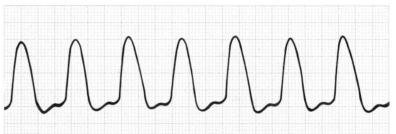

(b) Catheter in right ventricle.

Pulmonary Artery Pressure (PAP)

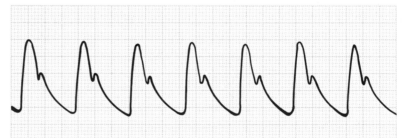

(c) Catheter in pulmonary artery.

Pulmonary Artery Wedge Pressure (PAWP)

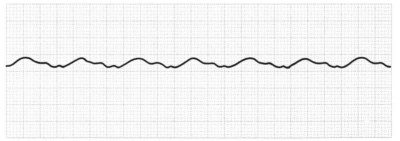

(d) Catheter is wedged in pulmonary capillary.

4   If the client moves, reposition and rebalance the transducer. For each inch away from the correct level, there is a 2-mm Hg error in the pressure reading.
5   Take cap off the balancing port of the dome to expose the diaphragm to atmospheric pressure.
6   Push monitor button to zero and check if monitor reading is zero. If so, the transducer is balanced to atmospheric pressure.
7   If the monitor does not have an automatic zero button, balance the transducer by turning the zero knob on the monitor until the reading is zero.
8   Check that the oscilloscope shows a flat wave at the zero line.
9   Cap the balancing port.
10 The monitor and transducer are now ready to be calibrated.

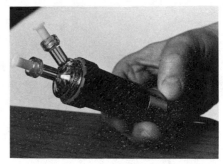

Use upright arm on transducer dome for balancing.

INTERVENTION: Calibrating the Transducer and Monitor

1   Press the zero button on the monitor.
2   Press the test/calibration button.
3   Turn the sensitivity knob until reading is 100 mm Hg on the digital readout, or until reading is appropriate for the equipment being used.
4   Transducer and monitor are calibrated when reading is at 100 mm Hg.

INTERVENTION: Balancing and Calibrating the Oscilloscope

1   Open transducer's balancing port to air.
2   Press the zero button on monitor.
3   Watch for baseline to register zero on the oscilloscope and then close balancing port.
4   Select a pressure range for the modality you are monitoring and press the scale button. Choose a low pressure of 100 mm Hg for central venous pressure or left atrial pressure, or 200 mm Hg for arterial blood pressure.
5   Press the test/calibration button and observe the oscilloscope for the waveform. The waveform should be visible at the pressure range selected (100 mm Hg or 200 mm Hg). Adjust the sensitivity knob on the monitor so the waveform reaches the pressure range.

▶ Method for calibrating a Hewlett-Packard electrical monitor.

EVALUATION

EXPECTED OUTCOMES

1   Catheter line remains patent. *If not*, follow these alternative actions:
    ANA: Flush the line using the pigtail on the flush line.
    ANA: Attempt to aspirate clotted blood through the line by pulling back on plunger of syringe.
    ANA: Notify physician if unable to clear line.
2   Pulse waveforms and readings are within normal findings. *If not*, follow these alternative nursing actions:

ANA: Deflate balloon on pulmonary artery catheter completely. Ask client to cough to help free catheter.

ANA: Test flush the catheter line.

ANA: If condition persists, notify physician to reposition line.

ANA: Assess client for other signs and symptoms indicative of a change in clinical condition.

UNEXPECTED OUTCOMES

1 Difficulty with obtaining wedge.

ANA: Anticipate or call physician to reposition catheter.

ANA: Anticipate chest x-ray.

ANA: Flush catheter using pigtail from flush line.

ANA: Recalibrate and balance transducer.

ANA: Instruct client to move arm, cough, deep breathe, or change position.

ANA: Anticipate use of fluoroscopy to determine placement of catheter.

2 Damping of waveform (waveform tracing appears to be in wedge position without balloon inflated).

ANA: Instruct client to cough and deep breathe; change client's position.

ANA: Flush catheter using pigtail from flush line.

ANA: Remove dressing — make sure tubing is not kinked.

ANA: Check that pressure bag is at 300 mm Hg. Change as necessary if leaks are detected.

ANA: Check to make sure transducer dome is not loose.

ANA: Check all connections for secure fit.

ANA: Check that stopcock is not turned in the wrong direction.

3 Dysrhythmias due to irritation of cardiac muscle.

ANA: Check tracing for position. If right ventricle tracings are observed, call physician because the catheter has most likely moved into the right ventricle.

ANA: Suspect intracardiac knotting of the catheter. (Rare occurrence; generally at time of insertion.)

ANA: Prepare for major arrhythmias and/or cardiac arrest.

ANA: Notify physician at once.

4 Infection occurs at site of insertion.

ANA: Prepare to aid in removal of catheter and insertion of new catheter, if required.

ANA: Prepare to culture tip of catheter and send to lab.

ANA: Change dressing, and apply antiseptic ointment.

ANA: Observe for signs and symptoms of phlebitis.

ANA: Remind physician to change site every 72 hours. (This is ideal — many times it's 7 to 10 days.)

5 Pulmonary ischemia or infarction occurs.

ANA: Keep wedging time short because prolonged wedging causes infarction.

6 No pressure tracing.

Causes of Elevated Pulmonary Artery Pressure

1 Right ventricle failure: liver enlargement, neck veins increase, sacral edema.
2 Tricuspid/stenosis/regurgitation
3 Constrictive pericarditis
4 Left ventricle failure/pulmonary hypertension
5 Volume overload

Causes of Elevated Right Ventricle Pressure

1 Pulmonary hypertension
2 Pulmonary valvular stenosis
3 Right ventricle failure
4 Constrictive pericarditis
5 CHF
6 Ventricular septal defect

ANA: Suspect clot in catheter (damping is an early sign). Try to aspirate; never flush.

ANA: Check stopcocks to make sure they are not turned wrong way.

ANA: Check that dome on transducer is tight.

7 No pulmonary wedge pressure tracing.

ANA: Suspect that catheter is not advanced far enough. Chest x-ray may be ordered to check placement of Swan-Ganz.

ANA: Reposition client.

ANA: Suspect possible balloon rupture.

ANA: Check and deflate balloon. Balloon may have caused the catheter to wedge. If you cannot inflate the balloon, it may be wedged.

ANA: For a brachial insertion of the catheter, reposition client's arm to float the balloon out of a smaller capillary.

ANA: For a larger vessel insertion site, instruct the client to cough, deep breathe, or change position.

8 Balloon rupture occurs.

ANA: Check pressure tracing.

ANA: Inflate balloon slowly if you suspect a ruptured balloon.

ANA: Allow passive deflation of balloon through stopcock.

ANA: Prepare for replacement line.

9 Intracardiac knotting.

ANA: Prepare to aid in removal of catheter because a change in pulse wave pattern indicates change in catheter position.

10 Client experiences anxiety and fear.

ANA: Reassure client and significant others.

11 Unusual or radical change in pulmonary artery and pulmonary artery wedge readings.

ANA: Clear transducer of air or blood.

ANA: Recalibrate and balance equipment.

ANA: Check connections.

ANA: Check if level of transducer is at level of right atrium.

ANA: Flush system.

12 Catheter whip (artifact seen in pulmonary artery tracing secondary to interference or turbulent blood flow).

ANA: Reposition and cough and deep breathe client.

ANA: Check patency by flushing catheter with pigtail from intraflow.

Guidelines for Pulmonary Artery Wedge

1 Pulmonary embolism: increased PA systolic
2 Pulmonary hypertension: increased PA systolic
3 Hypovolemic shock: decreased PA diastolic, MPWP
4 Cardiogenic shock: decreased PA diastolic, MPWP
5 Left heart failure: increased PA diastolic, MPWP
6 Right heart failure: increased CVP, increased PA systolic
7 Mitral stenosis: increased diastolic
8 Mitral insufficiency: increased diastolic
9 Pericardial disease: increased systolic, increased diastolic

Charting

- Size of Swan-Ganz catheter inserted
- Placement and technique used to insert catheter (cutdown or percutaneous)
- Pressure readings obtained
- Expected outcomes and nursing interventions completed
- Client's response and tolerance of the procedure

INTRA-AORTIC BALLOON PUMP

Circulatory assist devices have been in operation since the beginning of cardiac surgery. The underlying principle of circulatory assist devices, specifically the intra-aortic balloon pump (IABP), is to improve the function of the left ventricle.

In disease states such as left ventricular failure, myocardial infarction, unstable angina, massive pulmonary emboli, or postcardiopulmonary

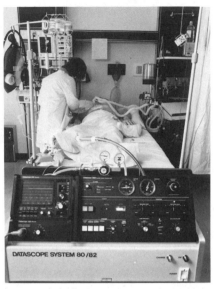

Intra-aortic balloon pump control console located near the bedside.

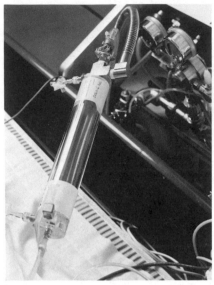

Safety chamber for intra-aortic balloon pump.

bypass, the injured heart cannot pump all the blood delivered to it. The remaining blood causes dilatation and hypertrophy of the heart and results in increased heart wall tension and increased myocardial oxygen consumption. Inotropic drugs alone cannot always increase perfusion of the myocardium, increase cardiac output, or assist in the perfusion of the coronary arteries. When an auxiliary pumping mechanism is employed, the myocardium, specifically the left ventricle, can function more efficiently even in a diseased state without creating excessive demands that could cause further deterioration. The intra-aortic balloon pump is such an auxiliary counter-pulsation device.

The intra-aortic balloon pump is an internal device that assists myocardial oxygenation and pump perfusion through a nonocclusive balloon that inflates and deflates cyclically. Inflation occurs during diastole, which begins at the closure of the aortic valve, and deflation occurs just prior to left ventricular ejection. Balloon inflation causes a retrograde and antegrade blood flow and a subsequent increase in mean arterial pressure. The force of blood is propelled into the coronary and systemic vasculature, causing an increase in tissue perfusion. As the balloon deflates just before systole, a relatively negative intra-aortic pressure is created. This pressure change decreases afterload, so that the LV contracts against a lower resistance. Therefore, the LV can pump more blood (increased cardiac output) while requiring less oxygen. As the amount of blood pumped increases, the preload will decrease to a more normal level.

The intra-aortic balloon is a single, double, or triple lumen balloon, mounted on a catheter, and is available for adults in 20-cc, 30-cc, and

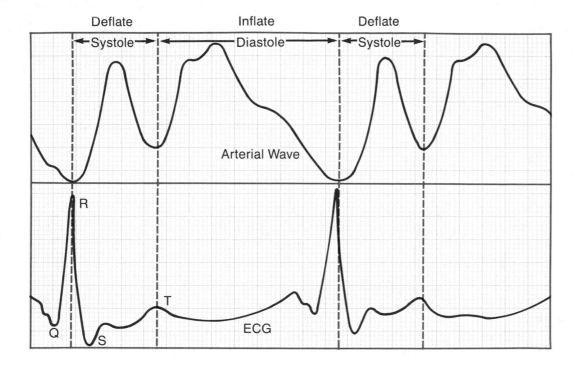

Diagram illustrates relationship between the ECG strip and the arterial pressure during inflation and deflation of the balloon.

40-cc sizes. The balloon, made of a nonthrombogenic material, is inflated with helium or carbon dioxide via a gas-propelled console. Balloon size is chosen so that the balloon when inflated occludes no more than 85 percent of the aorta.

The triple-chambered intra-aortic balloon is used most frequently. During inflation, the center chamber inflates first followed by the proximal and distal ends.

The intra-aortic balloon is usually inserted through an arteriotomy cutdown into the left femoral artery and threaded distal to the left subclavian artery and proximal to the renal arteries. Balloons which can be inserted percutaneously are also available.

The inflation-deflation sequence of the device is automatically triggered by a continuous electrocardiogram. Synchronization is usually timed according to the client's own R wave. The pump is capable of following heart rates as low as 30 BPM and as high as 160 BPM. Inflation actually occurs, however, on or shortly after the T wave, and deflation occurs either on the downslope of the P wave or at the time of the QRS. 60-Hz filter and sensitivity devices are usually incorporated to screen an electrical artifact or inhibit false triggering. Two simultaneous ECGs are done for client safety. In addition, an arterial pressure waveform is necessary since inflation is also timed directly at 60 M/sec, or prior to the dicrotic notch of the arterial pressure waveform. Deflation is timed to occur just prior to the systolic upstroke of the pressure waveform. A ratio of inflations to R wave is expressed in terms of a ratio: 1:1 (one inflation per R wave), 1:2 (one inflation per two R waves), 1:3, 1:4 and 1:8 (usually used in the weaning mode).

Complications Associated with Improper Timing of the Inflation-Deflation Sequence

- Compromised left ventricle
- Early aortic valve closure and decreased stroke volume due to premature balloon inflation
- Aortic blood volume falls rapidly during diastolic when late balloon inflation occurs
- Retrograde blood flow from the carotid and coronary arteries back into the aorta occurs with premature balloon deflation
- Increased resistance to left ventricle ejection occurs with late balloon deflation

727

A piston pump drives either helium or carbon dioxide to inflate the balloon. Helium, because it is a lighter gas, allows for faster inflation and deflation time. The machine is equipped with a continuous monitoring mechanism for gas pressure. The electronic component of the IABP has three divisions: monitoring, timing, and control. The monitoring division "reads" the client's ECG, the timing division triggers pumping, and the control division provides data to operate inflation-deflation valves. Contraindications to insertion of counterpulsation devices are an incompetent aortic valve, thoracic aortic aneurysm, severely atherosclerotic iliac or femoral arteries, or irreversible brain damage.

ACTION: MONITORING CARDIOVASCULAR COMPETENCY WITH AN INTRA-AORTIC BALLOON PUMP

ASSESSMENT

1   Determine baseline hemodynamic data.
2   Carefully assess ST segments and T waves obtained in 12-lead electrocardiogram.
3   Assess both lower extremities and femoral arteries.
4   Measure distal peripheral pulses and leg circumferences.
5   Evaluate baseline laboratory data and ensure availability of blood or platelets if needed.
6   Assess need for placement of other hemodynamic equipment, arterial line, Swan-Ganz catheter, pacemaker wires.
7   Determine pre-insertion cardiac output.
8   Assess respiratory status as client's position during pumping will be relatively immobile.
9   Evaluate baseline neurological check.

PLANNING

GOALS

- Myocardial contractility is increased.
- Adequate cardiac output is maintained.
- Coronary artery perfusion is increased.
- Peripheral perfusion is increased.
- Diastolic augmentation is accomplished.
- Afterload reduction is obtained.
- Fear, anxiety, and client discomfort are decreased.
- Inflation-deflation timing is correct and maximum counterpulsation is attained.

EQUIPMENT

- ECG machine
- IABP machine
- IABP catheter
- Emergency cart with defibrillator

Rationale for Action

- To decrease the work of the myocardium by decreasing ventricular ejection resistance
- To increase cardiac output by decreasing ventricular emptying resistance
- To increase coronary artery perfusion
- To increase peripheral perfusion
- To augment diastolic intra-aortic pressure

- Lidocaine 1 to 2 percent
- Sterile alcohol wipes
- Sterile drapes
- Sterile gown, gloves, mask, and cap
- Suture with needle attached
- Surgical balloon pump insertion or cutdown tray
- Suction equipment
- Operating room lights
- Skin antiseptic solution (povidone-iodine)
- 10-cc and 60-cc syringes with #18- and #25-gauge needles
- Heparin 1000 U/cc
- Sterile towels
- Two sterile basins
- Sterile saline for irrigation
- Antiseptic ointment
- Sterile pressure dressings
- Standby fluoroscopy

INTERVENTION: Preparing the Client for Intra-aortic Balloon Pump Insertion

1 Explain rationale for procedure to client.
2 Obtain signed consent.
3 Sedate client if ordered.
4 Prepare IABP machine according to manufacturer's instructions.
   a Determine gas or pressure gauge reading.
   b Calibrate or balance as necessary.
   c Select timing and pump ratio.
   d Attach ECG and arterial line to cables.
5 Connect IABP cable to ECG monitor. Choose monitor lead where R waves are dominant. Check amplitude of R wave. R wave should be at least 0.125 mv for proper sensing.
6 Obtain and record hemodynamic parameters, including cardiac output, pulmonary artery pressure, pulmonary artery wedge pressure, right atrial pressure, and arterial systolic and diastolic readings.
7 Prep groin by shaving and scrubbing skin with antiseptic solution.
8 Adjust lights.
9 Program the IABP machine using specific orders for individual client.
10 Administer heparin as ordered about three minutes before the physician begins the arteriotomy.
11 Check pressure gauge and gas tanks.
12 Zero and calibrate pressure channels.

INTERVENTION: Inserting the Intra-aortic Balloon Pump

1 Open sterile gloves.
2 Wipe lidocaine vial with alcohol swab when physician is ready.
3 Administer heparin prior to arteriotomy.
4 Place inflated balloon in sterile basin filled with sterile saline to check for leaks.

IABP Continuous Monitoring Modalities
- Pressure waveforms (arterial and pulmonary artery)
- Sequence of balloon counterpulsations
- ECG configurations and dysrhythmias

Fifteen-minute to one-hour monitoring modalities
- Blood pressure
- Pulse
- Respirations and breath sounds
- Temperature—rectal
- Pulmonary wedge pressures
- Intake and output
- Lab values as ordered
- IVs
- Gas deliverance volume
- Distal peripheral pulses
- Client's tolerance to procedure

Four-hour monitoring modalities
- Arterial blood gases (pO_2, pCO_2, pH)
- Cardiac output
- Hematocrit, white blood count, platelets
- Blood clotting tests
- BUN, creatinine

729

Arterial pressure waves
Normal arterial pressure tracing
1 Ventricular ejection after aortic valve opens.
2 Ejection period.
3 Peak of systolic phase.
4 Closure of aortic valve and beginning of diastole.
5 End of diastole.

Correct balloon timing
1 Peak of systole.
2 Balloon inflates at area of the dicrotic notch. A rise in diastolic pressure occurs after the balloon inflates.
3 Balloon deflates at the end of diastole and reduces the aortic diastolic pressure.
4 Reduction in systolic pressure following deflation.
5 Normal end diastolic pressure is higher when there is no balloon deflation.

Waveform indicates early balloon inflation which causes early aortic valve closure and thus a partially-filled ventricle.

Normal Arterial Wave Pressure

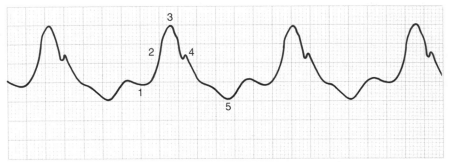

Correct Balloon Timing

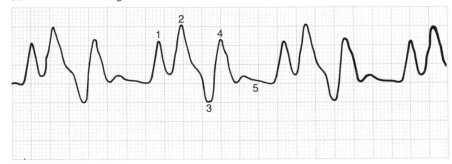

Early Balloon Inflation

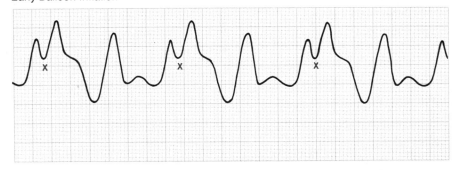

5 Evacuate air completely from balloon by aspirating with a 50-cc syringe.
6 Maintain sterile area.

Physician's Actions

a Physician (and others in the sterile field) don sterile mask, cap, gown, and gloves.
b Client is draped at insertion site.

Late Balloon Inflation

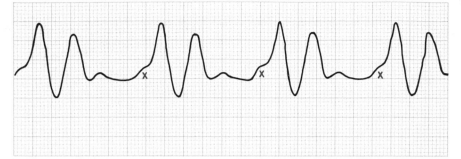

Waveform indicates late inflation leading to poor arterial perfusion.

Early Balloon Deflation

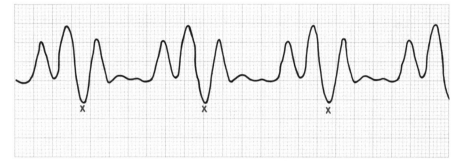

Waveform indicates early deflation leading to decreased afterload reduction.

Waveform indicates late deflation leading to increased aortic pressure which produces a heavier work load on the myocardium.

Late Balloon Deflation

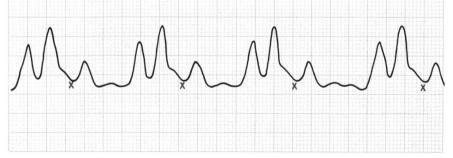

c If gloves are packaged with powder physician washes powder off in a sterile basin as the powder could cause clotting.

d Balloon is tested by injecting with 50 cc of air.

e Lidocaine is aspirated with a #18-gauge needle and skin is injected with a #25-gauge needle.

f Cutdown is completed using a side arm graft.

g Balloon is inserted. A side arm graft is sutured to the arteriotomy and to the exposed catheter.

h Placement of balloon is checked using fluoroscopy or chest x-ray.

i Balloon is sutured in place.

j Physician may initiate pumping by setting volume to one-half of balloon volume, turning machine on, and increasing volume to maximum balloon volume.

7 After balloon is sutured in place, connect balloon to safety chamber. Evacuate any air with syringe.

8 Ensure tight connections.

9 Client is made as comfortable as possible while keeping affected leg straight at all times.

10 Begin balloon pumping action by turning on pump. Select 1:1 pumping ratio.

11 Check inflation/deflation timing. Adjust timing as necessary according to the arterial pressure.

12 Apply sterile antiseptic ointment to insertion site.

13 Apply sterile pressure dressing.

EVALUATION

EXPECTED OUTCOMES

1 Timing is correct for the inflation-deflation sequence for maximum counterpulsation effect. *If not*, follow these alternative nursing actions:

ANA: Observe oscilloscope to determine where balloon is inflating in cardiac cycle. It should be inflating at the closure of the aortic valve and deflating immediately before systolic ejection.

ANA: Observe monitor for presence of PVCs because they can cause early balloon deflating. Treat arrhythmias as ordered.

2 Hemodynamic improvement of the cardiovascular system occurs. *If not*, follow these alternative nursing actions:

ANA: Observe for signs of poor perfusion, mental confusion, poor urine output, and weak peripheral pulse.

ANA: Notify physician to alter balloon pressure to increase the peripheral blood volume.

ANA: Evaluate client's position; it may interfere with blood flow if client is bending at waist.

3 Client is less fearful or anxious. *If not*, follow these alternative nursing actions:

ANA: Provide adequate rest, sleep, and reassurance.

ANA: Reorient client to his or her environment.

ANA: Allow client time for verbalization.

ANA: Anticipate and provide for client's needs.

ANA: Incorporate client's family or significant others in his or her care.

UNEXPECTED OUTCOMES

1 Client develops elevated T waves.
ANA: Change ECG leads as the machine may sense the peaked T as an R wave.
ANA: Evaluate client for signs of hyperkalemia.

2 ECG shows 60-cycle interference.
ANA: Check all electrical equipment in proximity to client and machine. Disconnect one at a time until the source is found.

3 Ineffective balloon pumping.
ANA: Check balloon position.
ANA: Maintain correct body alignment, i.e., leg not flexed, limit client movement.
ANA: Check timing sequence.

4 Ischemic limb or absent pulses distal to insertion site.
ANA: If condition occurs immediately after insertion, monitor continuously for capillary refill and function.
ANA: Notify physician of changes in condition of limb.
ANA: Place antiembolic stockings on client.
ANA: Prepare to remove balloon and perform an embolectomy.
ANA: Administer heparin as ordered.

5 Balloon ruptures with subsequent gas embolism or gas leak.
ANA: Remove catheter from machine, attach 50 cc syringe and aspirate all remaining gas.
ANA: Notify doctor immediately.

6 Decreased urinary output occurs.
ANA: Check position of catheter as it may be occluding renal artery.
ANA: Evaluate peripheral pulse to determine adequacy of pumping.

7 Thrombocytopenia occurs.
ANA: Check platelet count as ordered.
ANA: Anticipate blood or platelet transfusion.
ANA: Evaluate other laboratory values and notify physician of abnormal findings.

8 Hemorrhage from insertion site.
ANA: Apply direct pressure on site and call physician immediately.

9 Embolus forms on balloon or graft.
ANA: Administer heparin as ordered.
ANA: Anticipate removal if indicated.

10 Pulmonary complications occur.
ANA: Provide vigorous pulmonary toilet.
a Institute chest physiotherapy.
b Suction client.
c Turn client without flexing affected leg.
d Elevate head slightly (no greater than 30 degrees).

11 Infection occurs at graft site.
ANA: Maintain strict aseptic technique.
ANA: Keep insertion site dry.
ANA: Maintain antibiotic therapy if ordered.

Charting

- Size of intra-aortic balloon
- Complications that occur with insertion
- Client's response and tolerance to procedure
- Results of the monitoring modalities

12 Assist curve cannot be seen, or curve is damped.

ANA: Check balloon and safety chamber for kinks.
ANA: Check gas flow.
ANA: Check position of balloon via chest x-ray.
ANA: Anticipate balloon removal and insertion of new balloon.
ANA: Anticipate aspiration of balloon.

CARDIAC PACEMAKERS

A pacemaker is a device that provides electrical stimulation to the heart muscle in order to maintain an effective rhythm. It takes over the initiating and the maintaining function of the heart rate when the natural pacemaker fails.

Pacemakers have two primary parts — the pulse generator and the electrodes. When temporary pacing is desired, the pulse generator is external. When permanent pacing is desired, the pulse generator is placed internally. Conditions such as heart block and persistent bradycardia usually require permanent placement. Since the monitoring function is not utilized under these conditions, this text will focus primarily on the temporary pacemakers.

The temporary pacemaker is inserted in severe bradycardia or sinus arrest situations. Temporary conditions such as toxic drug reaction or inferior wall myocardial infarction also may require a temporary pacemaker. The temporary pacemaker is a device that provides a low-voltage electrical stimulus to the endocardial surface of the right atrium or ventricle (transvenous method) or into the ventricle itself (transthoracic or epicardial method).

All methods of temporary pacing utilize a pulse generator with rechargeable or replaceable batteries. This battery is the source of the low-

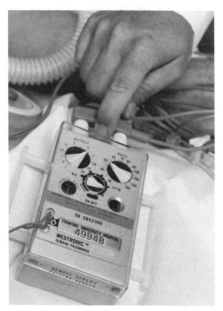

External temporary demand pacemaker.

Electrode wires from the client are connected to the pacemaker using both a positive and negative terminal.

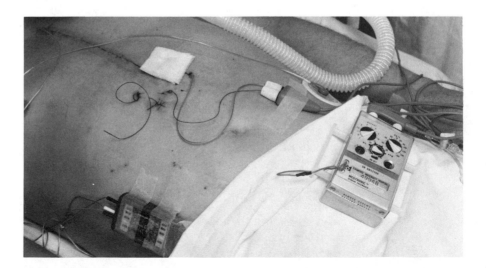

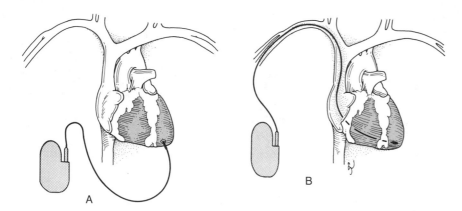

(a) Transthoracic pacemaker (b) Transvenous pacemaker

voltage output. In addition, all methods use some type of electrode or impulse conductor. These electrodes may be either unipolar or bipolar and differ in sensitivity. Unipolar (single-pole) catheter electrodes have a single cathode tip and are more sensitive to the client's generated impulses. The catheter electrode wire fits into the negative output terminal on the generator. The bipolar (two-pole) catheter electrodes have both an anode and cathode at the tip and fit into both positive and negative output terminals on the generator. The pace rate determines the rate of beats per minute (BPM) provided by the generator.

Initiation of temporary pacing by attaching electrode wires to an external generator source may be accomplished by the following routes:

Transvenous: pacemaker wires are threaded percutaneously through the subclavian or femoral vein or through a cutdown venotomy in the brachial or external jugular vein. With either method, the wire is advanced through the vena cava, right atrium, and tricuspid valve and positioned at the apex of the right ventricle on the endocardial surface. The wire is then attached to the generator.

Transthoracic: a needle is advanced through the chest wall into the right ventricle. The catheter wire is then threaded through the needle, the needle is removed, and the proximal end of the catheter wire is attached to the generator. Pacemaker wires are frequently inserted in this manner during cardiac surgery. The catheter electrodes are directly attached to the epicardial surface. Instead of being connected to the generator, the proximal ends of the wires are brought out through the chest wall, covered, and are then available for use if necessary.

There are three modes of temporary pacemaker therapy. Pacing differs according to the presence and/or function of a sensing mechanism. The first mode is a fixed or continuous rate (asynchronous). This type of pacemaker delivers an uninhibited impulse at a continuous set rate regardless of the client's underlying rhythm, so it does not have a sensing mechanism. The intervals between stimuli are unchanged even if ectopic or natural beats occur. This type is the simplest; however, its major drawbacks are its competition with the client's own heart rate and

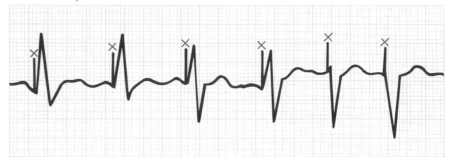

ECG tracing showing pacemaker spike.

the fact that in competition, the stimulus occurs during repolarization, thus pacing during the heart's vulnerable period.

Demand (synchronous) is the most frequently used. This type fires or stimulates the heart only when the heart's natural pacemaker does not function at predetermined rates. The atrial synchronous pacemaker senses the atrial impulse following a normal P-R interval. If the P wave fails to arrive at a set time, the pacemaker takes over. The ventricular inhibited pacemaker senses QRS waves and immediately discharges an impulse if the client's ventricular rate falls below the preset rate. This method is noncompetitive and is the most common; however, electromagnetic interference suppresses pacemaker function.

A third mode is AV sequential. Catheter electrode wires are placed in the atria and ventricles. The wires sense in both places and fire in both places. It is a complex mechanism and not as reliable as the other pacer modes.

In terms of pacemaker effectiveness, the nurse should be familiar with ECG monitoring and interpretation. Pacemaker spikes should be seen in relation to their appropriate ECG waveform. In addition, providing an electrically safe environment is essential.

ACTION: MAINTAINING CARDIOVASCULAR COMPETENCY WITH A PACEMAKER

Rationale for Action
- To provide temporary cardiac electrical stimulation for conditions resulting in alterations of heart rate or function
- To prevent bradycardia
- To improve cardiac function thereby improving cardiac output
- To provide a treatment modality for those cardiac dysfunctions impervious to drug therapy
- To assist in the treatment of existing or impending cardiac arrest situations

ASSESSMENT

1 Evaluate findings from a 12-lead ECG.
2 Assess vital signs.
3 Auscultate heart sounds.
4 Evaluate client's general appearance for pallor, cyanosis, and edema.
5 Assess for signs of low cardiac output.
   a Dizziness.
   b Weakness.
   c Altered level of consciousness.
   d Low blood pressure.

6 Determine client's and family's level of understanding of procedure and reinforce knowledge base as needed.

7 Ensure placement of an intravenous route for administration of fluids and drugs during an emergency.

PLANNING

GOALS

- Client's cardiac rate and rhythm are maintained through use of a pacemaker.
- Client is prepared psychologically and physically for insertion of the pacemaker.
- Pacemaker is inserted without complications.
- Dysrhythmias subside and cardiac output improves.

EQUIPMENT

- Emergency cart with defibrillator
- A bolus each of lidocaine, atropine, and isoproterenol
- External pacemaker pulse generator
- Pacing catheter electrodes
- ECG monitor
- Client cable
- Rubber glove
- Skin antiseptic solution (povidone-iodine)
- Sterile gloves and gown, mask and cap
- Sterile towels
- Lidocaine 1 to 2 percent
- Alcohol wipes
- Syringe
- #18- and #25-gauge needle
- Suture with attached needle
- Sterile 4 × 4s
- Sterile skin antiseptic ointment
- Tape
- Cutdown tray

INTERVENTION: Assisting the Physician with Pacemaker Insertion

1 Describe the procedure to the client and/or family and answer any questions.

2 Provide sedation as necessary. (Valium is frequently used.)

3 Connect client to a continuous ECG monitor.

4 Place the client in a supine position with head of bed flat. If client is hypovolemic, the bed may need to be in Trendelenburg.

5 If either the subclavian or external jugular vein is to be used, place a towel roll under the client's shoulders to provide better exposure of the insertion site.

6 Open the sterile gloves.

Physician's Actions

a Physician dons mask, cap, sterile gown, and gloves.
b Insertion site is cleansed with sterile antiseptic solution.
c Area is draped with sterile towels.
d Top of lidocaine is cleansed with alcohol wipe.
e Lidocaine is aspirated with #18-gauge needle, and skin is injected with #25-gauge needle.
f Insertion is accomplished (transvenous method via cutdown or percutaneously, or transthoracic method). Catheter electrode wires are positioned, and skin sutures are applied.

7 Continuously observe the ECG during the insertion. (Observe for PVCs — assess number per minute.)
8 Connect the pacing electrode to the appropriate outlet terminal (unipolar to negative and bipolar to both the positive and negative terminals).
9 Turn on power switch on external pacemaker.
10 Set rate according to physician's orders.
11 Set milliamperes (MA) by determining threshold. To do this, observe the ECG while slowly increasing the MA from its lowest setting to a point where a QRS complex is detected following each stimulus. Multiply the threshold level according to hospital policy (usually two to four times) to adjust the MA setting.
12 Set sensitivity mode according to physician's order.
13 Secure all connections. Make sure covering is over pacemaker. Put plastic cover back over pacemaker.
14 Place external pacemaker and exposed wires in a rubber glove to ensure insulation if required by hospital policy.
15 Apply sterile antibiotic ointment and sterile dressings to insertion site and *tape securely*.
16 Order chest x-ray following insertion.
17 Obtain 12-lead ECG.

EVALUATION

EXPECTED OUTCOMES

1 Client's cardiac rhythm is stabilized. *If not*, follow these alternative nursing actions:
ANA: Check sensitivity setting (if too high, P or T wave may be sensed; if too low, fixed rate pacing will occur).
ANA: Check MA setting (may be too high).
ANA: Check pace indicator for movement.
ANA: Check rate setting.
ANA: Check all connections.
ANA: Check catheter insertion site.
ANA: Check for battery depletion and change if necessary.

Clinical Alert

Observe for pacemaker failure.

1 Decreased urine output.
2 ECG pattern change.
3 Decreased blood pressure.
4 Cyanosis.
5 Shortness of breath.

ANA: Check for electrical artifact.

ANA: Insulate generator in rubber glove.

ANA: Obtain 12-lead ECG.

ANA: Anticipate replacement of pulse generator.

2 Pacemaker is inserted without complications. *If not,* follow these alternative nursing actions:

ANA: Check MA setting (may be too high).

ANA: Check sensitivity setting (may be too low).

ANA: Assess for signs of bleeding or shock due to trauma of insertion.

ANA: Observe for dysrhythmias due to irritability of conduction system upon insertion.

ANA: Anticipate cardiac emergency.

ANA: Obtain 12-lead ECG for diagnosis.

3 Client is prepared for pacemaker insertion. *If not,* follow these alternative nursing actions:

ANA: If client is frightened, reassure client that a pacemaker is not dangerous.

ANA: If client does not understand explanation of how the pacemaker or the heart functions, reexplain the procedure using illustrated learning aids.

ANA: Demonstrate the pacemaker and electrode and allow time for questions and further explanations.

ANA: Describe the insertion procedure specifically, allowing time for questions.

ANA: Orient your teaching to the client's intellectual and interest level.

UNEXPECTED OUTCOMES

1 Electrical interference.

ANA: Check electrical equipment for proper grounding.

ANA: Remove microwave ovens, TVs, electric razors, or other electrical equipment from vicinity of client.

ANA: Insulate generator, especially output terminals and exposed electrodes, in a rubber glove.

2 Infection or inflammation at insertion site.

ANA: Provide daily site care using strict aseptic technique.

ANA: Keep dressings dry at all times.

ANA: Monitor vital signs, especially temperature.

ANA: Instruct client to decrease extremity movement.

3 Diaphragmatic pacing.

ANA: Observe for hiccoughs or muscle twitching.

ANA: Change position of body.

ANA: Decrease MA.

4 Cardiac arrest.

ANA: Provide CPR, defibrillation, establish IV route, and administer drugs as required.

Client Teaching

Ascertain what client already knows and understands.

Determine client's ability and level of interest in learning about pacemaker.

Recognize client's fears and provide opportunity to talk about them.

Review facts: heart anatomy and physiology and pacemaker information. Use illustrations and audio-visual aids.

Clarify misconceptions and allay fears.

Describe insertion procedure.

Answer questions and provide additional opportunities to discuss impending procedure.

Charting

- Date and time of insertion
- Model and type of pacemaker used
- Type of catheter electrode wires
- Method of insertion
- Mode of pacing
- Pacemaker settings
- Client's tolerance of and response to treatment
- Vital signs
- Rhythm following pacemaker insertion
- Rhythm and strips of pacing obtained during insertion

5 Failure to capture.

ANA: Check client's heart rate. If less than the rate set on generator and if pace indicator shows firing, suspect failure to capture.

ANA: Check all connections.

ANA: Anticipate that pacer wires are dislodged.

ANA: Check battery.

ANA: Change position of extremity.

ANA: Turn client on left side; catheter may float back to epicardial wall.

ANA: Increase MA after checking threshold.

ANA: Obtain chest x-ray and 12-lead ECG.

ANA: Anticipate change of batteries, electrode terminals, or generator.

6 Battery depletion.

ANA: Have atropine and isoproterenol on stand-by.

ANA: Anticipate possible CPR.

ANA: Turn on power switch, and observe pace indicator. If there is little or no movement, replace battery immediately.

ANA: Record clock hours of battery usage (should be taped to back of generator).

ANA: Determine rate fluctuations.

ANA: Label each pacemaker with the date battery is inserted.

ANA: Store extra batteries in refrigerator, and put new battery in pacemaker before use.

7 Pericardial inflammation.

ANA: Auscultate for a pericardial friction rub.

ANA: Place in semi-Fowler's position to decrease pain.

8 Pneumothorax.

ANA: Auscultate lung sounds to make sure breath sounds are present in all fields.

ANA: Notify physician immediately.

ANA: Have chest tube and equipment ready for insertion.

ANA: Monitor vital signs.

MAINTAINING RENAL FUNCTION THROUGH DIALYSIS

Peritoneal dialysis is a method of separating substances by interposing a semipermeable membrane. The peritoneum is used as the dialyzing membrane and substitutes for kidney function during failure. This method is usually temporary and can be used for clients in acute, reversible renal failure. The most common circumstances under which this method would be used are decreased cardiac output due to myocardial infarction, cardiac arrhythmias, and cardiac tamponade. It could also be used when there is altered peripheral vascular resistance and hypovolemia.

Before the client is put on peritoneal dialysis, certain drugs are used in checking for renal failure. In most cases, mannitol is given because it has a large molecular size with great osmotic effect. This drug, given rapidly to obtain a higher blood level and, in turn, a filtered load, increases urinary flow. If urinary flow rate can be increased to 40 ml/ hour, the client is in reversible renal failure. If this medication does not work, the client may be given Lasix or Edecrin. If the client does not respond to either drug, a diagnosis of acute tubular necrosis is made.

The principle of peritoneal dialysis is diffusion and osmosis. While similar to hemodialysis, in this instance the peritoneum is the semipermeable membrane. The peritoneal membrane has two surfaces: the visceral surface that covers the abdominal organs, and the parietal surface that lines the abdominal cavity. In this method, the fluid is instilled into the peritoneal cavity between these two layers. The peritoneal membrane is impermeable to large molecules (such as proteins) but permeable to low molecular weight molecules (such as urea, sugar, and electrolytes). Fluids and solutes can cross this membrane via the process of osmosis, diffusion, and filtration.

Peritoneal dialysis cannot be used with clients who are diagnosed as having peritonitis, recent abdominal surgery, abdominal adhesions, or an impending renal transplant. For short-term use, however, it can be a life-saving intervention.

Hemodialysis, compared to peritoneal dialysis, is faster, more efficient, more expensive, and more technically difficult. This method consists of the diffusion of dissolved particles from one fluid compartment into another across a semipermeable membrane. This semipermeable membrane is a thin, porous cellophane-like substance. The pore size of the membrane permits the passage of low molecular weight substances, such as urea, creatinine, and uric acid, to diffuse through the pores of the membrane. Since water molecules are very small, they also move freely through the membrane. Most plasma proteins, bacteria, and blood cells are too large to pass through the pores of the membrane.

In hemodialysis the blood is in one fluid compartment and the dialysate is in another. The semipermeable membrane separates the blood from the prepared dialysate solution. The blood contains the waste products and flows into the dialyzer where it comes in contact with the dialysate. This exchange occurs due to differences in the diffusion rate across the membrane. A maximum gradient is established so that movement of these substances occurs from the blood to the dialysate.

The advantages of hemodialysis are that faster results may be obtained in an acute situation, it takes only three to five hours for each treatment (half that of peritoneal dialysis), and in an acute situation, a femoral catheter can be utilized.

ACTION: MAINTAINING RENAL FUNCTION
WITH PERITONEAL DIALYSIS

ASSESSMENT

1 Obtain baseline measurements of vital signs (especially blood pressure).
2 Assess for edema; measure abdominal girth.

Rationale for Action

- To remove excess fluid
- To remove end products of metabolism when the kidneys are nonfunctional
- To remove toxic substances from clients who have taken an overdose of drugs
- To control blood pressure

3 Check client's weight.

4 Assess renal function tests.

5 Examine dietary regimen:

    a Prior to dialysis, a low-protein diet is prescribed to reduce end products of protein metabolism.

    b During dialysis, protein restriction may not be necessary; diet should be high calorie, with limited sodium and potassium.

6 Evaluate client's abdomen for signs of infection or distention. Report any abnormalities to the physician.

7 Assess for signs of shock.

8 Auscultate breath sounds for rales and possible atelectasis.

9 Assess results of stool analysis for occult blood.

10 Assess condition of skin.

11 Review orders for solution to be used, number of cycles, and inflow, diffusion, and outflow times.

12 Verify signed consent form.

PLANNING

GOALS

- Specific symptoms decrease, and manifestations of renal failure diminish.
- Excessive fluid is reduced through use of peritoneal dialysis, and fluid balance is regulated.
- Creatinine and BUN levels are reduced.
- Asepsis is maintained throughout the procedure.
- Complications are detected early and treatment initiated promptly.

EQUIPMENT

- Sterile gowns, caps, masks, and gloves.
- Razor and blade
- Povidone-iodine solution
- Catheter insertion tray, with sterile drapes, catheter, trocar, connector, syringes, needles, sterile dressings, and sutures
- Local anesthetic, usually 1 percent Xylocaine without epinephrine
- Antimicrobial ointment
- Tape
- Dialysis machine (if available)
- Dialysis administration set
- Sterile, prewarmed dialysis solution
- Dialysis log

INTERVENTION: Assisting with Catheter Insertion

1 Explain procedure to client, reinforcing the physician's explanation and correcting any misconceptions.

2 Have client empty bladder to lessen the risk of bladder perforation.

3 Prime dialysate delivery system.
   a Check bottle labels against orders.
   b Check bottles for signs of contamination.
   c Connect dialysate bottle to administration set.
   d Clear air from inflow tubing and clamp line. If using an auto-
      mated delivery system, set controls according to the manufac-
      turer's directions.
4 Place client in supine position.
5 Shave abdomen between umbilicus and symphysis pubis.
6 Perform surgical scrub of shaved area.
7 Don sterile attire.
8 Hold bottle of local anesthetic so that physician can withdraw desired amount.

Physician's Actions

   a Physician dons sterile gown and gloves.
   b Abdomen is draped with sterile towels.
   c Local anesthetic is withdrawn and administered.
   d Insertion area is infiltrated and catheter inserted.
   e Trocar is removed.
   f Catheter is sutured in place.

9 Assess client's level of comfort and anxiety during procedure and
   relieve as necessary.
10 After physician has removed the trocar, connect the inflow tubing
   to the catheter.
11 Apply a sterile dressing following suturing of catheter.

Clinical Alert

Check bottles for broken seals or cloudy solution. Discard bottle if sterility is in question. Particularly note glucose and potassium concentrations.

INTERVENTION: Managing Peritoneal Dialysis

1 Inflow portion of cycle.
   a Open all clamps between the bottle of dialysate and the catheter.
   b Check that all clamps between the catheter and the drainage
      bottle are closed.
   c Make sure that the tubing is not kinked.
   d Note the time required to infuse the amount of solution ordered.
      Usually, it takes 5 to 10 minutes to infuse 1500 to 2000 ml.
   e Observe the client's breathing pattern and level of comfort.
   f Inspect the catheter insertion site for leakage or bleeding.
2 Diffusion (dwell) period: at the end of the infusion period, shut off
   the inflow line. Allow dialysate to dwell in abdomen 20 minutes.
3 Outflow phase:
   a Place the client in semi-Fowler's position.
   b Place bed in high position.
   c Open clamps between catheter and outflow bottle.
   d Allow dialysate to drain by gravity for 30 to 35 minutes.
   e Observe appearance of outflow fluid.
4 At end of cycle, calculate fluid balance.

▶ Method of calculation is as follows:
- The amount drained is subtracted from the amount infused.
- The result is described as positive or negative in relation to the peritoneal cavity.
- If the number is positive, fluid was retained in the cavity. If the number is negative, more fluid was drained out than instilled.

5 Throughout the cycle, monitor client status.
   a Vital signs.
   b Abdominal distention.
   c Mental status.
   d Check blood pressure and pulse every 15 minutes during the first cycle and every hour thereafter.
   e Check temperature every four hours.
6 Culture the outflow fluid from the first cycle and one cycle a day thereafter.

INTERVENTION: Maintaining Client on Peritoneal Dialysis

1 Monitor hydration status.
   a Check intake and output daily.
   b Record daily weight.
   c Check for edema.
   d Auscultate lungs for rales.
2 Evaluate electrolyte balance.
   a Check for leg cramping and diarrhea (signs of hyperkalemia).
   b Monitor ECG for tall, peaked T-waves and widening QRS segment (evidence of hyperkalemia).
   c Check potassium levels frequently.
3 Evaluate lung status at least every shift.
   a Perform deep breathing and coughing to prevent pulmonary complications.
   b Check for signs of pulmonary edema (dyspnea, restlessness, rales).
4 Examine site for possible infection (high temperature, leukocytosis, lethargy).
5 Monitor for any seizure activity: have padded side rails and tongue blade at bedside.
6 Check Chvostek's and Trousseau's signs frequently for indications of low calcium level.
7 Monitor diet: low potassium and sodium, high calorie, high bulk, and adjusted protein to complete amino acids (necessary to maintain positive nitrogen balance and replace protein lost through dialysis).
8 Maintain good skin care to prevent skin breakdown and pruritus.
9 Evaluate for signs of bleeding at catheter site, in stools and in urine; check hemoglobin and hematocrit frequently.
10 Monitor any medications. If iron is given as a supplement, have client take iron with meals.

▶ Perform site care daily, after each dialysis, or whenever site becomes wet or contaminated.

INTERVENTION: Caring for the Catheter Site

1 Remove old dressing with forceps.
2 Inspect site for infection or bleeding.
3 Use hydrogen peroxide to remove any dried blood or drainage.

4 Use povidone-iodine solution to clean around exit site.
5 Apply sterile pads around catheter at exit site and on top of catheter.
6 Tape dressing nonocclusively.

EVALUATION

EXPECTED OUTCOMES

1 Client tolerates procedure with minimal discomfort. *If not*, follow these alternative nursing actions:

ANA: Evaluate characteristics to differentiate dialysis-related pain from other types (for example, myocardial infarction).

ANA: If on inflow, reassure client that pain sometimes occurs.

ANA: Check that dialysate is at body temperature.

ANA: Promote effective fluid drainage.

ANA: Provide diversionary activities.

ANA: If persistent, consult with physician about decreasing infusion volume or instilling a local anesthetic through the catheter.

ANA: If accompanied by signs of peritonitis (abdominal rigidity, rebound tenderness, cloudy outflow fluid or fever), alert physician immediately.

2 Clear, straw-colored drainage is obtained. *If not*, follow these alternative nursing actions:

ANA: A slightly bloody outflow is normal at first. If condition persists, reassess catheter insertion.

ANA: Observe for signs of bleeding: petechiae, ecchymosis, or signs of blood in stool and urine.

ANA: Monitor hemoglobin and hematocrit to determine extent of bleeding.

3 Excessive fluid is reduced. *If not*, follow these alternative nursing actions:

ANA: Increase dialysate glucose concentration. The higher glucose level will "pull" more fluid across the semipermeable membrane (peritoneal cavity).

ANA: Make sure dialysate is body temperature when infusing. Cold fluid can promote vasoconstriction and increase fluid loss.

4 Creatinine and BUN levels are reduced. *If not*, follow these alternative nursing actions:

ANA: Make sure each dialysis cycle is only one hour long. To increase diffusion of BUN and creatinine across the peritoneal membrane, make sure the dialysate is allowed to stay in the abdomen no more than 20 minutes. Longer time periods cause equilibration of the BUN and creatinine on either side of the membrane so that BUN and creatinine are not reduced as necessary.

ANA: Warm the dialysate to body temperature to increase urea clearance.

ANA: Increase glucose, as ordered, in dialysate solution to increase urea clearance.

745

5 Asepsis is maintained throughout the procedure. *If not*, follow these alternative nursing actions:

ANA: Monitor client for signs of abdominal wall rigidity, abdominal palpation tenderness, cloudy dialysate outflow, and increased temperature.

ANA: Send daily cultures of dialysate outflow to monitor for peritonitis (a usual complication with repeated dialysis).

ANA: Instruct client on catheter care if peritoneal catheter is left in place between dialyzing procedures.

UNEXPECTED OUTCOMES

1 During catheter insertion, client experiences sudden pressure in bladder, rectum, or epigastrium.

ANA: Alert physician immediately, as these signs indicate malposition of catheter and require repositioning.

2 Inflow is slower than normal.

ANA: Check inflow tubing for kinks.

ANA: Lower bed position.

3 Outflow is slow or absent.

ANA: Check that outflow clamps are open.

ANA: Check for kinks in outflow tubing.

ANA: Check for and eliminate any air in drainage tubing.

ANA: Turn client from side to side.

ANA: Raise the head of the bed to a higher position.

ANA: Gently massage the abdomen.

ANA: Consult physician about possible blockage of catheter. He or she may probe catheter to dislodge fibrin plugs or reposition it to release a subcutaneous kink.

4 There is negative fluid balance at end of cycle.

ANA: Repeat outflow phase.

ANA: If negative balance is within limits specified by physician (usually 250 ml maximum), continue with next cycle.

5 Client experiences dyspnea.

ANA: Elevate head of bed.

ANA: Institute deep breathing and coughing exercises to prevent atelectasis.

ANA: If acute respiratory distress, immediately drain the fluid and notify the physician.

6 Client appears confused or lethargic; other signs of hyperglycemia are present during dialysis; signs of hypoglycemia are present after dialysis.

ANA: Check that dialysate glucose concentration on bottle label matches ordered concentration of glucose.

ANA: Be sure that dialysate is drained promptly at the end of the diffusion period.

ANA: Place diabetics on routine urine glucose and acetone tests.

ANA: Consult with physician about discontinuing dialysis slowly, giving the body time to readjust blood glucose and insulin levels.

7　Fecal-colored drainage or decreased drainage and diarrhea are present.

　　ANA:　Notify physician as these signs indicate possible bowel perforation. Surgical repair may be necessary.

8　Client experiences bladder fullness and increased urinary output, and there is decreased drainage.

　　ANA:　Notify physician as these signs indicate possible bladder perforation; surgical repair may be necessary.

9　Client on high glucose dialysate develops tachycardia or hypotension.

　　ANA:　Alert physician and implement changes in orders. A dialysate with lower glucose concentration will usually be ordered for future cycles to minimize recurrence of these signs.

10　There is leakage around catheter site.

　　ANA:　Change dressing as needed.

　　ANA:　Apply sterile plastic drape over skin.

　　ANA:　Weigh dressings to estimate fluid loss (1 gram = 1 ml).

Charting

- Predialysis weight and baseline assessment
- Time of catheter insertion
- Composition of dialysis solution
- Time of onset and termination of each cycle
- Number of cycles
- Amount of solution infused for each cycle
- Amount of fluid recovered for each cycle
- Cumulative fluid balance
- Appearance of outflow
- Postdialysis weight and clinical status

ACTION: MAINTAINING RENAL FUNCTION WITH HEMODIALYSIS

ASSESSMENT

1　Review dialysis orders.

2　Evaluate type of vascular access.

　a　Femoral vein catheter: used for immediate vascular access in life-threatening situations.

　b　Arteriovenous cannula (shunt): an external connection between an artery and vein.

　c　Arteriovenous fistula: an internal anastomosis between an artery and vein, present only in clients undergoing chronic hemodialysis.

3　Review chart and laboratory reports for factors that may alter management of dialysis.

4　Assess vital signs.

　a　Observe for shock and hypovolemia.

　b　Assess causes of hypotension: fluid loss; decreased blood volume, especially if hematocrit is low; or use of antihypertensive drugs between dialysis.

5　Check serum electrolytes frequently (pre-, mid-, and post-dialysis).

6　Weigh client before and after dialysis to determine fluid loss.

7　Complete physical examination for signs of fluid and electrolyte imbalances, e.g., edema.

PLANNING

GOALS

- Asepsis is maintained throughout the procedure.
- Creatinine and BUN levels are reduced and electrolyte balance remains in a satisfactory state.

Rationale for Action

- To remove byproducts of protein metabolism: urea, creatinine, and uric acid
- To remove excessive fluid by changing osmotic pressure (this is done by adding high concentrations of dextrose to dialysate)
- To maintain or restore body buffer system
- To maintain or restore level of electrolytes in the body
- To maintain a patent access site for hemodialysis
- To instruct the client in self care

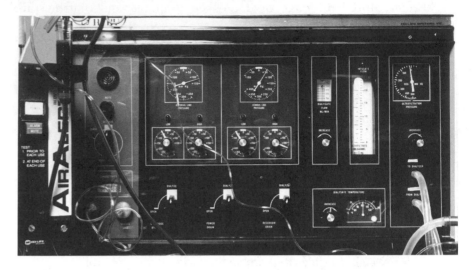

Hemodialyzer control unit.

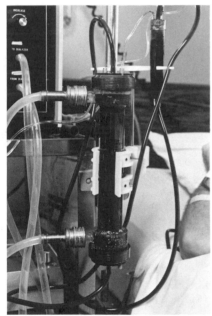

Blood flows down the hollow fiber dialyzer through small cellulose tubes utilizing a counter-current flow for removing exogenous waste materials. The dialysate fluid is pumped into the bottom of the coil and moves upward against the blood flow.

▶ Never initiate, monitor, or terminate dialysis without being thoroughly trained in routine and emergency procedures during dialysis.

- Excessive fluid is reduced.
- Toxic substances are removed and client's health status is improved.
- Access site remains patent.
- Client is able to care for self following client teaching.

EQUIPMENT

- Dialyzer (types are hollow fiber, parallel plate and coil)
- 500-ml bag of normal saline IV solution
- Macrodrop administration set
- 18-gauge needle
- Sterile masks and gloves
- Sterile gauze pads and alcohol swabs
- Hemostats, cannula ("bulldog") clamps
- Cannula separator, cannula-Teflon connectors, and infusion T connector
- Tape
- Sterile bowl and air pump
- Syringes and needles
- Heparin clotting rack and glass tubes
- Stop watch
- Hemastix
- Dialysis log

ADDITIONAL EQUIPMENT

For site care
- Masks
- Soap, water, and washcloth
- Hydrogen peroxide
- Sterile cotton applicators and alcohol swabs
- Antiseptic ointment
- Telfa pads
- Sterile gauze pads, tape, and flexible gauze roll

INTERVENTION: Performing Predialysis Procedures

1 Prepare dialysate bath composition as ordered.
2 Set up 500-ml IV of normal saline, macrodrop tubing, and large gauge needle on pole near bedside.
3 Set up heparin infusion pump on arterial line if constant heparinization is ordered.
4 Check location of nearest emergency power outlet in case routine power fails.
5 Prime the dialyzer and blood lines with saline.

INTERVENTION: Initiating Hemodialysis

1 Place blood lines at the same level as the bed.
2 Mask and wash your hands.
3 Unwrap the cannula dressing and discard it.
4 Put on sterile gloves.
5 Place sterile gauze pads under cannula connection to create a sterile field.
6 Clean cannula connection with an alcohol swab.
7 Clamp arterial cannula with a cannula ("bulldog") clamp.
8 Clamp venous cannula with a bulldog clamp.
9 Use a cannula separator to disconnect the cannulae.
10 Draw blood for predialysis blood samples as ordered by the physician. (These usually consist of electrolytes, BUN, hematocrit, clotting time, and any others necessary for the specific client.)
11 Insert sterile connectors into the disconnected cannulae.

Clinical Alert

The saline infusion must be available immediately in case of need for rapid reversal of hypotension or discontinuation of dialysis.

▶ If dialysate temperature or conductivity exceeds specified limits, the dialyzer will go into a "bypass" mode and dump the dialysate down the drain rather than allowing it to flow through the dialyzer. Dialysis with hot, hypertonic, or hypotonic solutions can cause hemolysis and death.

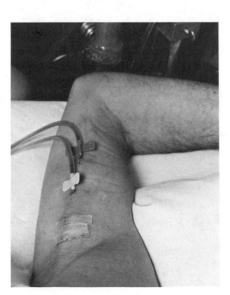

Needle placement for hemodialysis access site when client has an arteriovenous (A-V) shunt in place rather than external shunt.

12 Prime the extracorporeal circuit with blood.
  a Connect the dialyzer's arterial blood line to the arterial cannula.
  b Place the end of the venous line into a sterile basin. (The blood entering the extracorporeal circuit will displace the saline in the dialyzer into the bowl.)
  c Remove the venous blood line clamp.
  d Remove the arterial blood line clamp.
  e Remove the arterial cannula clamp. Do not remove the venous cannula clamp yet.
  f As blood enters the arterial drip chamber on the arterial line, add the prescribed dose of heparin prime.
  g Allow blood to circulate through the system until the saline in the venous drip bulb chamber is pink.
  h Clamp the venous blood line.
13 After priming the extracorporeal circuit, complete the circuit.
  a Wipe the venous cannula end with an alcohol swab.
  b Attach the venous blood line to the venous cannula.
  c Remove the venous blood line clamp.
  d Remove the venous cannula clamp.
14 Note the time of dialysis initiation.
15 Tape all connections securely; tape the tubing to the client's limb.
16 Add air to each drip chamber so that blood is about 1.2 cm below the top of the chamber.
17 Connect the pressure monitor lines to each drip bulb.
18 Set the alarm pressures.
19 Connect the air leak detector to the venous drip chamber.
20 Establish the specified blood flow rate (usually 200 to 250 ml/minute).
21 Test the dialysate outflow with a Hemastix. (Testing the outflow provides a double-check against the blood leak detector.)
22 Perform and record machine checks.
23 Check the client's blood pressure and pulse every two to five minutes while the dialyzer is filled and the blood flow rate is increased.
24 Increase the blood flow rate slowly to the specified rate. (The rate usually is 200 to 250 ml/minute.)
25 Obtain and record clotting times.
26 Increase negative pressure if ordered to establish ultrafiltration.

INTERVENTION: Managing Hemodialysis

▶ Keep the blood lines in clear view at all times (not under the covers!).

1 Maintain ordered clotting times of client and dialyzer.
  a Take clotting time about one hour before client comes off the machine. If less than thirty minutes, do not give protamine (heparin antagonist).
  b Keep clotting time at 30 to 90 minutes while on dialysis (normal six to ten minutes).
2 Assess client at least hourly for vital signs and potential complications.
3 Perform and record machine checks hourly.
4 Administer any ordered medications via the venous line.
5 Maintain dialysate temperature near body temperature.

INTERVENTION: Managing the Client on Hemodialysis

1 Limit fluid intake (400 cc over previous day's output); provide accurate intake and output.
2 Maintain diet: low sodium (20 to 40 g), low protein, high carbohydrate, high fat, and foods low in potassium and sodium.
3 Check vital signs for hypovolemia; check temperature for infection.
4 Auscultate lungs for signs of pulmonary edema.
5 Provide shunt care.
6 Observe level of consciousness—indicative of electrolyte imbalance or thrombus.
7 Administer antihypertensive drugs between dialysis if ordered.
8 Administer diuretics if ordered.
9 Administer blood if ordered (cellular portion only is needed because of low hematocrit).
10 Weigh daily to assess fluid accumulation.
11 Prevent use of soap (urea causes dryness and itching, and soap will just add to this problem).
12 Provide continued emotional support.
   a Allow for expression of feelings about change in body image.
   b Encourage expression of fears of death especially during dialysis.
   c Encourage family cooperation.
   d Give support for required change in life style.

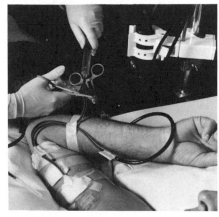

INTERVENTION: Terminating Hemodialysis

1 Reduce negative pressure to zero. Discontinue alarms.
2 Put on mask.
3 Remove tape and dressing to visualize cannula connectors.
4 Put on sterile gloves.
5 Place sterile pads under connectors.
6 Clamp arterial cannula and arterial blood line.
7 Separate cannula and tubing with cannula separator.
8 Connect IV of normal saline to arterial tubing.

When taking clients off hemodialysis, return as much blood from the machine to the client as possible by clamping the arterial tubing and allowing blood to flow into client via the venous site.

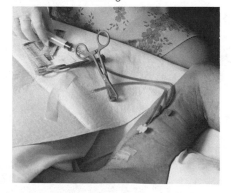

Rinse the access site tubing with normal saline before removing.

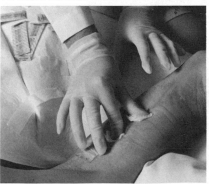

Apply pressure for at least five minutes to AV fistula site after needles are removed.

9 Release arterial line clamp and infuse about 150 ml to rinse tubing.
10 Clamp saline and arterial line.
11 Return blood remaining in extracorporeal circuit to client, using an air pump or more saline.
12 Separate venous line from venous cannula.
13 Insert cannula T connector into venous and arterial cannulae. Tape connections securely.
14 Remove venous cannula clamp and then arterial cannula clamp.
15 Perform site care, as explained in following intervention.
16 Measure and record postdialysis vital signs and weight.

▶ Perform site care every 24 hours whenever dressing is wet or contaminated or whenever sites have been exposed for observation or dialysis.

INTERVENTION: Caring for Cannula Site

1 Don mask and wash your hands.
2 Remove and discard old dressing.
3 Examine site for infection, bleeding, security of connections, and alignment of tubing.
4 Wash and dry skin under dressing area, except for immediate area of exit sites.
5 Using sterile cotton applicators and hydrogen peroxide, cleanse exit sites. Start at point closest to tubing exit from skin and work outward.
6 Use dry cotton applicators to dry exit sites.
7 Clean tubing with alcohol swabs, working from sites to connections.
8 Apply antimicrobial ointment if ordered.
9 Apply nonadherent gauze over sites if there is any bleeding or drainage; otherwise, apply sterile gauze pads.
10 Cover most of cannula tubing with gauze pad but leave a small loop visible for inspection.
11 Tape dressing to skin.
12 Use flexible gauze to wrap extremity securely but without constriction.
13 Tape end of gauze roll.
14 Place tape on dressing with the date, time, and your initials.
15 Attach bulldog clamps to dressing.

Clinical Alert
Clamps must be available immediately in event of cannula separation.

▶ With the physician's permission, blood can be drawn and medications can be administered through the infusion T. Use of the T may be preferable to venipuncture in other potential access sites, thus reducing possible infection or thrombosis.

INTERVENTION: Providing Routine Site Care Between Dialyses

1 Do not measure blood pressure on cannulated extremity.
2 Do not apply tourniquet on cannulated extremity.
3 Do not perform venipuncture above cannulation site.
4 Inspect, palpate, and auscultate the cannula every two hours or more often if the shunt is new or flow is poor.
5 Palpate pulses distal to the shunt and observe skin temperature and color every two hours at least.

EVALUATION

1. Access site remains clear of infection. *If not*, follow these alternative nursing actions:

   ANA: Culture exit sites separately.

   ANA: Notify physician. Client usually is placed on antibiotics to preserve access site.

2. There are no signs of fluid overload and/or electrolyte imbalance during dialysis. *If so*, follow these alternative nursing actions:

   ANA: Increase ultrafiltration.

   ANA: Check serum electrolyte values on fresh blood sample.

   ANA: Consult physician about possible changes in orders.

UNEXPECTED OUTCOMES

1. Decreased pulse, thrill, or bruit in shunt; blood in shunt very dark or separated into serum and red blood cells.

   ANA: Notify physician promptly of potential shunt clotting. Shunt will need to be aspirated, irrigated with heparin, or possibly vessel stripped of clots. (Success of declotting depends on speed with which it is instituted.)

2. Hemorrhage is observed from the shunt.

   ANA: Unwrap the dressing and examine the shunt. If cannulae have disconnected, immediately clamp with bulldog clamps. Then clean cannula tip, reconnect the cannulae, release the clamps, and notify the physician.

   ANA: If cannula has fallen out of vessel, stop bleeding with direct pressure or tourniquet above shunt. Summon physician immediately.

   ANA: Teach client how to control bleeding in case he or she is alone when bleeding occurs.

3. Hypotension occurs during dialysis.

   ANA: Anticipate possibility if antihypertensive or diuretic drugs were not omitted before dialysis.

   ANA: Administer normal saline into the venous line.

   ANA: Reduce pressure gradient if the client is on ultrafiltration.

   ANA: If hypotension is severe, consult physician about use of albumin, blood, or vasopressors.

   ANA: Before future dialyses, consult with physician about using smaller-volume dialyzer, less ultrafiltration, or intermittent normal saline doses to maintain blood pressure.

4. Bleeding occurs during dialysis.

   ANA: Administer protamine sulfate as ordered to return clotting time to desired range.

   ANA: If blood leak alarm sounds, observe dialysate. If no blood is apparent, check dialysate with Hemastix since air bubbles can cause false alarms.

   ANA: If bleeding or blood leak is present, discontinue dialysis.

5. Alarms sound during dialysis.

► The disequilibrium is believed to develop due to unequal rates of clearance of urea from bloodstream and brain. Urea retention in the brain results in hypertonic cerebro-spinal fluid, causing fluid to shift across the blood-brain barrier into brain tissues, producing cerebral edema.

Charting
- Predialysis assessment
- Time dialysis begun
- Dialysate used
- Any complications during procedure and actions taken
- Time dialysis terminated
- Postdialysis assessment

ANA: Before dialysis, thoroughly familiarize yourself with alarm sounds, functions, and troubleshooting maneuvers.

ANA: When alarms sound, quickly check for possible causes, such as obstructions or separations of tubing.

ANA: In an emergency such as clots, air emboli in venous line, or failure of bypass mode, clamp venous blood line tubing immediately.

6 Near the end of or following dialysis, dialysis disequilibrium syndrome develops.

ANA: Suspect dialysis disequilibrium if client develops confusion, seizures, headache, nausea, vomiting, and/or hypertension.

ANA: If these signs appear during dialysis, consult physician and implement possible orders to slow blood flow rate or discontinue dialysis.

ANA: Administer medications as ordered to control symptoms, for example, dilantin for seizures.

ANA: For future dialyses, consult with physician about possible orders regarding prevention, such as early dialysis before BUN rises excessively, shorter dialysis, or a change to the less-efficient peritoneal dialysis.

MONITORING THE FETAL HEART RATE

The traditional technique for counting the fetal heart rate involves listening with a fetoscope. This is called an intermittent evaluation since a sample of the fetal heart rate is used to make assessment about fetal health.

Two types of electronic fetal monitoring — external (EMS) and internal (IMS) — provide for a continuous data readout of both the fetal heart rate and the uterine contraction pattern. Each method has its place along a continuum of normal to high risk fetal status. Women who fall into higher risk categories are candidates for continuous electronic fetal monitoring. Use of continuous monitoring can be an invaluable aid to the obstetrical team in making a plan of care for the compromised, hypoxic fetus.

The most common method of obtaining an external recording of the fetal heart rate is with an ultrasound transducer, containing a transmitting and receiving crystal that picks up the motion of the fetal heart valves. The transducer is mounted in a capsule and held firmly on the maternal abdomen with an elastic strap. A special conductive jelly is applied to the transducer in order to provide proper sound transmission through the abdomen. External monitoring of uterine contraction is done with a pressure sensitive button, which is placed over the uterine fundus and held in place with a second elastic strap.

The heart rate sounds and uterine contractions are translated into electrical impulses. These, in turn, are reproduced on a printout strip on the fetal monitor. Both heart rate and uterine transducers may pick up extraneous sounds or movement. Fetal movement, maternal bowel

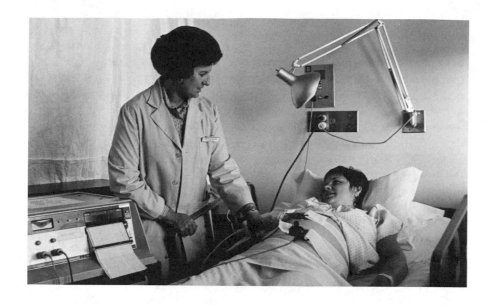

External fetal monitoring device.

sounds, or maternal coughing or vomiting should not be confused with the true reading.

It is important to note that external fetal heart rate tracing does not allow the nurse to assess fetal heart rate variability. Moreover, external uterine contraction monitoring does not quantify the strength of the contractions.

The EMS technique is noninvasive and can be done anytime during pregnancy as well as at any stage in labor. A woman in labor can easily move from bed to chair, sit up with legs over the side or even squat on the floor during second stage while wearing the EMS. It is important to note, however, that the long-term effects of the ultra sound fetal heart rate transducer are unknown.

The internal fetal monitoring is the most reliable, but it is also the most invasive. It is used when labor has begun, membranes are ruptured, the cervix is dilated at least 2 cm in order to apply the monitoring equipment, and the physician is available for insertion of the electrode.

A stainless steel spiral electrode is inserted just under the skin of the presenting part of the fetus. A special safety lock prevents penetration of the skin by more than 2 mm. These electrode signals are recorded on the printout strip on the fetal monitor. Beat-to-beat variability is accurately assessed by this method.

A fluid filled strain gauge catheter placed in the uterine cavity transmits uterine pressure to a transducer. This transducer converts the pressure into millimeters of mercury. Unlike the EMS, the internal uterine monitor gives a precise evaluation of contraction strength.

The woman in labor must remain in bed with this method of monitoring. She should be encouraged to turn from side to side and not to stay flat on her back. Maternal hypotension and placental insufficiency may be produced by the weight of the fetus compressing the aorta in the supine position.

Clinical studies have shown that there is positive association between a normal FHR tracing via continuous electronic monitoring and fetal outcome as measured by Apgar scores. However, the converse is not necessarily true. An abnormal FHR tracing is not always associated with a poor outcome. Abnormal tracings may mean that the fetus is in jeopardy only about half the time that they occur. This discrepancy was recognized in the late sixties and resulted in another assessment technique — fetal scalp blood sampling (FSBS).

The FSBS is a test where a small amount of blood is taken directly from the presenting part (if low enough in the pelvis to remain steady) and measured for pH. The physiological basis for this assessment is that a fetus who is truly in jeopardy, due to placental insufficiency, will not only have a decreased oxygen supply but also an increased carbon dioxide level. This increased carbon dioxide will cause respiratory acidosis and an increase in the pH (acid concentration of the blood). This can be measured in a very small quantity of fetal blood.

A pH of 7.25 or greater is normal for the fetus in labor. A normal pH correlates strongly with a positive outcome — a healthy fetus and an abnormal pH (below 7.25) correlates with a negative outcome. The FSBS is not only a useful tool but also a necessary adjunct to continuous electronic monitoring.

The widespread use of electronic fetal monitoring has caused consumers as well as providers to polarize opinions on the technique. Many feel that family centered maternity care and the joyful celebration of the normal birthing experience are threatened by the use of the technological advances of electronic fetal monitoring. Others cite fetal and maternal morbidity associated with internal monitoring (IMS) or the unknown consequences of use of ultra sound with external monitoring (EMS). Still others extol the decrease in perinatal mortality associated with the use of electronic monitoring. The National Institute of Child Health and Human Development has adapted the following guidelines for nurses, nurse-midwives, and physicians in order to promote family centered care regardless of the modality of fetal assessment:

1 Electronic fetal monitoring or any other technology should never be a substitute for clinical judgment. Electronic fetal monitoring is only one parameter of fetal assessment.
2 Proper use of both intermittent auscultation and continuous electronic fetal monitoring in both high and low risk clients should at the outset include a discussion with the client of her wishes, concerns, and questions concerning benefits, limitations, and risks of fetal monitoring. Women should have the opportunity to discuss the use of all forms of monitoring during the course of prenatal care and again upon admission to the labor suite.

Monitoring should be accompanied by supportive and knowledgeable personnel who are attentive to the client's expectations regarding the conduct of her labor. Hospital personnel should be cognizant of the potential impact of EFM upon family centered childbirth.

3   Periodic auscultation of the fetal heart rate (for 30 seconds every 15 minutes in the first stage of labor; every 5 minutes during the second stage; and immediately following a contraction) is an acceptable method of assessment of fetal condition for women at low risk of intrapartum fetal distress. Interpretation of auscultated FHR data should include an understanding of the relationship of FHR changes to uterine contractions.

4   The use of electronic fetal monitoring should be strongly considered in high risk clients. Some high risk situations may include: (1) low birth weight, prematurity, postmaturity, and intrauterine growth retardation; (2) medical complications of pregnancy; (3) meconium staining of the amniotic fluid; (4) intrapartum obstetrical complications; (5) use of oxytocin in labor; and (6) the presence of abnormal auscultatory findings.

    The medical record should reflect careful consideration of the benefits and risks to each individual including a discussion of the indications for EFM. Under certain circumstances, low risk clients and their physicians may choose to use electronic fetal monitoring.

5   Since unexpected risk factors may arise during labor in clients without prior evidence of risk, all hospitals and birthing centers providing maternity care should have the necessary trained staff and equipment to assess carefully the status of each fetus in labor and to take appropriate action.

6   In order that electronic fetal monitoring be used appropriately, the medical profession and others should encourage, through their various educational modalities, a thorough understanding of the principles and procedures of intrapartum fetal heart rate assessment, by all personnel responsible for the care of pregnant women. Special attention should be given to the benefits, limitations, and risks of each mode of assessment. Acquisition of expertise in the use of continuous fetal heart rate and intrauterine pressure data requires the opportunity for supervised practical training in the interpretation of monitor tracings, use of scalp blood sampling, and the integration of such data into the clinical setting.

7   The use of fetal scalp blood pH determination is strongly encouraged as a adjunct to electronic fetal heart rate monitoring.

8   Attention to the known potential hazards of EFM should accompany its use. Placement of the fetal scalp electrode and intrauterine pressure catheter should be performed with attention to aseptic and atraumatic technique. Prolonged supine position of the mother should be avoided, and maternal mobility should not be unnecessarily limited.

9   Hospital personnel should be cognizant of the potential impact of EFM upon family centered childbirth. Family centered care and indicated intrapartum fetal monitoring are not mutually exclusive. Maternity services should be encouraged to integrate concepts of family centered care with care of women who are electronically monitored.

Rationale for Action

- To assess the well-being of the fetus
- To monitor fetal heart rate
- To provide a measurement of uterine activity during labor
- To record the intensity of the uterine contractions during the oxytocin challenge test

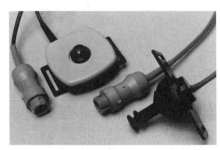

Tocotransducer and phonotransducer used for external fetal monitoring.

Types of External Fetal Monitors

- Abdominal electrodes: elicits fetal and maternal heart rates
- Phonotransducer: picks up fetal heart tones
- Ultrasonic transducer: picks up fetal heart tones
- Tocotransducer: monitors uterine activity

Fetal monitor with printout that records fetal heart rate on the left side and uterine activity on the right side.

ACTION: MONITORING FOR FETAL DISTRESS

ASSESSMENT

1 Evaluate client's and family's knowledge of rationale for fetal monitoring.
2 Identify client's concerns and answer questions about fetal monitoring before procedure is initiated.
3 Assess client's knowledge of procedure.
4 Evaluate position of fetus using Leopold's maneuver.
5 Identify which type of monitoring device is to be used.
6 Assess fetal heart rate: normal is 120 to 160 beats per minute.
7 Assess fetal monitor strip for early and late deceleration.

PLANNING

GOALS

- Fetal well-being is monitored throughout the client's labor.
- Client is well-informed of rationale for monitoring and procedure.
- Fetal heart rate and uterine activity are clearly displayed on monitor.

EQUIPMENT

For external monitoring system

- Tocotransducer and elastic strap
- Ultrasonic transducer or phonotransducer and elastic strap
- Conductive jelly (for ultrasonic transducer)
- Talcum powder
- Alcohol swabs, electrode paste, electrodes
- Fetal monitor with oscilloscope and printout graph

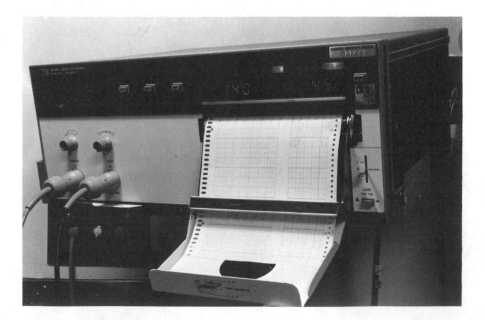

For internal monitoring system

- Sterile stainless steel spiral electrode with safety lock
- Catheter filled with sterile saline
- Transducer and cable
- Fetal monitor with oscilloscope and printout graph
- Leg plate and plate strap
- ECG paste

PREPARATION

- Identify client's knowledge of fetal monitoring
- Clarify and explain unclear aspects of fetal monitoring
- Show client the monitor and briefly explain how it functions
- Reassure and explain monitoring to significant others
- Gather equipment for specific type of monitoring

INTERVENTION: Monitoring Uterine Activity

1. Explain procedure to client.
2. Plug the tocotransducer into the monitor inlet labeled TOCO or UTERINE ACTIVITY.
3. Turn monitor on and press printout button.
4. Move the stylus to zero. The printout is divided into two parts. The uterine activity waveform is found on the right side.
5. Place the tocotransducer over the uterine fundus. (Locate fundus using Leopold's maneuvers.)
6. Position the tocotransducer in place with belt.
7. When client is free of contractions, tighten belt until the stylus on the monitor moves to the 50-mm Hg mark on the right side of the printout.
8. Turn control knob until stylus moves back to the 10-mm Hg mark.

▶ Powder belts first to avoid irritating client's skin.

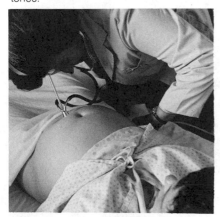

A fetoscope is used to listen for fetal heart tones.

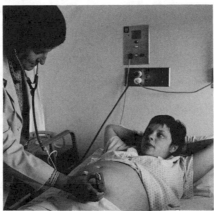

Doppler method of listening for fetal heart tones.

Uterine Contraction Waveforms

1 Early deceleration: 10 to 20 beat drop in rate usually within normal range of 120 to 160.
  a Occurs before peak or early contracting phase. Recovery as soon as acme of contraction has passed.
  b Uniform shape.
  c Indicate head compression—vagal stimulation results in decreased heart rate.
  d V-shaped appearance.
  e Not considered ominous.

2 Late deceleration.
  a Decrease in fetal heart rate of 10 to 20 beats/minute.
  b Occurs after peak or late contracting phase.
  c Uniform shape.
  d Usually indicates fetal distress.
  e Likely to appear in any situation where fetal-maternal exchange in placenta is reduced, resulting in hypoxia.

3 Variable deceleration: no uniformity in pattern.
  a Decrease in fetal heart rate occurs any time during contraction phase.
  b Usually below 120 beats/minute.
  c May indicate cord compression.
  d May occur when client pushes.
  e Must be evaluated carefully—may or may not indicate fetal difficulty.

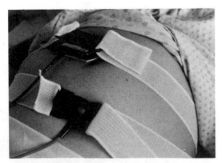

Examples of external fetal monitoring devices: a tocotransducer and a phonotransducer.

9 Test the tocotransducer by pressing down on the transducer. If the baseline recorder moves, the tocotransducer is functioning properly.

10 Record the frequency and duration of contractions as required by hospital policy.

INTERVENTION: Monitoring Fetal Heart Rate Using a Phonotransducer

1 Plug the phonotransducer cable into the monitor inlet marked PHONO.
2 Turn on monitor to evaluate if it is functioning properly.
3 Cleanse and dry client's abdomen.
4 Place the transducer over the site where the fetal heartbeat is the loudest (most common site is lower left quadrant of the client's abdomen).
5 Position transducer on abdomen with belt.
6 Watch that the heartbeat indicator light on the monitor flashes with each audible heartbeat and that the waveform appears on the oscilloscope.
7 Determine fetal heart rates from fetal heart rate waveform on printout.

INTERVENTION: Monitoring Fetal Heart Rate Using an Ultrasonic Transducer

1 Plug the ultrasonic transducer cable into the monitor inlet marked ULTRASOUND.
2 Turn on monitor to determine if it is functioning properly.
3 Apply conductive jelly to the transducer diaphragm and place transducer over site where the fetal heart rate is the loudest (use Leopold's maneuvers to determine fetal position).
4 Position transducer on abdomen with belt.
5 Watch that the heartbeat indicator light on the monitor flashes with each audible heartbeat and that the waveform appears on the oscilloscope.
6 Turn on recorder printout, and record fetal heart rate according to hospital policy.
7 Reposition transducer every hour to minimize skin irritation.

INTERVENTION: Monitoring Fetal Heart Rate Using Abdominal Electrodes

1 Determine position of fetus.
2 Cleanse client's abdomen with alcohol and allow to dry.
3 Apply the regular electrodes over the fetus's head and back and the suction electrode over the fetus's buttocks.
4 Attach lead wire with white clip to electrode over the head, and lead wire with green clip to electrode over the back, and the lead wire with black clip to electrode over the buttocks.
5 Plug electrode cable into the ECG inlet on fetal monitor.

6 Turn on monitor and assess maternal-fetal waveforms on the oscilloscope for adequacy.

7 Remove and replace electrodes if waveforms are inadequate.

INTERVENTION: Using an Internal Fetal Monitor

1 Gather equipment.

2 Assist the physician as needed with vaginal examination.

Physician's Actions

a Presenting fetal part is identified.

b The scalp electrode is mounted on the end of the drive tube, surrounded by guide tube.

c The electrode is retracted 2.5 cm from the mouth of the guide tube.

d The guide tube is placed inside client's cervix, and the tube is advanced until the electrode touches the fetal head. The drive tube is rotated one turn clockwise when electrode touches head.

e Handle is unlocked and removed from drive tube. The guide tube and drive tube are removed leaving the electrode wires exposed.

f At the end of the client's labor the electrode is removed by turning it counterclockwise.

3 After physician has inserted the scalp electrode, attach the electrode wires to the color-coded areas on the leg plate.

4 Lubricate and strap the leg plate on client's thigh.

5 Plug leg plate cable into ECG monitor inlet.

6 Turn monitor on and observe for ECG pattern on oscilloscope.

7 For a printout, press the monitor button that is used for activating the printout.

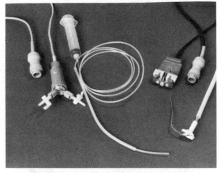

Fetal scalp electrode (right) and uterine pressure catheter and transducer (left) utilized for internal fetal monitoring.

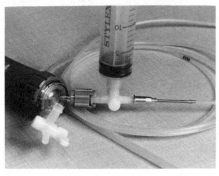

Flush catheter and dome of the transducer with distilled water to flush out air bubbles before using.

Fetal heart rate pattern is displayed in upper waveform segment. Intensity, rate, and duration of uterine contractions are shown in lower waveform pattern.

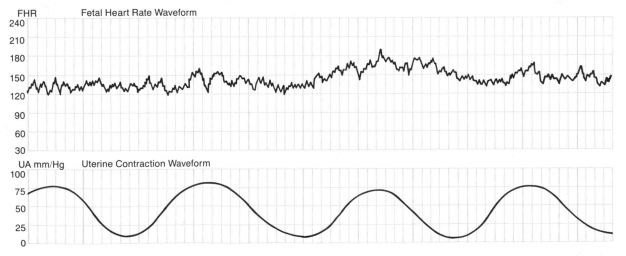

EVALUATION

EXPECTED OUTCOMES

1 Fetal heart rate and uterine activity are clearly displayed on readout. *If not*, follow these alternative nursing actions:

ANA: Check for sufficient amount of electrode jelly on leg plate. The jelly assists in conduction process.

ANA: Reposition leg plate on client's leg.

ANA: Check monitor and cables to detect any loose connections.

ANA: Check that stylet is not bent. If bent, it will not trace the pattern properly.

ANA: Evaluate fetal condition with Doptone to determine status of fetus.

2 Fetal well-being is monitored throughout client's labor. *If not*, follow these alternative nursing actions:

ANA: If unable to monitor client with internal electrode, check all equipment before changing to external monitoring device.

ANA: If unable to monitor client continuously, use Doppler procedure and assess fetal heart tones every 15 minutes.

ANA: If waveform interference, suspect change in fetus' position.

UNEXPECTED OUTCOMES

1 The scalp electrode falls out.

ANA: Obtain new setup. Old electrode will not be used due to chance of infection.

ANA: Assess whether fetal condition necessitates replacement of scalp electrode.

2 Fetal baseline data is variable.

ANA: Examine placement of monitor, check grounding and equipment.

ANA: If fetal heart rate is tachycardiac, assess hydration status of client. Turn client on right side and notify physician.

ANA: If fetal heart rate is bradycardiac, discontinue IV infusion of oxytocin. Position client on left side. Administer oxygen at 8 l/min via face mask. If bradycardia continues, prepare for C-section.

ANA: If decreased variability occurs, turn client to left side and administer oxygen.

Charting

- Time of vaginal examination and results of findings
- Time and type (spontaneous or artificial) of membrane rupture
- Character of amniotic fluid
- Type and time of monitor application
- Medications used
- Maternal vital signs
- Fetal heart tones
- Maternal position during monitoring
- Monitoring strip and evaluation of findings

CHAPTER 20
Coping with Crisis, Grief, and Death

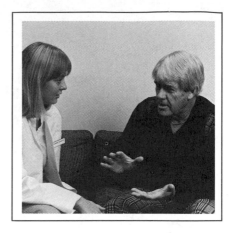

CRISIS SITUATIONS

The word *crisis* originates from the Greek word *krisis* meaning "turning point." The contemporary definition of crisis is a crucial situation, or turning point. Such a juncture in one's life cycle immediately affects the total being. When methods of dealing with stressful situations are not adequate, and the normal coping modes are not sufficient to resolve the situation, the individual is plunged into the chaos of conflict and indecision. Successful resolution of this crisis will occur with either a return to the precrisis state of being, a level of functioning below that of the crisis period, or psychological growth evidenced by increased competence and ability to cope. When an adult individual is in a crisis, it often precipitates such total involvement of the person that therapeutic intervention is required to sustain and assist the person to cope.

Crises can occur from any external or inner source, such as loss of a loved one or a relationship, impoverishment, disaster, unemployment, marriage, birth of a child, return of a loved one, adolescence, etc. A crisis can develop from stress, and stress can develop from any untoward or even a desirable event. Any change from normal living patterns can create stress. Stress develops into a crisis situation when the person is unable to cope with the stressful situation.

Individual responses to a crisis may vary, but a central theme of this state is a loss of control and an inability to cope. There may be a panic

Learning Objectives

Define a crisis and describe the precipitant factors.

List several behavioral responses to crises.

Outline the main characteristics of a crisis.

Identify the specific stages in the development of a crisis.

Discuss assessment techniques to identify a person in crisis.

Outline steps necessary to assist the client to manage crisis.

List the stages of the grief process.

State the main characteristics observed by a person experiencing grief.

Identify the factors that influence the outcome of the grieving process.

List at least two nursing interventions for each stage of grief.

Describe the phases of dying outlined by Elisabeth Kübler-Ross.

Discuss at least four nursing interventions that would assist the dying client.

episode that engenders a high level of anxiety, distortion of thought or perceptions, or even personality disorganization. If the latter occurs, you would observe increased motor activity, reduced sensory perception, and reduced ability to communicate leading to complete withdrawal and even loss of higher psychic functions. In addition to panic, there may be a reaction to acute grief that results in psychological and somatic symptoms leading to an inability to cope with activities of daily living.

We as individuals are typically in a state of balance, or homeostasis. This state is maintained by behavioral patterns involving interchange between the person and his or her environment. When problems or stress is encountered, the person employs learned coping mechanisms to deal with the stress. If the coping mechanisms work, a crisis does not develop. If, however, the problem becomes too great to be handled, a crisis situation emerges. The result is a major disorganization in functioning.

The major precipitating factors in a crisis are:
- Threat to individual security: loss or threat of loss.
- Situational crisis: actual or potential loss of job, relationship, etc.
- Developmental crisis, which may be any change, positive or negative.
- Two or more severe problems arising concurrently.

The main characteristics of a crisis situation are that it is initiated by a triggering event, such as those listed above, and the usual coping mechanisms are inadequate for dealing with the situation. The crisis is self-limiting, acute, and will last from a few days to a period of six weeks. The person is totally involved and hurts all over. This is a very dangerous situation for the person and intervention is essential.

There are specific stages in the development of a crisis situation. First, there is the initial perception of the problem, which causes a rise in tension and anxiety. The usual coping mechanisms are tried, and the usual situational supports are explored. The known methods prove unsuccessful and tension increases. The problem or stress remains and the person's functioning becomes disorganized. As anxiety increases, perception narrows, and the coping ability is further reduced. Resolution of the crisis occurs within six weeks with or without intervention.

When one is counseling in a crisis situation, it is important to remember that the main goal is simply to resolve the immediate crisis so that the individual can continue to function. Thus, the first principle is to be reality-oriented. This entails giving the necessary support, clarifying the problem, and providing adequate anticipatory guidance.

Anticipatory guidance involves being there and listening to the client. It includes providing the necessary information to assist the client to make decisions. For instance, the counselor may advise hospitalization if the external supports are not sufficient to enable the client to get through the crisis period without further loss of function. This is the moment that a person is most open for intervention; therefore, if appropriate intervention occurs, major changes can take place so that the crisis can be a turning point for the person and the individual emerges from the crisis situation functioning at a higher level than previously. This is the most positive result. An alternative outcome of intervention would be that the person survived the crisis period still able to cope with life and has accepted suggestions for future support.

GUIDELINES FOR MANAGING CLIENTS

Sets of interrelated factors can produce a crisis situation.

- An event that presents a threat (loss or threat of loss) to the individual and is a trigger.
- The threat is in a symbolic way linked to earlier ego-threats that resulted in vulnerability or conflict.
- The person does not have the ability to respond with adequate coping mechanisms.

The degree of stress experienced depends on such factors as stage of developmental growth, present and past environment, and the number of other emotional threats in existence.

- How previous developmental crises have been resolved acts as the basis for resolution of the present crisis.
- When the crisis period is experienced, the person immediately turns to the reintegration of former critical periods of life.

A person strives to maintain him or herself in a state of homeostasis through a constant series of adaptive maneuvers and problem-solving activities through which basic needs are fulfilled.

- Crisis results from a stressful precipitating event.
- Each individual develops his or her own style of coping with stressful situations.
- When faced with a problem that cannot be solved, inner tension and anxiety result in stress, which may evolve to a crisis.
- A crisis is any situation that causes a sudden alteration in the person's expectation of him or herself that lasts for at least several days, and that cannot be handled by the person with his or her usual coping mechanisms.
- The length of time for a crisis is short and self-limiting; that is, it will be resolved either positively or negatively within six weeks.

Intervention or counseling in a crisis situation is essential if the outcome is to be positive.

- The primary goal is to resolve the immediate crisis so that the individual can continue to function.
- The outcome goal is to return the individual to a precrisis level of functioning, not to resolve all problems.

- Since during the crisis period, the individual is most open for intervention, therapeutic intervention can result in a turning point for the person where he or she will function at a higher level following the crisis.

ACTION: INTERVENING IN CRISIS SITUATIONS

ASSESSMENT

1 Assess the client's psychological state and potential for loss of control.
2 Assess ability to cope with current crisis:
   a Level of anxiety manifested.
   b Distortion of thoughts or perceptions.
   c Degree of personality disorganization.
3 Evaluate behavior indicating client is experiencing a crisis:
   a Increased motor activity.
   b Reduced sensory perception.
   c Reduced ability to communicate.
   d Withdrawal or depression.
   e Symptoms of panic.
4 Assess presence of somatic symptoms.
5 Evaluate ability to go through activities of daily living.
6 Assess potential for suicide.
7 Assess need for hospitalization (either from lack of ability to function or danger of suicide).

PLANNING

GOALS

- Client who is in crisis is identified.
- Adequate assessment is completed.
- Client experiences relief of symptoms.
- Client is returned to precrisis level of functioning.
- Resolution of the immediate crisis occurs and client continues to function.
- Client learns new and more effective methods of coping with crises through professional support.

INTERVENTION: Identifying the Crisis Situation

1 Evaluate the period of disorganization.
   a Degree of disorganization.
   b Length of time situation has existed.
   c Level of functioning.
2 Identify the precipitant event.
   a Problem presented by the actual event triggering crisis.
   b Significance of the event to the individual.

Rationale for Action
- To intervene therapeutically
- To reduce anxiety in client to manageable level
- To prevent client from negative resolution of crisis period
- To assist client to set goals that can be realized
- To assist client to develop coping mechanisms to manage future crises

3 Identify past coping mechanisms.
   a Past history in experiencing similar situations.
   b Past history in coping with similar situations.
4 Evaluate situational supports.
   a Significant others.
   b Agencies.
5 Identify behaviors client is exhibiting due to crisis situation.
6 Establish a plan to assist client to deal with crisis.

INTERVENTION: Assisting the Client to Manage Crisis

1 Establish a rapid working relationship by listening and attending to client cues.
2 Remain with client in a crisis or have significant persons available.
3 Encourage the client to express feelings; avoid intellectual explanations or rationalizations.
4 Set firm limits and keep interaction goal-oriented.
5 Involve the client in formulating hypotheses of the underlying difficulty leading to the crisis period; clarify the problem.
6 Deal with target symptoms such as anxiety, depression, withdrawal.
7 Remain reality oriented, dealing with the "here and now" so that the client can accept reality.
8 Do not focus on weakness, pathology, or past crisis situations.
9 Outline with client a plan of action by which he or she may move in the direction of positive change.
10 Assist client to explore new ways of coping with problems to alleviate future crisis situations.
11 Explore external support systems and suggest new social networks that will provide support to the client.
12 Carry out a problem-solving process with the client so that he or she understands the crisis process and is more able to make decisions in the future.
13 Provide a plan of care for the client to follow to avoid crisis in the future.
14 Suggest follow-up procedures so that therapy may continue if advised.

EVALUATION

EXPECTED OUTCOMES

1 Assessment of client in crisis is completed. *If not*, follow these alternative nursing actions:
   ANA: If crisis is suspected, ask for assistance in assessment as this is a dangerous period and identification is important.
   ANA: Request validation from a colleague for identification of a crisis situation.
2 Client continues to function during crisis period. *If not*, follow these alternative nursing actions:

ANA: Evaluate situational supports to determine if they are adequate.

ANA: Request that client be hospitalized if support systems are not sufficient.

3 Client experiences relief of symptoms. *If not*, follow these alternative nursing actions:

ANA: Request that medication be administered temporarily during crisis period.

ANA: Request that specific anxiety-stress reduction methods, such as biofeedback, relaxation methods, etc., be utilized.

4 Resolution of crisis occurs with client returning to precrisis level of functioning. *If not*, follow these alternative nursing actions:

ANA: Since crisis is self-limiting, it will be resolved. If functioning level is lower, give client long-term assistance to work on changing behavior and integrating new coping mechanisms.

ANA: Suggest that client take courses in self-actualization to integrate new ways of coping with crises.

ANA: Suggest ways for client to develop more support systems outside of professional help.

UNEXPECTED OUTCOMES

1 Client attempts suicide as a means of coping with crisis.

ANA: Be aware of symptoms of possible suicidal behavior.

ANA: Recognize level of depression and potential for suicide (when depression begins to lift).

ANA: Determine presence of suicide ideation.

Ask questions such as "Do you wish you were dead?" "Do you think you might do something about it?" "What?" "Have you taken any steps to prepare?" "What are they?"

Important to recognize a continued desire to commit suicide.

ANA: Observe behavior closely for cues to potential suicide.

Listen to verbalization to determine what is meaningful for client.

Observe physical status so you can intervene if necessary (if client is not eating, sleeping, etc.).

Recognize ambivalence when client is considering suicide.

2 Client is hospitalized following suicide attempt.

ANA: Formulate a client care plan for suicidal client.

Provide safe environment to protect client from self-destruction.

Observe client closely at all times, especially when depression is lifting.

Establish supportive relationship, letting client know you are concerned for his or her welfare.

Encourage expression of feelings, especially anger.

Focus on client's strengths and successful experiences to increase self-esteem.

Provide a structured schedule and involve the client in activities with others.

Structure a plan for the client to use as a means of coping when next confronted with suicide ideation.

Charting

- Identification of crisis client is experiencing
- Assessment of client's psychological state
- Behavioral and somatic symptoms client is manifesting
- Coping mechanisms client is utilizing
- Situational supports available to client
- Interventions utilized to assist client to return to precrisis level of functioning
- Follow-up plan of care to prevent further crisis situations

Help the client plan for continued professional support after discharge.

ANA: When crisis period is over (usually self-limited at six weeks), provide follow-up care to avoid a repetition of crisis in the future.

THE EXPERIENCE OF LOSS: THE GRIEVING AND DYING PROCESS

Grief is an emotion experienced in relation to loss; it can also be viewed as a behavioral response to death and dying. Human beings experience loss as the emotion of grief and must withdraw from the painful stimulus to recuperate. Emotions allow us to experience our environment—they are the means of cognition. When we are grieving, we experience the emotion of grief; this experience is accompanied by a definite syndrome with somatic and psychological symptoms.

George Engle describes the classic progression of the grief process in stages. These stages may occur in order, or an individual may skip a stage, become locked in a particular stage, or even return to an earlier stage already worked through.

The first stage is *shock and disbelief*, denial and numbness. The first response upon learning of a death is shock and a refusal to accept or comprehend the fact. This reaction is followed by a stunned, numb feeling and does not allow the person to acknowledge the reality of death. This initial phase is characterized by attempts to protect oneself against severe stress by blocking recognition of the death.

Developing awareness is the second stage. Within minutes or hours the individual becomes acutely and increasingly aware of the anguish of loss. Anger may be present during this time and may be directed toward persons or circumstances held to be responsible for the death. Behavior that frequently accompanies this stage is crying and a regression to a more helpless and childlike state. The crying and regression appear to acknowledge the loss so conscious awareness is now present.

The third stage is *restitution*, where the various rituals of the culture, such as the funeral, attire, wake, particular folkways, and mores, help to initiate the recovery process. These rituals serve the function of emphasizing the reality of death and the very act of experiencing them assists the mourner to face the loss.

As the reality of death becomes accepted, the *resolution* of the loss begins. This stage involves a number of steps. First, the mourner attempts to deal with the painful void created by the loss of a loved one. At this time the thoughts of the mourner are occupied almost exclusively with the deceased. Then the mourner becomes more aware of his or her own body and bodily sensations. Finally, the mourner begins to talk about the dead person recalling the dead person's attributes and personality and reminiscing about the memories they shared. Resolving the loss is a long and painful phase that continues until the mourner remembers the positive aspects of the dead person.

The next stage that is frequently experienced is that of *idealization*. All hostile and negative feelings toward the dead person are repressed. As the process proceeds, two important changes are taking place: the recurring thoughts about the dead person bring a distinct image of the loss to mind and these memories serve to bring out the more positive aspects of the lost relationship. At the same time the mourner begins to assume certain admired qualities of the dead person through the mechanisms of identification or incorporation. The mourner may begin to dress, speak, or develop mannerisms or beliefs similar to the person who was lost. Often, many months are required for this process to be experienced, and as it dissipates, the mourner's preoccupation with the dead person lessens. It may be at this point that the person begins to reinvest intimate feelings toward other love objects.

The outcome of the mourning process usually takes a year or more. The clearest evidence of healing is the ability to remember the deceased comfortably and realistically, with both the pleasures and disappointments of the relationship. At this stage the obsession with the loss is ended and the person accepts the responsibility of living his or her own life.

Each individual who experiences loss will move through at least some of these stages as he or she attempts to cope with loss. The stages of grief are the means human beings have of moving through the loss to resolution.

Elisabeth Kübler-Ross has beautifully described the phases of dying, which mirror those of the grieving process. As a person learns of his or her own impending death, he or she will experience grief in relation to his or her own loss.

The first stage, as Dr. Ross views this process, is that of *denial*. The denial may be partial or complete and may occur not only during the first stages of illness or confrontation but later on from time to time. This initial denial is usually a temporary defense and is used as a buffer until such time as the person is able to collect him or herself, mobilize his or her defenses, and face the inevitability of death.

The second stage is often *anger*. The person feels violent anger at having to give up life. This emotion may be directed toward persons in the environment or even projected into the environment at random. Dr. Ross explains this reaction and the difficulty in handling it for those close to the person. "The problem here is that few people place themselves in the client's position and wonder where this anger might originate. Maybe we too would be angry if all our life activites were interrupted so prematurely."

The third stage is *bargaining*. The person attempts to strike a bargain for more time to live or more time to be without pain in return for doing something for God. Often during this stage the person turns or returns to religion.

Depression is the fourth stage. Usually, when people have completed the processes of denial, anger, and bargaining, they move into depression. Dr. Ross writes about two kinds of depression. One is preparatory depression; this is a tool for dealing with the impending loss. The second type is reactive depression. In this form of depression, the person is reacting against the impending loss of life and grieves for him or herself.

The final stage of dying is that of *acceptance*. This is when the person has worked through the previous stages and accepts his or her own inevitable death. With full acceptance of impending death comes the preparation for it; however, even with acceptance, hope is still present and needs to be supported realistically.

Many factors influence how individuals accept death. Personal values and beliefs about life; views of personal successes, both financial and emotional; the way they look physically when experiencing the dying process; their family and friends and their families' attitudes and reactions; their past experiences in coping with difficult or traumatic situations; and, finally, the health care staff who are caring for them during this process—all affect an individual's attitude toward dying.

GUIDELINES FOR MANAGING CLIENTS

The act of dying is fearful and traumatic even for those who have faced it and completed the grieving process.

- The dying client must cope with the physical symptoms of the dying process.
- The client must deal with the anxiety of moving from a known to an unknown state.
- The client must cope with the impending separation from loved ones.

A dying person faces impending death in one of three ways, even if he or she only realizes intuitively that death is near.

- Accepting it quietly and peacefully with inner strength.
- Exhibiting restless, irritable, angry, or hostile behavior to all those around.
- Becoming depressed, withdrawn, and fearful.

A dying person remains true to his or her personality, coping mechanisms, and general attitude toward life.

- A dying person will approach death in a manner similar to which he or she approached life.
- He or she will exhibit bravado, acceptance, strength, procrastination, disdain, or fear, just as in life.

The dying person often seeks identification and closeness with someone.

- Ability to resolve conflict of facing death depends not only on client's own strength but also upon his or her support systems: family, friends, and the health-care staff.

- Fear is reduced by knowing he or she is not to be left alone to experience this fearful process of dying.
- Adequate support requires the continued presence of a helping person with whom the dying client and his family can establish a meaningful relationship.

ACTION: INTERVENING IN THE GRIEF PROCESS

ASSESSMENT

Rationale for Action
- To assist the client who is experiencing the grief process
- To intervene therapeutically and provide support
- To allow the client to express feelings of loss openly
- To understand and tolerate client's behavior that is related to loss

1 Assess for presence of psychological symptoms.
   a Weeping.
   b Guilt.
   c Anger and irritability toward others and the deceased.
   d Depression.
   e Inability to initiate meaningful activity.
2 Assess for somatic symptoms.
   a Physical exhaustion.
   b Insomnia.
   c Restlessness and agitation.
   d Digestive disturbance.
   e Anorexia.
3 Evaluate client's complaints.
   a Sense of unreality.
   b Sense of detachment.
   c Lack of strength.
4 Assess stage of grief response client is experiencing.
   a Shock and disbelief.
   b Developing awareness.
   c Restitution.
   d Resolving loss.
   e Idealization.
   f Outcome of grieving process — positive or negative.
5 Assess for morbid reaction to grief.
   a Delay of reaction.
   b Distorted reaction: acquisition of symptoms that belonged to deceased, psychosomatic illness, or disease, etc.
   c Atypical grief syndrome manifested by distorted pictures of grief.

PLANNING

GOALS

- The client experiences support during the grieving process.
- Grief is allowed to be experienced rather than denied or ignored.
- The client moves successfully through stages of the grief process.
- Loss is accepted, resolution occurs, and the outcome of the mourning process is positive.

INTERVENTION: Understanding the Client's Experience of Grief

1   Understand the importance of the person lost as a source of support.
2   Evaluate the degree of dependency of the relationship — the more dependent, the more difficult is the task of resolution.
3   Identify the degree of ambivalence felt toward the deceased. When there are persistent hostile feelings, guilt may interfere with the work of mourning.
4   Evaluate the number and nature of other relationships the mourner has to depend on. Few meaningful relationships makes the willingness to give up the attachment to the deceased more difficult.
5   Check on the number and nature of previous grief experiences. Losses tend to be cumulative in their effects, and if previous losses have not been successfully worked through, they will only aggravate the current loss.
6   Evaluate the degree of preparation for the loss. For example, in terminal illness grief work may have begun long before the actual death of the person.
7   Evaluate the capacity to cope with loss. The physical and psychological health of the mourner at the time of the loss determines capacity.

INTERVENTION: Assisting the Client to Cope with Grief

1   The nurse must understand the grief process, the stages of grief, and natural responses to grief.
2   Denial stage:
    a   Allow client denial of grief to give client time to move through shock and to mobilize defenses.
    b   Encourage client to talk when he or she is ready to do so.
    c   Understand that shock and disbelief may be first response, and anticipate that behavior may be inappropriate or disturbed.
    d   Accept client's inability to face reality, and allow mood swings and expressions of happier times (which may seem inappropriate at this time).
3   Anger stage:
    a   Allow "acting-out" of feelings and verbalization of anger.
    b   Anticipate expression of anger toward others, loved ones, and the environment.
    c   Understand that unreasonable, insatiable demands are an expression of this stage of grief and attempt to meet the demands. Anticipate client's needs before demanded.
    d   Encourage client to take as much control as possible over care and environment. Avoid criticism and negative feedback at this time.
    e   Avoid false reassurance and false cheerfulness, which lead to distrust. Also, avoid diversion by introducing cheerful activities or stories. These actions lead client to believe you do not care about feelings.
    f   Explain and clarify all procedures and treatments to decrease misintrepretation and expansion of fears.

4 Bargaining stage:
  a Allow client to move through bargaining stage; listen to verbal expressions without judgment or pointing out reality.
  b Encourage client to talk about bargaining with God. This may assist client to cope with guilt and not lose faith.
5 Reactive depression stage:
  a Encourage verbalizations about loss, its meaning in client's life, and feelings about the loss.
  b Support client's self-esteem and understand that it will be affected with awareness of the loss.
  c Encourage and reassure as appropriate; do not give false reassurance at this stage but assist client to be realistic.
  d Be aware of own feelings of sadness and loss so that they do not interfere with therapy.
6 Preparatory depression:
  a Allow client to be quiet and silent in order to internalize feelings.
  b Remain with client and share on a nonverbal level.
  c Verbalize feelings to client when they are appropriate; do not deny yourself expressions of sadness or empathy (crying) when appropriate.
  d Limit association with cheerful insincere staff, friends, or family.
7 Resolution-acceptance stage:
  a Allow client to express whatever feelings are present, knowing that client has moved through the above stages and may now be feeling totally empty of emotion.
  b Spend quiet time with client, interacting on a nonverbal, nondemanding level.
  c Encourage client to make preparations for impending death by supporting requests to finish tasks and discussing options for plans to complete areas in his or her life.
  d Honor client's requests to be alone and do not overload with external information. Client may need a lot of quiet contemplation to prepare for death.
8 Show respect for cultural, religious, and social customs throughout stages of mourning.

EVALUATION

EXPECTED OUTCOMES

1 The client's experience of the grieving process is therapeutic. *If not*, follow these alternative nursing actions:
  ANA: Encourage the mourner to express feelings, especially tears.
  ANA: Attempt to meet the needs of the mourner for privacy, information, and support.
  ANA: If you cannot handle the grieving client, ask that another staff member take over.
2 Client moves through grieving process. *If not*, follow these alternative nursing actions:

ANA: Assist client to move from stage to stage by accepting his or her behavior without judgment.

ANA: Do not force attempts to speed up the grieving process, but allow client to move at own pace. Support client's attempts to work through grief.

3 Client accepts loss, and outcome of grieving process is positive. *If not*, follow these alternative nursing actions:

ANA: Understand that grief is cumulative and it is important to experience all of the stages to complete the process.

ANA: Suggest follow-up psychotherapy or group therapy as a way to cope with grief.

UNEXPECTED OUTCOMES

1 Morbid reaction to grief.

ANA: Recognize distorted symptoms and be accepting but firm with client.

ANA: Request further medication or psychotherapy for intermediate assistance.

2 Family cannot support grief of client or handle their own grief.

ANA: Know the general response to death by recognizing the stages of the grief process.

ANA: Understand that the behavior of the mourner may be unstable and disturbed.

3 Outcome of the grief process is prolonged and incomplete.

ANA: Be aware of factors that influence the outcome of grief.

Importance of the deceased in the life of mourner.

The degree of dependence in the relationship.

The amount of ambivalence toward the deceased.

The more hostile the feelings that exist, the more guilt that interferes with the grieving process.

Age of both mourner and deceased.

Death of a child is more difficult to resolve than that of an aged loved one.

Number and nature of previous grief experiences.

Degree of preparation for the loss.

Charting

- Stage of grief the client is experiencing and client's ability to cope
- Behavioral manifestations of grief
- Support systems available to client
- Complicating factors influencing the grieving process
- Suggestions as to what nursing measures seem to be most supportive

ACTION: ASSISTING THE CLIENT TO COPE WITH DEATH

ASSESSMENT

1 Assess the physical symptoms:
   a Evidence of circulatory collapse.
   b Variations in blood pressure and pulse.
   c Disequilibrium of body mechanisms.
   d Deterioration of physical and mental capabilities.
   e Absence of corneal reflex.
2 Assess the ability to fulfill basic needs without complete assistance.

Rationale for Action

- To assist the dying client to cope with the dying process
- To handle own feelings of loss and sadness that arise when caring for a client who is dying
- To provide support for the client and the client's family during the dying process
- To complete the actions necessary to care for the client who has died

3 Evaluate the nature and degree of pain the client is experiencing.

4 Assess for impending crisis or emergency situation.

5 Assess for psychosocial condition:
   a Need to establish a relationship for support.
   b Grief pattern and stage of grief the client is experiencing.
   c Need to express feelings and verbalize fears, concerns, etc.

6 Assess anxiety level, which may be expressed in physical or emotional behavior.
   a Sleep disturbance.
   b Palpitations.
   c Digestive complaints.
   d Anger or hostility.
   e Withdrawal.

7 Assess depression level that client may be experiencing.
   a High fatigue level or lethargy
   b Poor appetite, nausea, or vomiting.
   c Inability to concentrate.
   d Expressions of sadness, hopelessness, or uselessness.

In case of terminal illness, Euthanasia Council's "Living Will" can clarify your wishes. (Copies can be obtained by writing the Council at 250 W. 57th Street, New York, N.Y. 10019.)

TO MY FAMILY, MY PHYSICIAN, MY LAWYER, MY CLERGYMAN
TO ANY MEDICAL FACILITY IN WHOSE CARE I HAPPEN TO BE
TO ANY INDIVIDUAL WHO MAY BECOME RESPONSIBLE FOR MY HEALTH, WELFARE OR AFFAIRS

Death is as much a reality as birth, growth, maturity and old age—it is the one certainty of life. If the time comes when I, _____ can no longer take part in decisions for my own future, let this statement stand as an expression of my wishes, while I am still of sound mind.

If the situation should arise in which there is no reasonable expectation of my recovery from physical or mental disability, I request that I be allowed to die and not be kept alive by artificial means or "heroic measures". I do not fear death itself as much as the indignities of deterioration, dependence and hopeless pain. I, therefore, ask that medication be mercifully administered to me to alleviate suffering even though this may hasten the moment of death.

This request is made after careful consideration. I hope you who care for me will feel morally bound to follow its mandate. I recognize that this appears to place a heavy responsibility upon you, but it is with the intention of relieving you of such responsibility and of placing it upon myself in accordance with my strong convictions, that this statement is made.

Signed _____

Date _____

Witness _____

Witness _____

Copies of this request have been given to _____

_____

_____

_____

PLANNING

GOALS

- The client finds the internal resources to cope with impending death.
- The client is able to verbalize feelings, express needs, and communicate directly.
- Physical discomfort of the dying client is minimized.
- The client and the family are supported through the dying process.
- The final nursing actions are completed following death.

INTERVENTION: Assisting the Dying Client

1 Minimize the client's discomfort as much as possible.
   - a Provide warmth.
   - b Provide assistance in moving, and position client frequently.
   - c Provide assistance in bathing and personal hygiene.
   - d Administer the appropriate medications before the pain becomes severe.
2 Recognize the symptoms of urgency and/or emergency conditions and seek immediate assistance.
3 Notify the physician if there is an impending crisis and perform emergency actions until help arrives.
4 Encourage the client to do as much as he or she can for him or herself so that client does not just give up—a state that only reinforces low self-esteem.
5 Provide psychosocial nursing care for the client.
   - a Form a relationship with the dying client. Be willing to be involved, to care, and to be committed to caring for a dying client.
   - b Allocate time to spend with the client so that not only physical care is administered.
   - c Recognize the grief pattern and support the client as he or she moves through it.
   - d Recognize that your physical presence is comforting by staying physically close to the client if he or she is frightened. Use touch if appropriate and nonverbal communication.
   - e Respect the client's need for privacy and withdraw if the client has a need to be alone or to disengage from personal relationships.
   - f Be tuned into client's cues that he or she wants to talk and express feelings, cry, or even intellectually discuss the dying process.
   - g Accept the client at the level on which he or she is functioning without making judgments.
6 Provide the level of care that will encourage the client to retain confidence in the health care team.
7 Assist the client as he lives through the experience of dying in whatever way you are able to do so.

8 Support the family of the dying client.

  a Understand that the family may be going through anticipatory grief before the actual event of dying.

  b Understand that different family members will react differently to the impending death and support the different reactions.

  c Be aware that demonstrating your concern and caring will assist the family to cope with the grief process.

9 Be aware of your own personal orientation toward the dying process.

  a Explore your own feelings about death and dying with the understanding that until you have faced the subject of death you will be inadequate to support the client or the family as they experience the dying process.

  b Share your feelings about dying with the staff and others; actively work through them so that negativity does not get transferred to the client.

EVALUATION

EXPECTED OUTCOMES

1 Client finds internal resources to accept death. *If not*, follow these alternative nursing actions:

ANA: Provide extensive external support through relationship therapy, emotional support, and external system support.

ANA: Request consultation with local hospice chapter.

ANA: Allow client to respond and react naturally without expecting too much or making judgments.

2 Client is able to verbalize feelings and needs. *If not*, follow these alternative nursing actions:

ANA: Be very aware of cues so as to provide openings to talk regarding feelings.

ANA: Introduce topic yourself, if appropriate, so client can, if able, discuss feelings.

ANA: Anticipate needs so client will not have to ask.

3 Physical discomfort is minimized. *If not*, follow these alternative nursing actions:

ANA: Attend to all physical needs and, if necessary, request additional help.

ANA: Anticipate pain needs and administer medication before pain becomes too severe.

ANA: Request change in pain medication ordered if current dosage is not sufficient to keep client comfortable.

ANA: Introduce alternative method to control pain. (See Chapter 7 for methods of pain control.)

UNEXPECTED OUTCOMES

1 Nurse is unable to care for the dying client due to his or her own emotional reaction.

ANA: Request that other staff members take over as the objective is to be able to give good nursing care.

ANA: Request assistance from skilled professional to work through own feelings about death so that you will be able to cope with the next death experience.

2 Client loses confidence in the health-care team.

ANA: Attempt to ascertain exactly what occurred to cause client to lose confidence in the team.

ANA: Change staff that cares for client and be sure to choose experienced personnel who are equipped to cope with a dying client.

3 Client lingers on and does not fulfill expectation that death would occur in the near future.

ANA: Arrange for respite-supportive care for family who is having a difficult time coping.

ANA: Suggest hospice care for client if available.

ANA: If family desires, move client home and request physician's order for hospice mix or Brompton's solution (oral pain medication that family may administer).

4 Pain cannot be controlled adequately with ordered medication.

ANA: Request use of marijuana (either pill or pot) for pain relief.

ANA: Use alternative pain relief methods. (See Chapter 7 for methods of relieving pain.)

ACTION: PROVIDING POSTMORTEM CARE

ASSESSMENT

1 Verify that client has been pronounced dead by physician.
2 Complete your own assessment that client has no observable responses to stimuli.
3 Identify client by name and his or her belongings for labeling.

PLANNING

GOALS

- Death of the individual is confirmed and documented.
- Body is properly cleaned and prepared for family visiting and transfer to the morgue.
- Body and personal items are identified and labeled.
- Support is provided to the family as needed.

EQUIPMENT

- Bathing supplies
- Shroud or morgue bag
- Identification tags
- Protective pads, if necessary

Rationale for Action
- To prepare body for removal from clinical unit
- To protect the condition of the body for the purpose of respect for the deceased and his or her family during final viewing
- To document facts and time relating to death
- To identify and label client and client's belongings

- Rolls of gauze and abdominal pads, if necessary to secure limbs together
- Paper bags or plastic bags for personal belongings
- Guerney or specialized morgue cart

INTERVENTION: Providing Postmortem Care

1 If there are other clients or visitors in the room, carefully explain the situation and ask them to temporarily leave the room if possible.
2 Collect necessary equipment.
3 Follow hospital procedure regarding notification of various departments and personnel.
4 Maintain proper alignment of the body. Raise the head of the bed slightly to prevent pooling of fluids in the head or face.
5 If possible, place dentures in mouth to maintain original shape of face and mouth.
6 Remove any external objects causing pressure or injury to the skin, e.g., oxygen mask.
7 Following hospital policy, remove, cut, or secure any tubes, drains, or monitoring lines.
8 Following hospital policy, secure or replace dressings.
9 Cleanse the body as needed. A partial bath may be required to remove secretions, wound drainage, stains, etc.
10 Close the eyes. If necessary, use paper tape or gauze pads. You may do this after the family has visited the deceased.
11 Place protective incontinent pad under buttocks and between legs diaper fashion.
12 If family is to visit the deceased, provide clean linen and gown for client.
13 Remove equipment used for cleansing client.
14 If previously determined or requested by client or family, notify the appropriate clergy or religious support person.
15 After family and clergy have visited, label the body, attaching ID tags to the big toe, wrist, and morgue bag or as determined by standard procedure.
16 Tie limbs loosely together, using padding and gauze roll. Attach wrist and ankles, using proper alignment.
17 Place the body in the shroud or in morgue bag.
18 Label all personal belongings and place them in a bag.
19 Close doors to client's rooms and clear hallways in preparation to transfer the body to the morgue.
20 Transfer the body to the morgue on a guerney or special morgue cart.

EVALUATION

EXPECTED OUTCOMES

1 Postmortem care is completed by assigned staff member. *If not,* follow these alternative nursing actions:

▶ If the family is to visit the body, they may require support. Explain what the client looks like. You may want to accompany family members to the room. Privacy and quiet should be provided for the family during the visit. Remain nearby to offer emotional and physical support and to answer questions.

ANA: Request assistance from another staff member to complete procedure.

ANA: If you have difficulty in completing postmortem care, request consultation with appropriate therapist.

2 Client's personal items have been identified and labeled properly. *If not*, follow these alternative nursing actions:

ANA: Request family assistance to identify items.

3 Family is supported through grief process by staff. *If not*, follow these alternative nursing actions:

ANA: Attempt to work out own feelings about death so you will be able to support family during grief.

ANA: Request clergy or human support staff individual to be with and talk to family so that they receive necessary support.

UNEXPECTED OUTCOMES

1 Client is not identified properly when sent to the morgue.

ANA: Nurse should check identaband and shroud label before releasing client to mortician.

2 Family refuses to allow client to be released to the morgue.

ANA: Assess for denial or fear. If identified as fear, request grief consultant and give family time to work towards acceptance.

ANA: Assess for cultural restrictions; client may be released directly to mortician without going to morgue.

3 Donated organs are needed.

ANA: An explanation of this request to the family is essential. Provide support and an opportunity for questions. Sign or obtain signatures for consent form. Remove kidneys within one hour after death. Remove eyes within 6 to 24 hours after death.

ANA: Nursing staff should elicit information from family of terminally ill client about whether or not he or she wishes to donate organs.

Signed by the donor and the following two witnesses in the presence of each other:

_____   _____
Signature of Donor   Date of Birth of Donor

_____   _____
Date Signed   City & State

_____   _____
Witness   Witness

This is a legal document under the Uniform Anatomical Gift Act or similar laws.

For further information consult your physician or

National Kidney Foundation
116 East 27th Street, New York, N.Y. 10016

To ensure that your organs are donated efficiently, fill out and keep donor card with you at all times.

Charting

- The events leading to the actual death, i.e., termination of vital signs, etc.
- The exact time the physician was informed and death was pronounced
- When family members or significant others were notified
- Consent forms signed
- Condition of the body and postmortem care delivered
- Time the body and belongings were sent to the morgue

ANA: Examine reverse side of driver's license, or call mortician if burial plans have been made previously, to check on permission for organ donation through a living will.

4 An autopsy is necessary but permission has not been obtained.

ANA: The nurse and the physician must gently and clearly explain the need to the family in order to obtain consent. Providing comfort and support to the family is often necessary at this time.

ANA: If the medical examiner feels that an autopsy is necessary due to possible suicide, homicide, accident, potential malpractice, or death in the hospital within 24 hours of admission, an autopsy can be performed without consent. This must be explained to family.

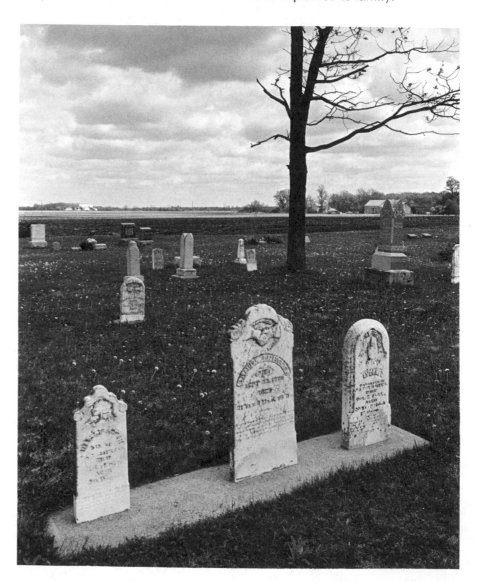

The End

BIBLIOGRAPHY

Abels, Linda. *Mosby's Manual of Critical Care*. St. Louis: The C. V. Mosby Company, 1979.

Adams, Nancy. "The Nurse's Role in Systematic Weaning from a Ventilator." *Nursing 79*, August 1979.

Aguilera, Donna. *Crises Intervention: Theory and Methodology*. St. Louis: The C. V. Mosby Company, 1978.

Allardyce, D. B., and Groves, A. C. "A Comparison of Nutritional Gains Resulting from Intravenous and Enteral Feeding." Surg. Gyn. and Obst. August 1974.

Altemeier, Wm. A. et al. *Manual on Control of Infection in Surgical Patients*. Philadelphia: J. B. Lippincott Company, 1976.

Amas, George. *The Rights of the Hospital Patients*. ACLU Handbook. Avon Books, 1975.

American College of Chest Physicians and American Thoracic Society Joint Committee on Pulmonary Nomenclature. "Pulmonary Terms and Symbols." *Chest*, 67: 583–593, 1975.

American Heart Association and National Academy of Sciences-National Research Council. "Standards and Guidelines for Cardiopulmonary Resuscitation (CPR) and Emergency Cardiac Care (ECC)." *JAMA* 244(5): 453–509, 1980.

American Journal of Nursing, "Fetal and Maternal Monitoring." December 1978.

American Journal of Nursing. "How to Work with Chest-Tubes." Vol. 80, No. 4, April 1980.

Anderson, Betty Ann, et al. *The Childbearing Family*, Vol. II, Pregnancy and Family Health. New York: McGraw-Hill Book Company, 1979.

Andreoli, Kathleen, et al. *Comprehensive Cardiac Care: A Textbook for Nurses, Physicians, and Other Health Practitioners*. 4th ed. St. Louis: The C. V. Mosby Company, 1979.

Arieti, Silvano, ed. *American Handbook of Psychiatry*, Vols. I, II, and III. New York: Basic Books, Inc., Publishers, 1974.

Armstrong, Margaret, et al. *McGraw-Hill Handbook of Clinical Nursing*. New York: McGraw-Hill Book Company, 1979.

Avco Corporation. *AVCO Intra-Aortic Balloon Pump: Model IABP: Operators Manual*. Cranbury, NJ: Hoffman-LaRoche, Inc., 1974.

Ayres, Stephen. "Pulmonary Physiology at the Bedside: Oxygen and Carbon Dioxide Abnormalities." *Cardiovascular Nursing*, January-February 1973.

Babson, S. G., et al. *Diagnosis and Management of the Fetus and Neonate at Risk*. St. Louis: The C. V. Mosby Company, 1980.

Bachm, Frank. "FHR Variability: Key to Fetal Well-Being." *Contempoary OB/GYN*, Volume 9, May 1977.

Baranowski, Karen, et al. "Vital Hepatitis — How to Reduce Its Threat to the Patient and Others." *Nursing 76*, May 1976.

Barber, Janet and Susan Budassi. *Mosby's Manual of Emergency Care*. St. Louis: The C. V. Mosby Company, 1979.

Barnard, Martha U., et al. *Human Sexuality for Health Professionals*. Philadelphia: W. B. Saunders Company, 1978.

Barry, Jean. *Emergency Nursing*. New York: McGraw-Hill Book Company, 1978.

Bates, Barbara. *A Guide to Physical Examination*. 2nd ed. Philadelphia: J. B. Lippincott Company, 1979.

Beckett, Peter, et al. *A Teaching Program in Psychiatry*, Vol. I, *Schizophrenia, Paranoid Conditions*, and Vol. II, *Psychoneurosis, Organic Brain Disease and Psychopharmacology*. Detroit: Wayne State University Press, 1969.

Beland, Irene, and Passos, Joyce. *Clinical Nursing*. 3rd ed. New York: Macmillan Publishing Company, Inc., 1975.

Bergersen, Betty S. *Pharmacology in Nursing*. 14 ed. St. Louis: The C. V. Mosby Company, 1979.

Bernheim, C. H., Block, E., and Atkins. "Fever: pathogenesis, pathophysiology and purpose." *Annals of Internal Medicine*, 1979,

Birchenall, Joan, and Streight, Mary Eileen. *Care of the Older Adult*. Philadelphia: J. B. Lippincott Company, 1973.

Bishop, B. "How to cool a feverish child." *Pediatric Nursing*, January/February, 1978.

Bistrain, B. R., and Blackburn, G. L. "Prevalence of Malnutrition in General Medical Patients." *JAMA* 235: 1567–1570, 1976.

Bleier, Inge J. *Workbook in Bedside Maternity Nursing*. 4th ed. Philadelphia: W. B. Saunders Company, 1979.

Bloom, B. S. ed. *Taxonomy of Educational Objectives, Handbook I: Cognitive Domain*. New York: David McKay Co., 1956.

Bolooki, Hooshang. *Clinical Application of Intra-Aortic Balloon Pump*. New York: Futura Publishing Co., 1977.

Bordick, Katherine. *Patterns of Shock: Implications for Nursing Care*. New York: Macmillan Publishing Company, Inc., 1965.

Borg, Nan, et al. *Core Curriculum for Critical Care Nursing*. Philadelphia: W. B. Saunders Company, 1981.

Borgen, Linda. "Total Parenteral Nutrition in Adults." *American Journal of Nursing*, February 1978.

Brink, Pamela J., ed. *Transcultural Nursing*. Englewood Cliffs, NJ: Prentice-Hall, Inc., 1976.

Britt, Michael, et al. "Severity of Underlying Disease as a Predictor of Nosocomial Infection." *JAMA*, March 13, 1978.

Brooks, Stewart. *Basic Facts of Body Water and Ions*. New York: Springer Publishing Company, Inc., 1973.

Brown, B. *New Mind, New Body*. New York: Harper and Row, 1975.

Brown, B. *Stress and the Art of Biofeedback*. New York: Harper and Row, 1977.

Broughton, Joseph O. "Chest Physical Diagnosis for Nurses and Respiratory Therapists." *Heart and Lung*, March-April 1972.

Broughton, Joseph O. "Understanding Blood Gases." Ohio Medical Products Article Reprint Library, August 1971.

Brunner, Lillian Sholtis, and Suddarth, Doris Smith. *Textbook of Medical Surgical Nursing*. 4th ed. Philadelphia: J. B. Lippincott Company, 1980.

Brunner, Lillian Sholtis, and Suddarth, Doris Smith. *The Lippincott Manual of Nursing Practice*. Philadelphia: J. B. Lippincott Company, 1978.

Budassi, Susan. "An Emergency Nurse's Guide to Drawing Arterial Blood Gases." *Journal of Emergency Nursing*, January-February 1977.

Budassi, Susan, and Barber, Janet. *Emergency Nursing: Principles and Practice*. St. Louis: The C. V. Mosby Company, 1981.

Bullough, Bonnie. *The Law and the Expanding Nursing Role*. 2nd ed. New York: Appleton Century Croft, 1980.

Burgess, Ann Wolbert, and Lazare, Aaron. *Psychiatric Nursing in the Hospital and the Community*. 3rd ed. Englewood Cliffs, NJ: Prentice-Hall, Inc., 1981.

Burnside, Irene Mortenson. *Nursing and the Aged*. 2nd ed. New York: McGraw-Hill Book Company, 1976.

Burrow, G. N., and Ferris, T. F. *Medical Complications During Pregnancy*. Philadelphia: W. B. Saunders Company, 1975.

Bushnell, Sharon Spaeth. *Respiratory Intensive Care Nursing*. Boston: Little, Brown & Company, 1973.

Butterworth, C. E. "The Skeleton in the Closet." *Nutrition Today*, March-April 1974.

Byrne, Judith. "Liver Function Studies, Part IV: Using Metabolism Tests to Investigate Liver Function." *Nursing 77*, December 1977.

Cannon, Christine. "Hands-On Guide to Palpation and Auscultation." *RN* 43 (3): 20– 24, 1980.

Cannon, W. B. *Bodily Changes in Pain, Hunger, Fear and Rage: An Account of Recent Researches into the Function of Emotional Excitement*. New York: D. Appleton and Co., 1929.

Cannon, W. B. *The Wisdom of the Body*. New York: Norton, 1942.

Carnevali, Doris, and Patrick, Maxine. *Nursing Management for the Elderly*. Philadelphia: The J. B. Lippincott Company, 1979.

Cataldo, C. B., and Smith, L. "Tube Feedings: Clinical Applications." Ross Laboratories, 1980.

Cazalas, Mary W. *Nursing and the Law*. Germantown, MD: Aspen Systems Corporation, 1978.

Chaffee, Ellen, and Lytle, Ivan. *Basic Physiology and Anatomy*. 4th ed. Philadelphia: J. B. Lippincott Company, 1980.

Cherniack, R. M., et al. *Respiration in Health and Disease*. Philadelphia: W. B. Saunders Company, 1972.

Chinn, Peggy L. *Child Health Maintenance: Concepts in Family Centered Care*. St. Louis: The C. V. Mosby Company, 1979.

Chrzanowski, Alexandria. "Intra-aortic Balloon Pumping: Concepts and Patient Care." *Nursing Clinics of North America*. 13:3, September 1978.

Ciuca, Rudy, et. al. "Passive Range-of-Motion Exercises." *Nursing 78*, July 1978.

Clark, Ann, and Affonso, Dyanne. *Childbearing: A Nursing Perspective*, (2nd Ed.). Philadelphia: F. A. Davis, 1979.

Cohen, Stephen. "Nursing Care of a Patient in Traction." *American Journal of Nursing*, October 1979.

Colley, Rita, and Wilson, Jeanne. "Meeting Patients' Nutritional Needs with Hyperalimentation." *Nursing 79*, May, June, and September 1979.

Comoss, Patricia M., et. al. *Cardiac Rehabilitation: A Comprehensive Nursing Approach*. Philadelphia: J. B. Lippincott Company, 1979.

Conway, Barbara. *Carini and Owens' Neurological and Neurosurgical Nursing*, 7th ed. St. Louis: The C. V. Mosby Company, 1978.

Craib, Alice, and Perry, Margaret. *EEG Handbook*, 2nd ed. Schiller Park, Ill.: Beckman Instruments, Inc., 1975.

Croushore, Theresa. "Postoperative Assessment: the Key to Avoiding the Most Common Nursing Mistakes." *Nursing 79*, April 1979.

Dickason, Elizabeth J., and Schultz, Martha Olsen. *Maternal and Infant Care*. 2nd ed. New York: McGraw-Hill Book Company, 1979.

Dison, Norma. *Clinical Nursing Techniques*. 4th ed. St. Louis: The C. V. Mosby Company, 1979.

Dossey, Barbara. "Perfecting Your Skills for Systematic Patient Assessment." *Nursing 79*, February 1979.

Doyle, Jeanne. "If Your Patient's Legs Hurt, the Reason May be Arterial Insufficiency." *Nursing 81*, April 1981.

Drauss, P., et. al. "The Other Side of Death—Good Memories and the Strength to Go On." *Nursing 78*, December 1978.

Dunphy, J. Englebert, and Way, Lawrence L. *Current Surgical Diagnosis and Treatment*. 5th ed. Los Altos, CA: Lange Medical Publications, 1981.

Dyer, Claire. "Burn Care in the Emergent Period." *J Emerg Nurs* 6(1): 9–16, 1980.

Engle, George L. "Grief and Grieving." *American Journal of Nursing*, September 1964. [a classic]

Erikson, Erik H. *Childhood and Society*. New York: W. W. Norton and Company, Inc., 1963. [a classic]

Ettinger, Bruce, and McCort, Dorothy. "Effects of Drugs on the Fetal Heart Rate During Labor." *JOGN*, Volume 5, No. 5, Sept./Oct. 1976.

Euland, K. "Cardiovascular Diseases Complicating Pregnancy." *Clinical Obstetrics and Gynecology*. Vol. 21, pp. 426–441, 1978.

Fagerhaugh, Shizuko. "How to Manage Your Patient's Pain . . . and How Not To." *Nursing 80*, February 1980.

Ferholt, Deborah. *Clinical Assessment of Children: A Comprehensive Approach to Primary Pediatric Care*. Philadelphia: J. B. Lippincott Company, 1980.

Fischbach, Frances. *A Manual of Laboratory Diagnostic Tests*. Philadelphia: J. B. Lippincott Company, 1980.

Fischer, Ruth. "Measuring Central Venous Pressure." *Nursing 79*, October 1979.

Food and Nutrition Board, National Research Council, National Academy of Sciences. *Recommended Dietary Allowances*. Washington, DC: 1979.

French, Ruth. *Guide to Diagnostic Procedures*. 5th ed. New York: McGraw-Hill Book Company, 1980.

Fuchs, Patricia. "Getting the Best out of Oxygen Delivery Systems." *Nursing 80*, December 1980.

Fuchs, Patricia. "Understanding Continuous Mechanical Ventilation." *Nursing 79*, December 1979.

Furman, Seymour. "Recent Developments in Cardiac Pacing." *Heart and Lung*, September-October 1978.

Galli, Nicholas. *Foundations and Principles of Health Education*. Santa Barbara: John Wiley & Sons, Inc., 1978.

Gardner, Ernest, et. al. *Anatomy: A Regional Study of Human Structure*. 4th ed. Philadelphia: W. B. Saunders Company, 1975.

Garvey, Judith. "Infant Respiratory Distress Syndrome." *American Journal of Nursing*, April 1975.

Gassner, Charles, and Ledger, William. "The Relationship of Hospital Acquired Maternal Infections to Invasive Intrapartum Monitoring Techniques." *American Journal of Obstetrics and Gynecology*. Volume 126, No. 1, September 1, 1976.

Gildea, Joan H. "Pre- and Postoperative Nursing Care." *American Journal of Nursing*, February 1978.

Gillies, Dee Ann, and Alyn, Irene Barrett. *Saunders Tests for Self-Evaluation of Nursing Competence*. 3rd ed. Philadelphia: W. B. Saunders Company, 1980.

Goloskov, Joan. "The Role of the Nurse in Qualitative Intracranial Pressure Determinations." *Journal of Neurosurgical Nursing*, March 1978.

Goodlin, Robert. "History of Fetal Monitoring." *American Journal of Obstetrics and Gynecology*, Volume 133, No. 3, February 1, 1979.

Grant, Harvey, and Murray, Robert. *Emergency Care*. 2nd ed. Bowie, MD: Robert J. Brady Company, 1978.

Greenberg, Diane. "Hyperbaric Oxygen: Exciting New Clinical Results." *RN*, September 1979.

Gresh, Cindy. "Helpful Hints You Can Give Your Patients with Parkinson's Disease." *Nursing 80*, January 1980.

Griggs, B. A., et. al. "Enteral Nutrition for Hospitalized Patients." *A.S.P.E.N. Monograph*, 1980.

Griggs, Barbara, and Hoppe, Mary C. "Nasogastric Tube Feeding." *American Journal of Nursing*, March 1979.

Guthrie, Helen Andrews. *Introductory Nutrition*. 4th ed. St. Louis: The C. V. Mosby Company, 1979.

Guyton, Arthur C. *Textbook of Medical Physiology*. 6th ed. Philadelphia: W. B. Saunders Company, 1981.

Haber, Judith, et. al. *Comprehensive Psychiatric Nursing*. New York: McGraw-Hill Book Company, 1978.

Hall, Joanne E., and Weaver, Barbara. *Nursing of Families in Crisis*. Philadelphia: J. B. Lippincott Company, 1974.

Hammond, Cecile. "ECG Made Easier than Ever." *RN*, October 1979.

Hammond, Cecile. "Plain Talk about Cardiac Monitors." *RN*, September 1979.

Hammond, Cecile. "Protecting Patients with Temporary Transvenous Pacemakers." *Nursing 78*, November 1978.

Hanlon, K. "Description and Uses of Intracranial Pressure Monitoring." *Heart and Lung*. 5:2, 1976.

Hathaway, Rebecca. "The Swan-Ganz Catheter: A Review." *Nursing Clinics of North America*. 13:3, September 1978.

Haughey, Brenda. "CVP Lines: Monitoring and Maintaining." *American Journal of Nursing*, April 1978.

Haverkamp, Albert, Thompson, Horace, McFee, John, and Certrulo, Curtis. "The Evaluation of Continuous Fetal Heart Rate Monitoring in High Risk Pregnancy." *American Journal of Obstetrics and Gynecology*, Volume 125, No. 3, June 1, 1976.

Hays, J. S., and Larson, K. *Interacting with Patients*. New York: Macmillan Publishing Company, 1965. [a classic]

Hemelt, Mary Dolores, and Mackert, Mary Ellen. *Dynamics of Law in Nursing and Health Care*. Reston, VA: Reston Publishing Company, 1978.

Henderson, Virginia, and Nite, Gladys. *Principles and Practice of Nursing*. New York: Macmillan Publishing Company, Inc., 1978.

Heymsfield, S. B., et. al. "Enteral Hyperalimentation: An Alternative to Central Venous Hyperalimentation." *Ann. Int. Med.* 90: 63–71, 1979.

Holloway, Nancy M. *Nursing the Critically Ill Adult*. Menlo Park, CA: Addison-Wesley Publishing Company, 1979.

Holmes, T. H., and Rahe, R. H. "Social Readjustment Rating Scale." *Journal of Psychosomatic Research* 11:213, 1967. [a classic]

Hudak, Carolyn M., et. al. *Critical Care Nursing*. 2nd ed. Philadelphia: J. B. Lippincott Company, 1977.

Huxley, Valerie. "Heparin Lock: How, What, Why." *RN*, October 1979.

Irwin, Betty. "Hemodialysis Means Vascular Access . . . and the Right Kind of Nursing Care." *Nursing 79*, October 1979.

Isacson, Laurey, and Schulz, Klaus: "Treating Pulmonary Edema." *Nursing 78*, February 1978.

Jensen, Margaret, et. al. *Maternity Care: The Nurse and the Family*. 2nd ed. St. Louis: The C. V. Mosby Company, 1981.

Johnson, Marion, and Quinn, Judith. "The Subarachnoid Screw." *American Journal of Nursing*, March 1977.

Jones, Cathy. "Glasgow Coma Scale." *American Journal of Nursing*, September 1979.

Juliani, Louise M. "Acute Glomerulonephritis." *Nursing 79*, September 1979.

Kalkman, Marion, and Davis, Ann. *New Dimensions in Mental-Health Psychiatric Nursing*. 5th ed. New York: McGraw-Hill Book Company, 1980.

Karones, Shelton B. *High-Risk Newborn Infants*. St. Louis: The C. V. Mosby Company, 1975.

Keithley, Joyce. "Proper Nutritional Assessment Can Prevent Hospital Malnutrition." *Nursing 79*, February 1979.

Kelso, I. M., et. al. "An Assessment of Continuous Fetal Heart Rate Monitoring in Labor: A Radomize Trial." *American Journal of Obstetrics and Gynecology*, Volume 131, No. 1, 1978.

Kessler, Diana. "The 12 Lead Electrocardiogram." *Journal of Emergency Nursing*, December 1979.

King, Quita, *Care of the Cardiac Surgical Patient*. St. Louis: The C. V. Mosby Company, 1975.

Kinney, M. R., et. al. *AACN's Clinical Reference for Critical-Care Nursing*. New York: McGraw-Hill Book Company, 1981.

Kintzel, Kay Carmen. *Advanced Concepts in Clinical Nursing*. 2nd ed. Philadelphia: J. B. Lippincott Company, 1977.

Korczowski, Marian M. "Strengthen the Nurse's Role in Nutritional Counseling." *Nursing and Health Care*, April 1981.

Koretz, R. L., and Meyer, T. H. "Elemental Diets—Facts and Fantasies." *Gastroenterology* 78: 393–410, 1980.

Kozier, Barbara, and Erb, Glenora L. *Fundamentals of Nursing: Concepts and Procedures*. Menlo Park, CA: Addison-Wesley Publishing Company, 1979.

Krebs, H. B., et. al. "Intrapartum Fetal Heart Rate Monitoring." *American Journal of Obstetrics and Gynecology*, Volume 133, No. 7, April 1, 1979.

Krizinofski, Marian T. "Human Sexuality and Nursing Practice." *Nursing Clinics of North America*, December 1973.

Krueger, Judith A., and Ray, Janis C. *Endocrine Problems in Nursing*. St. Louis: The C. V. Mosby Company, 1976.

Krupp, Marcus A., and Chatton, Milton J. *Current Medical Diagnosis and Treatment*. Los Altos, CA: Lange Medical Publications, 1980.

Krupp, Marcus, et al. *Physician's Handbook*. 19th ed. Los Altos, CA: Lange Medical Publications, 1979.

Kubler-Ross, Elisabeth. *On Death and Dying*. New York: Macmillan Publishing Company, Inc., 1969. [a classic]

Lamb, Joann. "Intra-Arterial Monitoring—Rescinding the Risks." *Nursing 77*, November 1977.

Langley, L. L., et. al. *Dynamic Anatomy and Physiology*. 5th ed. New York: McGraw-Hill Book Company, 1980.

Lipkin, Gladys B. *Psychosocial Aspects of Maternal-Child Nursing*. 2nd ed. St. Louis: The C. V. Mosby Company, 1978.

Long, Gail D. "Managing the Patient with Abdominal Aortic Aneurysm." *Nursing 78*, August 1978.

Luckmann, Joan, and Sorensen, Karen Creason. *Medical-Surgical Nursing: A Psychophysiologic Approach*. 2nd ed. Philadelphia: W. B. Saunders Company, 1980.

MacKinnan, Roger, and Michels, Robert. *The Psychiatric Interview in Clinical Practice*. Philadelphia: W. B. Saunders Company, 1971.

Malasanos, Lois, et. al. *Health Assessment*. 2nd ed. St. Louis: The C. V. Mosby Company, 1981.

Marlow, D. R. *Textbook of Pediatric Nursing*. Philadelphia: W. B. Saunders Company, 1979.

Marram, Gwen D. *The Group Approach in Nursing Practice*. St. Louis: The C. V. Mosby Company, 1979.

McCaffery, Margo. *Nursing Management of the Patient with Pain*. 2nd ed. Philadelphia: J. B. Lippincott Company, 1979.

McCalister, Donald, et. al. *Readings in Family Planning*. St. Louis: The C. V. Mosby Company, 1973.

McConnell, Edwina. "Ensuring Safer Stomach Suctioning with the Salem Sump Tube." *Nursing 77*, September 1977.

McConnell, Edwina. "Ten Problems with Nasogastric Tubes—and How to Solve Them." *Nursing 79*, April 1979.

Mead, Johnson. *Dialogues in Nutrition. Nutritional Care of the Critically Ill Patient: Selection of Appropriate Feeding Modalities*. Vol. 3, No. 2, 1979.

Meissner, Judith. "Measuring Patient Stress with the Hospital Stress Rating Scale." *Nursing 80*, August 1980.

Meltzer, Lawrence E., et. al. *Intensive Coronary Care: A Manual for Nurses*. 3rd ed. Bowie, MD: The Charles Press, 1977.

Mendels, Joseph. *Concepts of Depression*. New York: John Wiley & Sons, Inc., 1970.

Mereness, Dorothy, and Taylor, Cecelia. *Essentials of Psychiatric Nursing*. 10th ed. St. Louis: The C. V. Mosby Company, 1978.

Metheny, Norma M., and Snively, W. D. *Nurses' Handbook of Fluid Balance*. 3rd ed. Philadelphia: J. B. Lippincott Company, 1979.

Meyers, F. H., et. al. *Review of Medical Pharmacology*. 5th ed. Los Altos, CA: Lange Medical Publications, 1976.

Michael, Sharon. "Home IV Therapy." *American Journal of Nursing*, July 1978.

Millar, Sally. *Methods in Critical Care: The AACN Manual*. Philadelphia: W. B. Saunders Company, 1980.

Miller, Emmett, M. D. Relaxation Tapes, P. O. Box W, Stanford, California 94305.

Monk, Heather Boyd, "Screening for Glaucoma." *Nursing 79*, August 1979.

Mowinski, Bonnie. "Improving Your Management of DIC." *Nursing 79*, May 1979.

Narrow, Barbara W. *Patient Teaching in Nursing Practice, A Patient and Family-Centered Approach*. New York: John Wiley & Sons, Inc., 1979.

Neeson, Jean D., and Stockdale, Connie R. *The Practitioner's*

Handbook of Ambulatory Obstetrics and Gynecology. New York: Wiley, 1981.

Norris, Debra L. "What all Those Pressures Mean . . . and Why." RN, October 1981.

Nursing Grand Rounds. "The Nursing Care Plan: A Communication System that Really Works." Nursing 78, August 1978.

Nursing Photobook. Dealing with Emergencies. Horsham, PA: Nursing 80 Books, Intermed Communications, Inc., 1980.

Nursing Photobook. Giving Medication. Horsham, PA: Nursing 80 Books, Intermed Communications, Inc., 1980.

Nursing Photobook. Preventing and Correcting Tube and Cuff Problems in Artificial Airways. Horsham, PA: Nursing 80 Books, Intermed Communications, Inc., 1980.

Nursing Photobook. Providing Early Mobility. Horsham, PA: Nursing 80 Books, Intermed Communications, Inc., 1980.

Nursing Photobook. Assessing Your Patients. Horsham, PA: Nursing 81 Books, Intermed Communications, Inc., 1981.

Nursing Photobook. Giving Cardiac Care. Horsham, PA: Nursing 81 Books, Intermed Communications, Inc., 1981.

Nursing Photobook. Managing IV Therapy. Horsham, PA: Nursing 81 Books, Intermed Communications, Inc., 1981.

Nursing Photobook. Using Monitors. Horsham, PA: Nursing 81 Books, Inc., Intermed Communications, Inc., 1981.

Nurse's Reference Library. Diseases. Horsham, PA: Nursing 81 Books, Intermed Communications, Inc., 1981.

Nurse's Reference Library. Nurse's Guide to Drugs. Horsham, PA: Nursing 80 Books, Intermed Communications, Inc., 1980.

Nursing Skillbook. Helping Cancer Patients—Effectively. Horsham, PA: Nursing 78 Books, Intermed Communications, Inc., 1978.

Nursing Skillbook. Monitoring Fluid and Electrolytes Precisely. Horsham, PA: Nursing 79 Books, Intermed Communications, Inc., 1979.

O'Donnell, Bridgett. "How to Change Tracheotomy Ties—Easily and Safely." Nursing 78, March 1978.

Orthopedic Nurses Association, Inc. Manual of Orthopedic Nursing Care Plans. Atlanta, GA: May 1975.

Page, C. P., et. al. "Continual Catheter Administration of an Elemental Diet." Surg. Gyn. and Obst. 142: 184–188, 1976.

Parent, Bea. "Are In-line IV Filters Really Worthwhile?" Nursing 81, August 1981.

Payne, Dorris B. Psychiatric Mental Health Nursing. 2nd ed. Nursing Outline Series. Flushing, NY: Medical Examination Publishing Company, Inc., 1977.

Pellitteri, Adele. Nursing Care of the Growing Family: A Child Health Text. Boston: Little, Brown & Company, 1977.

Peplau, Hildegarde. "Talking With Patients." American Journal of Nursing, 1960. [a classic]

Perez, R. H. Protocol for Perinatal Nursing Practice. St. Louis: The C. V. Mosby Company, 1981.

Petrillo, M., and Sanger, S. Emotional Care of Hospitalized Children. 2nd ed. Philadelphia: J. B. Lippincott Company, 1980.

Petty, Thomas L. Intensive and Rehabilitative Respiratory Care. Philadelphia: Lea and Febiger, 1974.

Physician's Desk Reference to Pharmaceutical Specialities and Biologicals. Oradell, NJ: Medical Economics, Inc., 1978.

Polk, Hiram, Jr. "Prevention of Surgical Wound Infection." Annals of Internal Medicine, 89 (Part 2), 1978.

Pritchard, Jack A., and MacDonald, Paul C. Williams Obstetrics. 16th ed. New York: Appleton-Century Crofts, 1980.

Proctor, Diane, et al. "Temporary Cardiac Pacing: Causes, Recognition, Management of Failure to Pace." Nursing Clinics of North America. Vol. 13, No. 3, September 1978.

Promisloff, Robert A. "Administering Oxygen Safely: When, Why, How." Nursing 80, October 1980.

Pumphrey, John B. "Recognizing Your Patients' Spiritual Needs." Nursing 77, December 1977.

Rambeau, J. L., and Miller, R. "Nasoenteric Tube Feeding." Practical Aspects, Hedeco, 1979.

Rau, Joseph and Mary. "To Breathe or Be Breathed: Understanding IPPB." American Journal of Nursing, April 1977.

Redman, Barbara Klug. The Process of Patient Teaching in Nursing. 4th ed. St. Louis: The C. V. Mosby Company, 1980.

Reeder, Sharon, et al. Maternity Nursing. 14th ed. Philadelphia: J. B. Lippincott Company, 1980.

Rettig, Fannie M. "Appraisal of Intracardiac Monitoring." AORN, April 1979.

Reusch, Jurgen. Therapeutic Communication. New York: W. W. Norton & Company, Inc., 1961. [a classic]

Reynolds, Janis I., and Logsdon, Jann B. "Assessing Your Patient's Mental Status." Nursing 79, August 1979.

Rodman, Morton J., and Smith, Dorothy. Pharmacology and Drug Therapy in Nursing. 2nd ed. Philadelphia: J. B. Lippincott Company, 1979.

Rosenberg, Jack. "New Sophistication in Assessment: Finding the Therapeutic Window." RN, July 1980.

Sagar, Diane, and Bomar, Suzanne. Intravenous Medications: A Guide to Preparation, Administration and Nursing Management. Philadelphia: J. B. Lippincott, 1980.

Sanderson, Richard. The Cardiac Patient, a Comprehensive Approach. 2nd ed. Philadelphia: W. B. Saunders Company, 1981.

Satir, Virginia. Conjoint Family Therapy. Palo Alto, CA: Science & Behavior Books, Inc., 1967. [a classic]

Saxton, Dolores, and Haring, Phyllis. Care of Patients With Emotional Problems. St. Louis: The C. V. Mosby Company, 1979.

Saxton, Dolores, and Hyland, Patricia. Planning and Implementing Nursing Intervention. St. Louis: The C. V. Mosby Company, 1975.

Scherer, Jeanne C. Introductory Clinical Pharmacology. Philadelphia: J. B. Lippincott Company, 1975.

Schroeder, J., and Darly, E. Techniques in Bedside Hemodynamic Monitoring. St. Louis: The C. V. Mosby Company, 1976.

Schumann, Lorna. "Commonsense Guide to Topical Burn Therapy." Nursing 79, March 1979.

Scipien, Gladys, et. al. Comprehensive Pediatric Nursing. New York: McGraw-Hill Book Company, 1979.

Selye, Hans. The Stress of Life. New York: McGraw-Hill Book Company, 1965. [a classic]

Shafer, Kathleen Newton, et. al. Medical Surgical Nursing. 6th ed. St. Louis: The C. V. Mosby Company, 1979.

Shields, Donna. "Maternal Reactions to Fetal Monitoring." American Journal of Nursing, Volume 78, December 1978.

Shils, M. E. Defined Formula Diets for Medical Purposes. Chicago: American Medical Association, 1977.

Shils, M. E. "Enteral Nutrition by Tube." Cancer Research. 37: 2432–2439, 1977.

Shils, M. E., Bloch, A. S., and Chernoff, R. *Liquid Formula for Oral and Tube Feeding*. 2nd ed. New York: Memorial Sloan Kettering Cancer Center, 1979.

Shils, M. E., and Coiro, D. *Nutrition Assessment of the Cancer Patient: Report of a Pilot Study*. New York: Memorial Sloan Kettering Cancer Center.

Shipley, Susan. "Pitfalls and Perils of Intracardiac Monitoring." *AORN*, April 1979.

Shrake, Keven. "The ABC's of ABG's or How to Interpret a Blood Gas Value." *Nursing 79*, September 1979.

Silver, H. K., et al. *Handbook of Pediatrics*. 13th ed. Los Altos, CA: Lange Medical Publications, 1980.

Smith, Carol. "Abdominal Assessment: A Blending of Science and Art." *Nursing 81*, 11(2): 42–49, 1981.

Smith, Rae. "Invasive Pressure Monitoring." *American Journal of Nursing*, September 1978.

Smith, Sandra. *Sandra Smith's Review of Nursing for State Board Examinations*. 3rd ed. Los Altos, CA: National Nursing Review, Inc., 1982.

Solnick, Robert L., ed. *Sexuality and Aging*. Los Angeles: Ethel Percy Andrus Gerontology Center, 1978.

Spitz, Phyllis, and Sweetwood, Hannelore. "Kids in Crisis." *Nursing 78*, March 1978.

Stroot, Violet R., et. al. *Fluids and Electrolytes: A Practical Approach*. Philadelphia: F. A. Davis Company, 1977.

Suitor, Carol W., and Hunter, Merilly F. *Nutrition: Principles and Application in Health Promotion*. Philadelphia: J. B. Lippincott Company, 1980.

Sumner, Sara. "Refining Your Technique for Drawing Arterial Blood Gases." *Nursing 80*, April 1980.

Swift, Nancy. "Why the MS Patient Needs Your Help." *Nursing 79*, September 1979.

Tecklin, Jan S. "Positioning, Percussing, and Vibrating Patients for Bronchial Drainage." *Nursing 79*, March 1979.

Timmons, Joan. "Breath Sounds." *J. Emergency Nursing*, 6(6): 16–19, 1980.

Torosian, M. E., and Rambeau, J. L. "Feeding by Tube Enterostomy. Surg. Gyn. and Obst. 150: 918–924, 1980.

Travelbee, Joyce. *Intervention in Psychiatric Nursing. Process in the One-to-One Relationship*. 2nd ed. Philadelphia: F. A. Davis Company, 1979.

Traver, Gayle. "Assessment of Thorax and Lungs." *American Journal of Nursing*, March 1973.

Traver, Gayle. "Symposium on Care in Respiratory Disease." *Nursing Clinics of North America*, March 1974.

Tucker, Susan Martin, et. al. *Patient Care Standards*. 2nd ed. St. Louis: The C. V. Mosby Company, 1980.

Tucker, Susan Martin. *Fetal Monitoring and Fetal Assessment in High-Risk Pregnancy*. St. Louis: The C. V. Mosby Company, 1978.

Turner, Jeffrey S., and Helms, Donald B. *Contemporary Adulthood*. Philadelphia: W. B. Saunders Company, 1979.

U.S. Department of Agriculture. *A Daily Food Guide: The Basic Four*. Rev. ed. Washington, DC: Government Printing Office, 1979.

Van Meter, Margaret. "Keeping Cool in a Code." *RN*, 44(3): 29–35, 1981.

Vasey, Ellen. "Writing Your Patient's Care Plan . . . Efficiently." *Nursing 79*, April 1979.

Vaughan, Victor C. R., et. al. *Nelson Textbook of Pediatrics*. 11th ed. Philadelphia: W. B. Saunders Company, 1979.

Wade, Jacqueline. *Respiratory Nursing Care: Physiology and Techniques*. 2nd ed. St. Louis: The C. V. Mosby Company, 1977.

Waechter, Eugenia, et. al. *Nursing Care of Children*. Philadelphia: J. B. Lippincott Company, 1976.

Wasserman, Edward, and Slobody, Laurence B. *Survey of Clinical Pediatrics*. 7th ed. New York: McGraw-Hill Book Company, 1980.

Waterson, Marian. "Teaching Your Patients Postural Drainage." *Nursing 78*, March 1978.

West, John. *Respiratory Physiology—The Essentials*. Baltimore: Williams & Wilkins Company, 1974.

White, Sara. "Fluids and Electrolytes: Heading Off the Risks." *RN*, November 1979.

Whitman, Gayle. "Intra-aortic Balloon Pumping and Cardiac Mechanics: A Programmed Lesson." *Heart and Lung*, November-December 1978.

Widmann, Frances. *Goodale's Clinical Interpretation of Laboratory Tests*. Philadelphia: F. A. Davis Company, 1979.

Wiener, Matthew B., et. al. *Clinical Pharmacology and Therapeutics in Nursing*. New York: McGraw-Hill Book Company, 1979.

Williams, Emily. "Food for Enough: Meeting the Nutritional Needs of the Elderly." *Nursing 80*, September 1980.

Williams, Robert H., ed. *Textbook of Endocrinology*. 6th ed. Philadelphia: W. B. Saunders Company, 1981.

Williams, Sue Rodwell. *Essentials of Nutrition and Diet Therapy*. 4th ed. St. Louis: The C. V. Mosby Company, 1981.

Wilson, Holly Skodal, and Kneisl, Carol Ren. *Psychiatric Nursing*. Menlo Park, CA: Addison-Wesley Publishing Company, 1979.

Wing, Kenneth. *The Law and The Public's Health*. St. Louis: The C. V. Mosby Company, 1976.

Wood, Lucile A., ed. *Nursing Skills for Allied Health Services*. Philadelphia: W. B. Saunders Company, 1979.

Woods, Nancy Fugate. *Human Sexuality in Health and Illness*. St. Louis: The C. V. Mosby Company, 1979.

Worthington, Laura. "What Those Blood Gases Can Tell You." *RN*, October 1979.

Yalom, Irvin D. *The Theory and Practice of Group Psychotherapy*. 2nd ed. New York: Basic Books, Inc., 1975.

Yarborough, Mary G. "Training Needs of the Infection Control Nurse." *Annals of Internal Medicine*, November 1978.

Young, Shelley. "Understanding Intracranial Pressure." *Nursing 81*, February 1981.

Yura, Helen, and Walsh, Mary B. *The Nursing Process: Assessing, Planning, Implementing, Evaluating*. 3rd ed. New York: Appleton-Century Crofts, 1978.

Ziegel, Erna, and Cranley, Mecca. *Obstetric Nursing*. 7th ed. New York: Macmillan Publishing Company, Inc., 1978.

INDEX

Heart failure, 185, 626, 657
    causes of, 626
    intervention for treating, 627
    physiology of, 626–627
Heat
    action and intervention for applying, 242, *380–385, 385–390*
    relieving pain by applying, interventions for, 385, 389
    production and conservation of, of the body, 376–378
Heat application table, *389*
Heat cradle, 389
    intervention for, 386
Heat lamp, *389*
    intervention for, 386
Heating blanket, by using a cooling blanket, 394, *395*
Heating pads, 389
    action and intervention for applying, *385–390*
Heat-sensitive tapes, used to record temperature, 143
Height, pediatric assessment of, 211
Heimlich manuever, *648*
    alternate procedure, 653
Hemastix, *408*
Hemiplegia, sign of, 169
Hemispheres, of brain, *175–176*
Hemodialysis, 741
    action and intervention for maintaining renal function with *747–754*
Hemolytic reactions to blood transfusions, manifestations and interventions, *198*
Hemorrhage, 135
    action and intervention for controlling, *631–634*
    assessment guide to, *629*
    causes of, 625
    effect on blood pressure, 146
    intervention for treating, 625–626
Hemothorax, defined, 621
    site for, *596*
Hemovac suction, intervention for maintaining, *132*
Heparin
    in arterial lines, 706
    safety precautions, 23
Heparin lock, 475
    intervention for performing venipuncture with, 480
Hernia repair, skin preparation for, *676*
Hewlett-Packard electrical monitor, 723
Hexachlorophene antiseptic, used with surgical scrub, 123
High-Fowler's position, described, 71
High-iron diet, 522

High-polyunsaturated fat diet, 521
High-protein diet, 520
High-protein preoperative diet, 523
High-residue (roughage) diet, 523
Hip joints, flexion of, *330*
Histamine, effect on blood pressure, 147
History, health
    elements of a complete, 166–167
    importance of, in identifying contagious clients, 121
Hodgkin's disease, 119
Hoffman Colles frame, *358*
Holistic approach to health, 3–4, 34
Holistic stress model, 231
Holmes and Rahe stress scale, 223
Homeostasis
    defined, 246
    maintenance of, 3–4, 699
Hood, intervention for using oxygen, 570, 575–576
Hordeolum (sty), 177
Hormones, 237, 287
Hosiery. *See* Elastic hosiery
Hospital. *See* Health care unit
Hospital environment. *See* Environment
Hot moist applications and packs, intervention for 381–382
Hot water bottle, 389
    intervention for applying, 387
Household system, measurement, 279, 280
Hoyer lift, *323*
H.S. care-hour of sleep care, described, 72
Humidifiers. *See* Oxygen therapy *and* Nebulization
Humidity, in hospital environment, 7–8
Humoral immunity, defined, 139
Hydration
    assessment of, 470
    body sites for, *470*
    indications of, *471*
    See also Fluid and electrolytes
Hydrogen in concentration, 703
Hydrostatic pressure, defined, 655
Hydrothorax
    ANA, 536
Hygiene, personal
    assessment of, during mental assessment, 191
    providing, in health care unit, 33–34
Hyperalimentation dressing and tubing, intervention for changing, *533–534*
Hyperemia, defined, 70
Hyperextension, defined, 372
Hypermotility
    causes of, 430
    effect of, 429
Hyperopia, 177

Hyperpigmentation, 174
Hyperpnea, 162
    diagram of, *157*
    nursing action for, 157
Hypertension, 160
    nursing action for, 161–162
    range of, 161
    signs of, 173
Hypertonic enema, 439
Hyperventilation, process of, 547, 548
    See also Hypernea.
Hypnotics, 283
Hypocalcemia, causes of, signs of, and treatment for, *506–508*
Hypochloremia, causes of, signs of, and treatment for, *506–508*
Hypochondria, 192
Hypoglossal nerve, 176
Hypoglycemic diet, 519–520
Hypokalemia, causes of, signs of, and treatment for, *506–508*
Hypomagnesemia, causes of, signs of, and treatment for, *506–508*
Hypomotility
    causes of, 430
    effect of, 429
Hyponatremia, causes of, signs of, and treatment for, *506–508*
Hypospadias, 189
Hypotension
    blood pressure indication of, 147
    nursing action for, 160–161
    range of, 160
    signs of, 173
Hypothalamus, 175
    function of, 141, *375–376*
Hypothermia
    classifications of, 394
    control of, 152
    described, 142
    uses for, 394
Hypothermia blanket, action and intervention for using, *393–397*
Hypoventilation, 158. *See also* Bradypnea
Hypoxea,
    cause of, 142
    control of, 564–565

IABP. *See* Intra-aortic balloon pump
Ice application, intervention for using, 391
Icterus. *See* Jaundice
Ideas of reference, 192
Ideation, 192
Identification
    bracelet, issuing a, 16
    of deceased client, 781
Ileal conduit, 423–425

Review of Nursing, *See Sandra Smith's Review of Nursing for State Board Examinations*, 3rd edition, 1982
Rh-negative status, evidence of, 202
Rhonchi, 184
Ribs, assessment of, 181
Right subclavian vein, 532
Right ventricular pressure, causes of elevated, 724
Rights, client's, providing information to client regarding, 17
Rights, in drug administration, 250
Robinson Catheter, 133–134
Role playing, 92
Roman Catholic, 195
Room, health care, appearance and cleanliness of, 9
Rotating tourniquet, 627, 635, 642
    action and intervention for applying, *636–638*
Rotation, defined, 372
Ruptured membranes, 199

Sacrum, in assessment for hydration, 470
Safe environment, 9–12
    action and intervention for providing a, 20–26
Safety, instruction for adults, 11–12
Safety belt, intervention for applying, 346
Safety precautions
    for dye injection studies, 295
    intervention for surgical, 675, 682–683
    for using oxygen, 571
Saline, used in eye care, 63, 64
Salves. *See* Ointments
Scales, types of, 471
Scalp
    pediatric assessment of, 213
    See also Hair care
Scan
    bone, 301
    brain, 302
    lung, 301–302
    See also CAT scan
Scanning. *See* Radiographic procedures
Scaphoid, 187
School-age children
    physical assessment of, 207
    safety instruction for, 11
Scrub, surgical hand, intervention for completing, 123
Scultetus binder
    alternative intervention, 351
    intervention for applying, 349–*350,* 351
Secondary bottle and administration set, intervention for using, 490
Secretion of isolation clients, disposing of, 128

Sedatives, 284
Selye, Dr. Hans, 219, 225
Selye's general adaptation syndrome, 221–223, 225
Semiconscious clients, intervention for providing oral hygiene to, 51
Semi-Fowler's position, 71, *327*
Semilunar heart sounds, assessment of, 185
Semi-prone position, 327
Sensation
    assessment of, 174
    physical pain, 238
Sensory function, physical assessment of, 171, 194
Sepsis
    defined, 139
    infusion-related, 120
Septicemia, nosocomial, 120
Serum albumin, in blood component therapy, 503
Serum sodium, in assessment for hydration, 471
    See Fluid and Electrolytes
Serums, 283
Set point, 142, 375
Sexual relations, 204
Shampoo board, 58
Shampooing hair
    equipment needed for, 56
    intervention for, 57–58
Shaving
    equipment needed for, 56
    intervention for, 58
    intervention for surgical, 675–676
Shearing force, defined, 70
Sheets for bedmaking, types of, 72
Shivering, process of, 377
Shock, 626
    causes of, 626
    from stress, 221
    interventions for treating, 626
Shoulder, rotation of, *331*
Shrink bandage, intervention for applying, *353–354*
Side, turning the client on, intervention for, *326*
Side rails, 22
Sigmoid colostomy, described, 432
    See ostomy
Signaling system
    call light, 26
    in client's room, 10, 16–17
Silence, as a therapeutic tool, 82
Sim's position, *680,* 309, *327*
Sinoatrial (SA) node, defined, 655
Sinus arrhythmia, 162
Sinuses, 256
    pediatric assessment of, 213

Sitz bath, intervention for, 383–384
Skeletal muscles, physiology of, 317–318
Skeletal system. *See* Musculoskeletal system
Skeletal traction
    intervention for applying, to Stryker frame, 366
    intervention for assessing, *356–357*
Skin, 117–118
    action and intervention for applying medications to, *252–257*
    action and intervention for assessing, 52–54
    assessment of breast, 182
    care of, 328
    intervention for care of, between dialysis, 752
    newborn assessment of, 207–208
    pediatric assessment of, 21
    physical assessment of, *173–175*
    physiology of, 173
    problems, 33–34
    terminology relating to care of, 69–70
    tone, newborn assessment of, 208
Skin barriers, used with fecal ostomies, types of, *448*
Skin care tray, interventions for using, *137*
Skin color, assessment of, 173–175
Skin medications, intervention for preparing, 253
Skin traction, intervention for assessing, *355–356*
Sleep, client care prior to, 72
Sling, intervention for applying, 347–348
Small intestine, anatomy and physiology of, *427–429*
Smoking, in health care facility, 23, 25
Snellen chart, pediatric assessment of, 213
SOAP or SOAPIER notes, 105–106
Soap-suds enema, 440
Sociocultural dimension of environmental adaptation, 13–14
Sociocultural-religious factors, nutritional assessment of, *517*
Sodium, *465, 506–508,* 512
    foods high in, 522
    for prenatal clients, 203
    imbalance, 506
    restrictions, 522
Soft diet, 524
Solutions
    calculation of drug, 281–282
    enema, 439, 440
    types of, 281
Sorenson Intraflo, *712*
Sound levels, comfortable in hospital environment, 8–9
Source-oriented narrative charting, 100, 101
Source-oriented systems charting, 100–*101*

Vitamin C, sources of, 543
Vitamin D, source of, 7
Vitamin control, diets for, intervention for providing, 522
Vitamins, 282, *511–512*
Vivonex, used in IV infusion, 539, 541, 542
VMT. *See* Video matrix terminal, 106, *107*
Voice, pediatric assessment of, 212
Voiding. *See* Urination
Volume, air, judging depth of, 145–146
Volume of air. *See* Tidal volume
Volume control set, intervention for using, *489–490, 499*
Volume incentive spirometer
action and intervention for using, 553
types of, 553
Volume respirator, *605*

Walker, intervention for ambulating with, *333*
Warm, dry heat, action and intervention for applying, *385–390*
Warmer, infant, 386–387
Washing hands. *See* Hand washing
Waste disposal, safety precautions in, 12

Water
essential to client's well-being, 12
essential for life, *511*
Water, body physiology of, 463–464
Water bed, described, 71
Water-seal drainage system
action and intervention for monitoring, *598–603*
intervention for establishing and maintaining closed, *595–597*
Water-soluble vitamins, *511*
foods rich in, 522
Weak pulse, 144, 162
Weighing clients, action and intervention for, *471–472*
Weight
antepartum assessment of, 197
in assessment for hydration, 471
makeup of, 463
nutritional assessment of, 517
pediatric assessment of, 211
Wet cast, intervention for caring for, 340–341
Wheals, 175
Wheezes, 184
"Windmill" exercise, 233

Winged tipped needles, 475
intervention for performing a venipuncture with, *478–480*
Wounds
action and intervention care of for, *128–135*
culture, intervention for obtaining, 133
fever, 152
healing phase of, 131
hemorrhage, 135
infection, 692–693
inhibitors of healing of, 132
Wrist, rotation of, *331*
Wrist restraints, intervention for using, *345–346*

Xanthalasma, 177
Xylocaine, used in amniocentesis procedure, 314k

Yeast sensitivity, treatment for, 426
Y-set, 497
administering blood through, 500–501

Z-track method, *269*